D0946758

CLINICAL DIAGNOSIS

THE HIPPOCRATIC OATH

I swear by Apollo, the Physician, by Asclepius, by Hygeia, by Panacea, and by all the gods and goddesses, making them my witnesses, that I will carry out, according to my ability and judgement, this oath and this indenture. To hold my teacher in this art equal to my own parents, to make him partner in my livelihood; when he is in need of money to share mine with him; to consider his family as my own brothers, and to teach them this art, if they want to learn it, without fee or indenture. I will use treatment to help the sick according to my ability and judgement, but never with a view to injury or wrong-doing. I will keep pure and holy both my life and my art. In whatsoever houses I enter I will enter to help the sick, and I will abstain from all intentional wrong-doing and harm. And whatsoever I shall see or hear in the course of my profession in my intercourse with men, if it be what should not be published abroad, I will never divulge, holding such things to be holy secrets. Now if I carry out this oath, and break it not, may I gain forever reputation among all men for my life and for my art; but if I transgress it and forswear myself, may the opposite befall me.

Translation by
WILLIAM HENRY RICH JONES
(1817–1885)

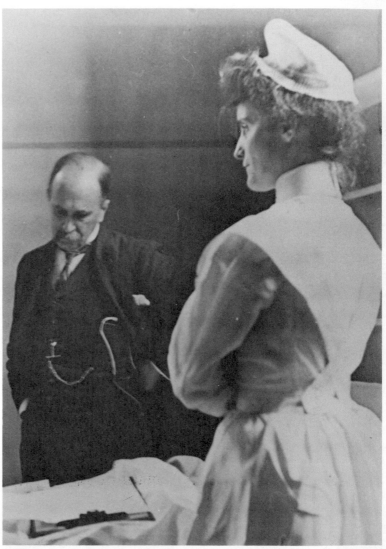

Osler

CLINICAL DIAGNOSIS

A PHYSIOLOGIC APPROACH

FOURTH EDITION

Richard D. Judge, M.D.

Clinical Professor of Internal Medicine (Cardiology), The
University of Michigan Medical School, Ann Arbor; Chief,
Cardiopulmonary Exercise Laboratory, Saint Joseph Mercy
Hospital, Ann Arbor

George D. Zuidema, M.D.

Warfield M. Firor Professor and Director, Section of
Surgical Sciences, The Johns Hopkins University School of
Medicine; Surgeon in Chief, The Johns Hopkins Hospital,
Baltimore

Faith T. Fitzgerald, M.D.

Associate Professor of Medicine and Associate Dean,
University of California, Davis, School of Medicine, Davis

With illustrations by
Mary Ann Olson and Leslie H. Arwin, M.D.

*We must turn to nature itself,
to the observations of the body
in health and disease to learn
the truth.*

HIPPOCRATES OF COS
(460?–377? B.C.)

Little, Brown and Company
Boston

Quotation on page 447 from *Now We Are Six* by A. A. Milne. Copyright, 1927, by E. P. Dutton & Co., Inc., Renewal copyright, 1955, by A. A. Milne. Reprinted by permission of the publisher, E. P. Dutton.

The head of Hygeia, Greek goddess of health, on the cover was originally part of a statue that stood outside the Temple of Athena in Tegea, Peloponnesus, Greece, in the fourth century B.C. Its style suggests the influence of the sculptor Praxiteles. The drawing was made by *Gerald P. Hodge,* Professor of Medical and Biological Illustration, The University of Michigan, Ann Arbor.

CONTENTS

CONTRIBUTING AUTHORS

Robert D. Currier, M.D.
Professor of Medicine (Neurology) and Chairman, Department of Neurology,
University of Mississippi School of Medicine, Jackson

Faith T. Fitzgerald, M.D.
Associate Professor of Medicine and Associate Dean, University of California, Davis,
School of Medicine, Davis

John C. Floyd, Jr., M.D.
Professor of Internal Medicine, Division of Endocrinology and Metabolism,
The University of Michigan Medical School, Ann Arbor

Bruce J. Genovese, M.D.
Clinical Instructor of Internal Medicine (Cardiology), The University
of Michigan Medical School, Ann Arbor; Medical Director, Coronary Care Unit,
Saint Joseph Mercy Hospital, Ann Arbor

Robert A. Green, M.D.
Professor of Internal Medicine, Pulmonary Division, The University of Michigan
Medical School, Ann Arbor

James R. Hayward, D.D.S., M.S.
Chief, Department of Oral and Maxillofacial Surgery, The University of Michigan
School of Dentistry, Ann Arbor; Director of Oral Surgery, The University of
Michigan Hospital, Ann Arbor

John W. Henderson, M.D.
Professor Emeritus of Ophthalmology, The University of Michigan
Medical School, Ann Arbor

Richard D. Judge, M.D.
Clinical Professor of Internal Medicine (Cardiology), The University of Michigan
Medical School, Ann Arbor; Chief, Cardiopulmonary Exercise Laboratory,
Saint Joseph Mercy Hospital, Ann Arbor

Theodore M. King, M.D., Ph.D.
Director, Department of Gynecology and Obstetrics, The Johns Hopkins University
School of Medicine, Baltimore

George H. Lowrey, M.D.
Professor Emeritus of Pediatrics, University of California, Davis, School of Medicine, Davis

Peter J. Lynch, M.D.
Professor and Chief, Section of Dermatology, and Associate Head, Department of Internal
Medicine, University of Arizona Health Sciences Center, Tucson

Muriel C. Meyers, M.D.
Professor Emeritus of Internal Medicine, The University of Michigan
Medical School, Ann Arbor

William W. Montgomery, M.D.

Professor, Department of Otolaryngology, Harvard Medical School, Boston; Surgeon in Otolaryngology, Massachusetts Eye and Ear Infirmary, Boston

Lee H. Riley, Jr., M.D.

Professor and Director, Department of Orthopedic Surgery, The Johns Hopkins University School of Medicine, Baltimore

Gerhard Schmeisser, M.D.

Professor of Orthopedic Surgery, The Johns Hopkins University School of Medicine, Baltimore

Ralph A. Straffon, M.D.

Head, Department of Urology, The Cleveland Clinic Foundation, Cleveland

Ron J. Vanden Belt, M.D.

Clinical Assistant Professor of Internal Medicine (Cardiology), The University of Michigan Medical School, Ann Arbor; Chief, Department of Internal Medicine, Saint Joseph Mercy Hospital, Ann Arbor

John G. Weg, M.D.

Professor of Internal Medicine and Physician-in-Charge, Pulmonary Division, The University of Michigan Medical School, Ann Arbor

George D. Zuidema, M.D.

Warfield M. Firor Professor and Director, Section of Surgical Sciences, The Johns Hopkins University School of Medicine; Surgeon in Chief, The Johns Hopkins Hospital, Baltimore

PREFACE

Although the term *physical diagnosis* seems to have become obsolete, the subject itself remains as important today as it was 50 years ago, and there is undeniably a continuing need for a well-structured introduction to the methods of clinical examination. Yet, when dealing with such fundamentals as history taking and physical examination, one might justifiably question the need for innovation. Shouldn't the same rules apply to today's physician as applied to his or her grandfather?

We believe the answer is clearly no. In the first edition of our textbook the approach to clinical examination was significantly modified, while the traditional emphasis on bedside examination was preserved. In subsequent editions, including this fourth edition, we have augmented these modifications to keep the content as up to date as possible. Modern instrumentation has improved our understanding of basic human physiology and pathophysiology. We have emphasized a combination of grouping by physiologic systems and classic regional orientation. We have integrated this approach with an illustrated step-by-step logical sequence of physical examination. Clinical medicine enters today's medical curricula at an earlier stage than before, which prompted a further segmentation of the material into units that correlate with various basic sciences, including sections on technique of examination and normal findings that interlock with anatomy and physiology. Cardinal symptoms and abnormal findings can be correlated with pathology and microbiology. With firm understanding of the fundamental pathophysiologic bases of clinical diagnosis, the student can learn not only **what** physical findings to seek in any case, but (and more important) **why**. The increasing importance of resuscitation and the growing incidence of trauma led to a greater emphasis on methods of examining the acutely ill or acutely injured patient.

Automation and data processing have modified the approach of history taking and record keeping. The problem-oriented medical record appears in Chapter 23.

Also, this fourth edition contains numerous new illustrations, as well as brief sections on special techniques of examination. We have continued to enlist contributing authors from a variety of surgical and medical subspecialties. Because of the changes in the format, some material by certain authors has been redistributed in the text to clarify maximally its relationships to closely aligned system examinations. We also solicited and have been enlightened and enriched by the many suggestions made by our student colleagues who have used the previous editions of this text. In particular, Ms. Carol Kastan and Mr. Jeffrey Milliken, students at The University of Michigan Medical School, have made original and invaluable contributions to the text.

In the last analysis, however, no book on the subject of clinical examination can be a substitute for bedside experience. Clinical examination, by its very nature, must be a matter of self-education on the wards and in the clinics. We hope the beginning student will find this text useful in the development of a clinical vocabulary and in reviewing methods of examination before starting practical work on the wards with a tutor. Later, as an upperclassman, he or she may wish to review certain sections while serving a clinical clerkship. Finally, the practicing physician may find a few pearls buried within these pages, for the art of medicine is seldom if ever mastered, even by the expert.

We wish to thank Alden and Vada Dow and Dorothy Dow Arbury for their spiritual and material support. Our appreciation is extended also to Dr. and Mrs. Michael Schmidt for their perceptive critique of earlier editions and to Ms. Mary Ann Olson and Dr. Leslie H. Arwin, who produced the illustrations for this text. The physician who appears in most of the drawings is Dr. Marilyn Tsao.

R. D. J.
G. D. Z.
F. T. F.

SECTION I

INTRODUCTION TO THE HISTORY AND PHYSICAL

CHAPTERS

Faith T. Fitzgerald
Richard D. Judge

If you would learn to do a thing, you go to one who does it well; you watch, you listen and your first attempts are made under supervision. The teaching of medical practice began and has continued until recent times under such a simple system of apprenticeship.

SIR THOMAS LEWIS
(1881–1945)

INTRODUCTION

This text has but one purpose—to start you on your way to becoming a clinician. It is an introduction to the technique of diagnosis. Until now, as a student, you have been a "receiver." School has focused on providing you with knowledge and experience and your achievements were duly rewarded. Now you take your first step as a "giver," for to practice medicine is to serve. There are no grades behind the closed door of the examining room—only you and your patient. From here on you must evaluate yourself. At this moment you are beginning a lifetime of self-education. Your success or failure in making the adjustment of the next year or two will determine to a large extent the kind of physician you will be 20 years after graduation.

There is a German aphorism that says, "Only as a physician does one become a physician." You cannot learn the art or science of medical practice from this or any other book. You cannot learn it in the library. You must learn it at the bedside. To function there requires some basic skills: how to talk to sick people, what to ask, how to touch them, what to look for. These techniques are not mastered in a year or in a lifetime of practice; but the method can and must be mastered—as rapidly as possible—for with the preclinical sciences it forms the foundation on which you will build your clinical superstructure.

To think of "physical diagnosis" as a separate discipline is erroneous. One cannot compartmentalize the history and physical. The diagnostic process is a continuum that begins invariably with a set of accurate observations. These may be verbal, physical, or laboratory—usually a blend of all three. To separate them is entirely artificial. The clinician does not cease to communicate with the patient, nor does he stop observing after the physical examination. His bedside impressions continue to guide indefinitely both the diagnostic and the therapeutic program. Sound medical practice in the modern era requires bedside observation as never before, for here we apply the scientific facts learned in the classroom and translate them into action. It is here also that compassion and understanding in medicine are primarily expressed.

THE PHYSICIAN

A man of moderate ability may be a good physician if he devotes himself faithfully to the work.

OLIVER WENDELL HOLMES, SR.
(1809–1894)

We physicians are relative newcomers to the realm of science. Western medicine was a combination of mysticism and empiricism for many centuries. The kind of accurate observation that characterizes true science has always been a part of the process, but this part was relatively minor until the eighteenth century.

The art of medicine without science is quackery. On the other hand, the scientific method is not inconsistent with a humanitarian attitude. Humanity and science are quite compatible.

From the patient's point of view, there is no substitute for interest, acceptance, and especially empathy on the part of the physician. These factors may indeed be more important to the patient in selecting a physician than pure scientific ability, for these are the qualities that communicate to him that his doctor is trying and wants to help. The patient will reveal his serious problems only to someone who he feels is accepting him unconditionally. In most instances, therefore, it is wise to conceal any moral judgments you might have about the attitudes or behavior of your patient. Try to avoid betraying feelings of surprise, disdain, or hopelessness by a facial expression or a passing remark.

Empathy is a very desirable characteristic for the physician to possess. It is an appreciative perception or the ability to feel as another is feeling. One way to achieve empathy is to ask yourself "How would I feel if it were me?" As you progress in your clinical experience and become more *technically* adept, never forget the *personal* needs of the patient for your compassion and understanding. In expressing concern for the patient, however, the doctor must maintain a significant degree of detachment, for sympathetic attachment destroys objectivity. If objectivity is surrendered, judgment becomes biased. This is part of the rationale behind the universal rule that under ordinary circumstances a physician should avoid caring for family members.

Empathy requires sensitivity, which each of us has in variable measure. The question often asked is "How does one develop sensitivity?" One answer, of course, is to look beyond medicine to philosophy, art, or religion. Time spent in cultivating an appreciation for music or poetry may lead in a very direct way to the type of sensitivity and perception that increases diagnostic acumen in the examining room. There is a solid basis for this assertion. Great writers, composers, and artists are geniuses at observing. For this reason alone they are worthy of study. A physician who develops an appreciation for subtle differences in form, color, harmony, or cadence is learning something indispensable. For him, art is also a means of educating the senses. An individual who is familiar with a grace note will have little difficulty with a split second sound.

Charles Darwin, in his autobiography, states the following:

. . . and if I had to live my life again, I would have made a rule to read some poetry and listen to some music at least once every week; for perhaps the parts of my brain now atrophied would thus have been kept active through use. The loss of these tastes is a loss of happiness, and may possibly be injurious to the intellect, and more probably to the moral character, by enfeebling the emotional part of our nature.

As a student you will approach the bedside with a certain amount of anxiety and dread. Do not be concerned about your initial awkwardness; this is natural. Try to "break the barrier" as quickly as possible. Fix your attention on your ultimate role and start to work. Remember that as a practicing physician you will be regarded as an expert with considerable authority and influence over the lives of your fellowmen. What self-confidence you display will greatly affect your patient's confidence

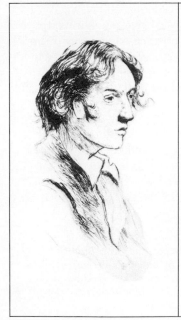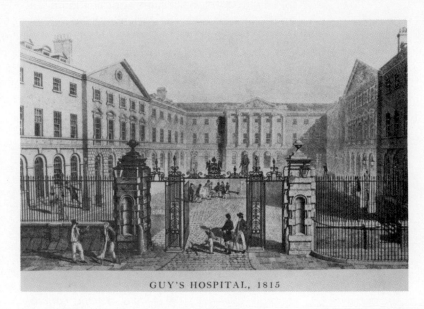

GUY'S HOSPITAL, 1815

FIGURE 1-1
John Keats was only 26 years old when he died of tuberculosis. During his short adult life, he was a medical student at Guy's Hospital for 5 years. He passed his qualifying examinations but never practiced. (Used by permission of the Easton Press, Norwalk, Conn.)

in you. As Galen put it, "He heals the best in whom the most people have the greatest confidence." Your age, sex, personal appearance, voice, attitude, and personality all influence the patient's behavior toward you. It is important, therefore, that you begin by learning all that you can about yourself. Only by developing your individual talents along lines that are natural to you, will you present a genuine image. Of course, there are innumerable approaches. One physician may use a touch of humor, another a friendly sincere attitude, another a dignified reserve, and so on. Whatever seems natural is usually the most effective. Nevertheless, the knack of really "reaching" the patient requires thoughtful practice regardless of the route selected. Study the approaches of your teachers who seem to have this ability. Later you can work the best of their techniques into your own personal approach to patients.

The complete list of desirable characteristics for a physician would be too long to include here. Honesty and integrity are always mentioned. Of course they are indispensable, but a foolish honesty can undermine confidence, and it can also be exceedingly cruel. Honesty must be tempered by compassion and practiced tactfully. The hardest three words for the physician to say are "I don't know." It is one of the stiffest tests of honesty. If you come upon a fellow physician who is so proficient that he never needs to say "I don't know," beware!

One last characteristic of the physician will be mentioned: The physician must be critical. Doubt is the foundation of scientific medicine. Therefore you must endeavor to develop the same critical attitude at the bedside that an investigator uses in the laboratory. By preserving critical judgment in your reasoning, in your reading, and in everything you do, you are less likely to become complacent. Complacency, more than anything else, will stymie your growth, and the lessons of medicine must be learned and relearned throughout a lifetime of practice.

In summary then, if you wish to be known as a "good physician" 20 years after graduation, you should be:

1. A good observer
2. A good communicator
3. A good critic
4. A good decision maker
5. A good student—now and later

THE CLINICIAN'S JOB

The term scientific cannot be denied to an accurate observation at the bedside, if it is conceded to a similarly accurate observation made by means of the microscope; nor can it be denied to a correct description of a process observed in a patient, while conceded to the correct description of a process observed in a rabbit or guinea pig. The clinic is scientific, not merely in so far as it utilizes chemical or physical methods and technique, but primarily because it represents a determined, fearless, and painstaking effort to observe, to explore, to interpret, to unravel.

ABRAHAM FLEXNER
(1866–1959)

A *physician* may be a scientist, teacher, philosopher, author, or administrator. A *clinician* is the "bedside" physician who cares for patients directly. A significant part of the clinician's job is deeply interrelated with the individual patient and the patient's personal life. The clinician does not treat a disease; he treats patients who are ill. The clinical phenomena caused by an illness include subjective sensations called *symptoms* and objective changes called *signs.* In practice, symptoms must be dredged from a morass of information and misinformation, and signs must be disentangled from a welter of confusing anatomic and physiologic variables. Here, then, is another important aspect of the clinician's job.

But the essence of the clinician's job is even more fundamental. The primary responsibility of the clinician is to make decisions. Every telephone call, every patient visit, every ward round, every laboratory report demands a rapid succession of decisions, many of which entail shattering consequences. Often the clinician must decide on the basis of limited or incomplete data; he is usually short of time and under considerable pressure. All kinds of decisions confront him, both diagnostic and therapeutic: What shall we do? What shall we say? When shall we proceed?

Many irrational factors inevitably become involved in the decision-making process, since emotional interaction between patient and physician is always a contributing element. The clinician must identify and try to understand these factors. He must learn to know himself and why he acts as he does; he must learn to know his patients and why they act as they do.

THE PATIENT

One who is ill has not only the right but also the duty to seek medical aid.

MAIMONIDES
(1135–1204)

The term *patient* is derived from the Latin word *pati,* "to suffer." A person becomes a patient by seeking medical aid.

Biörck has suggested an interesting idea. He has pointed out that there are really three patients: (1) the patient as he is, (2) the image of the patient in the physician's mind, and (3) the patient on the record. Each may differ in significant respects, but the clinician is involved with all three. The physician may never know the real patient—that is, the patient as he really is in his home and at his work. In addition, the real patient may withhold information, at times critical and important information. Some of this information may become apparent only through the chart; for example, a past history of a high uric acid level or elevated fasting blood sugar level. On the other hand, the chart may hold important facts about previous illness that have been forgotten by the "real" patient. The image of the patient in the physician's mind is often a mixture of the real patient and the patient on the record, modified by the effect of the doctor's own personality. This interplay is complex and changes from day to day as the chart thickens and the physician and patient (we hope) get to know each other better.

THE STUDENT

The very first step towards success in any occupation is to become interested in it.

SIR WILLIAM OSLER
(1849–1919)

All physicians ideally should be lifelong students of medicine. Even if modern medical information were, in its vast array, conquerable at any time, the data still would be substantially different 10 years hence. The student must fall early on into the habit of continual self-education—of questioning, integrating, and correlating the information acquired on the wards with the science that forms the basis for understanding clinical events.

The medical student at first exposure to the patient on the wards is in a difficult situation. Because the student is not yet equipped to diagnose and treat patients, he tends to feel that the intrusions made upon the patient's time and person are unjustified. The student interrupts the patient's nap or dinner, asks embarrassing questions for hours on end, and awkwardly pokes away at him. And from all of this, there is no evident concrete benefit to the patient. If, as is the case, the ruling moral dictum of medicine is "First, do no harm," how is this approach justified?

Medical training is an apprenticeship. There is no better way to learn than at the bedside, and there are no better teachers than the patients themselves. In every doctor's life there is a first patient—one to whom little advantage is returned for his pains; the skill necessary to give benefit is acquired only through multiple contacts with many patients.

But the patients *may* benefit. Many will delight in student visits. Sickness is a lonely condition. Student-doctor rounds may be the high point of the patient's week. And although the student lacks skill, he *does* have something to offer: time, interest, concern, and sympathy. The student may allow the patient, at a time when illness may have robbed him of a sense of social worth, to fulfill his need for self-value by participating in the education of a physician. The patient may take great pride in *his* students, and in himself for having taught them.

The student honors his patient-teachers in several ways. A student-physician must be honest about his limitations of knowledge, and must be respectful and well-groomed. A patient may find it difficult to tell the "doctor" that the latter's personal appearance or hygiene is offensive. Patients expect their doctors to look and act like doctors and are generally fairly conservative in their concepts of a physician's appearance. From the very beginning the student must also be rigorously protective of the patient's confidentiality. One may never divulge information about a patient to any person or agency without that patient's permission. Except when discussing the patient with other physicians for the purpose of teaching or learning (which ought not to occur in public places, such as elevators or restaurants), keep silent!

Above all, use every opportunity that presents itself to increase knowledge, skill, and understanding. Your patients deserve a superior physician.

THE MEDICAL HISTORY AND PHYSICAL

Clinical judgment depends not on knowledge of causes, mechanisms or names of disease but on a knowledge of patients. The background of clinical judgment is clinical experience: the things that clinicians have learned at the bedside in the care of sick people.

ALVAN R. FEINSTEIN
(1925–   )

The history, physical examination, and formulation of diagnosis and therapy are the basic tools of the physician. In this workup the patient's problems are described and evaluated, and plans are made for alleviating them. It is at the same time the most routine and the most difficult of the physician's functions.

There are many techniques for doing a history and physical. The basic form matters less than the substance. The ultimate criterion for an excellent history and physical is whether, upon their completion, one has a good idea of all the significant things that are bothering the patient. The history should be accurate, complete (although not lengthy), understandable, and coherent; and although this seems obvious, the history is extraordinarily tough to do right.

The medical history, the cornerstone of the physician's logical structure, serves many purposes.

1. **Establishing contact.** This frequently is referred to as "developing rapport" and involves getting to know and understand the patient and his environment. It is the first step in history taking and the first step toward making the diagnosis.

2. **Eliciting valuable diagnostic information.** It has been demonstrated that an experienced physician can closely predict the final diagnosis in most of his patients based on a careful history alone.

3. **Giving focus to the physical examination.** The history is the first signpost on the road to diagnosis. It puts the physician on guard and makes him particularly watchful for certain physical findings. Every intelligent physician modifies his examination according to historical findings.

4. **Gaining insight into the functional status of the patient.** Severity of the patient's symptoms is especially useful as an early index of the seriousness of the illness. It points the way to the case's subsequent disposition (i.e., emergent, urgent, or routine).

5. **Indicating appropriate laboratory studies.** Isolated symptoms or historical facts often require special laboratory follow-up. For example, food-relieved epigastric discomfort might prompt an upper gastrointestinal x-ray even in the absence of any associated physical findings. A history suggestive of angina deserves study by electrocardiogram, even though no auscultatory abnormalities may be present on physical exam.

9

6. **Initiating therapy**. The seeds of future therapy are sown during the history. Make no mistake; the patient is sizing you up. Whether he accepts your recommendations or throws away your prescription is, in part, being decided at this time.

TECHNIQUE OF INTERVIEWING

A doctor who cannot take a good history and a patient who cannot give one are in danger of giving and receiving bad treatment.

PAUL DUDLEY WHITE
(1886–1973)

Interviewing, like medicine itself, is partly an art and partly a science. It is a skill that is mastered not from a book but from experience in the examining room. The routine outline presented in this chapter lists the various topics that must be covered in a complete medical history. By following such an outline you assure yourself that the history you take is complete. Yet no instructor can teach you how to frame your questions effectively. This skill you must discover for yourself. The psychological relationships involved in the interaction between physician and patient during this process of history taking are far more complex than a simple outline might imply. Before proceeding to the mechanics of medical history taking, let us consider a few of the general principles that are common to all types of information-gathering interviews and apply them to the problem at hand.

As a physician you will have several fundamental objectives during the medical interview. These will include motivating the patient to communicate, controlling the interaction, and measuring the significance of the patient's responses.

Not all patients are suffering, but all are anxious. This we know from the personal experience of being patients ourselves. The patient may not recognize his anxiety —indeed he may deny it; but anxiety is not only normal, it is the expected reaction. This is true for the simple periodic health checkup as well as for the potentially serious illness. Part of this anxiety stems from a natural fear of disease with its many implications. Most patients are anxious about the physician as well. Will he be competent? Will she be friendly? Will he cause discomfort? Will she find something serious? When the patient and physician are of different sexes, there is bound to be some tension involved in discussing such matters as bowel function or in examining the genital area or the rectum.

A confident, gentle approach will do much to minimize these anxieties. The experienced clinician will frequently discuss them openly with the patient during the course of the interview, particularly when the patient seems excessively worried. Some early reassurance may be necessary during history taking. In fact, therapy may begin during history taking in the form of calming the excited patient. However, in attempting to calm the patient you should avoid implying that "there is nothing to be worried about" until you are convinced that that is true. Obviously, if serious disease eventually is discovered, you will have lost a certain amount of credibility.

The patient's anxiety may find expression in many ways other than simple agitation. Anger is a frequently used defense. The angry patient is a common and difficult problem, and you must avoid the temptation of meeting such anger with hostility of your own. On the other hand, you cannot ignore it. One helpful approach is to get the angry patient to discuss his hostility. The physician usually finds that the real source of anger is not the result of something that he himself has done. Even when it is, once out in the open the hostility tends to be lessened, particularly if the physician is wise enough to be reasonable and to take action to rectify the situation. There will be some patients, of course, who continue to be hostile despite your efforts to assuage them. As a student, it is wise to alert your supervising tutor or resident to the problem. Try to avoid direct confrontation with these patients without some guidance from a more experienced physician.

Another expression of the patient's anxiety may be extreme dependence. This can be very trying and requires great patience. You should make every effort to maintain a matter-of-fact relationship with overly dependent patients, and you should guard against displaying anger or exasperation. The seductive patient is an even more difficult problem, but fortunately such patients are very rare. Changing the subject at such times is usually all that is necessary.

If a patient begins to cry during the interview—and this will happen frequently —it is a mistake to feel that it is always necessary to rush in and try to stop the tears. More often it is preferable to remain as objective as possible and to try to communicate the fact that the patient should not be embarrassed by the outbreak and that you understand why he or she is upset. Wait for the storm to pass. Afterward you may want to explore the reasons for the patient's reaction, particularly if the patient is of a background that would suggest that a stoic rather than an emotional response would be typical.

Each patient will behave differently under the pressures of the examining room, and it is the obligation of the physician to try to understand why the patient feels the way he does. Only those of us who have been seriously ill ourselves can really understand the patient's point of view. Each of us has only one life, and an illness is a very serious event in the course of that life. It is therefore reasonable to consider experiences connected with an illness extremely significant and thus often fraught with emotion. Keep in mind that the patient's behavior in your presence may provide a unique opportunity to obtain a degree of insight into his personality, since it may typify his behavior with others. By analyzing this pattern as you go along, you may be able to obtain very important information. The patient occasionally reveals more about himself through his behavior than through anything he tells you.

The patient usually is motivated by a desire for relief from his symptoms. This is a very sound positive force, which favors a successful outcome. The major intrinsic deterrent is his fear of the consequences of his illness. This factor can produce a conflict that tends to make him an unreliable reporter. The physician himself introduces an extrinsic factor, namely, the effect of his own appearance, attitude, and pattern of questioning. By being calm and sympathetic and by showing genuine interest, you as a physician tend to minimize the forces that prompt the patient to distort or withhold information. A critical factor in this regard is the way in which you formulate your questions. For example, patients will respond almost universally in a biased manner to a question that conveys the possibility of serious consequences. This is not necessarily due to conscious falsification of information; rather, the response is simply affected by his subconscious fears. After you have created an atmosphere in which the patient feels safe in communicating openly and without fear of being judged, you can further motivate him by involving him more deeply in the topic at hand. As the patient forgets himself and focuses on the problem, more delicate areas can be explored without fear of his withdrawal.

Even if the physician and the patient were able to develop a relationship in which all sources of bias and all barriers to communication were eliminated, the problem of memory would still be an important limiting factor. The patient cannot tell the physician about something he has forgotten. Remembering and forgetting are subject to a number of well-known influences: intelligence, emotion, organic disturbances such as trauma or metabolic upset, and falsification. The ability to remember may be modified by the pertinence of the information, by interference from other factors, and by repression or distortion. In everyday life, forgetting to perform a task can at times be traced back to some conflict, while remembering events in vivid detail may correlate with positive emotional experiences or at least experiences that the individual considers significant. At Guy's Hospital, a consultant once elicited incredibly detailed information from a patient. When she left the room the consultant turned and said, "Whatever it was that happened to her on that day I'm not sure, but she considers it terribly important. She remembers everything!"

Direct questions may help to improve the patient's recall by reminding him of information that he has forgotten to volunteer. The review of systems is designed to bring out accessory symptoms that were overlooked during the presenting illness. When you run up against an important memory block, you may try two tricks to help the patient remember. One is to lead the discussion around the general area with the hope that some correlation will help to bring back the forgotten material. A second method is to put the subject aside (into the "subconscious oven") for a while, and then return and repeat the question in slightly different terms. You may be surprised to have the patient say "Now I remember. . . ."

Tension more often develops with patients of the opposite sex and with certain subjects, such as sex, alcoholism, mental illness, epilepsy, and venereal disease. When you sense that your patient is agitated, you might just as well desist, since the possibility of receiving distorted or falsified responses is very great indeed. This is the time for an explanation or a change of subject. If the area is critical, you must of course try again, at which time you can explain the importance of the information. If the patient remains abnormally defensive, do not fret. You have uncovered a very important fact. It is probably somehow related to the rest of the problem.

Because of the limitations of time, the interview should deal almost exclusively with relevant information. You, the physician, therefore must control the process. You begin by taking the initiative. You introduce yourself. You place the patient in a comfortable position. Since privacy is indispensable, relatives and friends are courteously excused except when the patient is a child or when an interpreter is needed. To "break the ice" a moment or two spent on some irrelevant subject helps the patient to compose himself. The business of history taking begins in earnest with an introductory question, such as "How may I help you?" or "What seems to be bothering you?" The physician makes it clear at this point that the patient has his undivided attention. This may be done by some gesture such as leaning forward, setting aside his pen, or by establishing eye contact.

Eye contact is a valuable method of controlling the interview situation. It establishes a sense of communication with the patient. It also helps the physician to concentrate on what he is being told and minimizes the patient's tendency to ramble. By carefully watching the patient's facial expression, the physician can sense immediately whether his questions are being understood. Needless to say, staring hypnotically at him will make the patient unbearably self-conscious and this should be avoided. With very shy patients, eye contact should be used with discretion since it can be detrimental. When properly used, however, it can be a major influence in the interview.

STRUCTURE OF THE MEDICAL HISTORY

It is of the highest importance in the art of detection to recognize out of a number of facts, which are incidental and which are vital.

Sherlock Holmes, as quoted by
Sir Arthur Conan Doyle
(1859–1930)

When taking or recording a medical history (and doing a physical exam), a reproducible, orderly approach is best. It ensures completeness and provides a structure on which to display the infinitely variable histories that patients may give.

The classic approach to the history and physical is outlined below. (A pocket copy for your reference is provided in the pocket inside the back cover of this book.)

THE HISTORY

1. **Biographical data**. Use the patient's stamp or clinic card if possible, including name and number. Add the date of admission or interview and the time at which you took the history. (The time of the history is important if clinical events change. It can be used as a baseline with more meaning if the reader knows when it was taken. This is particularly true in patients with rapidly changing clinical events, such as cardiac or neurologic disease.)

2. **Source of history and estimate of reliability**. The source should be very brief and might contain no more than "the patient," "old records," "the patient's wife," or whatever. If the source is unreliable (e.g., because of confusion), say so here.

3. **Chief complaint**. Statement of the chief complaint can be given in the patient's own words (using quotation marks liberally). Or you may with justice restructure what the patient has said to make it clearer, but without altering the basic meaning. Beware of inserting a premature diagnosis in the chief complaint, as it may lead you astray: Use symptoms rather than someone's opinion of what is wrong. The chief complaint should include age, race, sex, the complaint, and duration of the complaint. For example: "This 63-year-old white man presents with 'headache' for 3 days." There may be multiple chief complaints. For example: "This 34-year-old black woman has had nausea, vomiting, abdominal pain, and a rash for a week." Include in the chief complaint any major underlying illness of which you are aware, that is of such importance as to lead to immediate understanding of the chief complaint. For example, if the woman mentioned above has known diabetes, the sentence would be restructured to read "This 34-year-old black woman with known diabetes has had nausea, vomiting. . . ." Adults should be referred to as men and women, not males and females (the latter is dehumanizing, not being species-specific).

4. **History of present illness (HPI)**. The history of present illness (HPI) is the most challenging part of the clinical examination and requires more skill than the physical examination. It should be recorded as a paragraphic, orderly, logical, and grammatically correct description of the features of the chief complaint(s), written in full sentences. Think of it rather as a short story or a mystery story in which positive and negative clues contribute to a total understanding of the sequential events that have led to the patient's coming to you. The HPI should include *all* information referable to the system(s) involved in each major complaint. For example, for a cardiovascular complaint (angina), a *past history* of rheumatic fever belongs in the HPI, as do a *family history* of heart disease, a *social history* of severe work stress, and the entire cardiovascular *review of systems,* including all negatives.

In recording the present illness, you are more than a scribe, more than a simple recorder of information. It is your job to take the patient's story, examine it, probe it, and order and clarify it to the point where it most clearly describes the most likely illness or illnesses involved. This requires an ever-increasing familiarity on your part with the classic presentations of disease. Early on (and even later) in your career, it would be wise for you to take an initial history, do a physical, and then go immediately to a major textbook to read about the pathophysiology and clinical presentation of the disorder you suspect. Then go back to the patient to ask the additional questions and do the points of physical examination that you had, through ignorance, not known to ask and do before.

At the end of the HPI, the reader or listener should have a very good idea of the patient's status. Often the diagnosis will be quite clear at this point; sometimes it will be apparent that you do not know the diagnosis, but you will have explored many alternative possibilities in your mind.

The difficulty for the beginner is in eliminating irrelevant material, condensing and concentrating relevant findings into usable forms, and systematically arranging these findings into logical clusters or patterns. As you become more knowledgeable about disease, what to keep and what to throw away in the HPI becomes easier to determine. *All* abnormalities may *not* be related to the patient's current illness, and thus are recorded in the past history or review of systems.

The HPI may be long or short, depending on the nature of the illness, and it should be carefully scrutinized for excess verbiage, which should then be removed. Trivial pieces of information that have no bearing on the real complaint can be culled from the HPI. For example: "The patient was well until April 1982, when, while walking down the street on a sunny day, with the birds singing overhead, she experienced pain in her chest." Write instead, "This woman was well until April 1982, when, while walking easily, she had chest pain."

You will save both time and trouble by leaving out the stultified English so characteristic of medical workups. You may omit such statements as "The patient noted," or "The patient states that he was . . . at that time." It will be assumed, unless otherwise specified, that what is in the history is what the patient stated or noted. Similarly, "at that time" can usually be omitted and the history still will make sense. If not, use "then," which is shorter. "The patient" is more readily (and more humanely) referred to as "he, she, or Mr."

Minimize abbreviations, because they tend to be unintelligible. Since they are impossible to avoid altogether, however, we have listed some of the more common ones in Chapter 23.

If the patient has multiple problems, you might wish to describe them in paragraphs under separate problem headings, such as

    a. **Heart disease** (and then fully describe that chronologically)

    b. **Renal failure** (and then fully describe that chronologically)

This is generally easier than trying to write them all up together.

With the exception of the HPI, the remainder of the history and the physical may be written in truncated, staccato, incomplete sentences. The same caution about abbreviations should stand throughout, however.

5. **Past history (PH)**
   a. **Childhood illnesses** (e.g., measles, mumps, chickenpox, rheumatic fever, scarlet fever).
   b. **Adult illnesses**. Generally, record any for which the patient was hospitalized. Append dates if possible.
   c. **Trauma**. Major trauma (e.g., fractures) should be listed with dates and sequelae, if any.
   d. **Surgery**. Operations, with dates and, if known, the hospitals in which each procedure was done.
   e. **Allergies**. Describe not only what the patient is allergic to, but also the manifestations of that allergy. Drug allergies are especially important.
   f. **Medications**. Even if these have been included in the HPI, they should be listed, using both generic and brand names, with dose and frequency. If the indication for the medication is neither obvious nor stated elsewhere, include that here as well.
   g. **Travel**. Especially outside the continental United States.
   h. **Habits**. This generally refers most prominently to smoking, drinking, the use of illicit drugs, and bizarre diets.
   i. **Immunizations**. Particularly important in pediatric patients. Include measles, mumps, DPT, polio. Influenza, tetanus, and pneumococcal vaccination histories are more important in older patients.

6. **Family history (FH)**. You may do this by outlining a family tree or by simply listing blood kin, either living or dead, giving their ages and any health problems they may have had. Look especially for possible genetic disease if your patient's history of present illness is suggestive (certain forms of arthritis, kidney disease, and endocrine disease run in families.) In blacks, seek specifically a history of sickle cell anemia. In all patients, ask about heart disease, hypertension, diabetes, and cancer.

7. **Social history (SH)**. What you really want to know here is "who is this person who is sick?" Illness is really a limitation of function rather than the histopathologic process by which that function is compromised. An individual's response to sickness is in large part determined by his or her cultural background, social standing, educational and economic status, the opinions of the family about the sickness, and the individual's anticipation of functional compromise. In the SH, you will want to know about these features.

8. **Review of systems (ROS)**. You will find that doing the review of systems, which is an exercise in completeness, will become easier if you have asked all the necessary questions in the HPI and included the individual's positive and negative replies in the HPI. Then you are left with the important but not immediately applicable data about current other system function and malfunction. If your patient has a chief complaint involving the gastrointestinal system, the review of the GI system should logically be included in the history of present illness. Similarly, if the patient has diabetes, much of the ROS will be included in the HPI as pertinent positives and negatives, since diabetes may involve almost any system. Then, when you come to write this section, under each systemic subsection you will simply say "See HPI."
   a. **General**. Fever, chills, weight change, anemia.
   b. **Head**. Headaches, dizziness.
   c. **Eyes**. Acuity, diplopia, blurring, pain, discharge.
   d. **Ears**. Acuity, past infections, tinnitus, pain, discharge.
   e. **Nose**. Epistaxis, discharge, odd odors.
   f. **Throat and mouth**. Dental repair, sore tongue, frequent sore throats.
   g. **Chest**. Cough, pain, shortness of breath, wheeze, hemoptysis, production of sputum (amount, appearance). Last chest x-ray. Last skin test for TB. Breast masses, pain, discharge.

h. **Cardiovascular.** Chest pain, palpitations, shortness of breath, orthopnea, history of heart murmur, of heart attack, of rheumatic fever as a child, claudication, Raynaud's phenomenon.

i. **Gastrointestinal.** Appetite, nausea, vomiting, diarrhea, constipation, change in character of stool (calibre, consistency, color), jaundice, dark urine, abdominal pain, hematemesis, melena, hematochezia, heartburn. Any laxative or antacid use?

j. **Genitourinary.** Hesitancy, dribbling, difficulty starting stream, dysuria, frequency, urgency, gross hematuria, nocturia, incontinence. Any history of venereal disease? Sores on genitals? Any history of urinary tract infections?

k. **Menstrual.** Menarche, menopause. Interval between periods, duration of periods, regularity. Amount of flow. Any pain? Date of last period. Number of pregnancies, abortions, term deliveries. (A shorthand you may use is G = gravida, P = para, A = abortus. Thus, a woman pregnant four times with three live children and one miscarriage would be designated "G4P3A1.")

l. **Neuromuscular.** Syncope, vertigo, weakness or paralysis, numbness or tingling, seizures, psychiatric difficulties, "moodiness," arthritis, edema, cyanosis.

m. **Skin.** Rashes, hives, eczema, bruising.

THE PHYSICAL EXAMINATION

Though of less diagnostic help than a well-taken history, a pertinent physical is obviously very important. You will find the physical examination more interesting if you direct it to the elucidation of those points touched upon in the history. For example, if you suspect that your patient has infective endocarditis, you should look for physical hints of this disease when you do the examination. Then, instead of writing "eyes normal," you will say "no conjunctival petechiae, no Roth's spots." You will specify either that there are no murmurs or that one is present. You will look at the fingers and specify whether or not there is clubbing, splinter hemorrhages, Osler's nodes, or Janeway lesions. You will specify whether or not there is splenomegaly. Knowing that all these physical features correlate with your diagnostic suspicion makes the physical more than a routine and will help you to bolster your diagnostic acumen.

For patients who have potentially rapidly changing disease, it is important to put down the time at which your physical examination was performed.

DATE:

TIME:

1. **General appearance.** Well or poorly developed or nourished. Color (black, white, jaundiced, pale). In distress (acutely or chronically)?

2. **Vital signs.** Blood pressure (which arm or both, orthostatic change). Pulse (regular or irregular, orthostatic change). Respirations (labored or unlabored, wheeze). Temperature (axillary, rectal, or oral). Weight. Height.

3. **Skin, hair, and nails.** Pigmentation, scars, lesions, bruises, turgor. Describe or draw rashes.

4. **Nodes.** Any cervical, supraclavicular, axillary, epitrochlear, inguinal lymphadenopathy? If so, size of nodes (in cm), consistency (firm, rubbery, tender), mobile or fixed.

5. **Head**. Scalp, skull (configuration), scars, tenderness, bruits.
6. **Eyes**
   a. **External eye**. Conjunctivae, sclerae, lids, cornea, pupils (including reflexes), visual fields, extraocular motions.
   b. **Fundus**. Disc, blood vessels, pigmentation.
7. **Ears**. Shape of pinnae, external canal, tympanic membrane, acuity, air conduction versus bone conduction (Rinne's test), lateralization (Weber's test).
8. **Nose**. Septum, mucosa, polyps.
9. **Mouth and throat**. Lips, teeth, tongue (size, papillation), buccal mucosa, palate, tonsils, oropharynx.
10. **Neck**. Suppleness. Trachea, larynx, thyroid, blood vessels (jugular veins, carotid arteries).
11. **Chest and lungs**
    a. **Inspection**. Contour, symmetry, expansion.
    b. **Palpation**. Expansion, rib tenderness, tactile fremitus.
    c. **Percussion**. Diaphragmatic excursion, dullness.
    d. **Auscultation**. Rales, rhonchi, rubs, wheezes, egophony, pectoriloquy.
12. **Heart**
    a. **Inspection**. Point maximal impulse, chest contour.
    b. **Palpation**. Point maximal impulse, thrills, lifts, thrusts.
    c. **Auscultation**. Heart sounds, gallops, murmurs, rubs.
13. **Breasts**. Symmetry, retraction, lesions, nipples (inverted, everted), masses, tenderness, discharge.
14. **Abdomen**
    a. **Inspection**. Scars (draw these), contour, masses, vein pattern.
    b. **Auscultation**. Bowel sounds, rubs, bruits.
    c. **Percussion**. Organomegaly, hepatic dullness.
    d. **Palpation**. Tenderness, masses, rigidity, liver, spleen, kidneys.
    e. **Hernia**. Femoral, inguinal, ventral.
15. **Genitalia**
    a. **Male**. Penile lesions, scrotum, testes. Circumcised?
    b. **Female**. Labia, Bartholin's and Skene's glands, vagina, cervix. Bimanual of internal genitalia.
16. **Rectum**. Perianal lesions, sphincter tone, tenderness, masses, prostate, stool color, occult blood.
17. **Extremities**. Pulses (symmetry, bruits, perfusion). Joints (mobility, deformity). Cyanosis, edema. Varicosities. Muscle mass.
18. **Back**. Contour spine, tenderness. Sacral edema.
19. **Neurologic**
    a. **Mental status**. Alertness, memory, judgment, mood.
    b. **Cranial nerves** (I–XII).
    c. **Cerebellum**. Gait, finger–nose, heel–shin, tremors.
    d. **Motor**. Muscle mass, strength, deep tendon reflexes. Pathologic or primitive reflexes.
    e. **Sensory**. Touch, pain, vibration. Heat and cold as indicated.

THE LABORATORY STUDIES

The sequential recording of laboratory data (the least important of the information you have gathered to date because laboratory data only serve to confirm or deny what you have found on history and physical) is best done in orderly fashion.

1. **Hemogram** (hematocrit, hemoglobin, white count, differential and peripheral blood smear).
2. **Urine analysis**.
3. **Serologies** (electrolytes and other indicated studies).
4. **X-rays**. Describe these, rather than just noting that they are "WNL." Be specific in your descriptions.
5. **ECG**. This also should be recorded in a logical manner. In order, one notes the rate, the rhythm, intervals (PR, QRS, QT), axis, P wave configuration, QRS configuration, T wave configuration, abnormal configurations, interpretations.

   Only by reading the ECG in the preceding way (which gives much more information than "abnormal ECG" or "within normal limits") can a reader compare a cardiogram taken at a later time with the one that was present during your workup.

Include in the laboratory findings only those data that pertain to your patient. There is no intrinsic virtue to any lab study. If laboratory data disagree with clinical judgment, you would probably be correct in ignoring the laboratory data.

IMPRESSIONS

It is an old maxim of mine that when you have excluded the impossible, whatever remains, however improbable, must be the truth.

Sherlock Holmes, as quoted by
SIR ARTHUR CONAN DOYLE
(1859–1930)

It is in this section that you take the information that you have gleaned from the history, the physical examination, and laboratory studies and resynthesize it into a cogent explanation of your patient's status, along with your best advice as to how to further understand it, and what to do about it.

List your impressions (or the patient's problems) in the order of their importance to the patient and to you. Under each impression write a description of the rationale behind the diagnosis and what you plan to do about it. This description may take many forms, including the problem-oriented approach or one of the more traditional forms (e.g., differential diagnosis). The problem-oriented medical record (POMR) attempts to provide an ongoing system by which data, problems, plans, and follow-up are ordered in a logical sequence that, according to its promoters, lends itself to analysis more readily than does the classic history and physical. Which form you use may not really matter so long as the description is clear and complete. A single-paragraph summary is often included at the end.

Examples of both the traditional and POMR approaches to the history and physical are presented in Chapter 24. (A complete review of the POMR may be found in Weed, L. L., *Medical Records, Medical Education, and Patient Care.* Chicago: Case Western Reserve University Press, 1981.)

PROGRESS NOTES

As you follow your patient each day, new information will have to be recorded. This information may consist of new history (remembered by patient, family, or brought to light by the arrival of a medical record), new events occurring in hospital, changes in physical examination (the pertinent features of which must be repeated *at least* once a day, and often more frequently), and consultative or laboratory data. To this new information you should append any changes in diagnosis or therapy that you have instituted and the reasons why. Progress notes must be brief, relevant, and always dated and timed (things may change rapidly in hospital). They must, of course, be legibly signed. An example of progress notes follows.

9/18/82   5 P.M.   Hospital day #3

Mrs. Worth feels better on penicillin therapy, instituted yesterday at 10 P.M. Her myalgias and headache are less and her appetite improved. Her temperature has fallen from a high of 102°F orally at 3 A.M. today.

P.E. T (PO) 99°F, pulse 78 and regular, BP 130/85. R 12 and unlabored. She has no splinting (an improvement over yesterday evening). Her chest is clear to percussion.

Auscultation shows scattered inspiratory rales at the left base, unchanged from 9/17/82.

Lab from this morning shows wbc = 7800 with a normal differential.

Chest x-ray this noon shows no change in her fluffy left lower lobe infiltrate.

Sputum cultures of 9/15/82 are growing *D. pneumoniae.*

Impression: Pneumococcal (left lower lobe) pneumonia improving on penicillin therapy.

Plan: Continue procaine penicillin G (6 million units IM bid).

John Smith
(MS III)

(John Smith)

ORAL PRESENTATIONS

Physicians teach each other medicine mainly by the "case method." Simply put, doctors orally describe the history, physical examination, and laboratory findings on their patients so that listening doctors can learn (and teach) about the patient's problem. The oral presentation may be brief or lengthy, depending on the circumstance in which it is given. The least formal presentations occur when students or physicians chat with their colleagues over dinner about the interesting patient of the day: "I saw a 34-year-old woman with angina today. She'd had rheumatic fever as a kid. She's got a fantastic aortic insufficiency murmur. . . ." The most formal presentations are those given to the Senior Physician in formal rounds, when the student details chief complaint; history of present illness; past, social, and family history; and review of systems. The physical examination is described in its entirety, including pertinent negatives; and salient laboratory studies are detailed. The purpose of this exercise is to make as much information available to the Senior Physician as possible, so that he or she can knowledgeably discuss the case. Such a detailed presentation may take up to 10 minutes, but should never be much longer than that.

In either of these extremes, or in the multitude of variations between them, the oral presentation should be clear, logical, entertaining, and pertinent. Giving such a presentation takes considerable practice.

BEGINNING THE EXAMINATION

The best history taker is he who can best interpret the answer to a leading question.

PAUL H. WOOD
(1907–1962)

HOW TO TAKE THE HISTORY

Whether you use the problem-oriented or traditional method to record the medical history, accurate and complete data provide the substrate on which understanding your patients' problems depends.

Having made your patient as comfortable as possible and having set him at his ease (insofar as it is possible), you may find yourself floundering initially as to what questions to ask and how to ask them.

The physician's most effective tool for controlling the interview process is the way in which he frames his questions. The experienced physician uses all types of questions to gather information. In evaluating the responses, he is conscious of the possible introduction of bias into the interview by the question itself. Certain types of general questions are neutral and virtually free of biasing effects. Others may be strongly weighted in one direction or another. It is only when the physician is unaware of the potential distorting influence of this or that type of question that he is likely to get into trouble. Let us consider several basic types of questions.

The *neutral question* should be used whenever possible. It is structured so that it does not suggest that any particular response is more acceptable to the physician or more beneficial to the patient than another. A neutral question can be open or closed. The open neutral question simply establishes a topic: "Tell me more about your headaches." The closed neutral question incorporates several alternative answers in the question: "Are your headaches more likely to occur in the morning, afternoon, or evening?"

The *simple direct question* is always closed because it requires simply a yes or no answer: "Do your headaches upset your stomach?" Direct questions may or may not be neutral, depending on such factors as voice inflection, context, and previous questions. Although direct questions will speed the interview, too many of them tend to overwhelm the patient and put words into his mouth. They are indispensable but require moderation.

The *leading question* is one that tempts the patient to give one answer rather than another. Although it automatically introduces bias, it may yield special information unobtainable by any other means. This technique is particularly useful in testing the reliability of a series of questions by loading the final query: "Would you

21

say that your headaches come on only when you are feeling very tired?" Most physicians occasionally use leading questions.

The *loaded question* is usually interjected to study the reaction of the patient, since it is so heavily biased that the answer itself is unimportant: "Do you ever think you might be better off dead?" Such a question rarely if ever is needed under ordinary circumstances. It would be directed to a depressed patient only after laying considerable groundwork. This shock technique would be used primarily to assess his response to the suggestion of suicide.

Supplementary remarks are brief comments that are intended to stimulate the patient to proceed. They tell the patient that he is doing well and should continue. They may consist of a simple assertion such as "I see" or "Umm." A simple pause is sometimes an effective way of encouraging the patient to go ahead. Certain neutral remarks such as "Anything else?" "How do you mean?" and "Tell me more about that" have the same positive effect.

By using these different techniques selectively, you will gradually set a pattern that becomes intelligible to the patient. A head nod or an encouraging murmur is a reward that tells him that the topic is relevant and that he should continue. When the response is inadequate, you probe with a direct question. If the patient wanders too far afield, you may have to interrupt and change the subject. Interruption should be used only as a last resort, for if the patient's feelings are hurt, he will surely retreat. This must be avoided if possible. By carefully observing the effect of your remarks on the patient, your questions should improve as you proceed.

As you elicit your information, you simultaneously estimate its significance. You probe for precise temporal relationships and try to determine the relative severity of the various complaints. Certain symptoms considered extremely important by the patient may be discarded as irrelevant in the light of your insight and experience, while other symptoms that might be considered trivial by the patient are retained by you as significant. The interrelationships between symptoms must be determined as the interview proceeds, and you must decide whether any single complaint has more than one cause. This process of probing and measuring continues throughout the interview.

HOW TO RECORD THE HISTORY
It is often harder to boil down than to write.

Sir William Osler
(1849–1919)

During the interview, no attempt should be made to record the complete history in final form. There are several good reasons for this. First, it is literally impossible to do so; it distracts the patient and disrupts the procedure. Jotting down reminders, dates, ages, and numbers, however, is not only acceptable but indispensable. Second, the medical record is not meant to be a repository for raw data. The information must be suitably condensed, logically sequenced, and converted (as far as possible) into crisp, pertinent medical terminology before it is recorded. The procedure requires time and thought.

HOW TO DO THE PHYSICAL EXAMINATION

The trouble with doctors is not that they don't know enough, but that they don't see enough.

SIR DOMINIC J. CORRIGAN
(1802–1880)

A physical examination that follows a logical sequence maximizes both your efficiency and the patient's comfort. A minimum number of position changes, especially in the sick individual, is obviously desirable. Incidentally, a considerable amount of the historical review of systems can be done during the physical examination, as you touch upon each major area of the body.

Note **general appearance** (Chap. 4) as you take the history and when initiating the physical examination, usually with the patient sitting. **Vital signs** (Chap. 5) may be taken at this time, and a survey of the **skin** (Chap. 6) may be started.

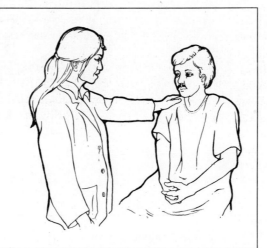

Examine the **head and neck** (Chaps. 8–10), including **cervical nodes** (Chap. 7). **Thorax** (Chaps. 11, 12), **breast** (Chap. 13), **supraclavicular** and **axillary nodes** (Chap. 7), and initial **cardiovascular examination**, including **upper extremity pulses** and **neck vein** observation (Chap. 12), are done next.

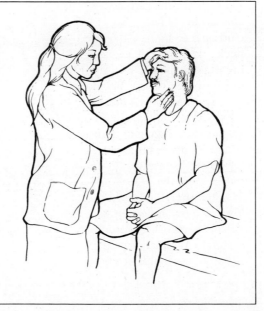

Examine the **posterior lung fields** (Chap. 11) and **back** (Chap. 17). A posterior palpation of the **thyroid gland** (Chap. 10) is often done. Observe the **skin** of the back (Chap. 6).

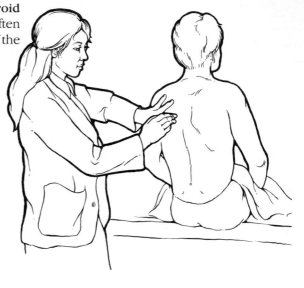

With the patient supine and the examiner on the right, continue **cardiac examination** (Chap. 12), including reexamination of the **neck veins**. Palpate the **breasts** (Chap. 13). Examine the **abdomen** (Chap. 14), including **kidneys** (Chaps. 14, 15) and **aorta** (Chaps. 12, 14). Palpate the **inguinal nodes** (Chap. 7) and **femoral pulses** (Chap. 12). Observe the **external genitalia** (Chaps. 15, 16). **Peripheral pulses in the lower extremities** (Chap. 12) and parts of the **musculoskeletal examination** (Chap. 17) are done in this position.

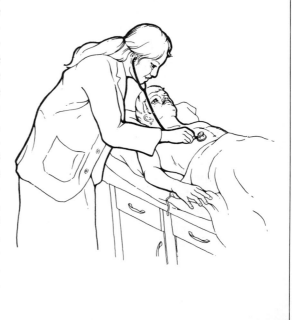

With the patient again sitting, examine the remainder of the **musculoskeletal system** (Chap. 17). As part of the **neurologic examination**, the cranial nerve, motor, reflex, cerebellar, and sensory examinations are done now (Chap. 18).

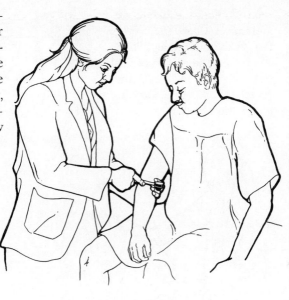

The patient stands for the rest of the neurologic examination (station and gait, Romberg's sign) (Chap. 18). In men, examine the **external genitalia**, including **hernia** (Chap. 15).

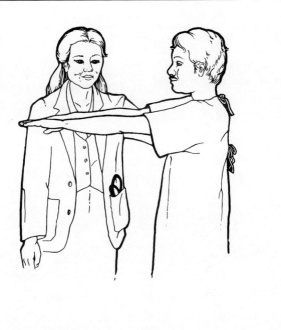

In women, the **pelvic examination** (Chap. 16) is done last, with the **rectal** (Chap. 14) conducted as part of this examination. In men, the **rectal** (Chaps. 14, 15) completes the physical.

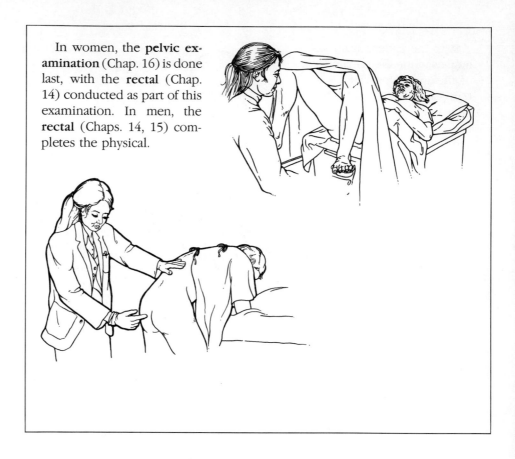

SECTION II
GENERAL EXAMINATIONS

It is a fraud of the Christian system to call the sciences human invention; it is only the applications of them that is human. Every science has for its basis a system of principles as fixed and unalterable as those by which the universe is regulated and governed. Man cannot make principles, he can only discover them.

THOMAS PAINE
(1737–1809)

1. Observe your patient, including skin.
2. Examine the hands.
3. Take the temperature.
4. Count pulse and respirations.
5. Take the blood pressure.
6. If the lymph nodes are enlarged, examine them all at this time. If not, do them regionally.

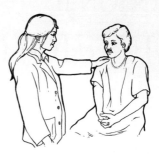

CHAPTER 4

GENERAL APPEARANCE

In all experimental knowledge there are three phases: an observation made, a comparison established, and a judgment rendered.

CLAUDE BERNARD
(1813–1878)

From the moment you meet your patient, and throughout the interview, you should be constantly observing him or her in an orderly and scientific way. The ability to observe accurately is a great asset in most fields of endeavor; it is indispensable in the practice of medicine. The physical examination is simply a series of observations.

Yet as Goethe said, "We see only what we know." The first step is to perceive. The second is to relate the sensory stimuli to relevant knowledge or past experience. Both abilities are indispensable, and both are irrevocably interdependent. From reading, from lectures and clinical experience, we accumulate the body of knowledge that gives significance to what we perceive. This background is concerned with more than the simple interpretation of findings; it is part of the act of observing. Let us consider an example.

An inexperienced student at the foot of the bed of a patient with clubbed digits is asked to describe anything he sees that might be significant. Rarely, he may point out the peculiar rounded appearance of the nails without being able to explain its significance. Far more often, however, the finding will go unnoticed. It does not register because it has no meaning for him. The lesson here is a simple one. In your eagerness to begin clinical work, do not lose sight of the importance of your preclinical scholarship. Without basic knowledge derived from careful study, you cannot expect to be an artful observer. You see only insofar as you understand. Medical observation is complex; it must therefore be deliberate and systematic. It requires concentration. An ill-timed distraction may cause an oversight; the oversight, a missed diagnosis. It is always helpful to focus your attention on one thing at a time. Looking at the hand is not enough. You must scrutinize in turn the nails, the skin texture, the color, the hair distribution, and so forth. Use of a disciplined system helps in this respect by limiting your field of observation. It makes you less susceptible to errors of omission.

The mental phase of observation may be both conscious and subconscious. What attracts us more than anything else is change. Like the continuous sound that is "heard" only when it suddenly stops, the physical abnormality captures our attention almost automatically. At this point we begin to think. We look more carefully. We may reposition the patient, have him breathe more deeply, or perform some other maneuver aimed at accentuating the finding or facilitating its analysis. We also begin to think ahead, for one finding may be a signpost that tells us to look carefully for other specific possibilities. One or two spider angiomas (indicating liver disease) noticed during history taking tells the experienced observer to watch particularly for an enlarged liver, palmar erythema, clubbing, splenomegaly, testicular atrophy, dilated abdominal veins, external hemorrhoids, hyperactive reflexes, or a flapping tremor. Of course, the first signpost on the way to diagnosis is the patient's history itself.

PREPARING THE PATIENT

The physical examination should be made as easy as possible for the patient, who usually expects it to be a relatively distasteful experience. If the physician is considerate and gentle, the patient should feel, when it is all over, that most of his or her fears on that score were unfounded. The ideal examining room is private, warm enough to avoid chilling, and free from distracting noise and sources of interruption. Adequate (preferably fluorescent or natural) light is essential. The examining table may be placed with its head against the wall, but both sides (particularly the right) and the foot should be accessible to the examiner.

The first crisis concerns the problem of undressing. In the outpatient department the patient disrobes while the physician is out of the room. It is always stressed that the patient must disrobe completely; it is folly to try to examine the heart through a nightgown or the abdomen through a slip. But it is equally true that respect for the patient's modesty is an important factor that greatly affects the subsequent physician-patient relationship. Tell the patient to leave on his or her underpants. They can be moved aside later, when necessary. This simple concession will not interfere with 90 percent of the examination, and it will greatly reduce anxiety. In addition, a sheet should always be available to drape the patient from the waist down. A towel or special gown may be used to cover the female chest (Fig. 4-1). This combination allows complete examination without prolonged, embarrassing exposure.

Begin and end the examination by washing your hands. When possible do this in the patient's presence. Your movements should be deliberate and methodical but always gentle. Your attitude should be basically objective but not serious. An occasional smile or distracting comment is a great help in relieving tension. Try to avoid surprise. Preface each maneuver with a simple direction or explanation. When the time comes to inspect the breasts, prepare the patient with a simple statement such as "Now we must remove this towel for a moment." The same is true for examining the abdomen. This gives a sense of purpose to your actions that practically eliminates embarrassment. The pelvic examination, of course, takes special preparation, and a female attendant should always be present if the examining physician is a man.

At times it will be necessary to cause the patient some discomfort. In these instances it is particularly important to explain the necessity of going ahead. For example: "I'm sorry if this hurts but it's important." The examiner should not hold back because of pain, but on the other hand he must balance the importance of the observation against the degree of discomfort and proceed as deftly as possible.

HISTORY

Changes in general appearance, especially gradual changes, may go unnoticed by the patient. It is often valuable to obtain a photograph of the patient from 1 or 2

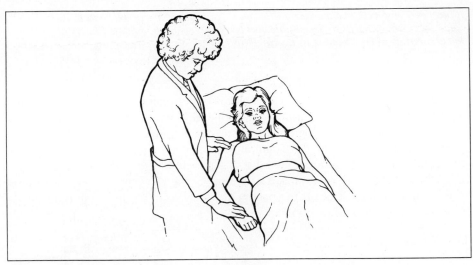

FIGURE 4-1
Woman draped for examination.

years before, to compare with current appearance. Most individuals, in our pound-conscious era, can tell you if they have gained or lost weight over recent months. If they cannot, old records (hospital charts, identification cards, some driving licenses) can be consulted for past weight.

Unaccustomed clumsiness or acquired "accident-proneness" may be the only historical clue to neurologic disease. Decrease in accustomed activity may signal progressive weakness.

Close friends, relatives, and neighbors may be more aware of changes in general appearance and activity than the patient. You should not hesitate to ask for their opinions and to incorporate these judiciously into your history.

PHYSICAL EXAMINATION

1. Observe your patient.
2. Examine the hands.

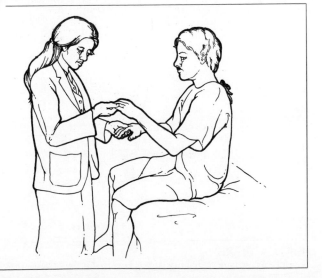

It has been observed, that the height of a man from the crown of the head to the sole of the foot, is equal to the distance between the tips of the middle fingers of the two hands when extended in a straight line.

PLINY THE ELDER
(23–79)

Even before the formal physical you will begin making observations that may alert you to disease. Throughout the history and physical, these cumulative observations form the basis for logical diagnostic deductions.

As the patient moves into the examining room, you might note the **gait**. Is it painful (antalgic)? Is there evident favoring of one side of the body, as in stroke? Is it rigid, bradykinetic, as in Parkinson's disease? Is the movement slow, the posture slumped, as in depression? Is the patient unsteady, as in weakness, middle-ear disease, or cerebellar dysfunction?

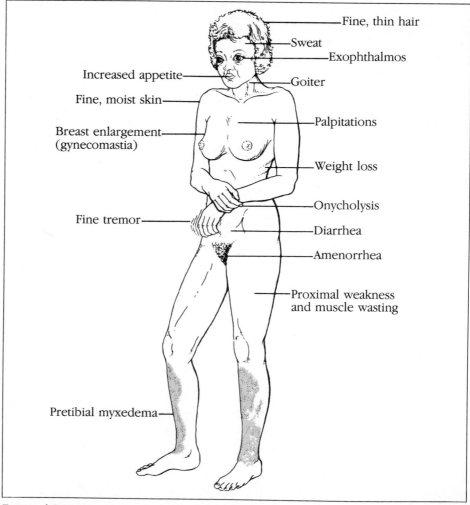

FIGURE 4-2
Hyperthyroidism. A diagnosis you can make by observation.

A wealth of information can be gained by **shaking hands** with the patient. Warm, moist hands may suggest hyperthyroidism (Fig. 4-2). Are they the painful, swollen hands of the arthritic? The cold, moist hands of the anxious patient? The calloused hands of the manual laborer or the softer fingers of the scholar? Is the ring loose, as with weight loss, or tight, as with edema?

When the patient speaks, does the tone of his **voice** suggest the hoarseness of laryngeal cancer; the weakened, thickened, and lowered voice of hypothyroidism; the "vocal ataxia" or "scanning speech" of multiple sclerosis or cerebellar disease? Is slurred speech the result of central nervous system injury or oropharygeal pathology? Do an elderly person's dentures click, suggesting weight loss or dehydration, or are the ill-fitting dentures themselves a cause of weight loss? Are words "hard to find," as in the aphasia following some cerebral vascular occlusive events? Is the speech monotonal or emotionless as in certain psychiatric disorders?

The **face** has always been the mirror of the mind. It shows pain, fear, anxiety, and sadness. It is in the face that we first notice whether our patients are pale, ruddy, cyanotic, or icteric. Thickened features suggest hormonal imbalance—e.g., of the thyroid or growth hormone. Fullness may be a consequence of edema, obesity, or a result of excess corticosteroids. A malar flush may signal *lupus* or *mitral stenosis*. Shiny skin and tight features first alert us to possible *scleroderma*. Cranial nerve dysfunction may be manifested by ptosis, strabismus, or facial asymmetry.

Habitus refers to your patient's general shape—his or her body build. *Cachexia* is an extreme thinness and debility caused by some serious disease, such as cancer or chronic infection. Signs of recent weight loss, such as loose clothes, newly punched belt holes, and redundant skin folds and striae (stretch marks), clue the clinician to a loss of flesh or fat that may or may not have been noticed by the patient.

Simple *obesity* is a deposition of body fat in excess of some arbitrary standard and is partly culturally defined. Pathologic obesity is deposition of body fat to the point of physiologic compromise of the individual, who may have respiratory, cardiac, or orthopedic difficulty. In these conditions excess fat is apportioned generally around the body—face, trunk, buttocks, and extremities. Deposition of fat around the trunk, with thin extremities in which muscle wasting is evident, may suggest hypercorticosteroidism.

Develop the habit of closely observing the patient's **hands**; they are highly informative (see Tables 4-1 and 4-2 at the end of this chapter). It is said that when a physician was called to the harem to treat one of the sultan's wives, he was allowed to examine only the hand of the patient extended between the folds of a curtain. This procedure was not entirely without diagnostic value. One need only watch a concert pianist to recognize the close relationship between brain and hand. Speech is intimately associated with the hand, and gestures may convey more meaning than words. The types of rings (and other jewelry) have a special message. Nicotine stains also convey a certain impression, as does the general hygiene.

Observe the nails closely (Fig. 4-3). *Beau's lines* are transverse furrows that begin at the lunula and progress distally as the nail grows. They result from a temporary arrest of growth of the nail matrix occasioned by trauma or systemic stress. If all the nails are involved, a period of general catabolism, such as infection, childbirth, and toxicity, may be postulated (local nail trauma seldom involves more than one or

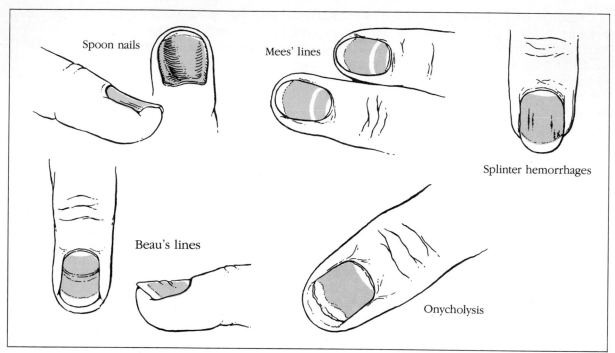

FIGURE 4-3
Some nail signs of systemic disease.

two digits). Knowing that the nail grows about 0.1 mm/day, one can, by measuring how far Beau's lines are from the cuticle, approximately date the stress. For example, if the line is 4 mm out, some serious event occurred about 40 days before.

Spoon nails (*koilonychia*) may occur in a form of iron deficiency anemia, as well as in a variety of other disorders (coronary disease, syphilis) and with the use of strong soaps.

Subungual splinter hemorrhages may provide a clue to bacterial endocarditis or *Trichinella spiralis* infestation in the febrile patient.

The nails may reflect metabolic disturbances. *Terry's nails* are the white nails with normal pink tips described in patients with cirrhosis. *Mees' lines* are paired, white, parallel transverse bands seen in individuals with hypoalbuminemia. *Lindsay's* (*half and half*) *nails,* in which the proximal portion of the nail is white and the distal 20–50 percent is red, are associated with renal failure. None of these is specific, but all give useful hints. *Onycholysis* or destruction of the nails, may be seen with hyperthyroidism, fungal nail infection, or in association with psoriasis. In the latter condition, a less severe change may be seen, namely, pitting of the nails.

Clubbing of the nails may occur in association with cardiovascular disease (congenital, cyanotic), subacute bacterial endocarditis, advanced cor pulmonale, pulmonary arteriovenous fistula, and pulmonary disease (inflammatory, bronchiectasis, abscess, empyema). One sees a bulbous enlargement of the distal portion of the digits (Fig. 4-4). The angle made by the proximal nail fold and the nail plate (Lovibond's angle) exceeds 180°. The etiology of clubbing is still uncertain, al-

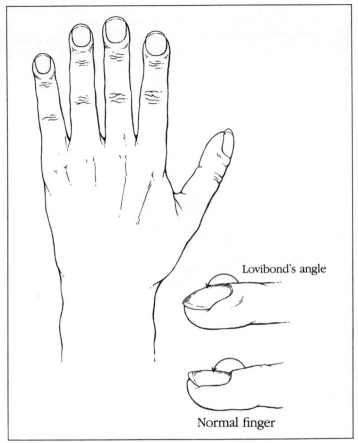

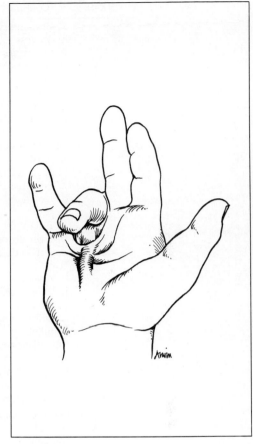

Figure 4-4
Clubbing.

Figure 4-5
Dupuytren's contracture.

though it is probably related to increased blood flow through multiple arterio-venous shunts in the distal phalanges (Table 4-3).

Extreme redness (erythema) of the palm is common in cirrhosis of the liver and in women who have borne children. Pallor of the palm, especially the creases, sug-gests anemia. *Dupuytren's contracture,* a fibrosis and contraction of the palmar fas-cia, is seen with liver disease, trauma, epilepsy, and simple aging (Fig. 4-5).

Table 4-3. Some Causes of Clubbing

I. Symmetric clubbing
  A. Cardiovascular disease
    1. Congenital, cyanotic
    2. Subacute bacterial endocarditis
    3. Advanced cor pulmonale
    4. Pulmonary arteriovenous fistula
  B. Pulmonary disease
    1. Inflammatory

TABLE 4-3. (Continued)

        a. Bronchiectasis
        b. Abscess
        c. Empyema
     2. Pneumoconiosis
     3. Neoplasm
        a. Carcinoma, primary
        b. Pleural mesothelioma
     4. Interstitial fibrosis
  C. Extrathoracic disease
     1. Gastrointestinal
        a. Sprue
        b. Ulcerative colitis
        c. Regional enteritis
        d. Dysentery
     2. Hepatic
        a. Biliary cirrhosis
        b. Liver abscess
        c. Amyloidosis
     3. Toxic
        a. Arsenic
        b. Phosphorus
        c. Alcohol
        d. Silica or beryllium
     4. Familial
     5. Miscellaneous
        a. Chronic pyelonephritis
        b. Syringomyelia
        c. Chronic granulocytic leukemia
        d. Hyperparathyroidism
II. Asymmetric clubbing
  A. Unidigital
     1. Median nerve injury
  B. Unilateral
     1. Aneurysm of innominate artery
     2. Recurrent subluxation of shoulder
  C. Unequal
     1. Anomalous aortic arch
     2. Reverse patent ductus

Arthritic changes in the hands will be discussed more fully under the joint examination.

Examine, by quick but thorough observation, the **entire body** of your patient before you begin a regional examination. Overall *hair distribution,* for example, not only differs according to age and sex (Fig. 4-6) but may signal disease (Table 4-4).

"Educated" observation may lead to a suspicion of diagnosis even before the patient speaks, as evidenced particularly in the endocrine disorders illustrated in Figures 4-7 through 4-10.

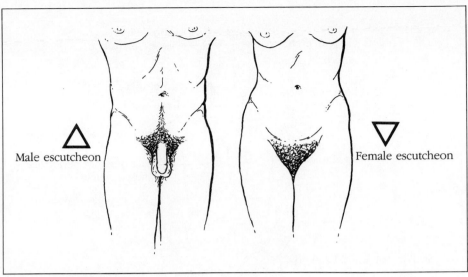

Male escutcheon   Female escutcheon

FIGURE 4-6
Normal sexual hair distribution in adult men and women. Changes may signal hormonal abnormalities.

TABLE 4-4. Some Causes of Hirsutism

Racial and familial

Puberty, pregnancy, menopause

Drugs
  Phenytoin
  Diazoxide
  Corticosteroids
  Progestagens
  Androgens
  Minoxidil

Endocrine abnormalities
  Adrenal hyperplasia
  Adrenal adenoma or carcinoma
  Stein-Leventhal syndrome
  Ovarian tumors
  Pituitary tumors

Congenital sex anomalies

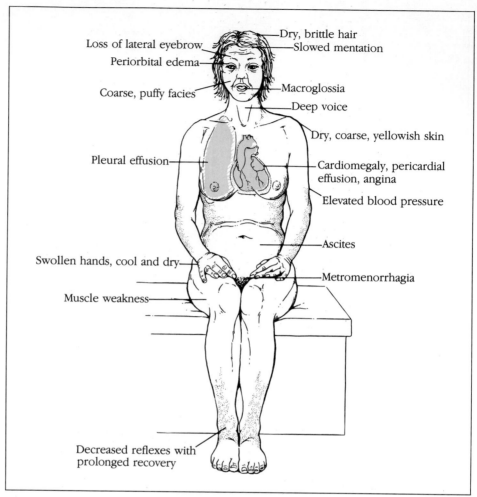

FIGURE 4-7
Myxedema. A diagnosis you can make by observation.

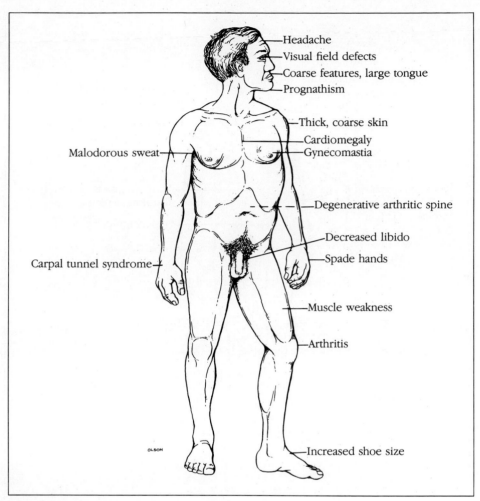

FIGURE 4-8
Acromegaly. A diagnosis you can make by observation.

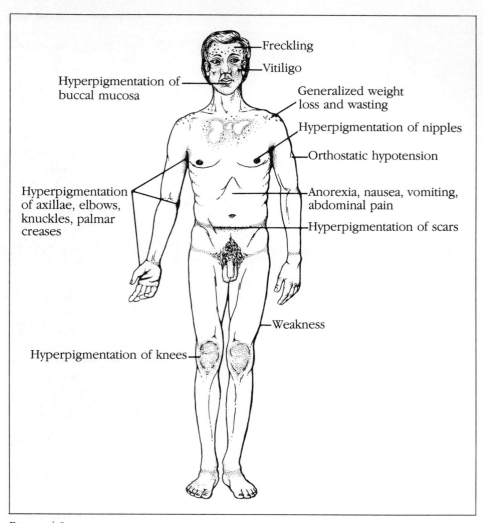

FIGURE 4-9
Adrenocortical insufficiency (Addison's disease). A diagnosis you can make by observation. Hyperpigmentation does *not* occur with pituitary adrenal insufficiency.

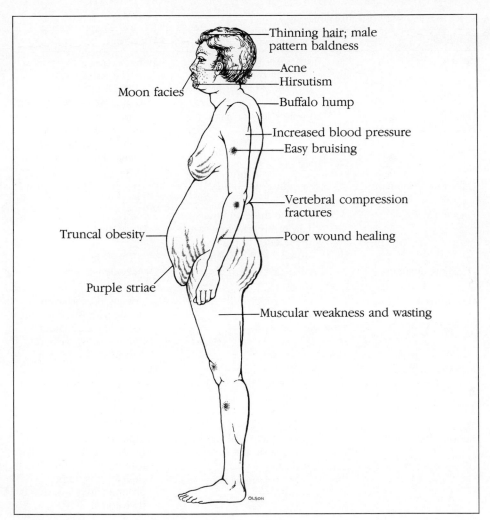

Thinning hair; male pattern baldness

Acne

Hirsutism

Buffalo hump

Increased blood pressure

Easy bruising

Vertebral compression fractures

Poor wound healing

Muscular weakness and wasting

Moon facies

Truncal obesity

Purple striae

FIGURE 4-10
Adrenocortical excess (Cushing's syndrome). A diagnosis you can make by observation.

TABLE 4-1. Glossary of Nail Pathology

Condition	Description	Occurrence
Beau's lines	Transverse lines or ridges marking repeated disturbances of nail growth	Systemic diseases, toxic or nutritional deficiency states of many types, trauma (from manicuring)
Defluvium unguium (onychomadesis)	Complete loss of nails	Certain systemic diseases such as scarlet fever, syphilis, leprosy, alopecia areata, and exfoliative dermatitis
Diffusion of lunula unguis	"Spreading" of lunula	Dystrophies of the extremities
Eggshell nails	Nail plate thin, semitransparent bluish-white, with a tendency to curve upward at the distal edge	Syphilis
Fragilitas unguium	Friable or brittle nails	Dietary deficiency, local trauma
Hapalonychia	Nails very soft, split easily	Following contact with strong alkalis; endocrine disturbances, malnutrition, syphilis, chronic arthritis
Hippocratic nails	"Watch-glass nails" associated with "drumstick fingers"	Chronic respiratory and circulatory diseases, especially pulmonary tuberculosis; hepatic cirrhosis
Koilonychia	"Spoon nails"; nails are concave on the outer surface	In dysendocrinisms (acromegaly), trauma, dermatoses, syphilis, nutritional deficiencies, hypochromic anemias, hypothyroidism
Leukonychia	White spots or striations or rarely the whole nail may turn white (congenital type)	Local trauma, hepatic cirrhosis, nutritional deficiencies and many systemic diseases
Mees' lines	Transverse white bands	Hodgkin's granuloma, arsenical and thallium toxicity, high fevers, local nutritional derangement
Moniliasis of nails	Infections (usually paronychial) caused by yeast forms (*Candida albicans*)	Frequently in foodhandlers, dentists, dishwashers, gardeners
Onychatrophia	Atrophy or failure of development of nails	Trauma, infection, dysendocrinism, gonadal aplasia, and many systemic disorders

TABLE 4-1. (Continued)

Condition	Description	Occurrence
Onychauxis	Nail plate is greatly thickened	Mild persistent trauma, systemic diseases such as peripheral stasis, peripheral neuritis, syphilis, leprosy, hemiplegia, or at times may be congenital
Onychia	Inflammation of the nail matrix causing deformity of the nail plate	Trauma, infection, many systemic diseases
Onychodystrophy	Any deformity of the nail plate, nail bed, or nail matrix	Many diseases; trauma; or may be caused by chemical agents (poisoning, allergy)
Onychogryposis	"Claw nails"—extreme degree of hypertrophy, sometimes with horny projections arising from the nail surface	May be congenital or related to many chronic systemic diseases (see onychauxis above)
Onycholysis	Loosening of the nail plate beginning at the distal or free edge	Trauma, injury by chemical agents, many systemic diseases
Onychomadesis	Shedding of all the nails (defluvium unguium)	Dermatoses such as exfoliative dermatitis, alopecia areata, psoriasis, eczema, nail infection, severe systemic diseases, arsenical poisoning
Onychophagia	Nail biting	Neurosis
Onychorrhexis	Longitudinal ridging and splitting of the nails	Dermatoses, nail infections, many systemic diseases, senility, injury by chemical agents, and hyperthyroidism
Onychoschizia	Lamination and scaling away of nails in thin layers	Dermatoses, syphilis, injury by chemical agents
Onychotillomania	Alteration of the nail structures caused by persistent neurotic picking of the nails	Neurosis
Pachyonychia	Extreme thickening of all the nails. The nails are more solid and more regular than in onychogryposis	Usually congenital and associated with hyperkeratosis of the palms and soles
Pterygium unguis	Thinning of the nail fold and spreading of the cuticle over the nail plate	Associated with vasospastic conditions such as Raynaud's phenomenon and occasionally with hypothyroidism

Source: T. J. Berry, *The Hand As a Mirror of Systemic Disease*. Philadelphia: Davis, 1963. Pp. 179–191.

TABLE 4-2. Outline of Physical Findings in the Hand

I. Variations in size and shape of hand
  A. Large, blunt fingers (spade hand)
    1. Acromegaly
    2. Hurler's disease (gargoylism)
  B. Gross irregularity of shape and size
    1. Paget's disease of bone
    2. Maffuci's syndrome
    3. Neurofibromatosis
  C. Spider fingers, slender palm (arachnodactyly)
    1. Hypopituitarism
    2. Eunuchism
    3. Ehlers-Danlos syndrome, pseudoxanthoma elasticum
    4. Tuberculosis
    5. Asthenic habitus
    6. Osteogenesis imperfecta
  D. Sausage-shaped phalanges
    1. Rickets (beading of joints)
    2. Granulomatous dactylitis (tuberculosis, syphilis)
  E. Spindliform joints (fingers)
    1. Early rheumatoid arthritis
    2. Systemic lupus erythematosus
    3. Psoriasis
    4. Rubella
    5. Boeck's sarcoidosis
    6. Osteoarthritis
  F. Cone-shaped fingers
    1. Pituitary obesity
    2. Fröhlich's dystrophy
  G. Unilateral enlargement of hand
    1. Arteriovenous aneurysm
    2. Maffucci's syndrome
  H. Square dry hands
    1. Cretinism
    2. Myxedema
  I. Single, widened, flattened distal phalanx
    1. Sarcoidosis
  J. Shortened fourth and fifth metacarpals (brachymetacarpalism)
    1. Pseudohypoparathyroidism
    2. Pseudo-pseudohypoparathyroidism
  K. Shortened, incurved fifth finger (symptom of Du Bois)
    1. Mongolism
    2. "Behavioral problem"
    3. Gargoylism (broad, short, thick-skinned hand)
  L. Malposition and abduction, fifth finger
    1. Turner's syndrome (gonadal dysgenesis, webbed neck, etc.)
  M. Syndactylism
    1. Congenital malformations of the heart, great vessels
    2. Multiple congenital deformities
    3. Laurence-Moon-Biedl syndrome
    4. In normal individuals as an inherited trait
  N. Clubbed fingers
    1. Subacute bacterial endocarditis
    2. Pulmonary causes
      a. Tuberculosis
      b. Pulmonary arteriovenous fistula

      c. Pulmonic abscess
      d. Pulmonic cysts
      e. Bullous emphysema
      f. Pulmonary hypertrophic osteoarthropathy
      g. Bronchogenic carcinoma
    3. Alveolocapillary block
      a. Interstitial pulmonary fibrosis
      b. Sarcoidosis
      c. Beryllium poisoning
      d. Sclerodermatous lung
      e. Asbestosis
      f. Miliary tuberculosis
      g. Alveolar cell carcinoma
    4. Cardiovascular causes
      a. Patent ductus arteriosus
      b. Tetralogy of Fallot
      c. Taussig-Bing complex
      d. Pulmonic stenosis
      e. Ventricular septal defect
    5. Diarrheal states
      a. Ulcerative colitis
      b. Tuberculous enteritis
      c. Sprue
      d. Amebic dysentery
      e. Bacillary dysentery
      f. Parasitic infestation (G-I tract)
    6. Hepatic cirrhosis
    7. Myxedema
    8. Polycythemia
    9. Chronic urinary tract infections (upper and lower)
      a. Chronic nephritis
    10. Hyperparathyroidism (telescopy of distal phalanx)
    11. Pachydermoperiostosis (syndrome of Touraine, Solente and Golé)
  O. Joint disturbances
    1. Arthritides
      a. Osteoarthritis
      b. Rheumatoid arthritis
      c. Systemic lupus erythematosus
      d. Gout
      e. Psoriasis
      f. Sarcoidosis
      g. Endocrinopathy (acromegaly)
      h. Rheumatic fever
      i. Reiter's syndrome
      j. Dermatomyositis
    2. Anaphylactic reaction—serum sickness
    3. Scleroderma
II. Edema of the Hand
  A. Cardiac disease (congestive heart failure)
  B. Hepatic disease
  C. Renal disease
    1. Nephritis
    2. Nephrosis
  D. Hemiplegic hand
  E. Syringomyelia
  F. Superior vena caval syndrome

TABLE 4-2. (Continued)

1. Superior thoracic outlet tumor
2. Mediastinal tumor or inflammation
3. Pulmonary apex tumor
4. Aneurysm
G. Generalized anasarca, hypoproteinemia
H. Postoperative lymphedema (radical breast amputation)
I. Ischemic paralysis (cold, blue, swollen, numb)
J. Lymphatic obstruction
  1. Lymphomatous masses in axilla
K. Axillary mass
  1. Metastatic tumor, abscess, leukemia, Hodgkin's disease
L. Aneurysm of ascending or transverse aorta, or of axillary artery
M. Pressure on innominate or subclavian vessels
N. Raynaud's disease
O. Myositis
P. Cervical rib
Q. Trichiniasis
R. Scalenus anticus syndrome

III. Neuromuscular effects
  A. Atrophy
    1. Painless
      a. Amyotrophic lateral sclerosis
      b. Charcot-Marie-Tooth peroneal atrophy
      c. Syringomyelia (loss of heat, cold and pain sensation)
      d. Neural leprosy
    2. Painful
      a. Peripheral nerve disease
        1. Radial nerve (wrist drop)
          a. Lead poisoning, alcoholism, polyneuritis, trauma
          b. Diphtheria, polyarteritis, neurosyphilis, anterior poliomyelitis
        2. Ulnar nerve (benediction palsy)
          a. Polyneuritis, trauma
        3. Median nerve (claw hand)
          a. Carpal tunnel syndrome
            1. Rheumatoid arthritis
            2. Tenosynovitis at wrist
            3. Amyloidosis
            4. Gout
            5. Plasmacytoma
            6. Anaphylactic reaction
            7. Menopause syndrome
            8. Myxedema
  B. Extrinsic pressure on the nerve (cervical, axillary, supraclavicular or brachial)
    1. Pancoast tumor (pulmonary apex)
    2. Aneurysms of subclavian arteries, axillary vessels, or thoracic aorta
    3. Costoclavicular syndrome
    4. Superior thoracic outlet syndrome
    5. Cervical rib
    6. Degenerative arthritis of cervical spine
    7. Herniation of cervical intervertebral disk
  C. Shoulder-hand syndrome
    1. Myocardial infarction

2. Pancoast tumor
3. Brain tumor
4. Intrathoracic neoplasms
5. Discogenetic disease
6. Cervical spondylosis
7. Febrile panniculitis
8. Senility
9. Vascular occlusion
10. Hemiplegia
11. Osteoarthritis
12. Herpes zoster
D. Ischemic contractures (sensory loss in fingers)
  1. Tight plaster cast applications
E. Polyarteritis nodosa
F. Polyneuritis
  1. Carcinoma of lung
  2. Hodgkin's disease
  3. Pregnancy
  4. Gastric carcinoma
  5. Reticuloses
  6. Diabetes mellitus
  7. Chemical neuritis
    a. Antimony, benzene, bismuth, carbon tetrachloride, heavy metals, alcohol, arsenic, lead, gold, emetine
  8. Ischemic neuropathy
  9. Vitamin B deficiency
  10. Atheromata
  11. Arteriosclerosis
  12. Embolic
G. Carpodigital (carpopedal spasm) tetany
  1. Hypoparathyroidism
  2. Hyperventilation
  3. Uremia
  4. Nephritis
  5. Nephrosis
  6. Rickets
  7. Sprue
  8. Malabsorption syndrome
  9. Pregnancy
  10. Lactation
  11. Osteomalacia
  12. Protracted vomiting
  13. Pyloric obstruction
  14. Alkali poisoning
  15. Chemical toxicity
    a. Morphine, lead, alcohol
H. Tremor
  1. Parkinsonism
  2. Familial disorder
  3. Hypoglycemia
  4. Hyperthyroidism
  5. Wilson's disease (hepatolenticular degeneration)
  6. Anxiety
  7. Ataxia
  8. Athetosis
  9. Alcoholism, narcotic addiction
  10. Multiple sclerosis
  11. Chorea (Sydenham's, Huntington's)

TABLE 4-2. (Continued)

12. Neurasthenia
13. Senility
14. Cerebellar lesions
15. Occupational neuroses
16. Hepatic coma
17. Posthepatitic disorder
18. Paresis
19. Cold, fatigue
20. Lesions of red nucleus
21. Toxicity (heavy metals, barbiturates)

IV. Color changes in the hand
  A. Cyanosis
    1. Congestive heart failure
    2. Raynaud's phenomenon
      a. Polyarteritis nodosa
      b. Buerger's disease
      c. Scleroderma
      d. Dermatomyositis
      e. Systemic lupus erythematosus
      f. Arteriosclerosis
      g. Cervical rib
      h. Tumors or aneurysms encroaching on the brachial plexus
    3. Polycythemia
    4. Obliterative vascular disease
      a. Scalenus anticus and related syndromes
      b. Ball valve thrombus
    5. Syringomyelia (Morvan's disease)
    6. Systemic lupus erythematosus
    7. Dermatomyositis
    8. Drug effects
      a. Acetanilid
      b. Coumadin ("purple toes and fingers")
      c. Phenolphthalein
    9. Acrocyanosis (cold, wet, swollen hand)
    10. Congenital heart disease
    11. Arteriovenous aneurysm
    12. Myxedema
    13. Hemosiderin deposits in congestive heart failure in children
    14. Cor pulmonale
    15. Scalenus anticus syndrome
  B. Pallor
    1. Anemia
    2. Aortic insufficiency ("paradoxic pallor")
    3. Raynaud's phenomenon sequence
    4. Vasospasm—fingertips
      a. Tobacco
      b. Anxiety
      c. Vasomotor instability
  C. Rubor
    1. Pellagra (dorsum)
    2. Polycythemia
    3. Systemic lupus erythematosus (fingertips)
    4. Dermatomyositis
    5. Erythromelalgia (see causes under "increased temperature")
    6. Pink disease (acrodynia, Swift's disease, erythredema)
    7. Lymphocytic leukemia ("l'homme rouge")

  D. Pigmentation overlying the veins of the dorsum
    1. Hodgkin's disease
  E. Diffuse melanosis
    1. Addison's disease (black freckles)
    2. Melanosarcoma
  F. Slate-gray pigmentation
    1. Argyria
  G. Yellow palms
    1. Pernicious anemia
    2. Carotinemia
    3. Laborer's callus
  H. Depigmentation
    1. Vitiligo
    2. Pinta
    3. Postdermatitic
    4. Scleroderma
    5. Dermatomyositis
  I. Purpuric spots
    1. Osler's disease (familial hemorrhagic telangiectasia)
    2. Peutz-Jeghers syndrome
    3. Subacute bacterial endocarditis
    4. Thrombocytopenic purpura
    5. Blood dyscrasias

V. Subungual hemorrhages
  A. Rendu-Osler-Weber's (familial hemorrhagic telangiectasia)
  B. Rheumatic fever
  C. Subacute bacterial endocarditis
  D. Trichiniasis
  E. Blood dyscrasias associated with bleeding tendency
  F. Scurvy

VI. Physical findings in the palm
  A. Dupuytren's contracture
    1. Diabetes mellitus
    2. Epilepsy
    3. Cirrhosis
    4. Raynaud's disease
    5. Scalenus anticus syndrome
    6. Postmyocardial infarction
    7. Syringomyelia
    8. Normal persons
  B. Xanthomata
    1. Familial disorder
    2. Hypercholesterolemia
    3. Diabetes mellitus
    4. Nephrosis
    5. Biliary cirrhosis
    6. Chronic pancreatitis
    7. Von Gierke's disease
    8. Cobaltous chloride
    9. Myxedema
    10. Hand-Christian-Schüller disease
    11. Gaucher's disease
    12. Niemann-Pick's disease
  C. Palmar erythema
    1. Hepatic cirrhosis ("liver palms")
    2. Pregnancy
    3. Alcoholism
    4. Mitral insufficiency

TABLE 4-2. (Continued)

 5. Rheumatoid arthritis
 6. Polycythemia
 7. Diabetes mellitus
 8. Tuberculosis (acroerythrosis)
 9. Vitamin B deficiency
 10. Hyperestrogenism
 11. Beriberi
 12. Shoulder-hand syndrome
 13. Arsenical toxicity
 14. 3–5 percent of normal persons

D. Pain
 1. Burning sensations in hookworm infestation
 2. Alcoholic neuritis
 3. Neuritis from any cause
 4. Carpal tunnel syndrome (see median nerve)

E. Unusual formation or color of palmar creases
 1. Single transverse crease
  a. Mongolian idiocy
  b. Congenital sclerodactyly
 2. Blue creases
  a. Generalized purpura
 3. Pale, silvery or white creases
  a. Anemia (hemoglobin below 7 gm/100 ml)
 4. Dark brown or black creases
  a. Addison's disease
 5. Displacement of triradii
  a. Certain congenital cardiac malformations

F. Petechiae
 1. Blood dyscrasias
 2. Thrombocytopenic purpura
 3. Subacute bacterial endocarditis
 4. Scurvy
 5. Vitamin deficiency
 6. Premenstrual

G. Janeway lesion
 1. Subacute bacterial endocarditis

H. Osler's nodes
 1. Subacute bacterial endocarditis

I. Callus

VII. Temperature changes in the hand
A. Increased
 1. Arteriovenous aneurysm (unilateral finding)
 2. Aneurysm
 3. Hyperthyroidism
 4. Fever
 5. Hypermetabolic states
  a. Pontine hemorrhage

 6. Environmental heat
 7. Paget's disease of bone
 8. Erythromelalgia (primary or secondary)
  a. Hypertensive cardiovascular disease
  b. Gout
  c. Diabetes mellitus
  d. Rheumatoid arthritis
  e. Arteriosclerosis
  f. Polycythemia

B. Decreased
 1. Shock
 2. Hypothyroidism
 3. Agonal hand
 4. Arterial occlusion
 5. Ischemic contracture
 6. Syringomyelia
 7. Scleroderma
 8. Dermatomyositis
 9. Systemic lupus erythematosus
 10. Raynaud's phenomenon
 11. Environmental cold
 12. Neurasthenia
 13. Normal persons
 14. Peripheral vascular diseases
  a. Embolus
  b. Thromboangiitis obliterans
  c. Scalenus anticus and related syndromes
  d. Pulmonary hypertension
 15. Acrocyanosis

VIII. Capillary pulsations of fingertip and nail bed
(Quincke pulse)
A. Aortic insufficiency
B. Hyperthyroidism
C. High-output cardiac failure
D. Anemia
E. High fevers

IX. Inoculated infectious diseases which produce
chancre-like lesions on the hand
A. Sporotrichosis
B. Anthrax
C. Actinomycosis
D. Tuberculosis
E. Syphilis
F. Coccidioidomycosis
G. Tularemia
H. Leishmaniasis
I. Blastomycosis

Source: T. J. Berry, *The Hand As a Mirror of Systemic Disease*. Philadelphia: Davis, 1963. Pp. 193–204.

VITAL SIGNS

CHAPTER 5

It is better that a fever succeed to a convulsion, than a convulsion to a fever.

HIPPOCRATES
(460?–377? B.C.)

Because a heartbeat, breathing, and body warmth are the clinical signs of life (the absence of which signaled death in the era before the advent of modern laboratory aids such as the electroencephalogram), the so-called vital signs (pulse, respiratory rate, temperature, and blood pressure) continue to be the most frequently examined of all physical findings.

HISTORY

Abnormalities in vital signs touch on all disease states. Certain symptoms (e.g., sweats with fever) may form a patient's isolated initial complaint. Conversely, a significant abnormality in vital signs (e.g., high blood pressure) may be asymptomatic.

Because of the pervasive nature of variations in the vital signs in health and disease, history regarding subjective awareness of changes in pulse, respirations, and temperature is correlated with each patient's total picture, no matter what the chief complaint might be.

PHYSICAL EXAMINATION

1. Insert oral thermometer.
2. Count radial pulse.
3. Count respirations.
4. Take blood pressure, both arms.
5. Remove and read thermometer.

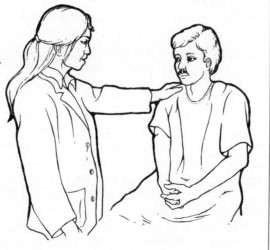

TEMPERATURE

The temperature is generally taken by placing the bulb of a well-shaken thermometer under the patient's tongue for 3 minutes. Newer instruments may allow the oral temperature to be recorded by thermistor in less than 60 seconds. The temperature

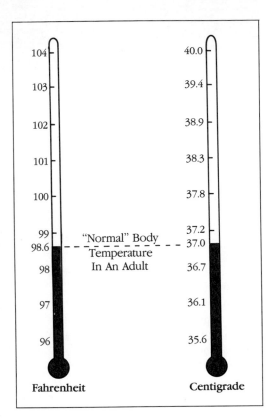

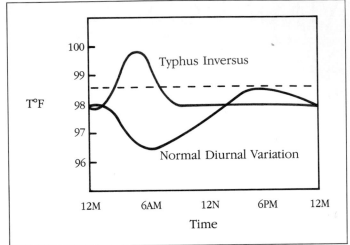

FIGURE 5-2
Nocturnal fever.

FIGURE 5-1
A comparison of the temperature scales commonly used in United States hospitals.

may be taken orally or rectally, and in the United States the Fahrenheit scale is usually used (Fig. 5-1). When fever is present the mercury column climbs quite rapidly (15 to 30 seconds) to within a few tenths of the final reading. Falsely low levels may result from incomplete closure of the mouth, breathing through the mouth, leaving the thermometer in place for too short a time, or the recent ingestion of cold substances. Falsely elevated levels may result from inadequate shaking down of the thermometer, previous ingestion of warm substances, smoking, recent strenuous activity, or even a very warm bath.

In most persons there is a diurnal (occurring every day) variation in body temperature of 0.5° to 2°F. The lowest ebb is reached during sleep, at which time the temperature may fall as low as 96.5° to 97°F. As the patient begins to awaken, the temperature slowly rises. The "fast starter" who jumps from his bed and reaches his peak efficiency early in the day usually has reached 98°F or more by the time he awakens and may peak to his maximum level of 98.6° to 99.2°F before noon. The "slow starter" often shows a lower temperature on rising and may not peak until late afternoon or early evening. His efficiency may be greatest later in the day.

There is a well-known temperature pattern in the menstruating woman that reflects the effects of ovulation. The morning temperature falls slightly just prior to menstruation and continues at this level until the midpoint between the two periods. There may be a further drop 24 to 36 hours prior to ovulation, and coincident with ovulation the morning temperature rises and remains at a somewhat higher

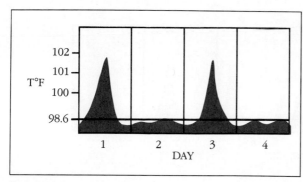

FIGURE 5-3
Intermittent fever.

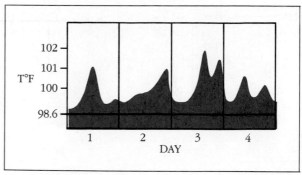

FIGURE 5-4
Remittent fever.

level until just before the next menses.

You will note that the upper limit of normal on the standard thermometer is 98.6°F. It must be remembered that this is an arbitrary value that applies primarily to patients at bed rest. Many normal people show higher levels when active, and on a hot summer day in the outpatient clinic, readings of 99.4°F are not at all uncommon in perfectly normal individuals. Even higher values can be recorded in children following hard play.

Rectal temperatures are usually 0.5° to 1°F higher than oral temperatures, but they tend to be less subject to alteration by the oral factors mentioned above and are generally more constant and reproducible. It is an error to believe that rectal temperatures are more accurate than oral temperatures in the sense that rectal temperatures are more reflective of "core" temperature than are oral readings. It is probably the case that the thermoregulatory centers in the hypothalamus are directed in their control of body temperature by temperatures that more closely approximate those in the anatomically neighboring mouth than those in the more distant rectal core. Axillary temperatures are so inaccurate that they will not be discussed further.

Fever is a temperature exceeding 100°F. It is one of the oldest and still most useful signs in clinical medicine. Pyrogens, both exogenous (e.g., endotoxin from bacterial cell walls) and endogenous (e.g., tumors, antigen-antibody complexes, thyroid hormone) act to "reset" the hypothalamic thermoregulatory centers at a higher "set point." The generation of heat to achieve this newly directed set point may be by the mechanism of violent muscular exertion—the shaking chill or "rigor." Attempts to dissipate extra body heat in febrile states are seen by the clinician as sweating (diaphoresis) and cutaneous vasodilation, the fever "flush." Increased body temperature of whatever origin increases heart rate and metabolic rate in general.

The *fever curve,* or pattern of fever, may give valuable clues to diagnosis. Most fevers follow the normal variation and are higher in the late afternoon, lowest in the predawn. Nocturnal fevers are said to occur more frequently with tuberculosis and other granulomatous infections (*typhus inversus fever pattern*) (Fig. 5-2).

Intermittent fevers, in which the temperature spikes upward during the day but on that same day falls back to normal or subnormal (Fig. 5-3), may be seen in ma-

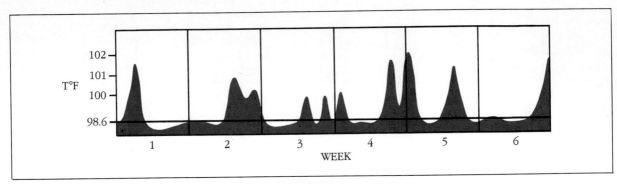

FIGURE 5-5
Relapsing fever.

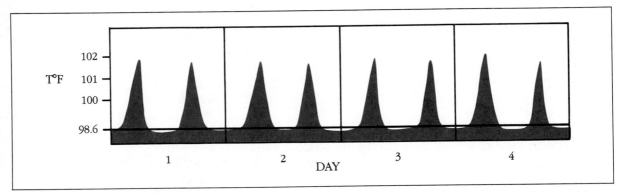

FIGURE 5-6
Double quotidian fever.

laria (the periodic occurrence of the fever is a clue to the species of parasite involved) and in sequestered abscesses. These same disorders may produce *remittent fevers,* in which the temperatures show marked rises and falls, but never fall to normal (Fig. 5-4).

Relapsing fevers, in which there are several days of fever followed by days during which the patient remains afebrile (Fig. 5-5), may occur with brucella infections or the Hodgkin's lymphoma (the Pel-Ebstein fever of Hodgkin's disease).

Double quotidian fevers, two spikes per 24 hours (as shown in Fig. 5-6), characterize miliary tuberculosis, gonococcal endocarditis, juvenile rheumatoid arthritis, mixed malaria, and kala-azar (leishmaniasis). The most common cause of double quotidian fever is probably aspirin therapy for a sustained fever.

Hypothermia, or an oral temperature of less than 94°F, may be missed if the examiner is unaware that most clinical thermometers do not go below 94°F. If you suspect a lower temperature, you must check it again with a special long thermometer or thermistor. Abnormally low temperatures may occur with severe brain injury, hypoglycemia, thiamine deficiency, starvation, exposure, sepsis, burns, hypothyroidism, hypoadrenalism, a variety of drug intoxications, and extremes of age.

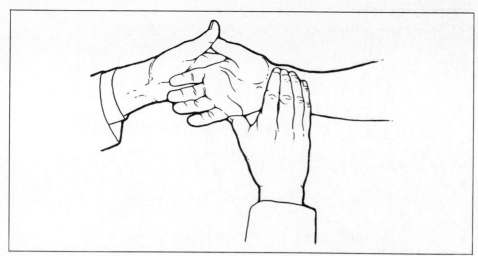

FIGURE 5-7
Palpating the radial pulse.

All these conditions have a common pathophysiology. They interfere either with central thermoregulation in the hypothalamus or with peripheral generation and retention of body heat.

PULSE

The radial pulse is best taken at the base of the patient's thumb (Fig. 5-7). If the examiner uses two or three fingers along the course of the artery, he or she may determine the pulse contour as well as the rate (see Chap. 12, Cardiovascular System).

Initially, and *always* if the pulse is irregular, the examiner should count the pulse for a full 60 seconds. If the pulse rate is between 60 and 100, and the rhythm is absolutely regular, many physicians will "shortcut" and count the pulse for 30 seconds, then multiply by two.

If the radial pulse is poor or irregular, the pulse may be taken by listening to or palpating the apex of the heart (the *apical pulse*). The normal resting pulse rate ranges from 60 to 100. It may be in the 50s in a conditioned athlete, or 100 or over in an excited patient. Rates less than 60 are often referred to as *bradycardia* (literally, "slow heart"), and rates over 100 as *tachycardia* ("fast heart").

The lability of the pulse rate is well known to all. Usually the rhythm is relatively regular. Occasional premature beats are so common that they are not necessarily considered abnormal. They are perceived as transient skips or breaks in rhythm. Sinus arrhythmia can be identified in most patients under the age of 40. It refers to a transient increase in pulse rate with inspiration, followed by a slowing with expiration. This phenomenon can be rather marked in some normal patients.

The pulse rate and rhythm should be recorded, and if abnormal contour is discovered, that too must be noted.

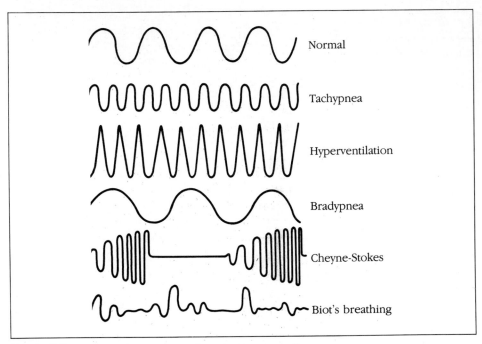

FIGURE 5-8
Patterns of respiration.

RESPIRATIONS

When man grows old . . . there is much gas within his thorax, resulting in panting and troubled breathing.

HUANG TI (the Yellow Emperor)
(2697–2597 B.C.)

Many physicians find it of value to count the respirations while appearing to take the pulse, since the natural tendency of the patient is to breathe awkwardly under observation. Normal respiratory rate is between 8 and 14 per minute in adults and is somewhat more rapid in children.

Note abnormalities of respiratory rate and rhythm (Fig. 5-8). Extremely slow respiration usually indicates central nervous system respiratory depression due to disease or drugs. Periodic or *Cheyne-Stokes respiration* occurs with serious cardiopulmonary or cerebral disorders. It is characterized by a periodic, regular, sequentially increasing depth of respiration followed by periods of apnea and is due to a loss of the normal fine-tuning of the respiratory centers to levels of arterial carbon dioxide. The PCO_2 rises during the apneic phases, stimulating vigorous breathing. As the patient breathes, however, he blows off so much carbon dioxide that apnea is induced until PCO_2 rises again. In contrast, *Biot's respiration* is irregularly irregular, almost spasmodic, with longer periods of apnea than of breathing; it is almost always associated with hypoventilation. It is generally associated with central nervous system disease. Deep slow breathing (*Kussmaul's respiration*) characterizes acidosis, in which state the physiologic response to increased metabolic acid in the blood is a compensatory "blowing off" of carbon dioxide. Extreme tachypnea is present during many acute illnesses. It may be due to chronic or acute pulmonary or cardiac disease or systemic disorders, such as shock, severe pain, and acidosis; although it may represent undue excitement or nervousness, especially when accompanied with sighing, an organic cause should be excluded.

The patient's preferred position is important. Can he lie flat comfortably? Patients with congestive heart failure prefer the sitting position, as do patients with pulmonary disease during acute attacks of infection or bronchospasm. Patients with pericarditis often sit and lean forward. Although cardiac patients often awaken dyspneic several hours after reclining (due to redistribution of excess blood volume into the lungs [paroxysmal nocturnal dyspnea]), people with large amounts of sputum frequently awaken shortly after reclining to clear retained secretions. Preference for lying on one side or the other may point to the localization of pathologic processes; secretions of foreign bodies may be aspirated into a specific area because of position.

BLOOD PRESSURE

At the moment the heart contracts, and when the breast is struck, when in short the organ is in its state of systole, the arteries are dilated, yield a pulse, and are in a state of diastole.

WILLIAM HARVEY
(1578–1657)

The normal adult blood pressure varies over a wide range. The normal systolic range varies from 95 to 140 mm Hg, generally increasing with age. The normal diastolic range is from 60 to 90 mm Hg. Pulse pressure is the difference between the systolic and diastolic pressures. Mean pressure can be approximated by dividing the pulse pressure by three and adding this value to the diastolic pressure. Routine measurements should be made with the patient sitting and recumbent. If you find an abnormality, compare the determination in both arms with the patient supine, sitting, and standing. Any reliable sphygmomanometer may be employed, but the bladder, or inflatable bag encased in the cuff, should be long enough to encircle the limb. In obese or very muscular patients, a leg cuff can be used.

Fit the cuff evenly around the upper arm, with the lower edge 1 inch above the elbow and the air bladder over the brachial artery. The palpation method is first employed to determine the systolic pressure (Fig. 5-9A). Rapidly inflate the cuff until the radial pulse disappears, and then deflate it slowly. The level at which the radial pulse first reappears is the systolic pressure. A gross estimate of the diastolic pressure is sometimes possible by palpation, for with further deflation of the cuff, the radial pulse assumes a bounding quality and then abruptly becomes normal. This point of change, when evident, roughly approximates the diastolic pressure. The auscultatory method is then employed to estimate both the systolic and diastolic pressures (Fig. 5-9B).

Place the stethoscope lightly over the brachial artery and inflate to 20 or 30 mm above the palpable systolic pressure. The highest level at which sounds are heard (phase 1 of Korotkoff) is the systolic pressure. With further lowering by decrements of 2 or 3 mm, the sounds are replaced by a bruit (phase 2) and then by loud, sharp sounds (phase 3). Finally the sounds suddenly become damped (phase 4), and a few millimeters below this they disappear. The point of complete disappearance of sound is considered the best index of diastolic pressure. Under hemodynamic con-

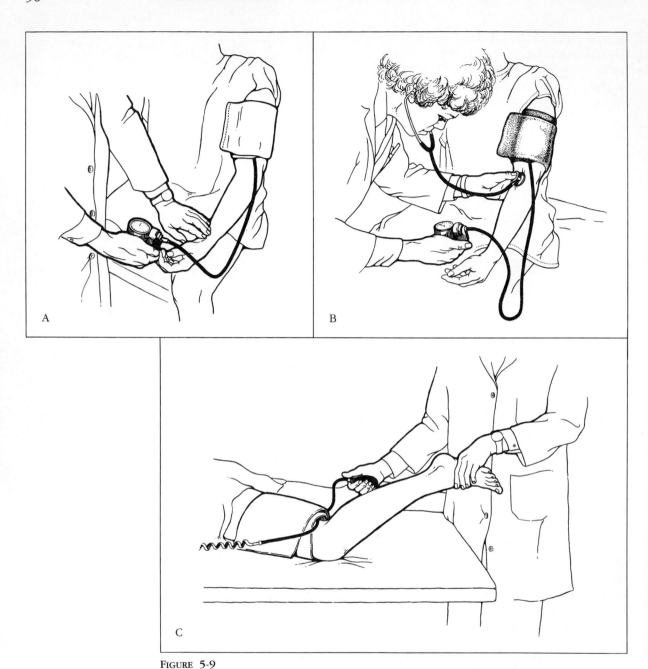

FIGURE 5-9
Blood pressure measurement. A. *By palpation.* Pump up the cuff to the point where the radial pulse is no longer felt. With decreasing cuff pressure, mark where the radial pulse reappears. This is the palpable systolic pressure. B. *By auscultation.* Auscultate the systolic and diastolic pressure over the brachial artery. C. *By palpation of blood pressure in the leg.* Palpate the dorsalis pedis pulse. Use a leg (oversized) cuff.

TABLE 5-1. Causes of Marked Asymmetry (>10 Torr Difference) in Blood
Pressure of the Arms

Errors in measurement
Thoracic outlet syndromes (e.g., cervical rib)
Embolic occlusion of an artery
Dissection of the aorta
External arterial occlusion (e.g., tumor, hematoma)
Atheromatous occlusion
Coarctation of the aorta
Marked difference in arm size (e.g., secondary to unilateral edema or withered arm)
Takayasu's arteritis
After Blalock-Taussig surgical procedure

ditions in which sound does not cease, the point of muffling should be taken as the
diastolic pressure, with the point of total disappearance recorded as well (e.g.,
140/60–0).

The pressure should be determined in both arms, at least on the initial evaluation. One may have a normal variation of up to 10 mm Hg (10 torr) between the
two arms (Table 5-1). When it is advisable to measure the blood pressure in the leg,
such as when a congenital narrowing (coarctation) of the aorta or dissecting aortic
aneurysm is suspected, the palpation method should be employed with the patient
prone (Fig. 5-9C). Apply the cuff to the calf or thigh and estimate the systolic level by
palpating the posterior tibial or dorsalis pedis artery. The systolic level in the leg is
normally equal to or higher than that in the arm (since it is never critical to measure the diastolic pressure in the leg, this practice is sufficient and accurate). Applying the standard cuff to the thigh and listening for sounds over the popliteal artery
in the average adult is not only mechanically difficult but also may result in falsely
elevated readings.

The patient's assuming an erect position may not necessarily affect the arm pressure taken at heart level. It is, however, not uncommon for the systolic pressure to
fall by 10 to 15 mm Hg on standing, and about half of the time the diastolic pressure
will rise slightly (by 5 mm Hg).

Orthostatic blood pressure changes should be sought in any patient in whom
there is suspicion of (1) *volume loss* (bleeding, dehydration), (2) *nervous system
dysfunction* (e.g., Parkinson's disease or diabetes, which may affect the autonomic
nerves), and (3) *drug therapy* (e.g., anti-hypertensive drugs have their therapeutic
effect by inducing orthostatic changes). Such orthostatic drops in blood pressure
should obviously be sought in patients who complain of dizziness on assuming an
erect posture.

Concomitant pulse rate must be measured with orthostatic blood pressure. Obviously, one who maintains a blood pressure of 120/80 only by increasing the pulse
rate 25 beats per minute on rising may be volume deficient, even though the blood
pressure does not drop noticeably.

Anxiety may raise the blood pressure, and multiple careful measurements over
time should be taken before applying the diagnosis of hypertension on an individual with modest elevations.

Low blood pressure (hypotension) may of course be present in shock states or may accompany cachexia, prolonged bed rest, dehydration, and adrenal insufficiency among other causes. In an asymptomatic patient with no other complaints, systolic blood pressures as low as 90 torr may be perfectly normal. Shock cannot be said to be present unless there is evident decreased regional blood flow (e.g., syncope, oliguria, and pallor). Decreased regional blood flow is associated with dizziness, visual blurring, sweating, and, at times, syncope.

Irregular rhythms, especially atrial fibrillation, may lead to wide variations in the measured blood pressure. The flow (stroke output) and peripheral resistance in these arrhythmias may be different from beat to beat. Several blood pressure determinations in this circumstance are useful to get an *average* reading.

The *auscultatory gap* is a silent period between the systolic and diastolic pressures that may be appreciated in some patients with hypertension. Using the palpation method prior to auscultation to determine systolic pressure, and carefully listening throughout the descent of the mercury column, will prevent underestimation of the systolic or overestimation of the diastolic pressure.

Widened pulse pressure is common to all conditions producing an *increased stroke volume.* Simple bradycardia widens the pulse pressure by raising the systolic pressure (e.g., 150/70) as do fever, anemia, and hypermetabolic states. These disorders all have in common an increased stroke volume. Incompetence of the aortic valve widens the pulse pressure due to lowering of the diastolic pressure (e.g., 150/30). With aging, the elasticity of the great arteries diminishes, producing an increase in the systolic pressure at times referred to as "systolic hypertension" (e.g., 165/80).

The following common errors in the determination of blood pressure should be recognized and avoided:

1. Discrepancies between the relative cuff size and limb size may result in false reading. For example, an obese arm yields falsely elevated pressures when measured with a normal cuff. In obese patients you may check the systolic level with the cuff on the forearm, palpating the radial artery. Similarly, a standard cuff on an emaciated arm or the small arm of a child may give falsely low values.
2. Applying the cuff too loosely will give falsely elevated values.
3. The anxious patient may have an elevated level. If it is high, always leave the cuff in place and recheck the blood pressure several times. Never rely on a single determination.
4. It is possible to fail to recognize an auscultatory gap. Sounds may disappear between the systolic and diastolic pressures and then reappear. If the cuff pressure is raised only to the range of the gap, the systolic reading will be falsely low. This error is eliminated by first determining the systolic level by the palpatory method.
5. Feeble Korotkoff's sounds may make your determination unreliable. In this event, deflate the cuff and have the patient elevate his arm, reinflating the cuff in this position. Then lower the arm and repeat. The sounds may be louder now because of diminished venous pressure. If they are not, you may have to settle for a palpable systolic pressure only.

SKIN

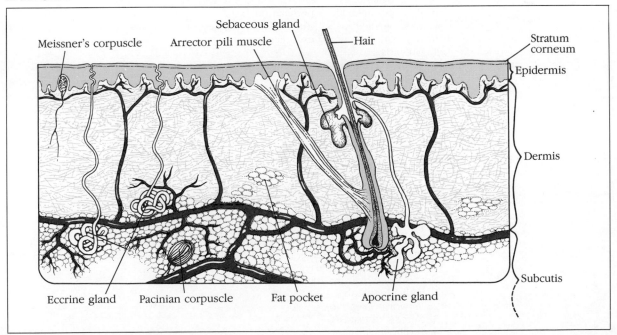

CHAPTER 6

The skin possesses the closest relations with the general economy, as shown by the observation that there are comparatively few so-called general diseases in which it . . . is not at some period involved in a slight or a marked degree.

LOUIS A. DUHRING
(1845–1913)

What portion of the physical examination could be easier than the examination of the skin? The skin is directly visible both in color and in three dimensions; it is directly palpable; and it is so thin that even the deepest cutaneous pathology is only a few millimeters away from the examiner. But this easy accessibility also creates some problems, in that it provides a great quantity of information, much of which is unimportant or unrelated to the patient's presenting problem. This abundance is complicated by the fact that we are so accustomed to viewing the skin that we really do not "see" it at all. Most of us, in performing the physical examination, consequently ignore all the information provided by the skin rather than make the effort to sort the important from the unimportant. This chapter is designed to assist the examiner in the sorting process.

ANATOMY

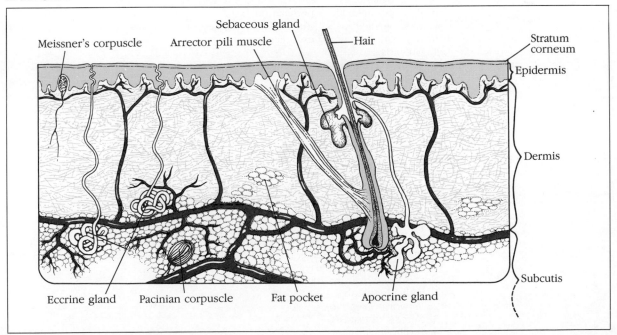

FIGURE 6-1
Cross section of the skin and appendages.

HISTORY

Two important **symptoms** signal cutaneous pathology: **pruritus** and **pain**. These two symptoms are related insofar as the respective sensations are both carried by the peripheral nervous system via its cutaneous branches.

Pain occurs under several sets of circumstances. Most commonly it appears when the skin around the nerves is no longer intact, exposing the sensitive nerve endings to the dry hostile environment outside the body. Pain may also occur as a direct effect of biochemical mediators in some kinds of cutaneous inflammatory reactions. Finally, pain may be the result of simple nonpenetrating external trauma. Usually these situations are clinically apparent; thus pain is more often a therapeutic problem than a diagnostic one.

Little is known regarding the pathophysiology of **pruritus,** but for the purpose of this chapter it suffices for us to know that itching is carried by the small nerve fibers of the skin. Generalized itching, and subsequent scratching, may occur in a variety of systemic diseases, notably in association with chronic disease of the liver and kidneys. It may also occur in patients with diseases of the hematopoietic system,

TABLE **6-1.** Pruritus

I. Pruritus with visible skin disease
   A. Excoriations present
      1. Eczematous skin disease (atopic/neurodermatitis, contact dermatitis, stasis dermatitis, anogenital pruritus, seborrheic dermatitis, dyshidrotic eczema)
      2. Scabies
      3. Dermatitis herpetiformis
      4. Psoriasis (scalp and intertriginous areas only)
      5. Superficial fungal disease (feet and intertriginous areas only)
      6. Pinworm infestation (perianal only)
      7. Psychogenic causes (prurigo nodularis, neurotic excoriation)
   B. Itching with little or no excoriation
      1. Urticaria
      2. Erythema multiforme
      3. Lichen planus
      4. Drug reactions*
      5. Pityriasis rosea
      6. Urticaria pigmentosa (mastocytosis)
      7. Pruritic papules of pregnancy
II. Pruritus without visible skin disease
   A. Associated with internal disease
      1. Uremia
      2. Liver disease (especially biliary cirrhosis and obstructive jaundice)
      3. Lymphoma (especially Hodgkin's disease)
      4. Polycythemia vera
      5. Pregnancy
      6. Miscellaneous (pruritus is often stated as being associated with diabetes mellitus, thyroid disease, parathyroid disease, and internal carcinomas, but most reports are anecdotal)
   B. Not associated with internal disease
      1. Pediculosis pubis
      2. Pinworm infestation
      3. Xerosis (asteatosis)
      4. Psychogenic causes

---

* Drug reactions generally result in urticaria or erythema multiforme.

especially Hodgkin's disease and polycythemia vera (Table 6-1). But most often, even after thorough examination, no explanation for generalized pruritus can be found. In these instances the functional disability that is often present may suggest a psychiatric cause.

Localized areas of itching are exceedingly common and, when unassociated with visible cutaneous disease, probably have no pathologic meaning. Many, if not most, kinds of visible cutaneous disease are associated with what is more or less pruritus. This pruritus causes a dual problem. First, the itching almost literally may "drive a patient crazy," causing serious interference with ability to function. Second, the concomitant scratching intensifies and continues the skin disease that was responsible for the itching in the first place. This itch-scratch cycle is one of the most vexing therapeutic problems in dermatologic disease.

Skin complaints may be the major symptoms in patients with more serious underlying disorders (Table 6-2). The bruising of coagulation defects, the painful skin

TABLE 6-2. Some Cutaneous Manifestations of Internal Malignancy

I. Cutaneous malignancy with frequent internal spread
   A. Melanoma
   B. Squamous cell carcinomas arising from old scars, x-ray–damaged skin, and mucosal surfaces
   C. Mycosis fungoides
   D. Kaposi's hemorrhagic sarcoma
II. Internal malignancy with extension or metastases to skin
   A. Breast carcinoma
   B. Leukemia and lymphoma cutis
   C. Miscellaneous manifestations (occasional metastases to the skin are seen with gastrointestinal, genitourinary, and pulmonary malignancies)
III. Pigmentary changes
   A. Hypermelanosis (especially with melanoma and polypeptide-secreting tumors)
   B. Acanthosis nigricans (especially with gastrointestinal carcinoma)
   C. Sign of Leser-Trelat (rapid appearance of multiple seborrheic keratoses)
   D. Peutz-Jeghers syndrome
   E. Jaundice (primary tumors of biliary tract and pancreas; liver metastases from other tumors)
   F. Purpura (mostly leukemias)
IV. Flushing and facial erythema
   A. Carcinoid
   B. Mastocytomas
   C. Pheochromocytomas
   D. Cushing's disease
V. Specific skin lesions sometimes signaling internal malignancy
   A. Dermatomyositis in adults
   B. Bullous disease in adults (pemphigus and pemphigoid)
   C. Bowen's disease on non-sun-exposed areas
   D. Arsenic keratoses of palms and soles
   E. Paget's disease of nipple or groin
   F. Basal cell nevus syndrome
   G. Urticaria and erythema multiforme of the chronic types
   H. Acquired ichthyosis (lymphomas)
   I. Exfoliative erythrodermatitis

nodules of rheumatic fever, the poorly healing skin ulcers of diabetes and sickle cell disease, and the yellowness of liver failure are but a few examples. In many ways it is very true that "the skin is the mirror of the body."

PHYSICAL EXAMINATION

1. Inspection
   a. General
   b. Specific
2. Characterize each abnormality by size, shape, quality, distribution of lesions.
3. Look specifically for skin findings associated with diagnoses suggested by history.

Examination of the skin is carried out through inspection and palpation. Inspection requires both adequate lighting and adequate exposure of the patient's skin. Bright, diffuse, overhead fluorescent light is the best way to achieve adequate lighting. Daylight and incandescent light can be used, but light from these sources is usually insufficiently bright and is too directional.

Proper exposure of the patient's skin for a general clinical examination requires the removal of clothing down to the underwear, over which may be worn a hospital examining gown of the type that opens at the rear. I cannot emphasize too strongly that inadequate exposure is almost always the fault of the examiner rather than that of the patient. In my professional lifetime I have met only a handful of patients who, because of modesty, were reluctant to disrobe sufficiently for proper examination. On the other hand, I have watched countless examinations in which the examiner, having failed to request proper exposure, attempted the shortcut of merely lifting the clothing for a quick peek underneath. The inadequacy of this approach is apparent. I have also seen examiners who, brusque and unthinking in their disregard for a patient's modesty, literally force a patient into a protective, covering response. This latter situation is most likely to develop in the handling of the examining gown. The following approach, which requires the use of a second sheet, is suggested.

First, with the patient sitting on the edge of the examining table, examine the exposed areas, including the scalp, hair, face, mouth, neck, arms, hands, and fingernails (Fig. 6-2). Place a second folded sheet such that it covers the waist. Ask the patient to pull the hospital gown out from under the covering sheet so that the gown is bunched over the breasts or shoulders, allowing examination of the abdomen, lower chest, anterior surface of the lower legs, feet, and toenails (Fig. 6-3). Ask the patient to stand with his back facing you and examine that (Fig. 6-4). Unfortunately, nonconsecutive viewing of the skin in a piecemeal fashion during the physical examination often leads to incomplete and inadequate information regarding the skin.

Most of us have acquired, on a nonmedical basis, significant knowledge regarding the appearance of normal skin, but this knowledge is probably insufficiently organized to be useful. This section will attempt to put that knowledge into appropriate perspective.

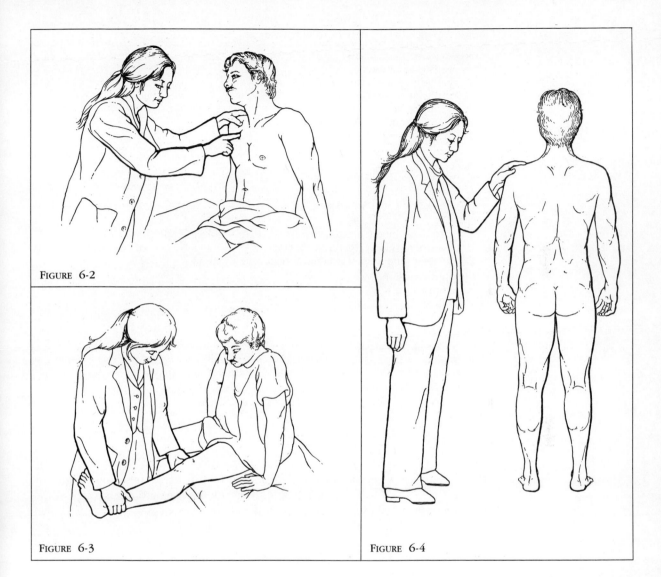

FIGURE 6-2

FIGURE 6-3

FIGURE 6-4

TABLE 6-3. Generalized Cutaneous Color Changes

I. Brown
   A. Addison's disease
   B. Hemachromatosis (may be gray-brown)
   C. Porphyria cutanea tarda
   D. Scleroderma
   E. Neurofibromatosis (café au lait spots)
   (See also Table 6-2)
II. Yellow
   A. Jaundice
   B. Anemia (especially pernicious anemia)
   C. Carotenemia (sclerae are not yellow)
   D. Quinacrine (Atabrine) usage
III. Gray
   A. Gold deposition (secondary to intramuscular gold therapy)
   B. Silver deposition (argyria)
   C. Phenothiazine usage (long-term, high-dose therapy)
IV. Hypopigmentation
   A. Albinism
   B. Vitiligo
   C. Pallor of anemia
V. Purpura
   A. Intravascular defects (e.g., thrombocytopenia, hemophilia)
   B. Vascular wall destruction (various types of vasculitis)
   C. Extravascular defects (steroid purpura, senile purpura, etc.)
VI. Red and blue hues (these color changes generally depend on vascular flow and are too variable and nonspecific to identify specific diseases)

COLOR

The range of color that can be considered normal is great and depends on many variables, such as race, nationality, and degree of sun exposure. Physiologically, skin color is derived from three major sources: (1) erythematous hues that come from oxygenated hemoglobin contained in the cutaneous vasculature, (2) brown hues that come from melanin pigment produced by the melanocytes of the epidermis, and (3) yellow hues that come from the natural color of nonvascularized collagen and from bile and carotene pigments. Cutaneous color changes, whether pathologic or physiologic, are related to changes in the balance of these three hues.

The range of normal skin color is wide, and the simple presence of one color or another is not necessarily significant; but the fact that the presenting color represents a change from what existed before is important. Changes in color may be generalized or localized. Small localized areas of color change are called *macules;* larger areas are called *patches.* The major kinds of color change include the following:

BROWN

Generalized darkening of melanin pigmentation is an important clue to some types of pituitary, adrenal (Fig. 6-5), liver, and other diseases (Fig. 6-6). Localized increase in melanin pigmentation may be seen in the brown macules or patches of café au lait spots, freckles, lentigines, nevi, and areas of postinflammatory hyperpigmenta-

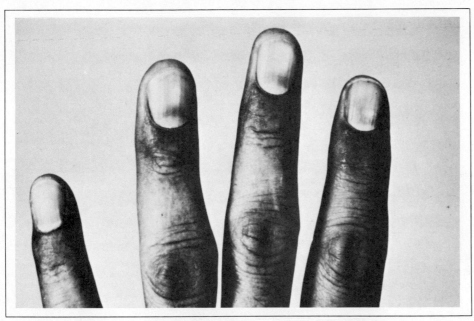

FIGURE 6-5
Hyperpigmentation of the fingers and nails in adrenal insufficiency (Addison's disease). Note accentuation of pigmentation at the knuckle folds.

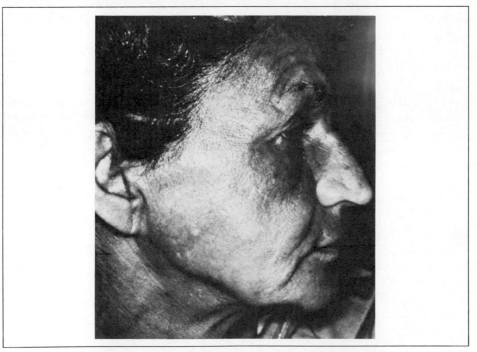

FIGURE 6-6
Hyperpigmentation in porphyria cutanea tarda.

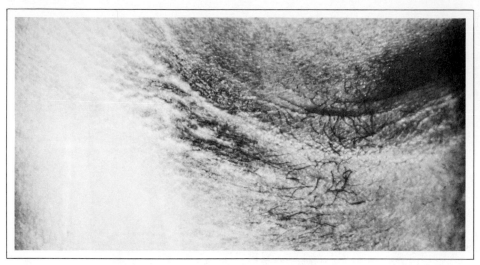

FIGURE 6-7
Acanthosis nigricans of the axilla.

tion. Acanthosis nigricans, a velvety black pigmentation in axillae and groin, associates with obesity, endocrine disorders, and certain tumors (Fig. 6-7).

WHITE
Absence of melanin gives the skin a white color. Generalized hypopigmentation may be seen in albinism, and localized areas of hypopigmentation may be seen in the macules or patches of vitiligo (Fig. 6-8), scars, postinflammatory hypopigmentation, and a variety of other cutaneous diseases.

YELLOW
Generalized yellowness of the skin due to an increase in cutaneous bile pigment may be seen in liver failure, in which case it is known as jaundice or icterus. More rarely, diffuse yellowness occurs in hypothyroidism and vegetarians as a result of increased carotene pigmentation. Finally, a pale yellow color may be seen in anemia, in which the contribution of the red oxygenated blood decreases, allowing accentuation of the normal yellow color of collagen. This latter phenomenon is particularly prominent in pernicious anemia and in anemia of chronic renal disease; in both, indirect bilirubin from hemolysis may contribute to the yellowness.

ERYTHEMA
Increased cutaneous blood flow, most commonly as a component of inflammation, leads to increasing redness of the skin. Thus, generalized erythema may occur with drug eruptions, viral exanthems, and urticaria. Localized inflammation and redness occur nonspecifically in a vast array of cutaneous diseases. Noninflammatory redness occasionally occurs due to an increased number of intravascular red blood cells (polycythemia).

OTHER COLORS
Rarely, some medications that are injected or ingested contribute their own color to the skin. Examples include the slate-gray color due to silver salts and the yellow

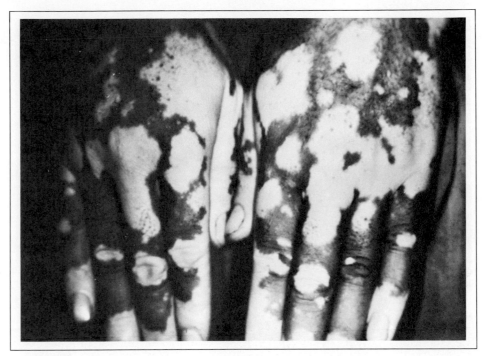

FIGURE 6-8
Vitiligo of the hands.

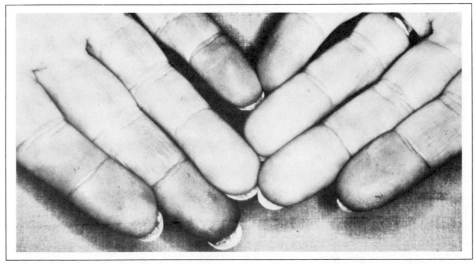

FIGURE 6-9
Cyanosis of the fingers in Raynaud's phenomenon.

color due to quinacrine. Cyanosis, the bluish color of unsaturated hemoglobin, may occur with decreased oxygen, decreased blood flow (Fig. 6-9), and certain drugs (nitrates).

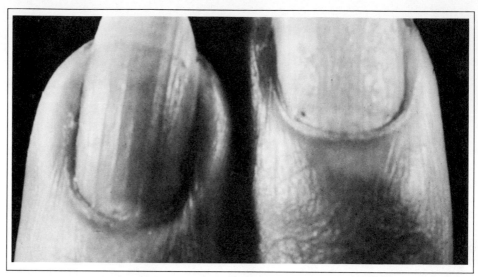

FIGURE 6-10
Pitting of the fingernails in psoriasis.

TEXTURE

The characteristic "feel" of skin depends on a number of physiologic processes. These include softness, as provided by the layer of fat cells which abuts the lower portion of the dermis; moisture, as provided by water diffusion through the skin and by sweating onto the surface of the skin; lubrication, as provided by the sebaceous glands; warmth, as provided by the circulation of internally warmed blood; and the presence or absence of roughness, depending on the amount of scale (keratin) produced by the epidermal cells. Balance among these factors depends on the patient's age, sex, and, of course, on the region of the skin being examined.

CHANGE IN TEXTURE

After puberty the scalp and face of most patients will feel oily (a condition known as seborrhea), but there are no pathologic states specifically associated with an increase in sebaceous secretion. On the other hand, decreased lubrication (dryness, chapping, or xerosis) is common after the age of 60 and occasionally occurs in younger people as a result of too-frequent bathing. Rarely, xerosis reflects a deficiency of thyroid or sex hormones.

As a result of thermal stimuli (such as fever or an overly warm examining room), patients may develop a palpable moistness of the skin associated with generalized sweating. Under emotional stimuli, localized sweating occurs on the forehead, palms, soles, axillae, and groin. Rarely, moist skin may be a reflection of the increased metabolic rate that occurs in hyperthyroidism.

Increased warmth of the skin occurs when an increase in cutaneous blood flow delivers body heat to the surface of the skin, where it is then lost by convection, conduction, and radiation. This may occur with fever or following exercise. Localized areas of increased warmth may accompany the increased blood flow seen with cutaneous inflammation. Coolness of the skin reflects decreased blood flow, such as is seen in the lower legs of patients with peripheral arteriovascular disease.

TABLE 6-4. Nail Changes*

   I. Nail pitting
     A. Psoriasis
     B. Alopecia areata
  II. Nail dystrophy
     A. Trauma
     B. Psoriasis
     C. Fungal infections
     D. Arteriosclerotic changes (toenails only)
 III. Curvature without clubbing
     A. Raynaud's phenomenon
     B. Scleroderma
 IV. Clubbing
     A. Chronic pulmonary disease
     B. Pulmonary malignancy
     C. Cardiovascular disease with cyanosis
  V. Onycholysis (Separation of nail plate from the nail bed)
     A. Candidiasis (moniliasis)
     B. Tetracycline (photo-onycholysis)
     C. Hyperthyroidism
     D. Trauma
 VI. White banding (Terry's nails, Mees' lines)
     A. Hypoalbuminemia
     B. Cirrhosis
     C. Renal failure
     D. Chronic arsenic exposure
 VII. Spoon nails (koilonychia)
     A. Iron deficiency anemia
     B. Familial, without associated disease
VIII. Transverse grooving (Beau's lines)
     A. Severe infection
     B. Myocardial infarction
     C. Trauma
 IX. Splinter hemorrhages (present in 20% of healthy individuals)
     A. Subacute bacterial endocarditis
     B. Trichinosis
     C. Collagen vascular disease
     D. Trauma

---

* See also Chapter 4.

Finally, the skin may lose its elasticity, or feel tough, when it is distended by edematous fluid, when the cutaneous fat is replaced by collagen (as in scleroderma), or when normal collagen is replaced by scar tissue.

MUCOUS MEMBRANES
Mucous membranes are characteristically pink in color and moist to palpation. Mottled brown or black melanin pigmentation may be present on the oral mucous membranes of black patients. Increased oral pigmentation may occur in adrenocortical insufficiency disease.

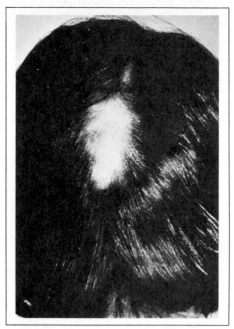

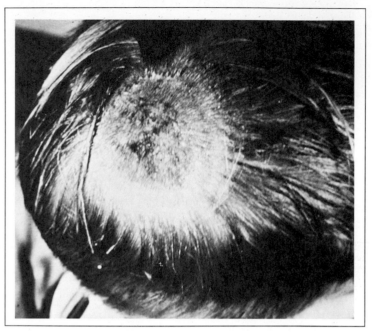

FIGURE 6-11
Alopecia areata. The area of hair loss is
sharply marginated, and the exposed scalp
appears normal.

FIGURE 6-12
Tinea capitis. A fungal infection of the scalp.

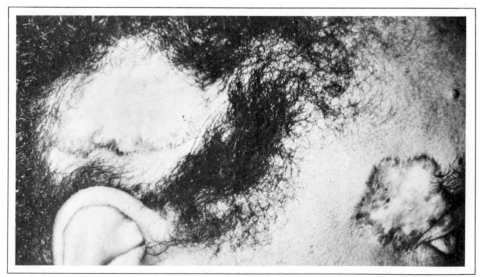

FIGURE 6-13
Discoid lupus erythematosus. Typical scarring plaques are found on the scalp.

HAIR

Normal hair distribution is well appreciated by most examiners and need not be considered here. However, it should be remembered that facial, axillary, and pubic hair depend on the presence of sex and other hormones and thus on both the sex and the age of the patient. Scalp hair should be specifically examined for length, texture, fragility, sheen, and the ease with which hairs can be manually removed from their follicles. Scalp hair normally grows about 0.3 mm per day or, in more practical terms, about 0.5 inch per month.

TABLE 6-5. Some Causes of Hair Loss

I. Generalized alopecia
  A. No underlying scalp disease
    1. Telogen effluvium (especially postpartum and after severe illness)
    2. Alopecia totalis
    3. Some cases of male and female pattern alopecia
    4. Thyroid disease
    5. Drug induced (mostly birth control pills and cancer chemotherapeutic agents)
    6. Congenital hair defects
  B. With underlying scalp disease
    1. Seborrheic dermatitis (hair loss is mild)
    2. Contact dermatitis (permanents, bleaches, and dyes)
II. Localized or patterned alopecia
  A. No scalp disease
    1. Alopecia areata
    2. Male and female pattern alopecia
    3. Trichotlllomania
    4. Secondary syphilis
    5. Traction alopecia
  B. With scalp disease
    1. Tinea capitis
    2. Lupus erythematosus (discoid type)
    3. Psoriasis (hair loss is mild)

SPECIFIC CUTANEOUS LESIONS

Thus far we have talked primarily about functional changes that occur in the normal components of the skin. In this section we will discuss structural changes, that is, the development of lesions that, strictly speaking, always represent cutaneous pathology. In some instances the pathology has little significance (e.g., nevi and senile angiomas), but the experienced examiner should consider the presence of any of these structural changes as potentially important until he has become familiar with those that can safely be ignored. The patient, of course, may be anxious about any skin lesion and should be assured that proper attention is being given to his fears. The most common structural changes are shown in Figure 6-14 and are discussed below.

NONPALPABLE LESIONS

These circumscribed flat changes in skin color are called macules (if less than about 1 cm in diameter) and *patches* (if larger). Freckles, for example, are macules, and large areas of hypopigmentation may be referred to as vitiliginous patches.

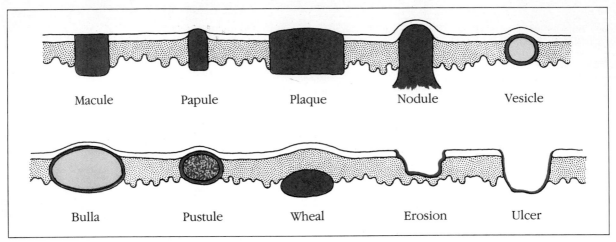

FIGURE 6-14
Most common structural changes in the skin.

PALPABLE LESIONS

These are localized lesions that have substance or mass, are always palpable, and are usually elevated above the surface of the skin. Small palpable lesions are called *papules,* and large papules are called *nodules.* A confluence of papules or nodules, resulting in a large flat-topped lesion, is called a *plaque.* The palpable substance of papules, nodules, and plaques occurs as a result of one or both of the following processes: (1) proliferation of the various cells normally found in the skin (e.g., inflammatory cells, metastatic tumor cells, leukemic cells); or (2) the accumulation of fluid within the skin. Fluid accumulating within the skin may be present in a diffuse fashion (e.g., a hive or wheal) or in a loculated fashion (as in a blister). Small blisters are known as *vesicles,* and large blisters are known as *bullae.* Vesicles or bullae that contain many polymorphonuclear leukocytes appear cloudy or white and are called *pustules.*

Extravasation of red cells into the skin (purpura) may present with red or reddish purple punctate lesions 1 to 5 mm in size (*petechiae*) or larger confluent bruises (*ecchymoses*).

EROSIONS AND ULCERS

Superficial loss of skin is called an erosion, whereas deep loss is termed an ulcer. In both situations the barrier function of the skin is lost, and serum, together with inflammatory cells, exudes to the surface as "weeping" or "oozing." When this exudate dries, it forms crusts. It is important to distinguish between the light gray flakes of scale and the yellow-brown friable granules of crusts, inasmuch as the former represents epithelial proliferation and the latter represents epithelial loss.

Erosions and ulcers arise in three major ways: (1) as a result of external trauma, most commonly scratching; (2) from the unroofing of vesicular or bullous lesions; or (3) from the necrotic effect of vascular ischemia. Ability to determine which of these three mechanisms is responsible for an ulcer greatly simplifies the preparation of a differential diagnosis.

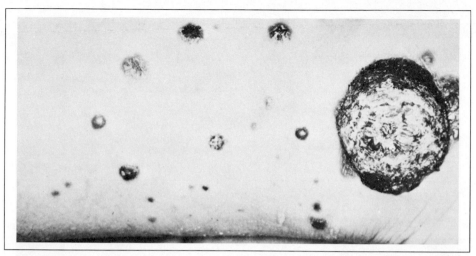

FIGURE 6-15
Malignant melanoma with satellite cutaneous metastases.

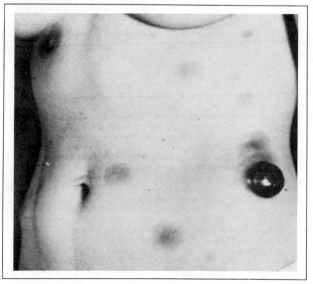

FIGURE 6-16
Lymphoma cutis. Each of the large nodules represents a cutaneous aggregation of atypical lymphocytes.

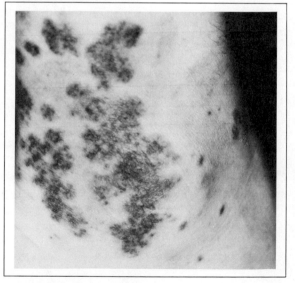

FIGURE 6-17
Purpura of the foot in vasculitis.

Once examiners have learned to recognize the kind of pathologic conditions described above and can use appropriate terms in their written or verbal descriptions, they are ready to formulate differential diagnoses. To assist the student in this task, many dermatology textbooks are arranged or organized according to the different patterns of cutaneous pathology; the student then may go directly from his own descriptions of the lesions to the appropriate textbook chapter.

Some characteristic lesions of the skin are illustrated in Figures 6-15 through 6-20.

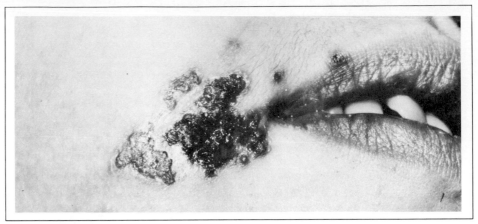

FIGURE 6-18
Impetigo. A crusted, weeping, infectious lesion common in children.

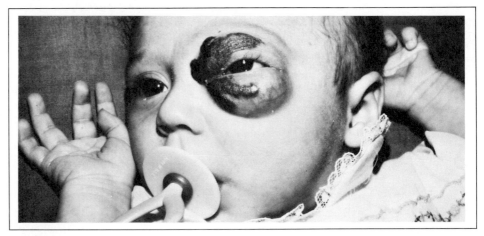

FIGURE 6-19
Hemangioma of the eye.

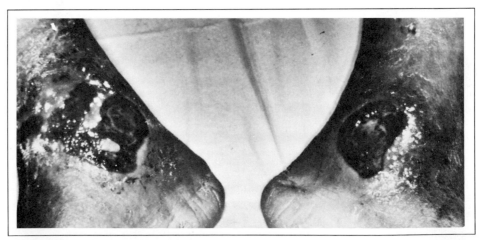

FIGURE 6-20
Bilateral stasis ulcers with surrounding dermatitis.

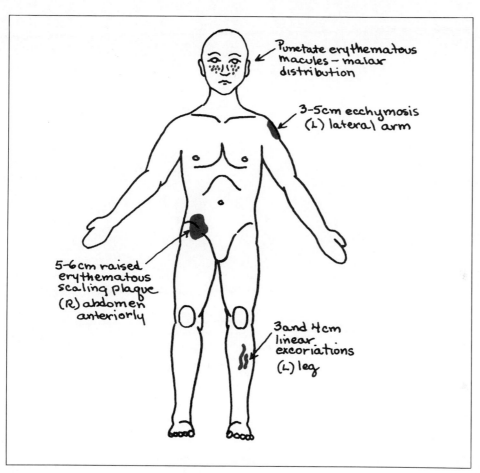

Punctate erythematous
macules — malar
distribution

3-5cm ecchymosis
(L) lateral arm

5-6 cm raised
erythematous
scaling plaque
(R) abdomen
anteriorly

3 and 4cm
linear
excoriations
(L) leg

FIGURE 6-21

In addition to describing the lesions by color, type, size, and distribution, the student (and those who read the workup) will find value in drawing the lesions, as illustrated in Figure 6-21.

CHAPTER 7

HEMATOPOIETIC SYSTEM

*She was very anaemic. Her thin lips were pale, and her skin was delicate,
of a faint green colour, without a touch of red even in the cheeks.*

W. SOMERSET MAUGHAM
(1874–1965)

In this chapter the major components of the hematopoietic system—the lymph
nodes, bone marrow, and circulating blood—will be considered as a unit. Physical
examination of the spleen, which is generally done as part of the abdominal examination, will be considered in Chapter 14. There is a sound basis for considering the
physical manifestations of diseases of the lymphoid and myeloid reticulum together. According to the monophyletic theory subscribed to by many authorities,
lymphocytes, granulocytes, monocytes, red blood cells, and platelets may be considered to arise from a single pluripotential mesenchymal precursor.

There are many important physical signs associated with hematologic disorders.
Some of these are due directly to changes in the reticulum of the lymph nodes,
spleen, or liver; others are indirect manifestations involving the skin, mucous membranes, ocular fundi, or bone. Although the final diagnosis almost invariably requires laboratory confirmation, the physical findings are of great value in directing
the physician's attention to the proper special studies.

ANATOMY

TABLE 7-1. Clinical Lymphadenopathy

Lymph Node	Region Drained	Causes of Enlargement
Submental	Lips, mouth, tongue	Oral infections, tumor
Submandibular	Face	Facial, oral infections, tumor
Preauricular	Ears, temporal scalp	Infection
Postauricular	Scalp	Scalp infections, injury
Occipital	Scalp	Viral, local infections
Superficial cervical	Ears, parotid	Infection, tumor
Deep cervical	Tongue, larynx, thyroid, trachea, esophagus	Infection, tumor
Supraclavicular	Neck, axillae, GI tract (left)	Infection, tumor
Inguinal	Lower extremities, pelvis	Infection, tumor
Axillary	Chest, upper extremities	Infection, tumor

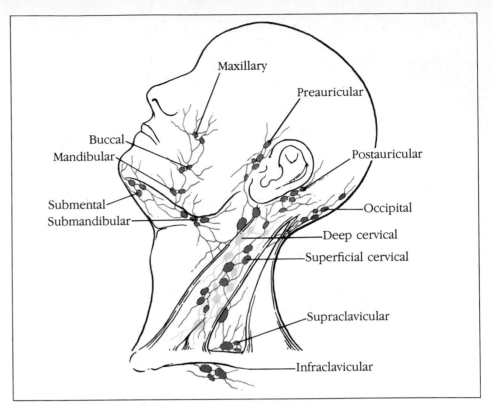

FIGURE 7-1
Cervicofacial and supraclavicular lymph nodes.

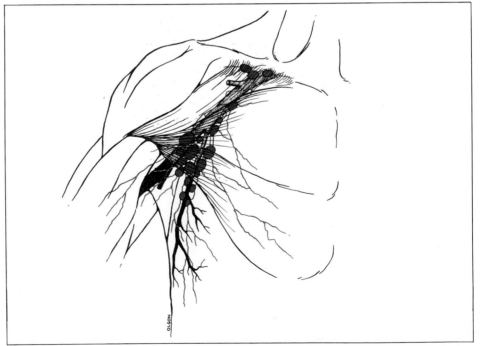

FIGURE 7-2
Axillary lymph nodes.

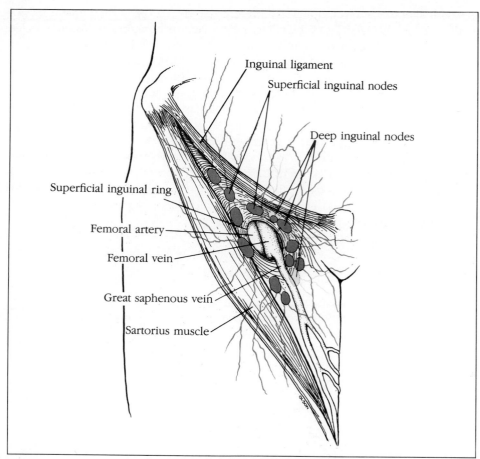

Inguinal ligament

Superficial inguinal nodes

Deep inguinal nodes

Superficial inguinal ring

Femoral artery

Femoral vein

Great saphenous vein

Sartorius muscle

FIGURE 7-3
Inguinal and femoral lymph nodes.

HISTORY

Symptoms arising from hematopoietic disease may originate from a *decrease* in the formed elements of the blood (anemia, thrombocytopenia, leukopenia) or an *increase* in these same cells (erythrocytosis, thrombocytosis, leukemia). *Systemic effects* of hematopoietic disease may arise directly from these alterations in absolute numbers (as with the weakness of anemia, or thrombogenic tendency of increased platelets) or indirectly in ways as yet poorly understood (the pruritus of lymphoma, for example). Some patients will complain only of the mass effect of enlarged lymph nodes or spleen.

Pallor, ease of fatigue, weakness, lassitude, shortness of breath on exertion, faintness, and vertigo are the important general symptoms of *anemia* of any cause. They are due chiefly to increased circulatory effort and, in part, to deficient oxygenation of the tissues, especially the brain. In an otherwise healthy individual, symptoms of anemia do not become conspicuous until the hemoglobin is lowered to half its normal value, unless there is a coincidental fall in blood volume, as in shock or hemorrhage.

The leukemias and lymphomas commonly give rise to anemia and thrombocyto-penia. In turn, epistaxis, gum bleeding, petechiae, purpura, or frank hemorrhage anywhere in the body may occur. Systemic symptoms include weight loss, fatigue, heat intolerance, night sweats, fever, and pruritus. Rapidly enlarging lymph nodes of any cause, with acute distention of the capsule, vary from "sore" to exquisitely tender. Slowly enlarging nodes produce no symptoms until they are large enough to result in mechanical difficulties. Enlarged mediastinal and hilar lymph nodes can compress the trachea, causing respiratory embarrassment with a dry "brassy" cough, progressive dyspnea, orthopnea, and cyanosis. In addition, obstruction to lymphatic and venous return can cause swelling of the face and neck (superior mediastinal syndrome). Enlarged retroperitoneal, periaortic, and perifemoral nodes can cause ascites and edema of the lower extremities. By encroachment on the stomach and intestine, massive splenic enlargement leads to early satiety, constipation, and/or diarrhea.

In both polycythemia vera and secondary polycythemia, total blood volume and blood viscosity are increased. In consequence, congestive heart failure, headache, hemorrhage, and thromboembolic phenomena are common.

PHYSICAL EXAMINATION

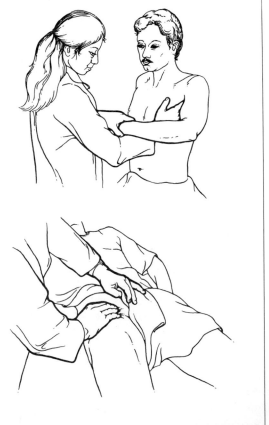

1. Palpate head and neck nodes.
2. Palpate epitrochlear and axillary nodes.
3. Palpate inguinal nodes.
   a. When looking specifically for lymphadenopathy, these examinations for regional nodes are done one directly after another. Otherwise, lymph node examination is often done as part of the regional examination of the head and neck, breast, abdomen, and extremities.
   b. Examination of the spleen is usually done as part of the abdominal examination (see Chap. 14).

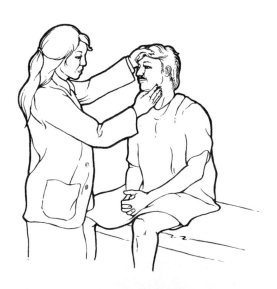

LYMPH NODES

Although there are more than 60 standard groups of lymph nodes listed by the anatomists, clinicians generally need to consider the palpable nodes in terms of only three regional groups: (1) cervicofacial and supraclavicular, (2) axillary and epitrochlear, and (3) inguinal and femoral. Needless to say, many groups of nodes lie beyond the reach of physical examination. Some of them can be evaluated by radiologic techniques; others, only surgically.

The standard examination of the lymph nodes requires only simple inspection and palpation. It is always useful to compare sides. Use the middle three fingers for palpation. Movements should be slow and gentle; your fingers should oscillate up and down, back and forth, and in a rotary motion.

In recording your findings, five characteristics should routinely be included: (1) location; (2) size, preferably giving the diameter in centimeters but at times using descriptive terms, such as split pea, bean, almond; (3) tenderness; (4) degree of fixation (e.g., movable, matted, fixed); and (5) texture (e.g., hard, soft, firm).

Normal lymph nodes are not palpable. However, nodes enlarged as a consequence of prior inflammation are frequently palpable. Cervical nodes up to 1 cm in diameter are almost always felt in children of up to 12 years of age. If these nodes are biopsied, they commonly show chronic hyperplastic lymphadenitis. Such nodes are usually 0.5 to 1.0 cm in diameter and are referred to as "shotty" (as in buckshot ammunition), which has come to mean firm, freely movable, and nontender. They are most common in the occipital region (from old scalp infections), axillae (infections of the hands), and the inguinal regions (old infections of the genitalia and feet).

In adolescents and adults, palpable inguinal lymph nodes are so common as to be almost the rule. At times, as a consequence of recurrent infections of the feet, they may be quite large without being of particular clinical significance. For this reason the inguinal region is a poor site for biopsy, since the nodes may be distorted by chronic lymphadenitis. Femoral lymph node enlargement is more commonly of pathologic significance.

CERVICOFACIAL NODES

Look for asymmetry. Is there any visible lymphadenopathy? Be methodical in your palpation, beginning above and posteriorly and proceeding downward as follows:

1. Occipital and postauricular
2. Submaxillary and submental
3. Downward along the sternocleidomastoid muscle (superficial cervical nodes)
4. Posterior triangle (lower end of deep cervical chain)
5. Supraclavicular

There are two satisfactory methods of palpation. With the anterior approach, the hand not used for palpation controls the head (Fig. 7-4). With the posterior approach, the neck is first flexed to obtain proper relaxation of the muscles, and corresponding zones on both sides are palpated simultaneously (Fig. 7-5). **Palpation must be light** or small nodes will escape notice.

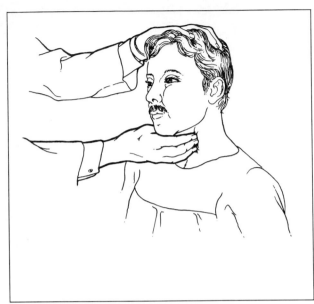

FIGURE 7-4
Palpation of anterior cervical nodes.

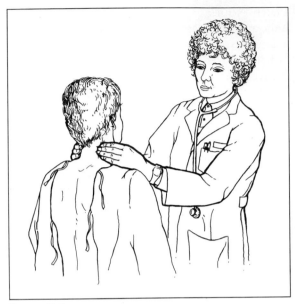

FIGURE 7-5
Palpation of posterior cervical nodes.

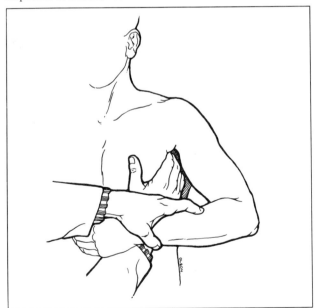

FIGURE 7-6
Palpation of axillary nodes.

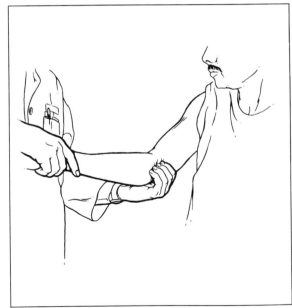

FIGURE 7-7
Palpation of epitrochlear nodes.

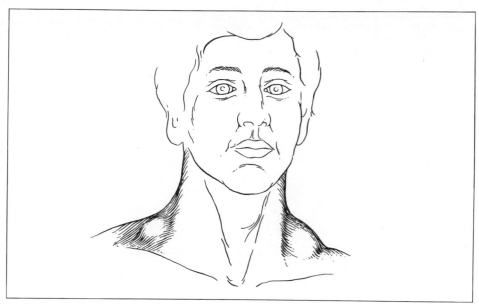

FIGURE 7-8
Hodgkin's disease.

AXILLARY AND EPITROCHLEAR NODES

The method of palpating the axilla is crucial. The patient may be either sitting or supine. In either case the arm must be supported (Fig. 7-6). Cup your hand slightly and reach as high into the apex of the axilla as possible. Now pull down, exerting gentle pressure against the thorax with the fingertips. Repeat several times, checking, in order, the lateral group (posterior), the central group, and the pectoral group. It is important not to abduct the arm too far, for this tenses the skin of the axilla, interfering with deep palpation and at times causing considerable discomfort to the patient. The epitrochlear nodes are palpated as shown in Figure 7-7.

INGUINAL NODES

With the patient supine, palpate the superficial inguinal and femoral nodes, using a rotary motion.

It is frequently impossible to determine whether a lymph node is normal or abnormal simply by its texture. Any node, regardless of how it may feel, may show typical granulomatous, neoplastic, or other changes on microscopic examination.

Localized lymphadenopathy is usually due either to inflammation or to neoplasm. Acute lymphadenitis causes enlarged, tender, rather soft nodes, which are sometimes assciated with induration and the red streaks of lymphangitis. The primary site of infection is usually obvious. Metastatic lymphadenopathy is usually stony, hard, nontender, and somewhat fixed to the underlying structures. From knowledge of anatomy, the physician must know the various patterns of lymphatic drainage in order to estimate the most likely site of a primary lesion when metastatic nodes are identified. For example, a left supraclavicular node, which is draining the thoracic duct, may signal an intra-abdominal malignancy (*Virchow's node*). Localized adenopathy may also result from chronic granulomatous processes, such as tuberculosis or Hodgkin's disease (Fig. 7-8).

TABLE 7-2. Some Causes of Generalized Lymphadenopathy

Lymphatic leukemia
Lymphoreticular malignancy
Secondary syphilis
Measles
Juvenile rheumatoid arthritis
Infectious mononucleosis
Plague
Tuberculosis
Sarcoidosis
Toxoplasmosis
Scabies
Cat-scratch fever
Amyloidosis
Serum sickness

Generalized lymphadenopathy is usually due to inflammation or neoplasm (see Table 7-2). Such nodes are soft, movable, and usually slightly tender. Many chronic systemic infections may at times produce generalized enlargement. The lymphomas are a common cause of generalized lymphadenopathy. Initially they may cause painless, progressive, discrete enlargement of the nodes. Involvement may at first be localized, but later it frequently becomes generalized, and the nodes may become firm, matted, and fixed. Leukemia may or may not produce generalized lymphadenopathy.

With the granulocytic forms of leukemia, lymphadenopathy is uncommon. With monocytic leukemia, lymphadenopathy is commonly associated with oropharyngeal infection and is most conspicuous in the cervicosubmandibular areas. Chronic lymphocytic leukemia often results in generalized lymph node enlargement and may be suspected by the feel of the nodes, which are usually 1 to 3 cm in diameter, nontender, elastic (rubbery), and freely movable. Other varieties of leukemia may produce variable degrees of lymph node enlargement. In acute leukemia, because of rapid enlargement, the nodes are frequently tender.

SPLEEN

Splenomegaly may signal disease of the hematopoietic system. Since the spleen is usually considered a part of the examination of the abdomen, the technique of that examination and the significance of abnormalities are treated in Chapter 14.

SKIN

Many hematologic disorders have cutaneous manifestations. *Pallor* and *coldness* of the skin may be present in patients with chronic anemia. The nail beds and conjunctivae are particularly helpful in estimating the significance of pallor, since many Caucasians normally are fair-skinned. *Rubor,* particularly of the face and neck, may be present in patients with polycythemia vera. There is often associated dilation of the superficial veins and venules, as well as suffusion of the bulbar conjunctivae (bloodshot eyes). *Cyanosis* may be associated with secondary polycythemia. *Icterus*

TABLE 7-3. Some Causes of Anemia

I. Decreased production
    A. Marrow suppression
        1. Toxins
        2. Chronic infections
        3. Uremia
        4. Hepatic disease
    B. Marrow destruction
        1. Fibrosis
        2. Toxins
        3. Infiltration (neoplasm, infection)
    C. Deficiency states
        1. Folic acid
        2. Vitamin B_{12}
        3. Vitamin B_6
        4. Iron
        5. Copper
        6. Zinc
        7. Phosphorus
    D. Defective hemoglobin synthesis
        1. Thalassemia
        2. Sickle cells
        3. Other hemoglobinopathies
II. Hemolysis
    A. Red cell defects
        1. Hemoglobin (e.g., sickle cell anemia, vitamin B_{12} deficiency)
        2. Membrane (e.g., spherocytosis)
        3. Energy systems (e.g., glucose 6-phosphate dehydrogenase deficiency,
           phosphorus deficiency)
    B. Red cell toxins
        1. Bacterial hemolysins (e.g., clostridial toxin)
        2. Antigen-antibody complexes (e.g., drug hemolysis)
        3. Erythrophagocytosis (certain tumors)
    C. Red cell parasitism
        1. Malaria
        2. *Borrelia*
        3. Babesiosis
III. Increased loss
    A. Gastrointestinal bleeding
    B. Uterine blood loss
    C. Pregnancy
    D. Hematuria
    E. Epistaxis
    F. Hemoptysis
    G. Trauma

(jaundice) may be a sign of rapid hemolysis. *Purpura* may be due to any of a number of deficiencies of the hemostatic mechanism. *Pruritus* (with certain lymphomas) may be intense, resulting in extensive excoriation of the skin. There may be primary invasion of the skin by lymphoma or leukemia, and almost any type of secondary dermatitis may develop with these two disorders (see Chap. 6).

MUCOSA

Glossitis and stomatitis are common with the deficiency anemias (Table 7-3). When

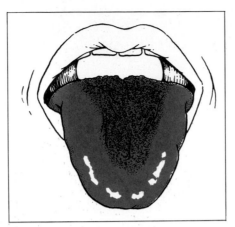

FIGURE 7-9
Tongue in pernicious anemia.

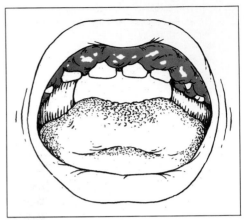

FIGURE 7-10
Gums in leukemia.

they are longstanding, atrophy of the glossal papillae occurs, making the tongue pale and smooth. The gums may bleed whenever there is a hemorrhagic tendency associated with a blood disorder. Gingival and mucosal ulcerations of the mouth and pharynx occur with leukemia, particularly with the acute forms. A characteristic plum-colored swelling of the gingivae may be the most prominent physical finding in monocytic leukemia; it can be almost pathognomonic. Necrotic mucosal ulcers and pharyngitis are important signs of agranulocytosis.

BONE

Bone tenderness commonly accompanies disorders of the blood-forming organs. Although the sternum is commonly tender to point pressure, exquisite tenderness may develop as a consequence of increased intramedullary proliferation of blood cells, as in the leukemias and regenerative anemias (e.g., hemolytic anemia). Localized bone tenderness may be due to localized invasion of bone by leukemia or other malignancies of hematopoietic tissue (e.g., multiple myeloma, Hodgkin's disease).

OCULAR FUNDI

Many hematologic disorders produce funduscopic signs, including retinal edema, hemorrhages, exudates, and dilation and tortuosity of the veins. These changes may be on the basis of hypoxemia, thrombocytopenia, stasis, capillary injury, or metabolic deficiencies. Abnormalities of the retina are further discussed in Chapter 8.

SECTION III
HEAD AND NECK

If nature had only one fixed standard for the proportions of the various parts, then the faces of all men would resemble each other to such a degree that it would be impossible to distinguish one from another; but she has varied the five parts of the face in such a way that although she has made an almost universal standard as to their size, she has not observed it in the various conditions to such a degree as to prevent one from being clearly distinguished from another.

LEONARDO DA VINCI
(1452–1519)

1. Examine regional lymph nodes and skin.
2. Inspect the head.
3. Examine the eye.
   a. Visual acuity
   b. External eye
   c. Pupils
   d. Extraocular movements
   e. Visual fields
   f. Fundi

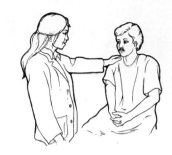

4. Examine the ear.
   a. External ear
   b. Auditory acuity
   c. Middle ear
   d. Sinuses
5. Examine the nose.
6. Examine the mouth and throat.
7. Observe the neck and check range of motion.
8. Palpate (cervical nodes)
   a. Trachea
   b. Thyroid
   c. Carotids

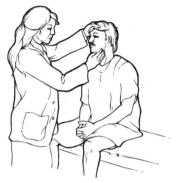

9. Auscultate the neck.
   a. Thyroid
   b. Carotids

EYE

CHAPTER 8

O loss of sight, of thee I most complain!
JOHN MILTON
(1608–1674)

Examination of the eyes gives clues to a variety of local and systemic disorders. The eyes may reflect central nervous system, metabolic, vascular, and infectious disease. Since the importance of vision to the patient can hardly be overestimated, this portion of the physical examination must be done with great care and tact.

ANATOMY

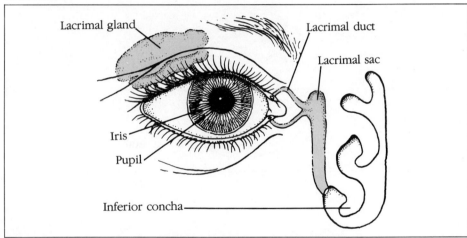

FIGURE 8-1
External eye and lacrimal apparatus.

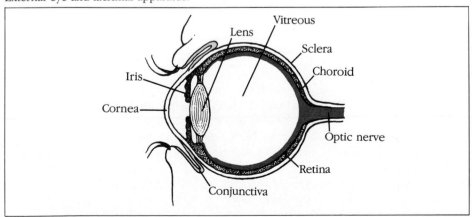

FIGURE 8-2
Cross-section of the eye.

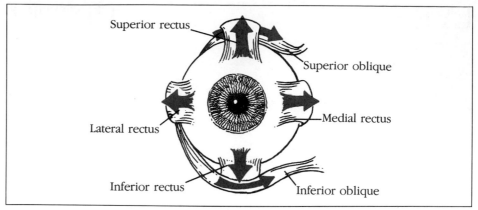

FIGURE 8-3
Extraocular muscles (right eye).

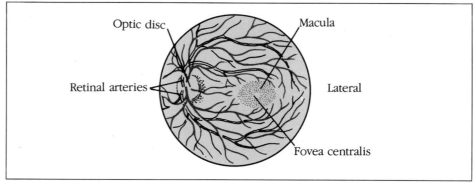

FIGURE 8-4
Ocular fundus (left eye).

HISTORY

The historical review of systems concerning symptoms of the eyes may be done as you do the physical examination. In addition to the symptoms listed below, be sure to record when the patient last had his eyeglasses refracted (some people buy their eyeglasses off the counter in the five-and-dime) and when he or she last had a glaucoma check.

PAIN

The complaint of pain in or about the eyes must be evaluated as to location, duration, type, and mode of onset. It may be related to a specific incident, as in the case of an injury to the eye. Pain in the eyes and forehead may be the result of uncorrected refractive error or ocular muscle imbalance, in which case it will often follow use of the eyes. Almost all patients with headache will ask whether the eyes are involved, but few headaches will be found to result from eye disease; on the contrary, a typical unilateral migraine headache, which will often include ocular pain on that side, is unrelated to eye pathology.

Very severe localized pain in one eye usually suggests surface disease, such as a foreign body or corneal ulcer. A dull throbbing pain is more typical of iritis or of acute glaucoma and may be worse when the patient is lying down. Deep pain in the orbit may not be associated with local signs but may indicate neighboring disease, such as sinus disease or intracranial sensory nerve involvement. Irritation of the meninges or increased intracranial pressure may produce orbital pain.

VISUAL LOSS

This may range from blurring of vision to complete blindness in one or both eyes. The earliest signs of double vision may be recognized by the patient only as a visual blur related to the overlapping images. A reduction in visual acuity can reflect systemic disease, such as early diabetes, where a shift to myopia may occur. The early symptoms of senile cataract may include visual blurring, especially for distance, and the ability to read without glasses ("second sight" due to myopia).

Sudden loss of vision usually signals retinal or optic nerve disease and may be related either to inflammation or to vascular embarrassment. Transient visual loss (amaurosis fugax) may signal occlusion (by atherosclerosis or emboli) or spasm of the great vessels of the neck or in the eye itself. Central visual loss must be distinguished from that of the peripheral areas; the patient is usually much more aware of loss of central reading acuity than of a peripheral narrowing of the visual field. *Reduced vision* is a significant finding and suggests either local or general disease, especially when loss has been sudden or when relatively recent glasses no longer aid. A reason must be sought for any instance of reduced vision. Causes can range from local ocular pathology (e.g., cataracts, retinal detachment, and vitreous or retinal hemorrhage) through optic nerve involvement as a part of neurologic disease. Sudden changes may suggest circulatory insufficiencies of various types, such as cerebral hemorrhage, major carotid occlusions, and the like. Poor vision in one eye may be noted in many patients who had a strabismus in childhood, with resulting suppression of central vision. Visual field defects of intracranial disease may be associated with complaints of visual loss, but the central acuity often may be normal and visual field examination necessary.

Any case of reduced vision, either unilateral or bilateral, demands an explanation.

DOUBLE VISION

Visual confusion is characteristic of the patient with double vision (diplopia). He will often close or cover one eye for relief. In certain cases of incomplete paralysis of an eye muscle, he may assume an unusual head position in order to maintain single vision; for example, head turning to the left, with the eyes directed to the right, in the case of a partial paralysis of the left lateral rectus muscle. Diplopia usually signifies either muscular or neurologic disease. A lack of parallelism of the eyes may not be associated with double vision when it is the result of a "lazy" or amblyopic eye dating from a muscle imbalance in childhood. Monocular diplopia usually indicates either corneal or lens changes.

PHOTOPHOBIA

Sensitivity to light varies considerably among normal individuals, but where it is significant there is usually disease of the cornea or of the anterior segment of the globe. In acute cases, a corneal foreign body, corneal ulcer, or iritis may be suspected, although old corneal scarring and vascularization may also produce a hypersensitivity to light.

TABLE 8-1. Differential Diagnosis of "Red-Eye"

	Conjunctiva	Iris	Pupil	Cornea	Anterior Chamber	Intraocular Pressure	Appearance
Acute glaucoma	Both ciliary and conjunctival vessels injected. Entire eye is red	Injected	Dilated, fixed, oval	Steamy, hazy	Very shallow	Very high	
Iritis	Redness most marked around cornea. Color does not blanch on pressure	Injected, swollen, muddy	Small, fixed	Normal	Turgid	Normal	
Conjunctivitis	Conjunctival vessels injected, greatest toward fornices. Blanch on pressure. Mobile over sclera	Normal	Normal	Normal	Normal	Normal	
Subconjunctival hemorrhage	Bright red sclera with white rim around limbus	Normal	Normal	Normal	Normal	Normal	

DISCHARGE

Material emerging from the eye as either watery or more viscid discharge usually suggests either conjunctival disease or difficulty in the lacrimal drainage system. In acute infections it may be more purulent and may collect on the lid borders. Where the lacrimal system is occluded, a flow of tears may be continuous, and mucus may collect in the tear sac so that pressure over this structure causes regurgitation of material into the eye. In allergic conjunctival disease the consistency of the discharge is stringy and tenacious. Tears may also be a part of the light-sensitivity response of a diseased eye.

REDNESS

Vascular congestion, or redness of the eyes, must be evaluated in terms of other findings and may represent infective or allergic conjunctivitis, inflammation of the iris, or acute glaucoma. The latter must be kept in mind as a diagnostic possibility in all cases of redness of the eye if precipitous blindness is to be prevented. In certain florid individuals, redness of the eye may not be significant unless other findings support the diagnosis of disease (see Table 8-1).

"EYE STRAIN"

This commonly used term is not sound from the medical standpoint and should not be used to denote the symptom of fatigue. "Strain" connotes damage, but eye use in itself never produces irreversible change. If there is discomfort with use of the eyes (asthenopia), a search should be made for refractive error or ocular muscular imbalance.

PHYSICAL EXAMINATION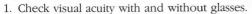

1. Check visual acuity with and without glasses.
2. Inspect.
   a. Lids
   b. Conjunctivae
   c. Corneas
   d. Sclerae
   e. Lacrimal system
3. Test pupillary responses.
4. Test extraocular movements.
5. Check visual fields by confrontation.
6. Perform funduscopy.
7. Check intraocular pressure.

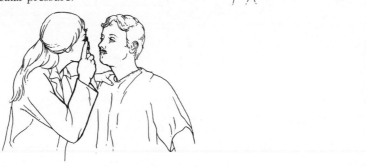

Visual Acuity

Accurate estimation of the patient's visual acuity is often mandatory. In cases involving head trauma or injury of the face or eyes, the vision should be measured, in case of future compensation or legal action, using Snellen's chart (Fig. 8-5). Seat the patient a measured 20 feet from the chart, cover one eye at a time, and ask him to read the letters starting from the top and reading down the chart. The last row in which he is able to read the majority of the letters should be recorded. The lower figure in the designation of visual acuity (20/**20**) represents the distance at which the normal eye would see the letter, and the upper figure (**20**/20) always refers to the distance (in feet) that the patient is seated from the chart. For example, the notation of 20/40 vision indicates the standard chart distance (20 feet) from the patient and the fact that the subject cannot read past the line that a normal individual would be able to read from 40 feet away. The numbers are in no sense a fraction.

Ask the patient to cover one eye and read down the chart, preferably with his distance glasses on. If he reaches the 20/30 row and misses two letters, the record notation is: 20/30−2. The cover is shifted to the other eye, and if he reads through the 20/40 row and reads only two letters in the next row, the record notation is: 20/40+2. The result is written "O.D. (right eye) 20/30−2: O.S. (left eye) 20/40+2." If glasses are worn, note "with correction"; if not, "without correction."

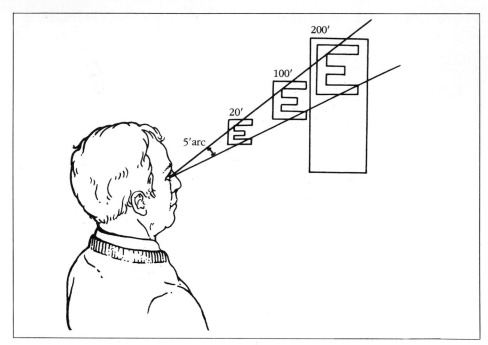

FIGURE 8-5
Measuring visual acuity.

If the patient cannot see any of the letters on the chart, gradually move him closer to it until he can read the large letter at the top. If this is 5 feet from the chart, write "5/200" (since the upper figure designates the distance of the patient from the letter). The designation "5/200" means the patient can see at 5 feet what a normal individual can see at 200 feet. If no letters can be read, hold up your fingers and ask him to count them; record the distance at which this occurs (e.g., "counts fingers at 2 feet"). If the patient cannot see (or count) your fingers, check his ability to see moving objects or the direction from which your flashlight beam is shining on his eye; record "moving objects" or "light projection." "Light perception" may be recorded if he is unable to recognize direction but knows that the light is on. Do not record the eye as blind unless no light is perceived.

In some cases it may be desirable to record the near vision. Special graded reading cards are available for this, but in a general examination ordinary newsprint will suffice for your records.

For general purposes a vision of 20/30 or better in each eye can be accepted as normal. Be sure that the patient is wearing his glasses if a refractive error is present. In normal individuals there usually is no more than a one-line difference between the vision of the two eyes. It is normal for persons over 40 years of age to begin to have near-vision difficulty because of presbyopia, and to require glasses for reading.

EXTERNAL EXAMINATION
Before and while you are checking the visual acuity, you should be observing the

TABLE 8-2. Some Eye Signs of Thyroid Disease

Eponym	Description	Appearance
Stellwag's sign (or stare)	Retraction of the upper lid due to spasm of levator palpebrae (in hyperthyroidism)	
Graves' exophthalmos	Protrusion of the eye(s) from the orbit (in Graves' disease)	
von Graefe's sign	Lagging of the lids upon looking downward, with visible sclera above the iris	

TABLE 8-3. Some Causes of Unilateral Exophthalmos

Graves' disease (may be asymmetric)
Orbital hemorrhage
Orbital cellulitis
Orbital tumor
Orbital vein thrombosis
Sphenoid wing meningioma
Carotid-cavernous fistula
Orbital von Recklinghausen's disease

patient's face and eyes along with his general physical characteristics. Clues to general disease may be evident in the facial and ocular expression, the state of the face and eyelids, the prominence of the eyes, and the alert or dull expression that they may convey.

The general appearance of the eyes and face may reveal a staring expression, with retraction of the upper lids and prominence of the eyeballs in hyperthyroidism (see Table 8-2). Unilateral prominence of an eye (proptosis) (Table 8-3) may indicate a space-occupying lesion of some type in the orbit, and bilateral prominence may be associated with thyroid abnormalities (which may also give unilateral proptosis), chronic lung disease, and genetic factors (American blacks

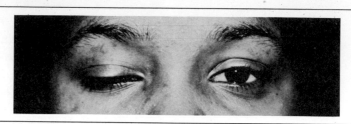

FIGURE 8-6
Congenital ptosis.

TABLE 8-4. Some Causes of Ptosis

Congenital
Paralysis of cranial nerve III
Cervical sympathetic paralysis (Horner's syndrome)
Myasthenia gravis
Inflammation of lid
Progressive external opthalmoplegia

may have more prominent eyes than whites do). Drooping upper lids may indicate extreme debility or neuromuscular disease. Partial ptosis can be a part of Horner's syndrome, with involvement of the cervical sympathetics (Table 8-4). More marked ptosis of an upper lid associated with decreased pupillary light reaction may be the earliest indication of oculomotor paralysis (Fig. 8-6).

Always remember the order in which observation of external findings should be made: lid, sclera, conjunctiva, lacrimal apparatus, cornea, iris, pupil, and anterior chamber. If each of these is thought of in turn, findings will not be overlooked.

EYELIDS

Note the appearance of the **eyelids** (Table 8-5). There may be changes in the skin, edema (Table 8-6), and differences in height of the palpebral fissures; a staring expression may be evident; or the upper lids may be pulled upward in a retracted position. Many structural variations may fall within the normal range. A slight difference in the palpebral fissures is not significant unless associated with unequal pupils. Differences in the depth of the upper lid fold may occur. Normal racial differences can be expected.

The appearance of the eyelids themselves may reveal systemic edema in advance of more noticeable changes elsewhere. The skin may be involved in either local or generalized dermatologic conditions.

Inversion (turning inward) of the lid border (entropion) causes irritation by abrasion of the lashes against the cornea and may be due to lid spasm or to contraction of scar tissue. Eversion of the lid border (ectropion) may result from scar tissue or from senile laxity and is associated with overflow of tears (epiphora).

SCLERAE

Yellowness of the **sclerae** may precede clinical jaundice of the skin in the hyperbilirubinemic patient. A "muddy" color to the sclerae is common in dark-skinned people and should be distinguished from jaundice. "Scleral" lesions include fibro-

TABLE 8-5. Some Lesions of the Lids

Name	Description	Appearance
Ectropion	Eversion of the lid margin	
Entropion	Rolling inward of the lid margin	
Hordeolum (stye)	Inflammation of an eyelash follicle	
Chalazion	Chronic granuloma of a meibomian gland	
Xanthelasma	Raised yellow cholesterol plaque at inner canthal area	
Dacryocystitis	Painful swelling of tear sac	
Blepharitis	Inflammation of the lid margin	
Epicanthal fold	Fold of skin across inner canthus	

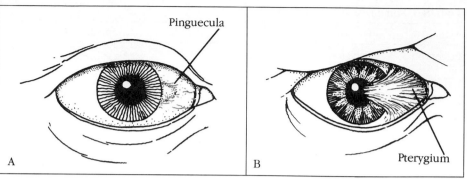

FIGURE 8-7
Lesions of the sclera. A. Pinguecula. B. Pterygium.

TABLE 8-6. Some Causes of Edema of the Lids

Local lesions of the lid or eye
Acute sinusitis
Acute allergic reactions
  Angioneurotic edema
  Urticaria
Dermatitis of the face
Cellulitis of the face
Measles
Mononucleosis
Hypoproteinemia
  Nephrotic syndrome
  Malabsorption
  Starvation
Congestive heart failure
Trichinosis
Thyrotoxicosis
Myxedema
Cavernous sinus thrombosis

vascular (conjunctival) proliferation which may encroach on the cornea (as pterygium) or may not (as pinguecula) (Fig. 8-7).

CONJUNCTIVAE

The **conjunctiva** covers the entire anterior eyeball (other than the cornea) and is reflected back onto the posterior lid surfaces. Its appearance (edema, pallor, vascular injection) should be noted. The palpebral conjunctivae and the fornices must be seen, since foreign bodies may lodge here. To examine the conjunctiva of the lower lid, place your index finger firmly over the midpoint of the lid just above the bone of the lower orbital rim and pull downward. This everts the lower fornix; changing the position of your finger will expose different areas.

In order to see the superior fornix and the conjunctiva of the upper lid, the eyelid must be everted (Fig. 8-8). Ask the patient to look downward, grasp the upper

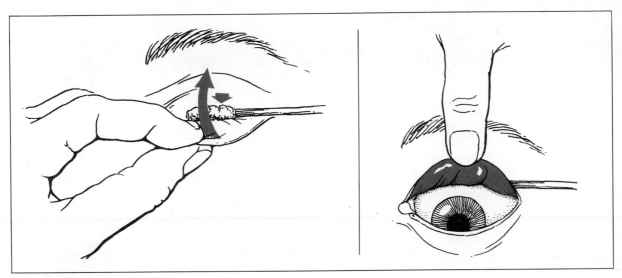

FIGURE 8-8
Technique of eversion of the eyelid.

lashes gently with the thumb and forefinger of one hand, use a cotton swab to form a fulcrum just at the upper border of the tarsal plate. By pushing down at this point and pulling upward on the lashes, you will evert the upper lid, exposing the posterior surface. As long as the patient keeps looking downward, the lid will remain in this position. After inspection, ask the patient to look upward, and the lid will flip over to its normal position.

There is considerable normal variation in the degree of vascularity of the conjunctivae. In general, the more florid the patient's complexion, the more he is apt to have reddened eyes. A small amount of discharge present in the inner canthus merely reflects the "wastebasket" function of the tear drainage mechanism and is to be expected, more so in patients with oily skin and greater meibomian secretions.

Almost all disease affecting the conjunctivae produces both injection of the vessels and discharge. In conjunctivitis of infectious origin the injection usually increases in the fornices, and secretions are present. More severe involvement produces small hemorrhages beneath the conjunctivae. Spontaneous ecchymoses may occur beneath the conjunctivae in otherwise healthy patients, and usually have no significance unless signs of a bleeding tendency are present elsewhere.

Boggy conjunctivae may occur in patients with systemic fluid retention, or as a manifestation of endocrine exophthalmos, local inflammation, or vascular stasis.

LACRIMAL DRAINAGE SYSTEM
Inspect the **lacrimal drainage system**. Observe the position and patency of the punctum at the inner end of each lid. The puncta should be turned backward slightly to contact the pool of tears in the inner canthus. Tears also should not spill over onto the cheek (epiphora). Gently palpate each lacrimal sac and note whether any material regurgitates back into the eye. Conjunctival inflammation that is greater in the inferior fornix may be associated with lacrimal obstruction or tear sac infection. A mass in the lacrimal gland may be a solid tumor or lymphoma.

TABLE **8**-7. Some Lesions of the Cornea

Name	Description	Appearance
Arcus senilis	Concentric gray depositions of lipid around the cornea. May or may not suggest hyper-lipidemia	
Band keratopathy	Horizontal band of subepithelial calcification, most marked at the periphery of the cornea (at 3 and 9 o'clock) and fading toward the center. Occurs in hypercalcemic states and in degeneration of the globe	
Keratoconus	Congenital condition but often not manifest until after puberty	
Keratitis	Inflammation of the cornea May be infective, toxic, or allergic	
Keratoconjunctivitis sicca	Defect in lacrimation leading to drying of conjunctiva and lens Associated with certain forms of arthritis	
Corneal ulcer	Acute or chronic lesion, due to trauma or infection	
Kaiser-Fleischer ring	Pericorneal deposition of copper salts seen in Wilson's disease, biliary cirrhosis, and chronic copper toxicity	

IRIS

Findings of the **iris** and pupil often are associated. An irregular pupil may be due to adhesions of the iris to the lens (synechiae) as the result of prior iritis. Congenital abnormalities, such as multiple or displaced pupils, must be differentiated from tears of the iris base due to prior trauma (iridodialysis). Localized elevation of the iris is immediately suspect for possible tumor, especially if darkly pigmented.

Iritis is a nonspecific inflammation of the iris. The patient notes throbbing pain and visual blurring. There is circumcorneal injection with a small pupil. The eye is usually quite soft to palpation and is tender.

CORNEA

Observe the **cornea**. It should be shiny and bright when illuminated by your flashlight. Any break in this clear continuity, such as scarring, vascularization, or ulceration, will dull the reflection. The size (horizontal diameter 9 to 11 mm) and curvature should be noted. In elderly patients a partial or complete white ring about the periphery of the cornea (arcus senilis) may be expected.

Pain in the eye is usually severe in acute disease of the cornea. Photophobia, manifested by the patient's evident discomfort in light, also occurs in most corneal diseases. In abrasions and ulcers of the cornea there is often increased redness of the globe around the corneal limbus. Loss of the bright surface reflection occurs in surface lesions, and at times a surface area of involvement will cast a shadow on the underlying iris if the flashlight is directed at the proper angle. Enlargement of the cornea is the most common finding in infantile glaucoma and is usually associated with clouding and photophobia. Edema of the cornea may be a part of local disease or of acute glaucoma.

Any vascularization or visible white scarring of the cornea is indicative of disease. A white arcus occurring around the limbus in younger individuals may indicate abnormality in lipid metabolism. A brown ring of pigment occurs around the corneal limbus in hepatolenticular degeneration (Wilson's disease) and is known as a Kayser-Fleischer ring (Table 8-7).

PUPILS

Remember that when you are looking at the pupillary opening you are also inspecting the **lens** of the eye, which is normally transparent.

Any visible clouding of the lens as seen through the pupil is indicative of cataract formation and may also be seen as a dark shadow against the light of the fundus in the beginning of the ophthalmoscopic examination. If the lens has been removed or is dislocated, the normal support of the iris will not be present and the iris will "flutter" with quick movements of the eye (iridodonesis).

Abnormalities of the position of the pupils and irregularities in shape or difference in size between the two (anisocoria) should be recorded (Table 8-8). The size of the pupils varies in normal individuals. Large pupils are generally found in myopic eyes, smaller ones in patients with hyperopia. A small difference in pupil size between the two eyes is usually not significant unless accompanied by abnormal reflexes or change in consciousness.

The presence of **pupillary reflexes** denotes integrity of cranial nerves II (optic) and III (oculomotor). Cranial nerve II must be intact to perceive and transmit the presence of light to the brainstem. Cranial nerve III must be intact to effect pupillary constriction (Fig. 8-9A). An easy mnemonic device for this is "In two, out three." Note that in cortical blindness (damage to the occipital visual cortex of the brain) the pupillary reflexes will be intact, but the patient will still be blind.

Shine your light quickly into one eye and observe the response of both eyes. The illuminated eye shows constriction of the pupil (direct light reaction), and the pupil of the other eye also constricts an equal amount (consensual light reaction).

TABLE **8-8**. Some Pupillary Abnormalities

Condition	Causes	Appearance
Anisocoria	Cranial nerve III paralysis Sympathetic paralysis Ocular disease (ciliary spasm)	 UNEQUAL PUPILS
Horner's syndrome (small pupil is the pathologic one)	Unilateral (generally) sympathetic paralysis, usually due to trauma or tumor along the sympathetic train in neck or brain	Ptosis Miosis Anhidrosis Pseudoexophthalmos
Dilated, fixed pupil (large pupil is the pathologic one)	CNS disease, cranial nerve III palsy, Adie's pupil	No direct or consensual reaction
Argyll Robertson pupil (small pupil is the pathologic one)	Syphilis, diabetes, CNS disease due to involvement of the Edinger-Westphal nucleus	Small, irregular pupil Reacts to accommodation but not to light
Miotic pupils	Drugs (pilocarpine or other para-sympathetic stimulants), sympathetic blockade, narcotics	 PINPOINT PUPILS
Mydriatic pupils	Drugs (atropine, catecholamines) Brain death	 FIXED AND DILATED
Irregular pupils Postsurgical	Iridectomy for cataract	
Postinflammatory	Syphilis, occular inflammation (synechial)	

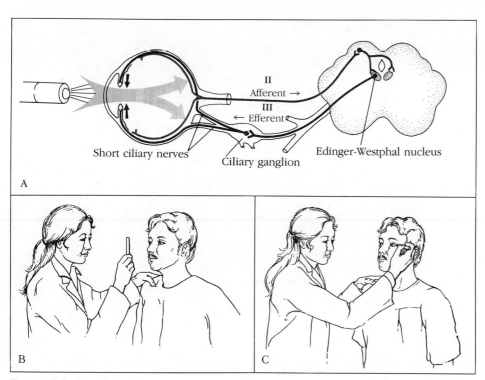

FIGURE 8-9
Pupillary reflex pathway. A. Physiologic pathways: The afferent (II) and the efferent (III) loops of the pupillary reflex pathway. B. Checking accommodation. C. Checking the light reflex.

Then shine the light into the other eye and observe the same reactions. Then ask the patient to look at his finger or an object (such as a pen) in your hand and move it directly toward his nose. With focusing for this near object, both pupils will constrict (the "near reaction," or "reaction in accommodation") (Fig. 8-9B).

Avoid confusing the light and near reactions by shining your light into the eye from the side rather than from directly in front of the patient (Fig. 8-9C). (Some patients, if the light is in front, will look directly at the light, and their accommodative pupillary response may be mistaken for an intact light reflex.)

The rapidity of response of the pupillary reflexes varies considerably in normal patients. Usually the presence of the response is sufficient, as long as it is equal in the two eyes. Older patients who do not accommodate well often show a normal slowing of the near reaction.

Loss of the pupillary light reflex is always important (Table 8-9). Where it is unilateral due to blindness, neither a direct reflex nor a consensual reflex will occur when the blind eye is tested. Where loss is bilateral in the nonblind patient, neurologic disease is usually present. One example is the Argyll Robertson pupil of central nervous system syphilis, in which the light reflexes are gone but the near reflex in accommodation is present. As the old clinical saw has it: An Argyll Robertson pupil is like a prostitute—it's accommodating but doesn't react.

Pupils that resemble the Argyll Robertson pupil may also occur in diabetes mel-

TABLE 8-9. Some Abnormal Pupillary Reflexes

Name	Finding	Suggested Condition
Amaurotic pupil	Light in affected eye gives no direct and no consensual reflex Light in normal eye gives both direct and consensual reflex	Blind eye, without light perception
Marcus Gunn pupil (afferent pupillary defect)	Light in affected eye gives minimal direct, normal consensual reflex Light in normal eye gives brisk direct and consensual reflex If, after the normal eye is checked, the light is quickly returned to the abnormal eye, the pupil of the abnormal eye appears to dilate (since the direct response is less constrictive than the abnormal eye's consensual response)	Optic nerve disease but not blindness
Hutchinson's pupil	Dilated, fixed, unresponsive to light	Neurologic disease (e.g., herniation, aneurysm impinging on cranial nerve III)
Adie's pupil	May be unilateral or bilateral Pupil shows minimal reaction to light, slow reaction to near vision Occurs in women 20–30 years old and is associated with decreased knee and ankle reflexes	Ciliary ganglion dysfunction

litus, midbrain lesions, myotonic dystrophy, and familial amyloid. In midbrain involvement, the pupils are enlarged, in contrast to the Argyll Robertson pupil.

A unilaterally fixed, dilated pupil may be the result of local trauma to the eye, but more often it is a serious sign in a patient with recent head injury, since it indicates beginning involvement of the oculomotor nerve. A miotic pupil associated with partial drooping of the upper lid may indicate disease of the cervical sympathetic on that side and is part of Horner's syndrome.

ANTERIOR CHAMBER

Observe the depth of the **anterior chamber**. There should be adequate clearance between the cornea and iris, with no irregularities in depth. The depth varies somewhat among normal persons, but if the iris appears to bulge forward and the space is very shallow, you should immediately think of the possibility of potential acute

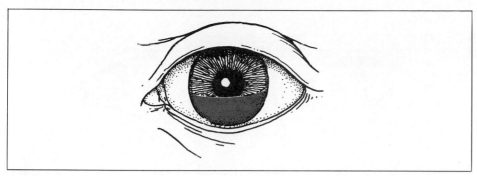

FIGURE 8-10
Hyphema.

glaucoma. Anything other than clear aqueous occupying the anterior chamber is abnormal.

Blood may be present after injury (hyphema) (Fig. 8-10), or pus may level out in the lower chamber in association with corneal infection (hypopyon). The chamber may be lost in perforating wounds with aqueous leakage.

EXTRAOCULAR MOVEMENTS

Seat yourself facing the patient and hold your flashlight in the midline between yourself and the patient, asking him to look directly at the light. Observe the position of the reflection of the light on each of his corneas with respect to the location of the pupils (corneal light reflex). Then cover one eye while he looks at the light. Remove the cover quickly and notice whether the eye moves in to regain fixation on the light (cover-uncover test). This may indicate a drift of the eye behind the cover, which can be indicative of muscle imbalance. Then shift the cover from one eye to the other and back again, always observing the movement that the uncovered eye makes to regain fixation (alternate cover test). If weakness or paralysis of one of the horizontal rectus muscles is present, a horizontal shift will occur. If one of the elevator or depressor muscles is involved, a vertical movement will be noted.

The maintenance of parallel eyes (and therefore of corneal light reflexes that are equally centered) occurs in most patients because of the fusion reflex, which makes binocular vision possible. If deviation of the eyes occurs behind the cover, which then recovers when both eyes are uncovered, you are dealing with *phoria,* a latent tendency to deviation that is held in check by fusion (Fig. 8-11A,B). If, on the other hand, the alternate cover test demonstrates shift that does not regain parallelism with removal of the cover, the muscle imbalance is called a *tropia* (Fig. 8-11C,D).

It is normal to find a small amount of horizontal shift of the visual axes with the alternate cover test, provided the eyes regain a parallel position as soon as the cover is removed. It is more common to find a small outward deviation (exophoria) than a minor inward deviation (esophoria). In both instances parallelism is regained. Usually any vertical shift behind the cover is abnormal.

In evaluating possible weaknesses of individual extraocular muscles and consequently their innervation (in most cases), it is helpful to use a system of "diagnostic

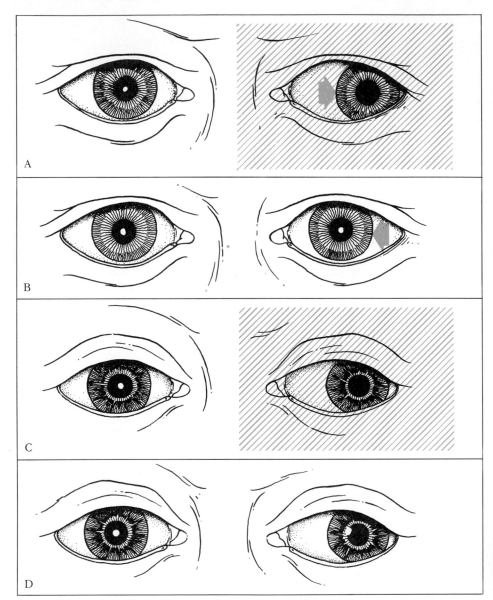

FIGURE 8-11
Alternate cover test. A and B. Exophoria. C and D. Exotropia.

positions of gaze" to unravel the complexities of movement of 12 muscles (6 on each eye) acting in concert (see Fig. 8-12).

In each of the diagnostic positions, two muscles are evaluated. The muscle pairs indicated are known as "yoked muscles," since they are yoked together by innervation to act in unison (see Table 8-10). Remember, the outturned eye is in position to evaluate the superior and inferior recti, and the inturned eye is in position to evaluate the obliques.

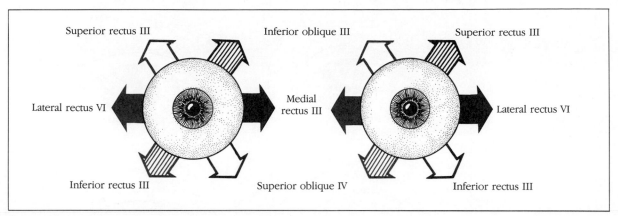

FIGURE 8-12
Extraocular movements and their controlling nerves.

TABLE 8-10. Yoked Muscles

Right Eye	Left Eye	Turn Eyes
Medial rectus	Lateral rectus	Left
Lateral rectus	Medial rectus	Right
Superior rectus	Inferior oblique	Up and right
Inferior rectus	Superior oblique	Down and right
Superior oblique	Inferior rectus	Down and left
Inferior oblique	Superior rectus	Up and left

Ask the patient to follow your light with his eyes, and observe him in each of these diagnostic positions: (1) up to the right, (2) directly to the right, (3) down to the right, (4) down to the left, (5) directly to the left, and (6) up to the left. Notice the position of the corneal light reflexes in each eye to make sure they are parallel. If the eyes go out of parallel in a certain position, the lagging muscle can be designated directly. In addition, ask the patient whether he sees two lights in any of the positions (diplopia, or double vision). This will give you a clue as to the muscle pair to be analyzed further.

Any lack of parallelism in the diagnostic positions of gaze is beyond the range of normal. Any tropia (constant deviation from parallel) is abnormal. A transient jerking movement of the eyes in the *extremes* of horizontal gaze (nystagmus) ordinarily falls within normal limits, though marked nystagmus is abnormal and suggests drug toxicity, thiamine deficiency, and congenital, vestibular or neurologic disease.

Paralysis of specific nerve supply to the extraocular muscles produces characteristic findings (Fig. 8-13). In abducens (cranial nerve VI) paralysis, the involved eye will be turned in toward the nose because of unopposed action of the normal medial rectus, and the esotropia will be greater when looking in the direction of normal action of the paralyzed muscle. The patient with an oculomotor (cranial nerve III) paralysis will have his eye turned down and out, with ptosis of the upper lid. Diplopia will not occur because of the closure of the lid. The patient with trochlear

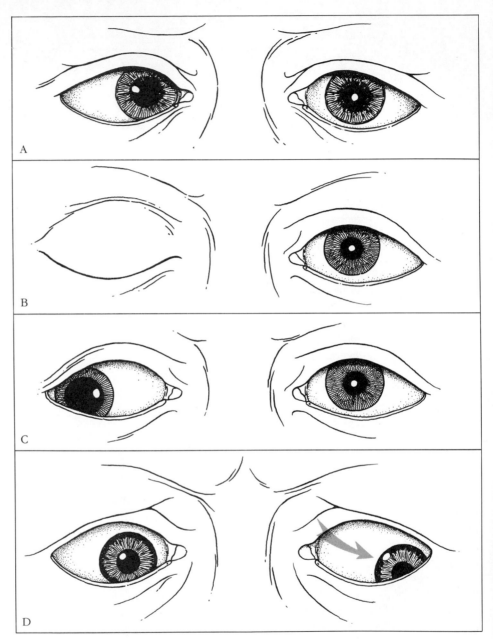

FIGURE 8-13
Extraocular motor palsies. A. Right VI palsy: Patient looks straight ahead; affected right eye turns nasally. B and C. Right III palsy: Lid closed and open. Eye is ptotic. If lid is lifted, affected eye turns out and down, with dilated pupil. D. Right IV palsy: Patient cannot look downward nasally.

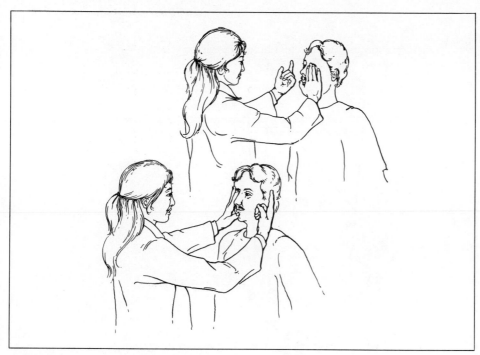

FIGURE 8-14
Visual fields by confrontation.

(cranial nerve IV) palsy will complain of difficulty with vision in the lower field, as in reading; if he has been able to maintain single binocular vision, his head will be tilted toward the shoulder opposite the side of paralysis.

Isolated involvement of ocular muscles may occur with certain neuromuscular diseases, may follow orbital or facial fractures, or may be part of the findings of the endocrine exophthalmos of thyroid disease.

VISUAL FIELDS BY CONFRONTATION

The visual fields may be grossly determined by confrontation. Facing the patient, have him stare fixedly into your eyes. Then cover the patient's left eye with your right hand. At his eye level bring your *wriggling* left index finger slowly from behind the right side of the patient's head into his view, and note where he first perceives it. Then check each of the four quadrants of his field (Fig. 8-14). In examining children, asking the patient to tell you how many fingers are seen in each quadrant may be helpful.

Since significant neurologic field defects often show a difference on either side of the vertical midline, the use of two red objects to test fields (such as the tops of two eye-drop bottles) may show subtle differences in color saturation, even though the visual confrontation test is normal.

To evaluate a central field defect, ask the patient to look at your nose and tell you whether a part of your face is missing. Now cover the patient's right eye with your left hand; using your right index finger, repeat this procedure for the left visual field.

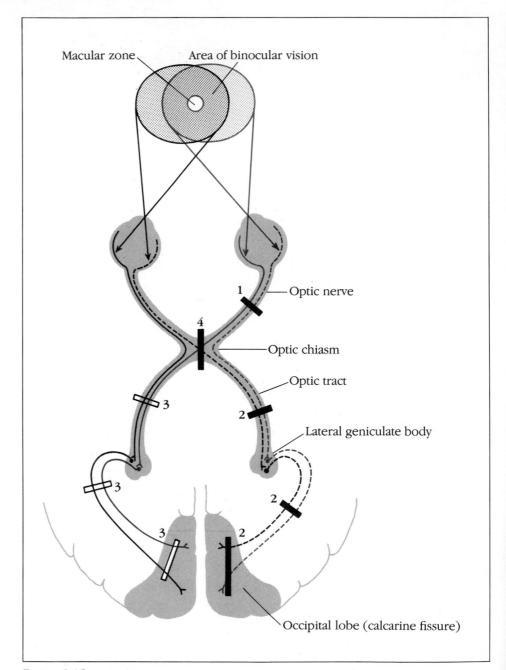

FIGURE 8-15
Normal pattern of the visual fields as represented in the optic pathways. Numbered lesions cause defects shown in Table 8-11 (complete lesions are indicated by solid bars and partial lesions by open bars).

TABLE 8-11. Abnormalities of Visual Fields

Condition	Causes	Appearance	
		Left	Right
1. Blind eye	Lesions of the optic nerve	○	●
2. Homonymous hemianopsia	Lesion contralateral optic tract, optic radiation, or occipital cortex	◐	◐
3. Homonymous quadrantanopsia	Partial lesion contralateral optic tract, optic radiation, or occipital cortex	◔	◔
4. Bitemporal hemianopsia	Lesion of the optic chiasm	◐	◐

Note: Conditions are caused by lesions shown in Figure 8-17 with corresponding numbers (1 through 4).

Abnormalities of the visual field are shown in Figure 8-15. If there is any suspected defect of visual fields (Table 8-11), a formal field examination by an ophthalmologist should be requested. Since visual field defects occur early in cases of uncontrolled chronic glaucoma, serial examinations are necessary to assess the response of the disease to treatment (see also Chap. 18, Nervous System).

FUNDUSCOPIC EXAMINATION

Evaluation of the ocular fundus will often aid in general physical evaluation of the patient. Constant practice with the ophthalmoscope is necessary and most rewarding.

Seat the patient comfortably and ask him to look straight ahead. Hold the instrument in your right hand and stand on the patient's right side. Examine his right eye with your right eye; the reverse holds for his left eye. A +8 lens (black numbers on the dial) is placed in the instrument aperture, and the pupil is observed from a distance of 6 to 8 inches. This illuminates the retina, and any opacity or obstruction to the emerging light will be seen as a dark spot or shadow against an orange-red background. Gradually move closer to the patient, holding his upper lid open gently with the thumb of your free hand, resting your hand on his forehead. The lens wheel of the ophthalmoscope is turned (toward zero on the dial) until the lighter color of the optic disc is seen just nasal to the center of the retina. Then refocus your instrument until details of the optic nerve head are seen clearly (Figs. 8-16 through 8-18).

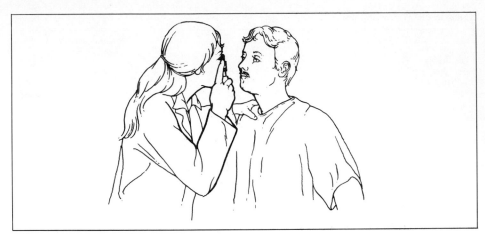

FIGURE 8-16
Ophthalmoscopy.

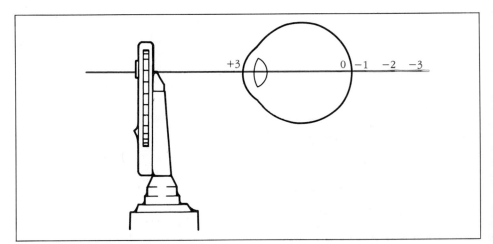

FIGURE 8-17
Sites of focus (with normal eyeball).

While dimming the lights is sufficient preparation for ophthalmoscopic examination in most patients, a mydriatic drop is occasionally useful. In the vast majority of patients a mydriatic drop may be used safely, but you must be aware of the possibility of inducing a rise in intraocular pressure (glaucoma) in a predisposed eye. This is more often the case in patients over 40 years of age. Always question the patient as to the previous diagnosis of glaucoma, observe the optic nerve head for abnormality, and, if there is any question, measure the intraocular pressure. The presence of a small corneal diameter with a shallow anterior chamber increases the possibility of glaucoma. After checking for these points, you may instill 1 drop of a mydriatic (among others, 0.5% Mydriacyl or 2.5% Neo-Synephrine) into one eye. If the patient remains well after 15 minutes, do the other eye. If this is done early in the physical examination, you may return to the funduscopic examination later.

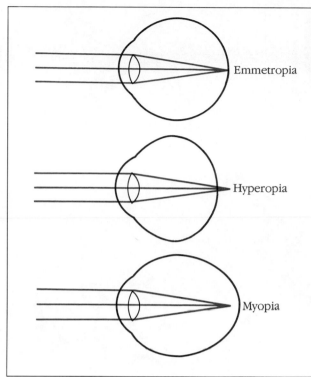

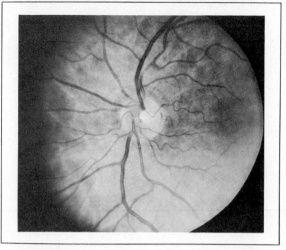

FIGURE 8-19
Normal ocular fundus.

FIGURE 8-18
Common defects in the optical system of the eye. Emmetropia is a normal-size orb. A shortened eyeball gives rise to hyperopia (farsightedness). An abnormally long eyeball may characterize myopia (nearsightedness). Adjustments should be made in the lens selection on the ophthalmoscope for these anatomic differences.

Note: If there is acute neurologic disease, especially a recent brain hemorrhage or head trauma, the observation of serial changes in the pupils is crucial in planning treatment. In order to avoid masking important changes, *do not* dilate the pupils.

You must follow a definite order of examination of the retina, always reserving the central or macular area until last. This avoids "dazzling" the patient early in the examination and will ensure better cooperation for prolonged viewing.

A blurred image of the fundus that will not clear with proper focus of the ophthalmoscope is usually due to clouding in the media of the eye (i.e., the cornea, lens, or vitreous). Vitreous haziness is present in intraocular inflammation. *Cataract* in the lens or *corneal scarring* may also blur visualization of the fundus. In an occasional patient with a high refractive error, the fundus may be difficult to see, and in this case you should attempt funduscopy through the patient's correcting lenses.

The blood vessels of the retinae (Fig. 8-20) emerge from and enter the disc in four main pairs. Examine the superior nasal vessels first, following them out as far as possible without having the patient turn his eye. This is followed in order by the

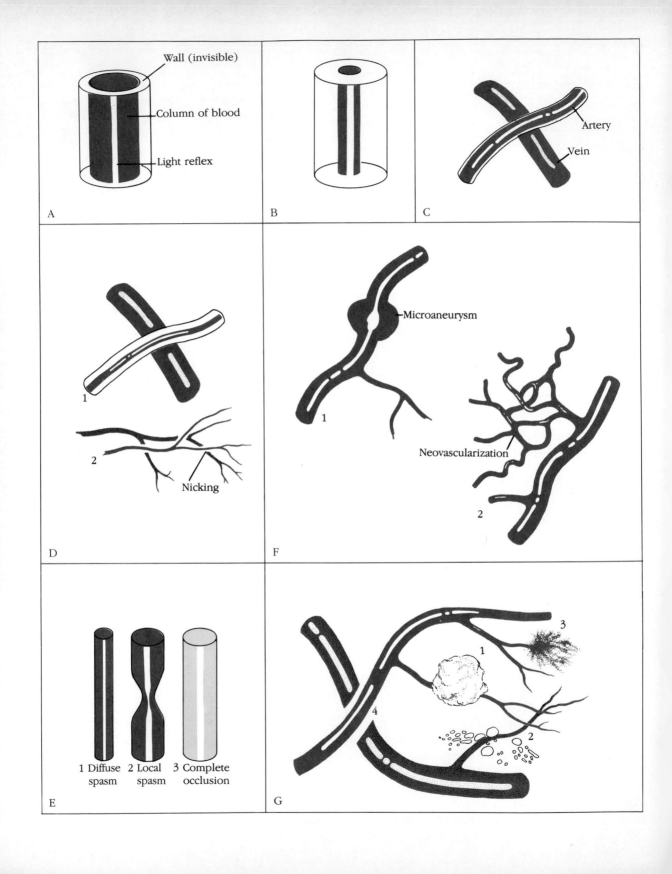

TABLE 8-12. Keith-Wagener-Barker Classification of Hypertensive Retinopathy*

Group	Description
I	Moderate arteriolar narrowing, often with focal spasm and accentuated arteriolar light reflex
II	Arteriolar narrowing, arteriovenous nicking Hard exudates and small hemorrhages
III	Marked arteriolar narrowing Retina appears wet, edematous Soft exudates and hemorrhages
IV	Signs in group III *and* papilledema

* It is always preferable for the examiner to *describe* fully the changes seen in the fundus rather than to classify them arbitrarily.

inferior nasal, inferior temporal, and superior temporal pairs. The retina adjoining each of these pairs is inspected at the same time. Then ask the patient to look up, up and in, directly toward the nose, down and in, straight down, down and out, directly outward, and then up and out. This covers eight successive overlapping zones of the peripheral retina, and each zone joins the margins of the more central retinal areas seen along with inspection of the vessels. The central retina and macular area are visualized last; ask the patient to look directly at the light if necessary. The foveal pit in the macula is seen as a small bright dot produced by light reflection from the indentation.

The position of the vessels on the nerve head may vary. The retinal vessels are usually gently sinuous in their courses, with approximate right angles at division points. They usually cross each other without noticeable indentations. The veins are somewhat darker than the arterioles and are about one-third wider. Both can be traced almost to the visible periphery in the eye with a widely dilated pupil.

Evaluation of the retinal vessels is helpful in assessing the patient with arteriosclerosis or hypertensive disease (Table 8-12 details a system for classifying hypertensive retinopathy). The normal retinal arteriole is seen only as a blood column. Where thickening of the wall occurs, a shinier reflection is noted. It may be copper-

FIGURE 8-20

Blood vessels of the fundus. A. Normal artery. B. Atherosclerosis. Note that light reflex *appears* broader (relative to the visible column of blood) in the sclerotic arteriole. Since arteriolar wall is not seen, early atherosclerosis is perceived as a narrowing column of blood and widened light reflex. C. Normal arteriovenous crossing. Note that arteriole is from two-thirds to three-fourths the size of the vein. D. Arteriovenous nicking. As the arteriolar wall thickens (1), it cuts off vision of the underlying vein. The obstruction (2) makes it appear as though there were a gap between the arteriolar column of blood and the underlying vein. E. Vasospastic disease. In hypertension, spasm may be complete and diffuse along the arteriole (1) or may be local or segmental (2). If atheroma has totally occluded the vessel, it appears whitish, the "silver wire" phenomenon (3). F. In diabetes, weakening of the arteriolar wall may give micro-aneurysms (1). New-vessel formation (neovascularization) (2) may, in this disease, be mistaken for hemorrhage unless careful observation is made. G. Soft exudates (1) are fuzzy, gray patches thought to represent infarcts in areas of arteriolar insufficiency. Hard exudates (2) are dense, gray localized infiltrates probably due to venous stasis. Hemorrhages (3) may occur as well as arteriovenous nicking (4).

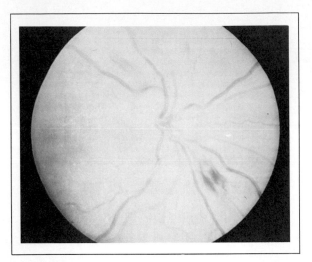

FIGURE 8-21
Hypertensive retinopathy with papilledema.

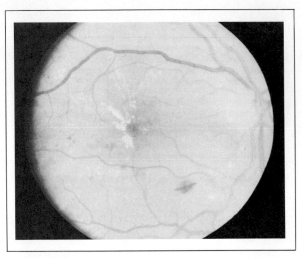

FIGURE 8-22
Diabetic retinopathy with hard exudates.

colored in less advanced sclerosis but will appear like a silver wire in advanced disease. This change is due to visibility of the vessel wall, and at times the wall itself may be seen along the edge of the blood column. In addition, where an involved artery crosses a retinal vein, it may indent the vein and even cause evidence of back pressure in the vein distal to the crossing (AV notching). The disappearance of the vein on both sides of the blood column representing the artery is a measure of thickening of the arteriolar wall.

With hypertension there is localized or generalized narrowing of the arteriolar blood column. This is identified by a change in the ratio of arteriolar to venule size. In tracing out the smaller branches toward the periphery, the arterioles will disappear earlier than the veins. In the more severe degrees of hypertension, leakage of the vascular walls will lead to hemorrhages and deposits in the retina, and papilledema may ensue (Fig. 8-21).

Hemorrhages and exudates in the retina are always important signs of disease (Figs. 8-22 through 8-26). The shape of the hemorrhage indicates the depth of the retina at which it occurs. Superficial hemorrhages are flame-shaped or splinterlike in contour and lie in the nerve fiber layer of the retina. They usually occur when venous back pressure is present, such as in occlusion of the central retinal vein or one of its branches, or in association with papilledema. In contrast, closure of the central retinal artery or a branch results in ischemic edema of the area involved; where the artery is completely closed, the retina is pale and edematous, with the thinner macular area shining through as a cherry-red spot. Hemorrhages that are located in the deeper retinal layers are rounder or blotchier in contour and are often associated with exudates (Fig. 8-24). These latter deposits represent residues of edema and of blood substances that are incompletely absorbed due to poor retinal circulation. Sharply defined yellow or white deposits should be distinguished from more fuzzy cotton-wool patches, which are small ischemic infarcts in the nerve fiber layer.

The association of hemorrhages and exudates occurs in advanced hypertension, severe renal disease, certain of the collagen diseases, diabetes, the blood dyscra-

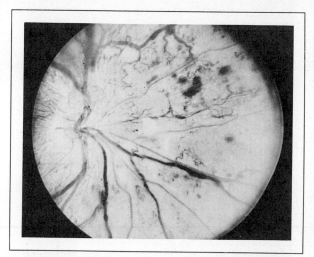

FIGURE 8-23
Neovascularization.

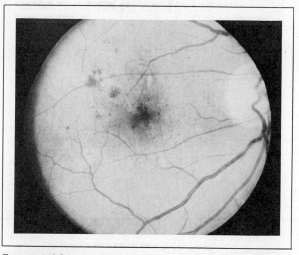

FIGURE 8-24
Deep retinal hemorrhage.

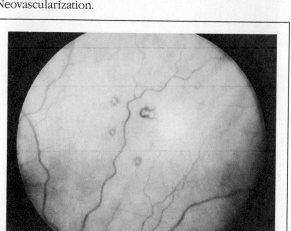

FIGURE 8-25
Roth spots.

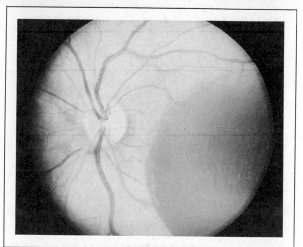

FIGURE 8-26
Preretinal hemorrhage.

sias, and retinal venous occlusions. The early hemorrhages of diabetic retinopathy may be punctate or clusterlike, since they are really venous microaneurysms (see Fig. 8-22). They are usually present only in the macular area and surrounding the posterior pole of the eye. A significant difference between the two eyes in hemorrhages and exudates may indicate carotid occlusive disease.

When round, blotchy hemorrhages occur that are noted to have whiter centers (Roth spots), one must think of blood dyscrasias or of the embolic lesions of subacute bacterial endocarditis (Fig. 8-25). When blood extravasates in front of the retina (preretinal hemorrhage) it will obscure the underlying details and may show a gravitational fluid level (see Fig. 8-26). Such bleeding is associated with sudden intracranial hemorrhage.

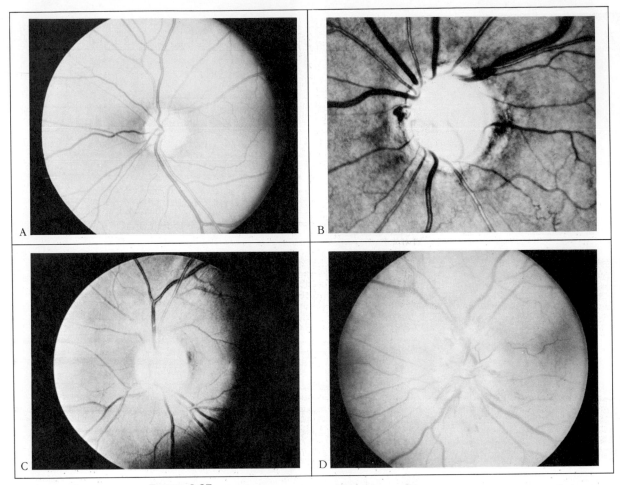

FIGURE 8-27
Optic disc. A. Optic atrophy. B. Glaucomatous cupping. C. Physiologic cupping. D. Papilledema.

Note that the background color of the fundus may be darker in brunettes, very light in blonds, and in the latter the deeper choroidal vessels may shine through. The healthy retina is transparent and produces no visible findings except for highlights, which often follow the expected pattern of the retinal nerve fibers.

Considerable variation in the size and shape of the *nerve head* may occur. If the disc is small the nasal border may be blurred. If the eye is myopic there may be an arc of retraction along the temporal side. The physiologic depression may vary from highly prominent to nonexistent. Pigment may be noted along the disc border.

Note the size, shape, color, margins, and physiologic depression of the optic nerve. Any elevation can be measured by focusing on the highest part of the disc. Then throw the light beam about two disc diameters nasally to the nerve head and refocus on the retina. Note the number of clicks as the lens wheel is turned to refocus; then read the difference directly from the dial.

Major abnormalities of the optic nerve are optic atrophy, cupping of the disc in glaucoma, and papilledema. In optic atrophy the color of the disc is paler than normal and may be chalky white in advanced cases (Fig. 8-27A). There may be associated superficial scar tissue or loss of substance, and usually there is resultant decrease in vision.

The cupping of the disc that occurs in glaucoma (Fig. 8-27B) consists of an exaggeration of the physiologic depression (Fig. 8-27C) on the temporal side that extends to the temporal border. The cup may be deep and is bluish white; the emerging retinal vessels may disappear behind the shelf at the edge of the cup, then emerge over the edge to reach the retina. Cupping of the disc is expressed as a ratio of the cup diameter to the horizontal disc diameter (C/D ratio). While no exact C/D value differentiates physiologic from abnormal, a ratio greater than 0.3 or an asymmetry between the two eyes should be viewed with suspicion.

Swelling of the nerve head (papilledema) (Fig. 8-27D) may be unilateral in localized optic nerve disease or bilateral in the choked disc of increased intracranial pressure. The amount of elevation should be measured with the ophthalmoscope for estimation of future change. Early papilledema is difficult to determine, but filling in of the physiologic depression, blurring of the margins of the disc, fullness of the retinal veins, and loss of spontaneous venous pulsation on the disc are early signs. Where the process is more advanced, superficial hemorrhages and exudates around the disc make diagnosis more certain.

Any area of retinal elevation is significant. A solid mass indicates tumor growth, usually arising in the choroid. If it has a dark color it is likely to be melanoma (Fig. 8-28), and if lighter, one must think of metastatic malignancy. When the elevation is transparent and wrinkled, retinal detachment must be considered.

Areas of localized chorioretinal scarring are recognized by irregular pigment deposition around a paler center (Fig. 8-29). If they are clear-cut and sharp in outline, no current inflammatory activity is suspected; but if they have fuzzy borders, hemorrhages along the margin, or associated clouding in the vitreous, an active process may be suspected. Irregular mottling of pigment and scar tissue change in the macular areas may be seen in older patients who are suffering from senile macular degeneration (Fig. 8-30), and associated decrease in central vision will be found.

INTRAOCULAR PRESSURE

The intraocular pressure should be considered in every complete physical examination, and many clinicians refer patients who are over 40 years of age to ophthalmologists for this essential yearly test. The Schiøtz tonometer measures the indentation pressure of the cornea by means of a central plunger fitted into a curved footplate, with movement of the plunger transmitted to a lever scale. The reading is translated into millimeters of mercury, and the range of normal is from 12 to 22 mm Hg. Make the patient comfortable in a reclining position, and instill one drop of a local anesthetic, such as 0.5% tetracaine, into each eye. When the eyes are anesthetized, direct the patient to look straight above him, fixating either on his extended finger or on a spot on the ceiling. Hold the instrument lightly in one hand, and separate the lids gently with the fingers of the other hand. Rest the footplate on the cornea and take the reading from the dial. A small rhythmic deviation in the pointer

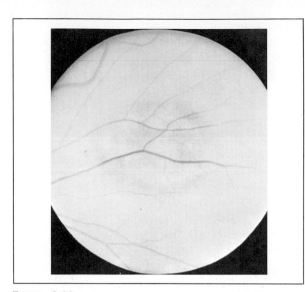

FIGURE 8-28
Choroidal melanoma.

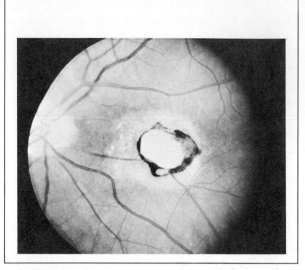

FIGURE 8-29
Chorioretinitis (congenital toxoplasmosis).

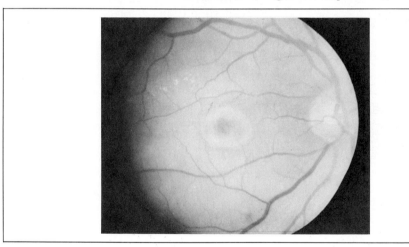

FIGURE 8-30
Macular degeneration.

is observed (transmitted pulse pressure) to ensure a proper reading. Repeat the procedure for the other eye. Care must be taken not to exert pressure on the lids, and the instrument must be kept meticulously clean. Any elevation in the intraocular tension is abnormal. Glaucoma is the greatest single cause of blindness in patients over 40 years of age and can be controlled by proper treatment if discovered early. Acute glaucoma is rare but is associated with pain in the eye, a steamy cornea, moderately dilated pupil, and systemic symptoms, such as severe headache, nausea and vomiting, and prostration. Abdominal symptoms have led to misdiagnosis of an acute abdomen in rare instances. The more common chronic glaucoma may cause only variable visual blur, minor headache, and peripheral visual loss or may be entirely silent. Clues here are indications of moderately elevated intraocular tension and early cupping in the optic nerve head. Tonometry and evaluation of the visual fields must be done.

HEAD

Nature has given man one tongue, but two ears, that we may hear twice as much as we speak.

EPICTETUS
(620?–120?)

Headache, alterations of hearing, nasal and sinus disorders, and oropharyngeal diseases are among the most common of patient complaints in practice. The seriousness of head and neck disorders that are detectable by careful history and physical examination ranges from the trivial (though discomforting) viral upper respiratory tract infection to the malignant tumor. Complaints of headache, tinnitus, nasal discharge, change in voice, sores in the mouth, and masses about the head and neck, though commonplace, are never treated lightly by the good physician.

The variety of structures in the head, though obviously integrally interconnected, will be presented separately in order to clarify the anatomy, history, and physical examination of each.

Ears

ANATOMY

The auricle usually forms a 30-degree angle with the side of the head. Its lateral surface is irregularly concave (Fig. 9-1). The concha of the auricle receives its sensory innervation, as does the external auditory canal, from the auricular branch of the trigeminal nerve and the vagus (Arnold's nerve). In contrast to that of lower

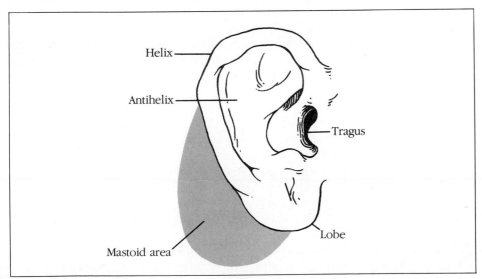

FIGURE 9-1
External ear (auricle).

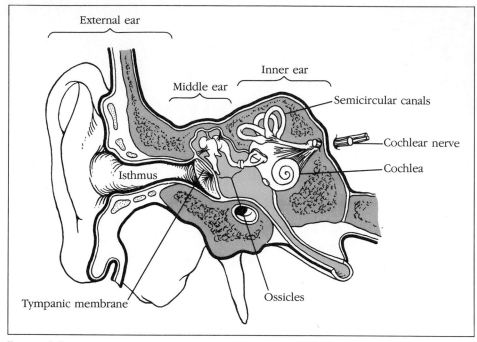

FIGURE 9-2
Cross section of the ear.

animals, the auricle of higher animals does not serve to direct and amplify sound. Its usefulness seems to be limited to "leading around little boys and hanging earrings."

The outer one-third of the canal contains hair follicles, sebaceous glands, and cerumen glands. At the junction of the middle and inner thirds of the canal is located a bony narrowing called the isthmus (Fig. 9-2).

The tympanic membrane is usually found on a slanted plane (Fig. 9-3). The anteroinferior quadrant is the farthest away from the examiner. This accounts for the triangle of light that is reflected anteroinferiorly from the umbo.

HISTORY

The historical review of systems concerning the ear may be done as you examine your patient. Remember that "**earache**," a common malady, may reflect pathology in the jaw (temporomandibular joint disease) as well as a problem with the ear. Wax (cerumen) in the ears is not a pathologic condition unless hearing is compromised by its buildup. Many patients poke sharp objects into their ears, such as hairpins and wooden sticks, to clean out the wax, risking injury to the drum. Children put things in their ears because they are children, and a complaint of decreased hearing in one ear in a child may follow the impaction of anything from bugs to peanuts in the ear canal. Ask specifically about a history of frequent childhood ear infections, ringing in the ears (tinnitus, which suggests disease or drug toxicity to cranial nerve VIII), and **discharge** from the ears. Any discharge should be classified as serous, mucoid, purulent, putrid, or sanguineous. A putrid, foul discharge may

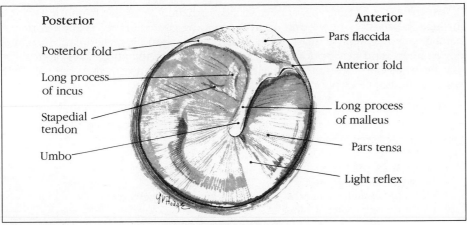

Posterior   **Anterior**

Posterior fold   Pars flaccida

Long process
of incus   Anterior fold

Stapedial
tendon   Long process
                                                        of malleus

Umbo   Pars tensa

                                                        Light reflex

FIGURE 9-3
Right tympanic membrane showing important landmarks.

TABLE 9-1. Common Causes of Hearing Loss

Conductive
    Blockage of the external canal by foreign body, wax, tumor, inflammation with swelling
    Middle ear disease (otitis media), acute or chronic
    Rupture of the tympanic membrane
    Otosclerosis (fixation of the ossicles due to bony overgrowth)
Sensorineural
    Toxins (e.g., aspirin, quinine, aminoglycosides, diuretics)
    Viral disease of the inner ear
    Syphilis
    Cerebellopontine tumor
    Congenital defect
    Ménière's disease
    Trauma to cranial nerve VIII
    Very loud noises, chronic or acute
    Aging
    Late otosclerosis

---

indicate mastoid disease with bone destruction. A sanguineous discharge can occur with acute otitis, but neoplasm or injury also are possible.

Vertigo is the specific sensation of the room spinning, rather than the less discrete "light-headedness" or dizziness. Vertigo often occurs with disease of the labyrinth and may be associated with nausea and vomiting.

Hearing loss is a frightening symptom for anyone. There are three basic types of hearing losses (see also Table 9-1):

1. *Conductive hearing loss* applies to any disturbance in the conduction of sound impulse as it passes through the ear canal, tympanic membrane, middle ear, and ossicular chain to the footplate of the stapes, which is situated in the oval window. As a general rule, a person with conductive hearing loss speaks softly, hears well on the telephone, and hears best in a noisy environment.

2. *Sensorineural hearing loss* applies to a disturbance anywhere from the cochlea, through the auditory nerve, and on to the hearing center in the cerebral cortex. A person with a perceptive hearing loss usually speaks loudly, hears better in a quiet environment, and hears poorly in a crowd and on the telephone. He often states that he hears but does not understand (i.e., hears sounds but they are garbled), which is indicative of poor discrimination.

3. *Mixed hearing loss* is a combination of conductive and sensorineural loss.

PHYSICAL EXAMINATION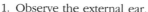

1. Observe the external ear.
2. Palpate the mastoid process.
3. Otoscopic examination of the ear canal and tympanic membrane.
4. Check hearing, Weber's, Rinne's.

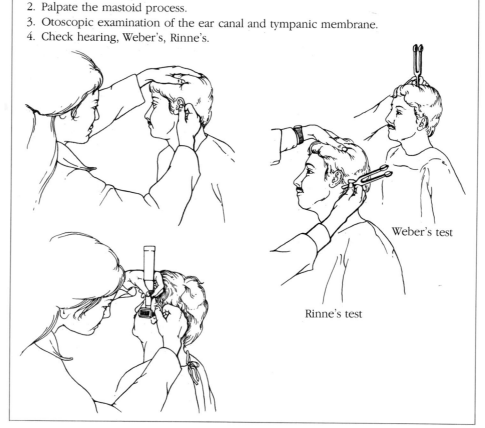

Weber's test

Rinne's test

Abnormalities in the **external ear** may reflect systemic disease, as in alterations of configuration or acuity associated with renal disease and mental retardation. Gouty tophi may occur on the pinna. Pigment or calcium deposition in the ears may give clues to other metabolic disorders.

Examine the lateral and medial surfaces of the auricle, and palpate the mastoid process. The auricle is commonly affected by frostbite, eczema, and sebaceous cysts. Tenderness in the external auditory canal usually indicates furunculosis or external otitis. The external canals may become obstructed by cerumen or foreign bodies, or by certain tumors, particularly exostoses, cysts, and malignant neo-

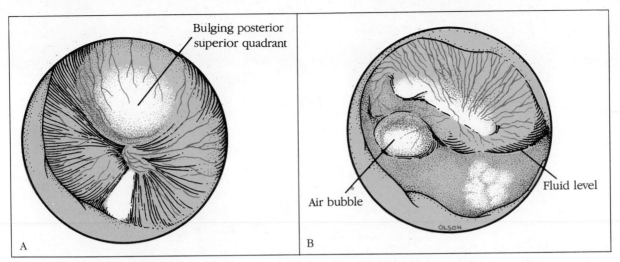

FIGURE 9-4
A. Acute otitis media. B. Serous otitis media. Both are shown in the left drum.

plasms. Exostoses (benign bony projections usually associated with prolonged swimming in cold water) are commonly found in the canal; however, these are rarely significant.

The ear canal and tympanic membrane are best examined with a head mirror and ear speculum. However, the battery otoscope is used by most non-otorhino-laryngologists and is adequate. It may be somewhat cumbersome when instrumentation is necessary. The pneumatic otoscope tests the mobility of the tympanic membrane and provides magnification. To obtain proper visualization of the canal and tympanic membrane, *the auricle must be pulled upward and backward.* In infants and small children, the auricle is pulled straight back. The reason for this is that the outer one-third of the canal is directed upward and backward, while the inner two-thirds is directed downward and forward.

The **tympanic membrane** mirrors past and present middle ear disease. With bulging, the landmarks become obscure, and there is usually some thickening and erythema, indicating acute otitis media (Fig. 9-4A). With retraction the landmarks are accentuated. This usually indicates obstruction of the eustachian tube or old scarring from past otitis. An amber-colored membrane indicates serous otitis media, and air bubbles or a fluid level can at times be seen (Fig. 9-4B). Perforations vary in size and usually point to old inflammatory disease (Fig. 9-5). They may be central (usually benign), anterior, or marginal. Pearly white cholesteatomas may occur in chronic otitis media.

WHISPERED AND SPOKEN VOICE TEST

The test is performed in a quiet room, with the examiner facing the ear to be tested. The other ear is blocked with the examiner's hand. A rough hearing test is then performed 1 foot from the patient's ear. If the patient cannot hear a whispered voice at 1 foot, he has at least a 30-decibel loss. This loss is 60 decibels if he cannot hear a spoken voice at 1 foot.

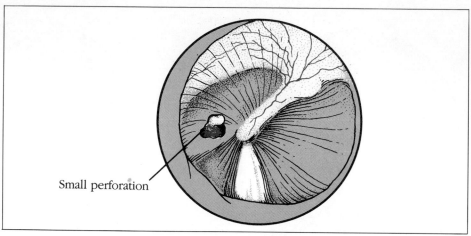

Small perforation

FIGURE 9-5
Perforated drum (right).

TABLE 9-2. Tuning Fork Tests

Hearing	Weber's	Rinne's
Normal	Midline	AC > BC bilaterally
Conductive loss	Lateralizes to affected ear	BC > AC affected ear AC > BC normal ear
Sensorineural loss	Lateralizes to normal ear	AC > BC both ears

AC = air conduction; BC = bone conduction.

WEBER'S TEST

This test is accomplished by placing the vibrating tuning fork on the vertex, forehead, or front teeth. With a conductive loss the sound lateralizes to the diseased ear. The reason is that the conductive loss is masking some of the environmental noise, and thus the cochlea is more efficient on the diseased side. The lateralization of the sound or vibrations to the better-hearing ear signifies sensorineural hearing loss in the poorer-hearing ear.

RINNE'S TEST

This test is a comparison of the duration of air conduction with that of bone conduction. The tuning fork is struck against a rubber object with maximum force so that the results will be consistent. It is first held against the mastoid bone. The fork is then held approximately 1 inch from the ear canal opening. Have the patient compare the loudness of the sound with the tuning fork 1 inch from the ear canal (air conduction) to the sound with the tuning fork pressed on the mastoid (bone conduction). Air conduction should normally be louder than bone conduction (AC > BC). Air conduction that is equal to or less than bone conduction indicates a conductive hearing loss.

Another good test is to strike the tuning fork lightly and compare the patient's air and bone conduction with your own. There are many other methods to test the hearing, such as electric audiometry, speech audiometry, and psychogalvanic skin resistance testing.

Nose

Know that I glory in this nose of mine,
For a great nose indicates a great man—
Genial, courteous, intellectual,
Virile, courageous.

Cyrano de Bergerac
Edmond Rostand
(1868–1918)

ANATOMY

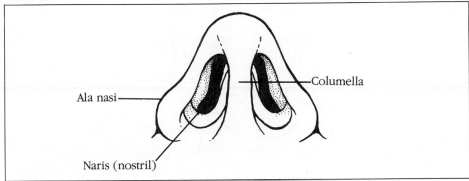

Figure 9-6
Frontal view of the nose.

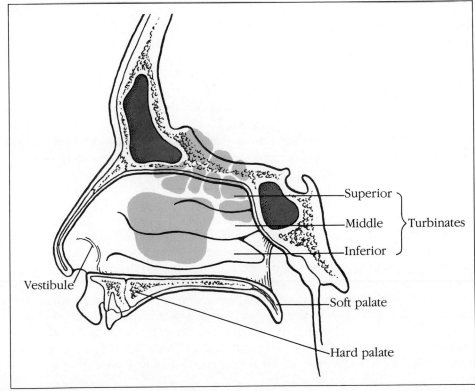

Figure 9-7
Lateral view of the nasopharynx.

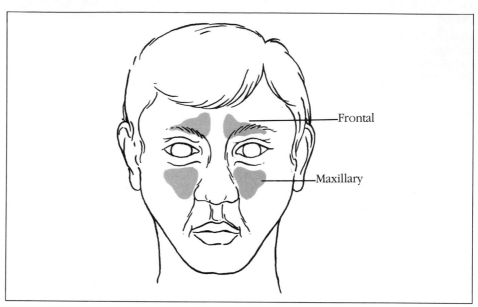

FIGURE 9-8
Paranasal sinuses.

HISTORY

Rhinitis, as in the common cold, is a frequent complaint. Inflammatory disease of the nose is usually on an infectious, allergic, or vasomotor basis. Nasal allergy results in sneezing, watery rhinorrhea, stuffiness, and epiphora. With infections, watery rhinorrhea suggests a viral etiology, while a thick purulent discharge points to probable superimposed bacterial infection.

Sinusitis rarely, if ever, causes generalized headache. More frequently there is pain and tenderness over the involved sinus. There are numerous orbital complications of sinus disease that are a first sign or symptom (for example, proptosis, pain, diplopia, epiphora, swelling of lid(s), and tumor mass). A purulent nasal discharge is frequently present. Fever and prostration may occur.

Nasal obstruction may be unilateral or bilateral. Unilateral obstruction suggests deviated septum, foreign bodies, or neoplasm. Bilateral obstruction is usually the result of rhinitis. In children, adenoid hypertrophy is a common cause of bilateral obstruction. A deviated septum, which is S-shaped, may actually obstruct both airways. Nasal polyps are another common cause of bilateral obstruction.

Perforation of the nasal septum may be on a traumatic or infectious basis. Anterior perforation occurs with tuberculosis, while posterior perforation is more common with syphilis. Other causes of septal perforation are lupus erythematosus and the use of catecholamine nasal sprays and cocaine. When **epistaxis** occurs it may arise posteriorly from a branch of the sphenopalatine artery or superiorly from an ethmoid vessel. By far the most common site of epistaxis, however, is the anterior septum (Kiesselbach's plexus), which is easily accessible to the examiner.

PHYSICAL EXAMINATION

1. Inspect the external nose.
2. With a nasal speculum examine:
   a. Vestibule
   b. Septum
   c. Nasal mucosa
   d. Turbinates
3. Palpate for sinus tenderness.
4. Transilluminate the sinuses (if tender).

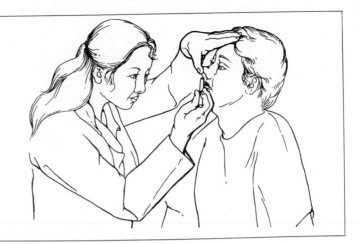

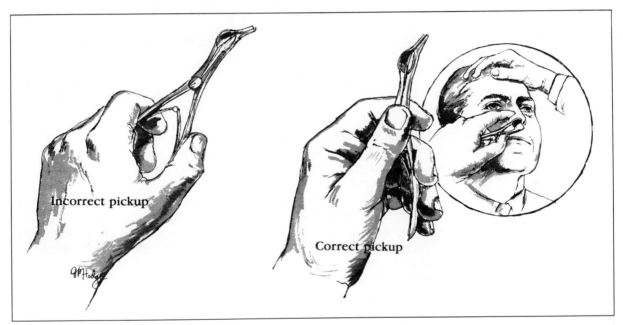

Incorrect pickup

Correct pickup

FIGURE 9-9
Use of the nasal speculum.

Begin by examining the **external nose**. The examiner may stand or sit beside and face the patient. Observe and palpate for any loss of structure or support. A nasal speculum is necessary for adequate **intranasal examination** (Fig. 9-9). Be sure not to overdilate the external nasal orifice or to touch the nasal septum with the tip of the speculum, for this will be quite painful. Observe the nasal vestibule; determine the adequacy of the airways. Observe carefully for a deviation of the nasal septum. Check the color of the nasal mucosa and determine whether the turbinates are normal, hypertrophic, edematous, erythematous, or atrophic. If you spray the nose with 0.25% Neo-Synephrine or 1% ephedrine solution and reexamine after a few

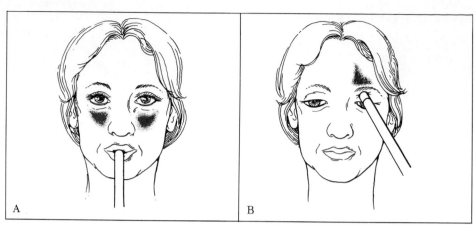

FIGURE 9-10
Transillumination of the sinuses. A. Maxillary. B. Frontal.

minutes, the posterior aspect of the nasal cavities and the superior nasopharynx can be visualized in most cases.

Examine the **sinuses** by *palpation* of the roof of the orbit, the ascending processes of the maxillae, and the canine fossae. Tenderness may be elicited, or masses may be palpated.

TRANSILLUMINATION OF THE SINUSES

Transillumination of the sinuses is used as a diagnostic tool for frontal and maxillary sinus disease (Fig. 9-10). The light is placed under the intraoral hard palate for the maxillary sinus and under the supraorbital rim for the frontal sinus. The test is not of true diagnostic value, for the frontal sinus is often underdeveloped. A sinus filled with clear fluid may transilluminate fairly well, but thickness of soft tissue and bone will interfere with transillumination. This test is used mostly to follow the patient's progress once a clinical and x-ray diagnosis has been made. Transillumination must be carried out in a dark room.

The **internal nose** is the conditioner for inspired and expired air. There are two openings posteriorly, known as choanae, which lead into the nasopharynx and are sometimes referred to as the *posterior nares*. Usually the sinus orifices cannot be visualized during routine rhinoscopy, for they are located in the meati and obscured from vision by the turbinates.

A mucous blanket of viscid secretion covers the entire lining of the nasal cavities. This functions to collect debris and bacteria from the inspired air. The mucous secretion is continuously carried to the nasopharynx by ciliary action. When it reaches the pharynx, it is either swallowed or expectorated.

As the air enters the nasal cavities it is warmed by heat from blood in the cavernous spaces in the turbinates. You will notice that one side of the nose remains more patent than the other at any given time. Blood entering and leaving the cavernous spaces is controlled by the autonomic nervous system. Air is also moistened as it enters the nasal cavities. The parasympathetic supply (vidian nerve) affects turbinate swelling and mucous secretion.

The *olfactory organ* is a small yellowish area on the roof of the nasal cavity and is very difficult to visualize by ordinary rhinoscopy. There are two theories of olfactory function: (1) the undulation theory—that energy waves, similar to light, impinge on the olfactory nerve endings; and (2) the chemical theory—that odorous substances initiate a chemical reaction in the olfactory epithelium.

Oral Cavity

Diseases enter by the mouth.
                    JAPANESE PROVERB

ANATOMY

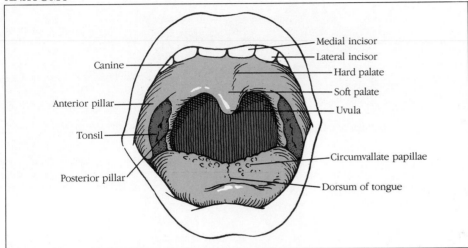

FIGURE 9-11
Anatomy of the mouth.

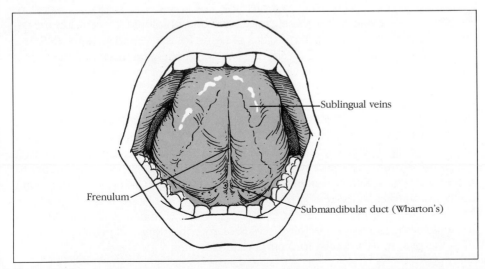

FIGURE 9-12
Sublingual view of the mouth.

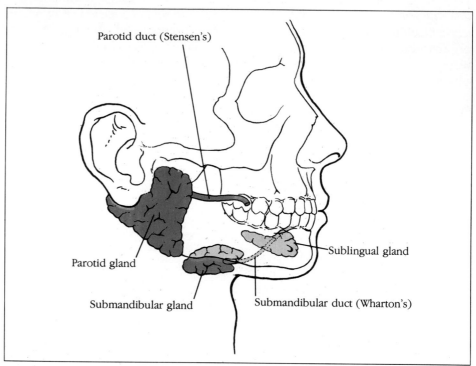

FIGURE 9-13
Salivary system.

HISTORY

The oral cavity is the most accessible body orifice and may reveal significant local diseases as well as signs of systemic diseases. Few areas of the body are exposed to the degree of continuous insult to which the oral tissues are subjected. Constant exposure to mechanical, thermal, chemical, and microbiologic stress makes the tissues of the oral region a significant index of tissue tolerance and systemic defense. Therefore, systemic diseases that reduce tissue tolerance often have oral manifestations. Reactive lesions to local injury also are common in the mouth.

MOUTH AND JAWS

The guidance of the patient's history is as important to the examination of the mouth as to that of any other part of the body. However, minor discomfort in the oral region is apt to be a common and transient experience. The fact that significant oral pathology may present only slight discomfort should stimulate the examiner to inspect this region with critical interest. Although the mouth and jaw region is commonly examined and treated by the dentist on a periodic basis, it is important for the physician to recognize the normal spectrum, the common abnormalities, and the oral manifestations of systemic diseases. Many conditions will prompt the referral of the patient to a dentist for appropriate treatment.

COMMON SYMPTOMS IN THE MOUTH

DRY MOUTH (XEROSTOMIA). A condition seen with atrophy of salivary glands in senility, disease states, radiation, and many drugs that decrease salivary function.

EXCESS SALIVA (PTYALISM). Responses of salivation to any mucosal irritation, heavy-metal toxicity, or pilocarpine-like drug action.

COMMON SYMPTOMS AFFECTING THE LIPS

ULCERS. Chiefly secondary to vesicular lesions of viral origin and to trauma.

NUMBNESS. In lower lip, deficit is due to anesthesia or damage to the inferior alveolar nerve in the mandible resulting from trauma, inflammation, or neoplasm.

DROOLING. Motor loss due to facial nerve paralysis, either peripheral or central.

SWELLING. Rather pronounced response to any inflammatory process; it is sometimes subtle, as in angioneurotic edema and other allergic phenomena.

COMMON SYMPTOMS OF THE TONGUE

COATED TONGUE. Thickening of mucosal keratin, with filiform papillae hypertrophy, is found in response to irritation and immobility and in association with poor oral hygiene.

BURNING TONGUE. Chiefly a psychogenic disorder.

ABNORMAL MOTILITY. Neuromuscular disorders of stroke and myasthenia gravis induce changes and may cause speech disturbance from faulty tongue action. A fixed, firm tongue may result from infiltration by scar tissue or malignant neoplasm, usually squamous cell carcinoma. Excess frenulum attachment may limit tongue motion (ankyloglossia).

COMMON SYMPTOMS AND SIGNS AFFECTING GUMS AND TEETH

GINGIVAL BLEEDING. Local inflammation and infection, or hemorrhagic disorders.

GINGIVAL RECESSION. Gingivae recessed to a low position on the roots of the teeth with increased age, as a result of trauma from incorrect brushing, and from chronic periodontitis conditions.

GINGIVAL SWELLING. A common sign of odontogenic infection, which also may produce sinus tracts draining dentoalveolar abscesses. Note: Enlargement of the gingivae may be seen in generalized form in conditions of chronic inflammation, pregnancy, endocrine disturbance, phenytoin medication (Dilantin), blood dyscrasias, and as a familial tendency to gingival fibromatosis.

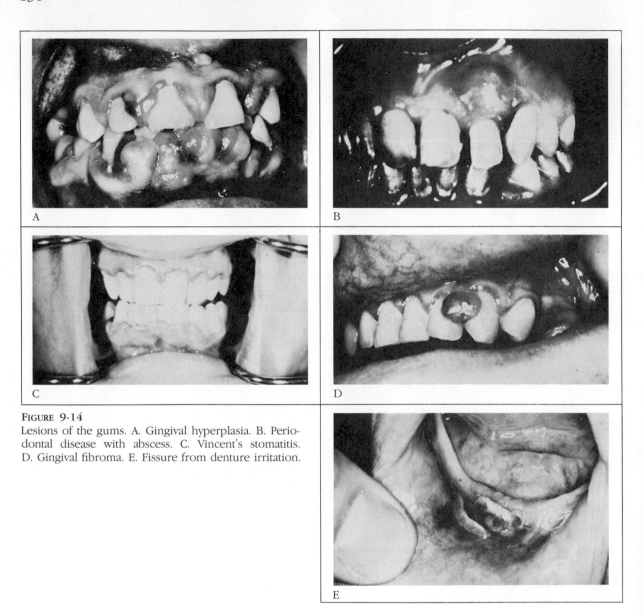

FIGURE 9-14
Lesions of the gums. A. Gingival hyperplasia. B. Periodontal disease with abscess. C. Vincent's stomatitis. D. Gingival fibroma. E. Fissure from denture irritation.

NASOPHARYNX

The nasopharynx may be the site of inflammatory, neoplastic, or congenital disease. Polyps and cysts are not uncommon. When there is obstruction, there may be a change in the quality of the voice since normal voice resonance is produced by the nasopharynx. The student should remember that inflammatory and neoplastic disease of the nasopharynx almost always produce obstruction of the eustachian tube orifice, which will result in hearing loss and otalgia. The resultant negative middle ear pressure causes transudation of serum into the middle ear space.

TABLE 9-3. Some Causes of Hoarseness

Traumatic
  Foreign body
  External injury to larynx
  Voice abuse (singer's nodes)
  Irritant gases (tobacco and other smoke)
  Aspiration (acid, alcohol)
Infectious
  Virus
  Diphtheria
  Syphilis
  Leprosy
Idiopathic
  Sarcoidosis
  Lupus erythematosus
  Cricoarytenoid ankylosis in rheumatoid arthritis
Neurologic
  Recurrent laryngeal nerve injury
  Bulbar palsy
  Myasthenia gravis
Other
  Weakness
  Myxedema
  Acromegaly

OROPHARYNX

"Sore throat" is among the most common of patient complaints and may suggest viral or bacterial infection, toxic irritation (as from smoking or thermal injury), trauma, or tumor.

Dysphagia, or difficulty in swallowing, may rarely result from neuromuscular dysfunction of the oropharynx as part of more systemic neurologic disease (e.g., diphtheria, polio, multiple sclerosis, botulism). More commonly, dysphagia is esophageal in origin.

The sensation of a *mass* in the throat can never be ignored, and tumor must be assiduously sought. Globus hystericus, or the feeling of a lump in the throat as a neurotic manifestation, is always a diagnosis of exclusion. Malignant and benign tumors may arise from the buccal mucosa, the tonsils, and the nasopharynx itself.

LARYNGOPHARYNX

The most common indication for careful laryngeal examination is *hoarseness* of more than 2 weeks' duration (Table 9-3). Hoarseness may occur as a result of acute inflammation (laryngitis). Hoarseness may also result from chronic laryngitis due to repeated infections, voice abuse, smoking, tuberculosis, or poor nasal respiration. Hoarseness may occasionally result from congenital abnormalities or benign tumors. It is an extremely important symptom of carcinoma of the larynx. Stridor, dysphagia, severe pain, halitosis, hemoptysis, and cervical adenopathy are advanced symptoms. Hoarseness may be the only early symptom.

Paralysis of the vocal cords causes hoarseness when incomplete. Cord paralysis indicates interruption of the recurrent laryngeal nerve on the same side. This can result from a large number of traumatic, operative, inflammatory, neoplastic, or vascular abnormalities. It is occasionally a symptom of central nervous system disease as well.

PHYSICAL EXAMINATION

1. Inspect the lips, gums, and teeth.
2. Inspect the buccal mucous membrane, including Wharton's and Stensen's ducts.
3. Inspect the hard palate, soft palate, and uvula with and without phonation.
4. Inspect the protruded tongue, both ventral and dorsal surface.
5. Palpate the intraoral structures, including salivary glands.
6. Gently percuss the teeth.
7. Palpate the temporomandibular joint and inspect the range of mandibular motion.
8. Do mirror examination of the nasopharynx (when suggested by symptoms).
9. Do mirror examination of the laryngopharynx (when suggested by symptoms).
10. A quick cranial nerve examination may be done at this time.

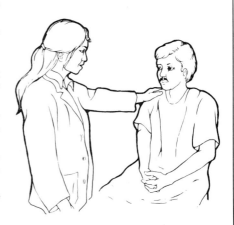

MOUTH AND JAWS

The examination of the mouth and jaws is carried out by inspection, palpation, percussion, and transillumination.

Seat the patient comfortably and, if possible, stabilize the head with back support.

Observe the symmetry in form and function of the **lips** in pursing action. The function of the lips in speech, oral intake, control of secretion, and contributing to facial expression is governed by the orbicularis oris muscles. Sensory nerve supply is abundant, and there is a rich blood and lymphatic supply. Accessory salivary glands under the inner aspect of the lips provide lubrication. Because the lips closely cover the hard tooth structure, they are easily injured.

The vermilion surface of the lips in the young shows slight vertical linear markings and a smooth pliable surface. Atrophic changes of the vermilion with age erase the striated pattern and lose the sharp definition at the mucocutaneous junction. Surface keratosis, induration, and ulceration in older individuals should suggest the changes of squamous cell carcinoma. Herpetic vesicles, or ulcers of the lip, are common. Fissures with inflammation at the angle of the mouth and loss of dental structures may be seen in the aged, and also may be a feature of nutritional deficiency. Superficial accessory salivary glands of the lip occasionally develop retention cysts (mucocele) (Fig. 9-15A) following injury. Congenital anomalies include

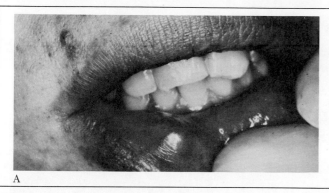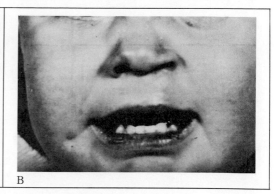

A   B

FIGURE 9-15
Lesions of the lips. A. Mucocele of the lip. B. Repaired cleft lip.

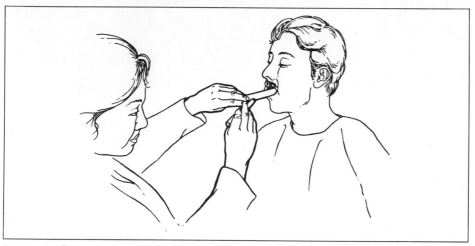

FIGURE 9-16
Examination of the mouth.

folds of the double lip and parasagittal scars in the upper lip from congenital cleft lip repair (Fig. 9-15B). The rich blood and lymphatic supply contributes to rapid edema collection with inflammation of the lips.

Ask the patient to remove any dental appliances. With the patient's mouth only slightly open, retract the lips and cheeks with the tongue blade, and with direct light inspect the inner lip and cheek surfaces and all recesses of the **gingivobuccal fornices** and **gums** (Fig. 9-16).

Attachment of the upper and lower lips in the midline to underlying bone is demonstrated in the normal frenula extending toward the attached gingiva. Posteriorly, similar frenula represent muscle attachments to the alveolar process of the jaws. Buccal mucous membrane inspection may reveal a horizontal white line extending from the commissure of the mouth to the retromolar pad, indicating the contact made by the occluding surfaces of the teeth. This may be a zone of hyperkeratotic reaction and shaggy superficial slough when cheek-biting habits are present. A generalized prominence of the posterior buccal mucosa with fairly large buccal fat-pad structures may be seen. There often are small yellow macules or papules

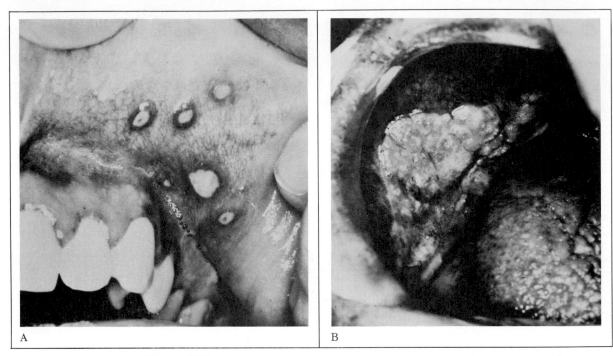

FIGURE 9-17
Lesions of the buccal mucosa. A. Aphthous stomatitis. B. Carcinoma of the buccal mucosa.

indicative of normal sebaceous gland deposition (Fordyce's spots). Recent trauma of the buccal mucosa may produce small spots of submucosal hemorrhage, and similar lesions are produced readily in patients with blood dyscrasias with bleeding tendency.

The **parotid duct orifice** (*Stensen's duct*) is found in the posterior mucosal surface of the cheek opposite the maxillary second molar. The posterolateral recess behind the tuberosity of the maxillary alveolar process requires mirror inspection for complete vision.

Next, ask the patient to open his mouth wide and tilt his head back so that the **hard and soft palates** can be seen. Depress the dorsum of the tongue with a blade and request "ah" phonation to observe midline uvula elevation and coordinated pharynx constriction. The **tonsils**, aggregated lymphoidal tissue between the anterior and posterior fauces, may be atrophic in adults or surgically absent. Painless enlargement is also common. Lesions of the tonsils include acute tonsillitis, chronic tonsillitis, peritonsillar abscess, tuberculosis of the tonsil(s), and lymphoma.

Morphologic and functional aspects of the hard and soft palates are quite different. The hard palatal vault is composed of underlying body processes of the maxilla covered by dense fibrous tissue and mucosa. In the anterior one-third of the hard palate, specialized ridges of normal palatal rugae are noted, with a midline anterior palatine papilla just behind the central incisor teeth. Cysts in this area are associated with the nasopalatine canal.

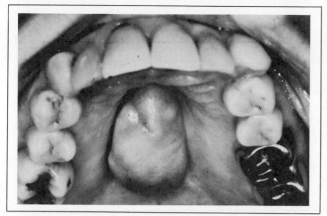

FIGURE 9-18
Torus palatinus.

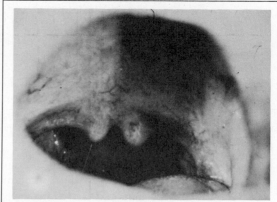

FIGURE 9-19
Bifid uvula.

The most common variation in hard palate structure is seen as a midline hard swelling or exostosis (torus palatinus) (Fig. 9-18). It occurs in 20 percent of the adult population. Such bony growths are benign and are significant only when the surface mucosa becomes ulcerated, or when dental prosthetic requirements necessitate their removal. The soft palate is muscular and has abundant submucosal accessory salivary glands. The normal central position of the soft palate is demonstrated by elevation and reflex.

Soft palate function is coordinated with the pharynx in a constrictor mechanism functioning as the velopharyngeal valve. These actions are essential for normal swallowing and speech.

The palatal vault beneath a maxillary artificial denture may indicate changes of nodular papillomatosis from irritation and altered function of the region. Congenital clefts involve both the hard and soft palates and may extend through the alveolar ridge between the canine and lateral incisor teeth. Degrees of original congenital deformity or scar tissue from surgical repair may be noted in these regions of potential cleft. A bifid uvula (Fig. 9-19) may be featured as part of a submucosal cleft palate, which usually includes hypernasal speech.

The chronic irritation of nicotine stomatitis may produce inflammation of the accessory salivary glands with red dilated orifices, in contrast to general white mucosal hyperkeratosis. Palpation of the posterior palatal vault with the gloved hand may reveal submucosal nodular swelling as the only sign of neoplasm in this region.

Inspect the **oral mucous membranes**. The oral mucosa has a rich vascular supply and a resilient, flexible epithelial surface. Except for the vermilion tissue of the lips, the oral mucosal surfaces are kept moist by numerous submucosal accessory salivary glands adding to the major salivary gland secretions.

Normal mucosal surfaces are pale coral pink. Bright red surfaces generally indicate the erythema of inflammation, while pallor indicates localized ischemia or generalized anemia. Cyanotic color changes may indicate local congestion or many systemic states that produce hypoxemia. The oral mucous membranes are normally pigmented with generalized and local melanin on the basis of race. Local deposits of brown pigment in the mucosa also are seen in some metabolic disturbances, such as hypoadrenalism (Addison's disease). Linear pigmentation of the terminal capillary beds of the gingival margin may indicate heavy-metal absorption, which may correlate with toxic symptoms. Localized bluish pigmentation in the gingival areas that is not related to underlying vascular abnormality may be due to the accidental implantation of metal dental filling materials.

The most frequent surface changes of the oral mucous membranes are ulcers and white patches. Increase in the layer of mucosal keratin produces white thickened patches. Candidal infection will also produce white plaques. Ulceration is indicative of trauma or secondary lesions following initial vesicles of viral or other primary disease lesions.

Swelling of the oral mucosa and submucosa may be found on the basis of inflammation, reactive hyperplasia, cysts, congenital deformities, and neoplasm, in that order of frequency. Many submucosal swellings are detected only by careful palpation.

The examiner should look for bleeding from any surface. Such a finding dictates great care in locating the source of bleeding and the tissue characteristics of the bleeding source (inflammatory or neoplastic).

Have the patient resume the original head examination position and protrude the **tongue**. Note here the symmetry and muscle coordination of midline protrusion as well as the dorsal surface characteristics of the tongue (Fig. 9-20). Complete the inspection of the oral cavity by retracting the patient's tongue laterally to view its posterior surface and the floor of the mouth. The importance of this maneuver lies in the frequency of malignancy in this area. Ask the patient to touch the hard palate with the tip of the tongue in open-mouth position. Observe the ventral surface of the tongue and structures in the anterior floor of the mouth. Tongue mobility and function are essential to speech, mastication, taste, and swallowing.

The specialized mucosa of the dorsum of the tongue presents palpillations of filiform, fungiform, and circumvallate types; at the posterolateral borders of the tongue, ridges of foliate papillae are noted. Many variations of the pattern of papillae are seen. Atrophy leaves a smooth-surfaced red appearance suggesting nutritional deficiency or pernicious anemia. Hypertrophy and hyperkeratosis of the filiform papillae may present a furred, hairy surface. Such a thick coat, which may be pigmented, is a condition associated with poor oral hygiene. A midline elevated area in the posterior dorsum of the tongue represents the congenital benign lesion of median rhomboid glossitis. A striking pattern of arcuate variations in papillary distribution is seen in transient forms in the benign condition known as geographic tongue. The dorsum of the tongue is deeply furrowed in a congenital morphologic variation in some 5 percent of the population. Macroglossia may be indicative of hypothyroidism as well as a number of inflammatory, cystic, congenital, and neoplastic variations (Table 9-4). Lesions that produce asymmetric tongue enlargement are hemangioma, lymphangioma, and neurofibroma.

Ventrally the **lingual frenulum** is noted at the midline attached to the gingiva at the symphysis of the mandible. The sublingual caruncles at the orifices of the submandibular ducts are noted and the flow of secretion is observed. The floor of the mouth may be the site of retention cysts of the sublingual glands, producing soft

TABLE 9-4. Macroglossia

Acute
 Injury with hemorrhage or edema
 Hemorrhage without injury (bleeding disorders)
 Toxic insect sting to tongue (e.g., bee sting)
 Angioneurotic edema
 Infections (streptococcal—Ludwig's angina)
 Pemphigus
Chronic
 Generalized enlargement
  Hypothyroidism (cretinism)
  Down's syndrome
  Acromegaly
 Local enlargement
  Irritation (e.g., by tooth)
  Tumor
  Gumma
  Tuberculosis
  Actinomycosis
  Calculus in sublingual salivary gland
  Angioma
  Lipoma
  Amyloidosis

---

translucent swellings. Occasionally a localized stone in the course of the submandibular duct (Wharton's) may be palpated and will produce obstructive symptoms. Exostosis of the mandible is seen as a hard mass projecting toward the floor of the mouth from the region of bone supporting the premolar teeth (torus mandibularis) (Fig. 9-21). Similar hard swelling may be noted in the midline of the mandible at the position of the genial tubercles, which are especially prominent when teeth are gone and the alveolar process has atrophied.

Begin palpation with a request for tongue protrusion, which is maintained by grasping the tongue between layers of gauze. With this control, use the index finger of the opposite hand, covered with a finger cot, to palpate gently but firmly the soft, smooth tongue surfaces. Release the tongue and continue palpation of the floor of the mouth. Palpate these sublingual structures, with the opposite hand supporting the submental and submandibular tissues. Bimanually palpate between oral mucosa and facial skin in the cheek and lip regions. Conclude palpation with the hard and soft palate areas. Note the flow and secretion quality from the orifices of the submandibular and parotid ducts.

The **submandibular gland** can be palpated directly under the ramus of the mandible about halfway between the chin and the angle of the jaw. It has a firm, irregular consistency. This gland can be more accurately palpated bimanually. Place the index finger of one hand on the floor of the mouth, between the lateral aspect of the tongue and the teeth. The other hand palpates the gland externally. The submandibular glands descend and become more prominent with advancing age; this is frequently misinterpreted as enlargement of the glands. The **parotid gland** is located anterior to and below the auricle. It normally extends from the sternomastoid muscle anteriorly to the masseter muscle (Table 9-5 presents some causes of parotid

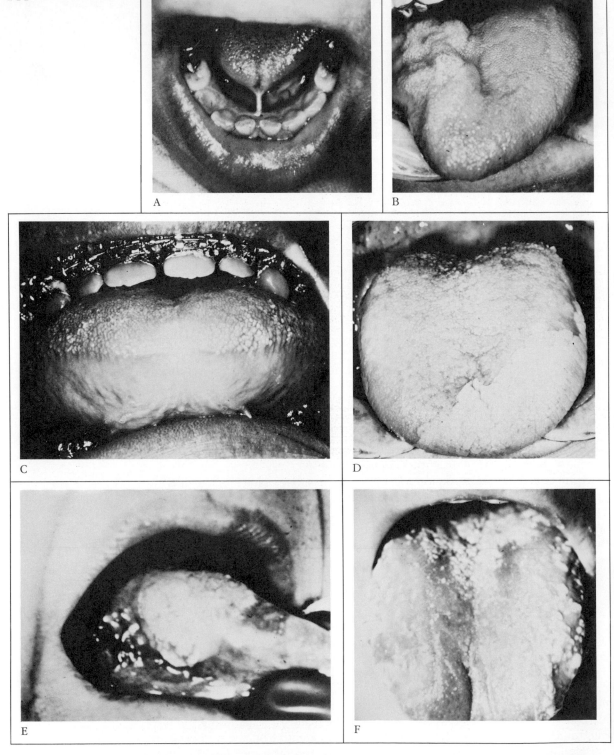

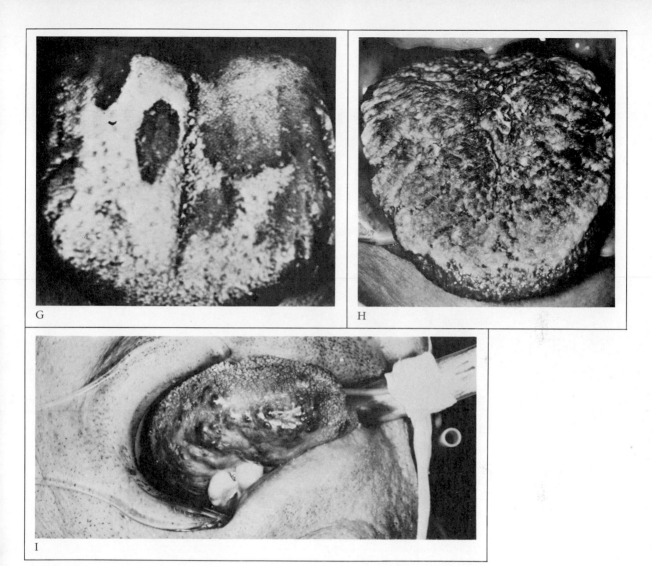

FIGURE 9-20
Some lesions of the tongue. A. Lingual frenulum (ankyloglossia). B. Right XII nerve paralysis. C. Macroglossia. D. Leukoplakia. E. Cancer of the tongue. F. Candidiasis. G. Geographic tongue. H. Black hairy tongue. I. Hemangioma of the tongue.

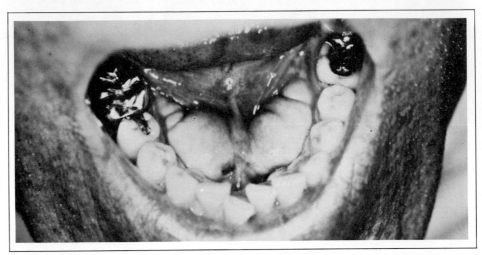

Figure 9-21
Torus mandibularis.

Table 9-5. Some Causes of Parotid Enlargement

Acute
  Infection
    Virus (especially mumps)
    Bacteria
  Recurrent mucus plugging Stensen's duct
  Calculi in Stensen's duct
  Trauma
Chronic
  Lead or mercury poisoning
  Iodides
  Thiouracil
  Lymphoma
  Lymphoblastoma
  Solid tumors of parotid
  Chronic alcoholism
  Diabetes mellitus
  Sarcoidosis
  Actinomycosis
  Chronic insufflation (trumpeter's parotitis)

enlargement). Unless abnormal, the numerous sublingual glands cannot be palpated with any degree of accuracy.

Examine the **gingivae**. The gingival tissues covering the alveolar process normally have a pale coral-pink color and slightly stippled surface. Normal gingivae attach to the teeth, and gingival projections fill the interdental spaces as papillae. Gingivitis is a common inflammatory reaction that may result from local factors of irritation and infection. The most common irritant to this region is the deposition of dental calculus around the necks of teeth. This hard deposit is particularly abundant in the anterior mandibular teeth and the maxillary molar teeth near the ori-

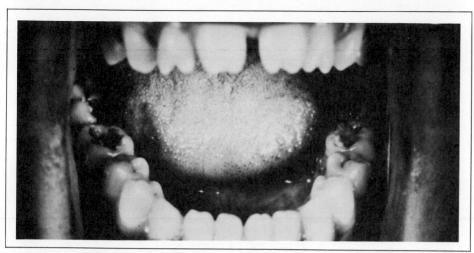

FIGURE 9-22
Hutchinson's incisors.

fices of the major salivary gland ducts. The epithelial attachment of the gingivae to the necks of the teeth is lost in the lesions of periodontal disease, with the production of pocket lesions adjacent to the teeth and loss of supporting soft tissue and bone (chronic periodontitis). The presence of pocket lesions and the level of gingival attachment are determined with a fine probe. A combination of painful gums with bleeding from the free gingival margins, pseudomembrane, and loss of interdental papillae is seen in ulcerative gingival stomatitis (Vincent's infection). Although the acute symptoms of this process may be attenuated by anti-infective medication, comprehensive dental treatment is required to eliminate the disease process. The most common localized gum inflammation is around the partially erupted third molar (pericoronitis). Local care and prompt removal of the third molar are usually required.

Examine the **teeth** for their form, function, and support in the jaws. Light percussion with a mirror handle may be helpful in localizing painful dental conditions. The normal white enamel surface of the crowns of teeth becomes dark with surface stains and also with devitalization of the pulp of teeth through trauma or disease. The crowns of teeth may be irregular in form because of congenital hypoplasia, may become reduced in length by attrition, and may be broken down by destructive phases of dental caries. The classic hypoplasia of incisors in congenital syphilis presents the notched and barrel-shaped Hutchinson's incisor (Fig. 9-22).

Normally the teeth are firmly anchored in the alveolar process by the periodontal membrane. Hypermobility of permanent teeth (adult) may be due to injury but is most frequently seen in advanced periodontal disease. Localized hypermobility of teeth should alert the examiner to consider alveolar bone destruction by neoplastic disease (primary or metastatic).

Observe the excursions of the mandible and occlusion of the teeth that determine the functional potentials of the masticating system. Palpate the condyles of the temporomandibular joint in motion by placing your fourth ("little") fingers in the external auditory canals during jaw excursions. The normal excursion of the jaws

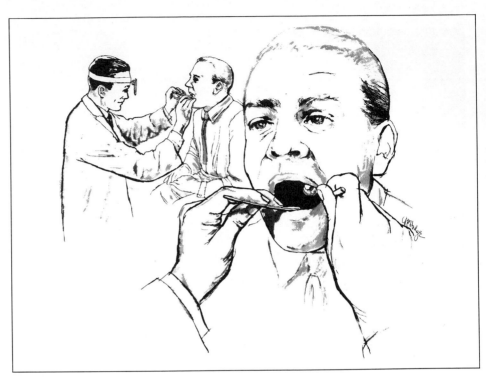

FIGURE 9-23
Technique of examination of the nasopharynx.

will admit the width of three contacting fingers of the patient's hand (3.5 to 4.5 cm). The excursions of the mandible should be smooth and gliding in type. Restriction of the mandible may be caused by disturbances in the temporomandibular joint, extra-articular restriction by scar tissue, trismus from spasm of the elevating muscles of mastication from any inflammatory cause, and the specific contractions of hysteria or tetanus. Findings of crepitus or pain may be indicative of disturbances in the temporomandibular joint.

NASOPHARYNX

Although it is not part of a routine physical examination, the student should familiarize himself with the technique of looking into the nasopharynx (Fig. 9-23). A size 0 through 3 mirror is used. The mirror is warmed by a flame, by being immersed in hot water, or by being held over an electric light bulb. If no heat is available, place a thick soapy solution on the mirror and wipe it off without rinsing. Both of these techniques prevent fogging of the mirror by the patient's breath. The patient sits directly in front of the examiner. The examiner's and the patient's heads should be at the same level. Ask the patient to sit erect and well back in the chair with his head projected slightly forward.

   Depress the tongue into the floor of the mouth with the left hand, making sure not to extend the tip of the tongue blade posterior to the middle third of the tongue. Light is reflected into the pharynx with a head mirror. Grasp the mirror

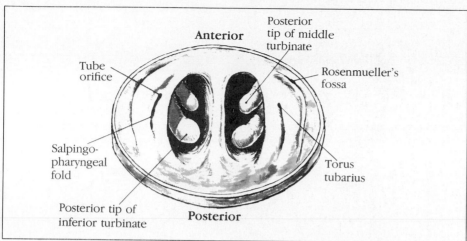

FIGURE 9-24
Mirror view of the nasopharynx.

with the right hand as one would hold a pencil and slip it behind and to one side of the uvula. Encourage the patient to breathe naturally and not to hold his breath; asking the patient to breathe through his nose or to hum often relaxes a tense palate and opens the nasopharynx for examination. Be careful not to touch the base of the tongue. When necessary, 2% tetracaine (not to exceed 80 mg) or 4% cocaine (not to exceed 20 mg) solution may be sprayed into the pharynx to control the gag reflex. Figure 9-24 shows the important landmarks.

The nasopharynx extends from the choanae to the inferior border of the soft palate. Looking anteriorly from the nasopharynx into the nose, the posterior border of the nasal septum dividing the two choanae can be seen. In each choana, the posterior tips of the middle and inferior turbinates can be visualized.

Adenoid tissue is present on the posterior wall (usually absent by age 16 years). This mass of lymphoid tissue is also known as the pharyngeal tonsil. The adenoid is connected with the palatine and lingual tonsils by a band of lymphoid tissue extending down the lateral pharyngeal wall. This entire lymphoid complex is known as Waldeyer's ring.

The mucous blanket passes from the nose into the oropharynx by way of the nasopharynx. Under normal conditions, the nasal mucosa produces approximately a quart of seromucous fluid a day. When this amount is decreased as a result of nasal or environmental factors, the mucous blanket becomes greatly thickened. It is then referred to as a postnasal drip, and the patient is quite conscious of this concentrated form of secretion. Smoking and air pollutants tend to thicken the mucus and intensify the symptoms of postnasal drip, which at times is seen as white or yellow strands or webs in the nasopharynx.

LARYNGOPHARYNX

Inspection of the laryngopharynx is not considered part of the routine physical examination. It should be done if the patient complains of prolonged hoarseness or change of voice. To examine the laryngopharynx, a size 4 through 6 mirror is used

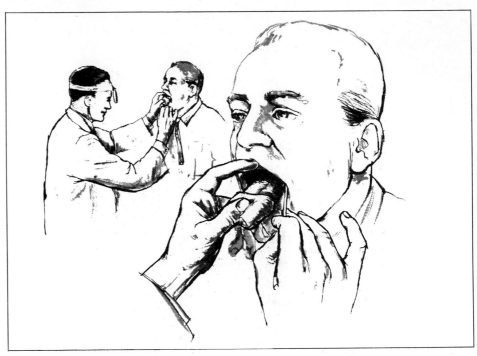

FIGURE 9-25
Technique of examination of the laryngopharynx.

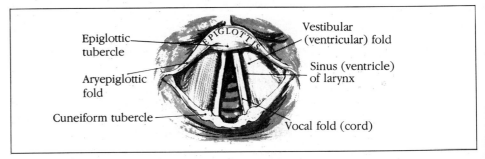

FIGURE 9-26
Mirror view of the laryngopharynx.

(Fig. 9-25). The mirror is prepared as described in **Nasopharynx**, above. Instruct the patient to sit erect, with his head projected slightly forward. Grasp the tongue with a piece of folded gauze. It is important that the thumb be on top of the tongue and the second finger be underneath the tip of the tongue. The index finger elevates the upper lip. Insert the mirror after testing the temperature on the back of the left hand. Place it in the oropharynx so that it elevates the uvula. Touching the lateral walls, tonsils, or back of the tongue will cause gagging. If the patient has a hypersensitive gag reflex, discontinue the examination and spray the pharynx with 2% tetracaine or 4% cocaine solution. Cetacaine spray is also useful and has a more rapid onset of anesthesia. Wait 4 or 5 minutes before resuming the indirect laryngoscopy.

First ask the patient to breathe quietly and not to hold his breath. Especially reassure the patient that you will not obstruct his airway. Then ask him to say "a-a-a-a-a" and "e-e-e-e-e." This will bring the larynx up and back to facilitate visualization. Observe the landmarks, listed below (see also Fig. 9-26).

1. Base of tongue—lingual tonsils
2. Epiglottis
3. Arytenoids
4. Aryepiglottic folds
5. True and false vocal cords

6. Trachea
7. Hypopharynx
8. Pyriform sinuses
9. Mouth of the esophagus

The intrinsic muscles of the larynx act on its cartilaginous framework to tense, relax, abduct, and adduct the vocal cords. This action can be observed during indirect laryngoscopy. The sphincteric action of the laryngopharynx can also be noted during swallowing. The trachea is guarded by three layers of sphincters: the epiglottis and aryepiglottic folds, the false cords, and the true cords.

Cranial Nerves

Before leaving the examination of the head, you may wish to complete the cranial nerve examination which has been partially done already as a normal component of examination of the eyes, ears, nose, and throat. Any historical suggestion of cranial nerve dysfunction would, of course, dictate a far more thorough cranial nerve examination than that outlined in Table 9-6.

TABLE 9-6. Quick Cranial Nerve Examination*

Cranial Nerve	Observation
I	Smell. Is there sense of smell? (seldom useful)
II	Vision.
III, IV, VI	Extraocular movements and pupillary responses.
V	Muscles of mastication. Ask the patient to clench his teeth, and feel the masseter contract.
VII	Facial muscles. Ask the patient to smile, and watch his face for symmetry.
VIII	Hearing.
IX	Muscles of soft palate and palatal symmetry. Watch motion when the patient says "Ah-h-h."
X	Muscles of pharynx and larynx. Is the patient hoarse? Is his swallowing normal?
XI	Trapezius muscles. Ask the patient to shrug his shoulders.
XII	Muscles of tongue. Ask the patient to stick out his tongue.

* Smell and see
 And look around,
 Pupils large and smaller.
 Smile, hear!
 Then say ah . . .
 And see if you can swallow.
 If you're left in any doubt,
 Shrug and stick your tongue right out.

NECK

*The enlargement of the thyroid, of which I am now speaking, seems to
be essentially different from goiter in not attaining a size at all equal to
that observed in the latter disease. Indeed, this enlargement deserves,
rather, the name hypertrophy.*

ROBERT JAMES GRAVES
(1795–1853)

Pain in the neck, a common joke, is not funny to those who have it. In addition to
disorders of musculoskeletal function, neck pain may accompany infection of the
meninges or intracranial bleeding—grave medical emergencies. Symptoms in the
neck may suggest pathology of the structures therein (thyroid, trachea, esophagus,
muscles), may signal disease in head or chest (nodes, referred pain, meningitis), or
may be a feature of systemic illness (tetanus, myopathies).

ANATOMY

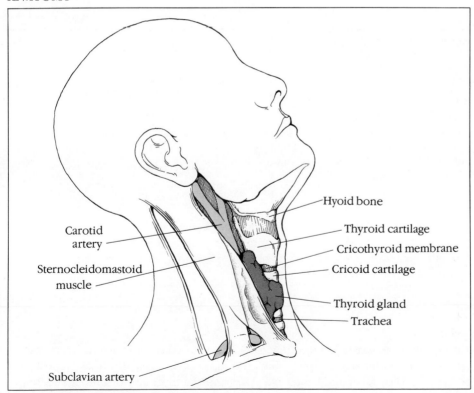

FIGURE 10-1
Structures of the neck identifiable by palpation.

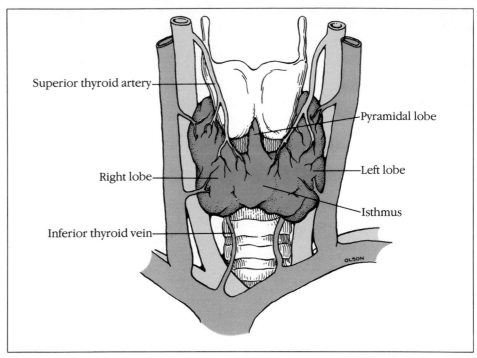

FIGURE 10-2
Anatomy of the thyroid gland.

TABLE 10-1. Some Causes of Cervical Muscle Spasm (Stiff Neck)

Exposure to cold, as with a draft
Strain (physical or emotional)
Abnormal positioning of the head for protracted periods (attending altered vision, poor sleeping posture, prolonged reading, etc.)
Enlarged lymph nodes, abscesses, tumors of the neck
Inflammation of muscles of the neck
Cervical spine arthritis or radiculitis (traumatic, inflammatory, infectious, neoplastic)
Meningitis (infective, irritative, neoplastic)
Muscle disease (parkinsonism, phenothiazines, myotonia)
Tetanus
Acute thyroiditis
Congenital wryneck (torticollis)

HISTORY

NECK

Cervical muscle spasm is a frequent cause of so-called tension headache, characterized by predominantly occipital pain. The rapid onset of a **stiff neck**, especially if accompanied by fever and headache,* is a symptom that calls for immediate evalua-

---

* Abrupt stiff neck with excruciating basilar headache ("the worst headache ever," according to the patient) warns of subarachnoid hemorrhages.

TABLE 10-2. Hyperthyroidism: Physiology and Pathophysiology

I. Physiology

> TRH = thyrotropin-releasing
>   hormone
> TSH = thyroid-stimulating
>   hormone
> T_3 = triiodothyronine
> T_4 = tetraiodothyronine

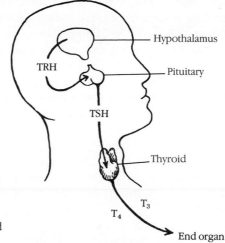

II. Pathophysiology
    A. Diffuse enlargement of the thyroid
       1. Graves' disease
       2. Activity similar to that of thyroid-stimulating hormone
          a. Choriocarcinoma
          b. Hydatidiform mole
          c. Hepatoma (rare)
          d. Pituitary adenoma secreting thyroid-stimulating hormone
    B. Nodular, enlarged thyroid
       1. Graves' disease
       2. Toxic multinodular goiter (Plummer's disease)
       3. Toxic uni-nodular goiter (functional thyroid adenoma)
    C. Tender, enlarged thyroid
       1. Subacute thyroiditis
       2. Hashimoto's thyroiditis (occasionally tender)
       3. Irradiation thyroiditis
       4. Iodine thyroiditis (Jodbasedow) (occasionally tender)
    D. Nonpalpable thyroid
       1. Factitious hyperthyroidism—excessive ingestion of thyroid hormone
       2. Struma ovarii
       3. Metastatic thyroid carcinoma
       4. Normal gland (may be nonpalpable)

tion for *meningitis* (other causes of stiffneck are given in Table 10-1). Neck pain may occur as one of the referred pain patterns in *acute myocardial infarction.*

Masses in the neck may be nodes (as with Hodgkin's disease, cancers of the mouth and throat, and thyroid cancer), infections (pharyngitis, tuberculosis [scrofula], actinomycosis), or cysts. Inflammatory or neoplastic disease of the salivary glands may present as a painless or painful neck mass.

THYROID

The thyroid gland may enlarge as a result of iodine deficiency or as a result of the action of certain goitrogens, with or without overt clinical evidence of thyroidal dysfunction. Neoplastic and inflammatory disease may also produce enlargement of the thyroid.

Thyrotoxicosis, the metabolic expression of overproduction of thyroid hormone(s), usually is accompanied by clinical thyroidal enlargement (Table 10-2) and weight loss, with disappearance of subcutaneous fat. Other symptoms of hyperthyroidism may include heat intolerance, easy sweating, increased emotional lability, tremulousness, palpitations, easy fatigability, diarrhea, and double vision (see Chap. 4).

Myxedema, the result of severe and often prolonged hypothyroidism, presents characteristic symptoms. The patient may feel "puffy" and complain of continual coldness. He may note a dry skin, hoarsening and deepening of the voice, thinning and increased brittleness of the hair, slowing of thought and movement, and chronic constipation (see Fig. 4-7).

It should be appreciated that these are descriptions of symptomatic, classic, or fully developed states of thyroid dysfunction in the adult. Hypothyroidism in the child may result in dwarfism, in which case body skeletal proportions tend toward the infantile.

PHYSICAL EXAMINATION

1. Inspect for symmetry, pulses, masses.
2. Check range of motion, passive and active.
3. Palpate nodes, trachea, carotids, thyroid.
4. Auscultate thyroid, carotids, supraclavicular arteries.

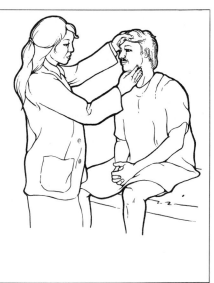

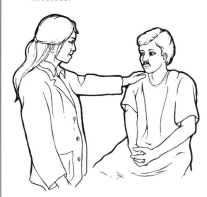

The glands in the neck had assumed the form of large, smooth, ovoid masses connected together merely by loose cellular membrane and minute vessels; when cut into they exhibited a firm cartilaginous structure, of a light colour and very feeble vascularity, but with no appearance of softening or suppuration.

THOMAS HODGKIN
(1798–1866)

NECK

With the patient sitting, inspect the neck for symmetry, pulsations, masses, and range of motion. Have the patient touch his chin to his breastbone. If he must open his mouth to do this, some degree of stiffness or pain in the neck is suggested. Touching the ear to the shoulder tests lateral flexion. Hyperextension of the neck tests mobility and, in addition, throws the thyroid gland and trachea into more

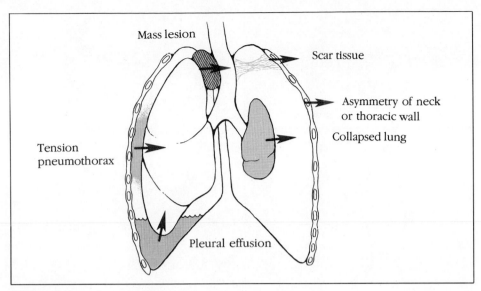

FIGURE 10-3
Causes of tracheal deviation.

prominent view. Hyperextension should not be attempted in an individual with severe rheumatoid arthritis, however, as this may cause serious harm because of involvement of axial cervical joints by synovitis. Both normal and abnormal structures are further evaluated by gentle palpation.

The **trachea** is midline, and any deviation to either side must be noted (Fig. 10-3). Such deviation may be caused by a pulling of the trachea to right or left, as by scar tissue, ipsilateral collapse of lung, or tumor; the trachea may be pushed to the contralateral side by a mass lesion in the neck or increased pressure in the chest (e.g., tension pneumothorax). The "tracheal tug" of aortic aneurysm is the pulsation of the aorta transmitted through the trachea, felt when the examiner palpates the cricoid cartilage and extends the patient's neck.

Palpation of the **lymph nodes** in the neck is systematically done (see Chap. 7) as part of the neck exam or, as you prefer, as a segment of general nodal examination.

Palpation of the **carotid pulses** should be done with gentle care (Fig. 10-4). Carotid pressure receptor reflexes may slow the heart if massage is too vigorous. Moreover, especially in the elderly, vigorous massage may occlude blood flow to the brain or break off an atheromatous plaque, sending the fragment as an embolus to the cerebral cortex and precipitating a stroke. Always ask the patient whether he is left- or right-handed and begin by palpating the ipsilateral carotid. Since there is crossed cerebral representation, the carotid serving the nondominant hemisphere should be palpated first. In this way, if embolism or occlusion results (fortunately, extremely rare), the nondominant hemisphere will be affected.

An aneurysm of the carotid artery may produce a striking pulsatile enlargement on one side of the neck. Any high-output state (aortic insufficiency, thyrotoxicosis, fever) may also result in dramatic pulsations of both carotids.

To auscultate the carotid in the neck, ask the patient to hold his breath (to stop

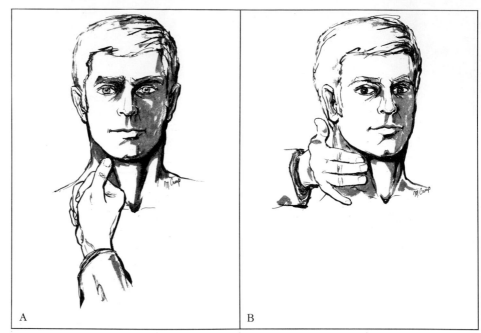

FIGURE 10-4
Technique of carotid palpation. A. Some examiners prefer to stand in front of the patient and use the thumb on the carotid artery for analysis of the arterial pulse contour. This also allows one to examine the neck veins easily without changing position while using the carotid pulse for timing purposes. B. Others prefer to use three fingers from behind or at the side of the patient.

airway sounds), and listen with the diaphragm of the stethoscope over each carotid. The supraclavicular fossae should be auscultated for bruits in the same way. Don't forget to tell your patient to begin breathing again after you've finished!

Venous pulsations in the neck, a valuable clue to cardiac function, are discussed in Chapter 12. They are observed both during examination of the neck (with the patient sitting) and again as part of the cardiac examination (with the patient supine).

Torticollis or wryneck causes deviation of the head to one side. This often very painful condition may be a consequence of drugs, congenital disease, muscle strain, or infection.

THYROID

The **thyroid gland** is examined by inspection and palpation. When it is located substernally it frequently is enlarged, in which case it may be detected by percussion of the chest at the manubrium (restrosternal dullness). Movement of the thyroid, produced by the act of swallowing, aids in its inspection and palpation. Sips of water allow repetitive swallowing. Face the patient and observe the base of the neck as he swallows. Repeat the observation with the patient slightly extending his neck. The normal thyroid gland usually is not visible. An enlargement may be evident as a subtle fullness that glides upward transiently on swallowing. Such movement is more easily appreciated when the neck is slightly extended and illuminated by obliquely directed natural light. Turn off the artificial light and raise the window shades.

The thyroid gland is frequently not palpable in normal patients. However, in the average asthenic individual it is felt as a vague layer of tissue that glides briefly beneath the fingers, rising slightly with swallowing. The isthmus can usually be felt as a soft transverse band below the cricoid cartilage.

The examiner may palpate the thyroid gland from a position in front of or behind the patient (Fig. 10-5). In either case, flexion of the patient's neck toward the lobe being examined results in relaxation of the corresponding sternocleidomastoid muscle, and this facilitates palpation. When the examiner is behind the patient, he lightly places the tips of the first two or three fingers of both hands on either side of the patient's trachea, slightly below the level of the thyroid cartilage. Both lobes are surveyed simultaneously as the patient swallows. A light, rotary motion of the examiner's fingers will help to delineate nodules and irregularities. Next, palpate each side separately. Flex the neck to the side being examined. The first two fingers of the left hand are used to palpate the right lobe, while the right hand is placed behind the sternocleidomastoid muscle to evert the gland as much as possible. The left lobe is similarly examined with the neck flexed slightly to that side. With each maneuver the patient is asked to swallow. Palpation should be gentle because vigorous pressure may cause soreness, choking, or cough, making further examination difficult.

Standing in front of the patient, examine the right lobe. Use the right thumb to displace the larynx and the gland to the side being examined. With the left first and second fingers placed behind the sternocleidomastoid muscle, attempt to palpate the underlying thyroid tissue between these fingers and the thumb of that hand. The left side is examined by exchanging the relative positions of the examiner's hands.

A variation of this technique that is useful for smaller goiters is to place the hand on the base of the neck and palpate the thyroid with the thumb. The right hand is used to examine the left lobe; the left hand, the right lobe. Patients appreciate this gentle approach.

Enlargement of the gland into the thoracic inlet may prevent palpation of the lower poles. An enlarged gland that has descended into the thoracic inlet may occasionally be made to rise into the neck and become visible when the patient performs the Valsalva maneuver. Percussible retrosternal dullness can also help in delineating such enlargement.

Auscultate the thyroid with the stethoscope. Because of the increased thyroidal blood flow that occurs with hyperthyroidism, a hum or systolic bruit—sometimes accompanied by a thrill—may be detectable over the gland. If there is a goiter or thrill, or historical suspicion of hyperthyroidism, examine the skin, which is classically warm and moist with a fine velvety texture. The eyes may protrude. The eye findings in thyrotoxicosis (Table 8-2) result from:

1. Retraction of the lids, which produces widening of the palpebral fissures, a staring expression, and lid lag.

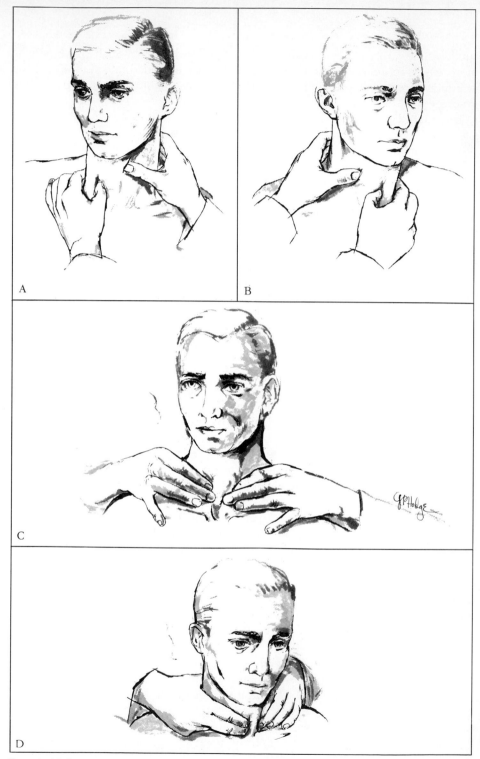

FIGURE 10-5
Examination of the thyroid gland. A. Anterior (lateral deviation to the right). B. Anterior (lateral deviation to left). C. Posterior. D. Lateral deviation posterior.

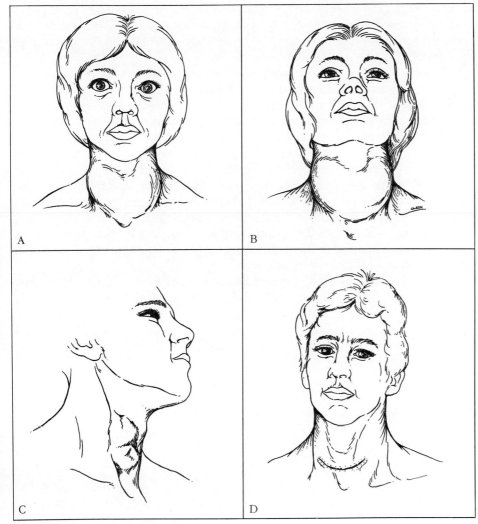

FIGURE 10-6
Thyroid abnormalities. A. Diffuse toxic goiter (Graves' disease). B. Diffuse nontoxic goiter. C. Nodular goiter. D. Thyroidectomy scar.

2. Swelling of the orbital contents, which produces forward displacement of the globe.
3. Swelling of the conjunctivae (chemosis), due in part to orbital swelling and in part to the effects of trauma to the exposed globe.
4. Weakness of the extraocular muscles, with limitation of upward gaze. Later, convergence and lateral movement may be impaired.

There may be a fine tremor of the hands, onycholysis, and exaggeration of the deep tendon reflexes in the **hyperthyroid** patient. The pulse rate is almost invariably elevated, and the pulse has a bounding quality. The pulse pressure is widened due to an elevation of the systolic pressure, the result of increased cardiac stroke volume. Cardiac arrhythmias are common. The heart sounds are loud and hyperactive (particularly the first sound), and a functional systolic murmur may be present. In Graves' disease, warmth and elevation of skin over the shins may occur (pretibial myxedema).

The most common cause of **hypothyroidism** in the United States is Hashimoto's thyroiditis, in which the gland characteristically is moderately enlarged bilaterally and is firm and bumpy to feel. Its upper and lower extents can easily be delineated by palpation. It is the feel of the gland that is so characteristic of this condition. If hypothyroidism is very long-standing or caused by iodine-131 treatment, the gland may not be palpable. The hypothyroid patient (see Chap. 4) presents a puffy face, particularly noticeable in the eyelids. The lips and tongue may be thickened. The speech is slow and the voice deep. The skin is thick and dry and frequently has a yellowish cast, with rough scaly texture and appearance. There may be thinning of the hair, which is coarse and brittle. The body temperature is usually subnormal. The pulse rate is slow. Blood pressure is usually normal but may be increased. Heart sounds are soft and muffled. The deep tendon reflexes are characteristically hypoactive, with a slow recovery phase.

Clearly some, all, or none of these findings may be present in any given individual with thyroid disease, depending on the severity of the disorder.

SECTION IV
CHEST

The physician observing a disease in different circumstances, reasoning about the influence of these circumstances, and deducing consequences which are controlled by other observations—this physician reasons experimentally, even though he makes no experiments.

CLAUDE BERNARD
(1813–1878)

Patient Sitting

1. Examine the regional lymph nodes and skin.
2. Inspect the thorax and accessory muscles of respiration.
3. Inspect and palpate the breasts.
4. Palpate the bony thorax, anterior and posterior.
5. Percuss the spine and costovertebral angle.
   Check for sacral and flank edema.
6. Check expansion and diaphragmatic excursion.
7. Percuss the chest. Check vocal fremitus.
8. Auscultate the lungs.
9. Inspect, palpate, and auscultate the precordium.

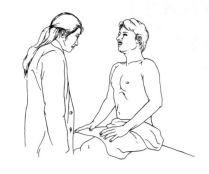

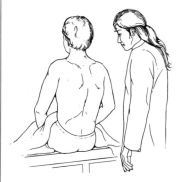
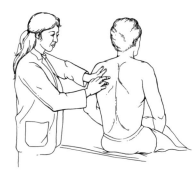
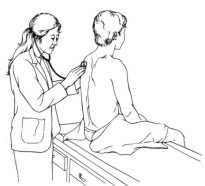

Patient Supine

10. Inspect the precordium.
11. Palpate the precordium and concurrently inspect the neck vein.
12. Auscultate the heart.
13. Palpate the breasts.

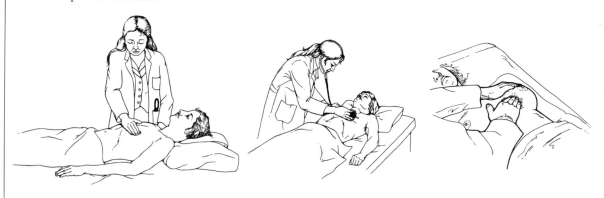

CHAPTER 11

RESPIRATORY SYSTEM

The crepitus rattle is the pathognomonic sign of the first stage of peripulmonary [lobar] pneumonia. It is perceptible from the very invasion of the inflammation; at this time it conveys the notion of very small, equal-sized bubbles, and seems hardly to possess the character of humidity.

RENÉ THÉOPHILE HYACINTHE LAËNNEC
(1781–1826)

Examination of the respiratory system consists primarily of examination of the chest.

To master physical diagnosis of the chest, it is only necessary to have good eyes, good ears, one stethoscope . . . a good roentgenographic unit, a ration of intelligence, a measure of determination and a mess of patients.*

Traditionally the four components of the examination are inspection, palpation, percussion, and auscultation. To these have been added a fifth—study of the chest roentgenogram, which is indispensable to the physical examiner—and a sixth—arterial blood gases. The student must sharpen perception to learn the normal and appreciate the abnormal findings. You must first learn what to look for; later, you must avoid the pitfall of prejudiced perception because of prior experience. Look for nothing specifically, yet see what is actually there. Develop a thorough, systematic routine that is the same for each patient you see. Think of the pathologic changes, rather than specific diseases, that may account for the abnormalities elicited. Diagnosis awaits the correlation of clinical, roentgenographic, and laboratory findings.

ANATOMY

Knowledge of the underlying anatomy of the lungs is essential to a properly conducted examination, because each bronchopulmonary segment must be checked. The sketches and roentgenograms with bronchopulmonary anatomy superimposed in Figures 11-3 through 11-6 may be helpful. The angle of Louis is a prominence in the sternum at the second chondrosternal junction; it is a helpful landmark for counting ribs and then identifying segments from which abnormal findings arise. Other helpful topographic aids are a series of imaginary lines, names of which are self-explanatory, projected onto the chest wall (Figs. 11-1, 11-2).

Record your findings by their relation to these lines, ribs, and interspaces. For example, rales may be heard 3 cm to the right of the midsternal line at the level of the fourth anterior intercostal space. Record the finding as such; later you will interpret the rales as arising from the medial segment of the right middle lobe.

* J. J. Waring. Physical examination, helps and hindrances. *Ann. Intern. Med.* 28:15, 1948.

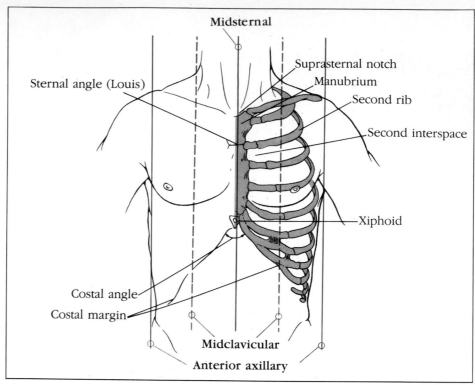

FIGURE 11-1
Landmarks on the chest wall (anterior).

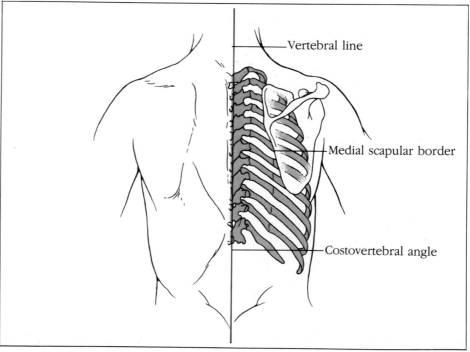

FIGURE 11-2
Landmarks on the chest wall (posterior).

The bronchopulmonary segments are outlined on the roentgenograms as they project on the surface of the lung and thus on the chest wall where their physical findings would present separately. The lines do *not* necessarily represent the roentgenographic projection of each entire segment. All projections on the external chest are drawn to correspond to the position in which the associated roentgenogram is taken. The continuous lines represent interlobar fissures; the interrupted lines represent segmental planes. The bronchopulmonary segmental nomenclature is dependent on the anatomy and nomenclature of the supplying bronchi.

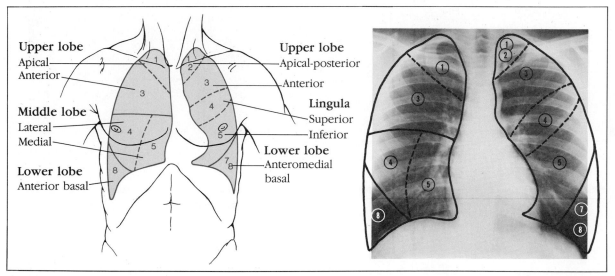

FIGURE 11-3
Segmental pulmonary anatomy (anterior).

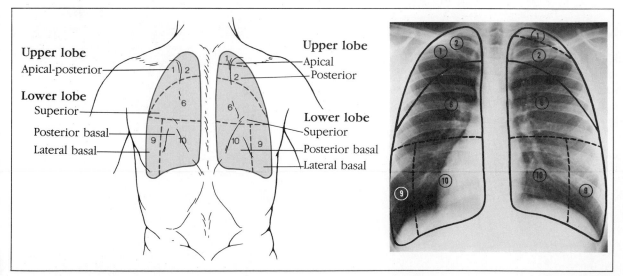

FIGURE 11-4
Segmental pulmonary anatomy (posterior).

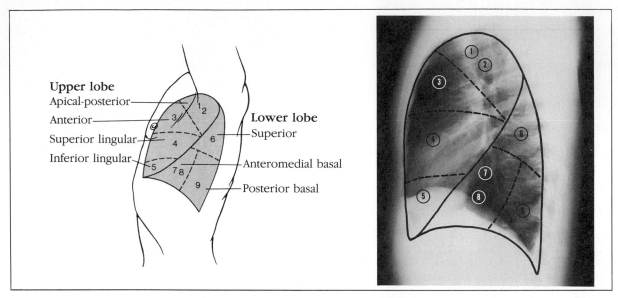

FIGURE 11-5
Segmental pulmonary anatomy (left lateral).

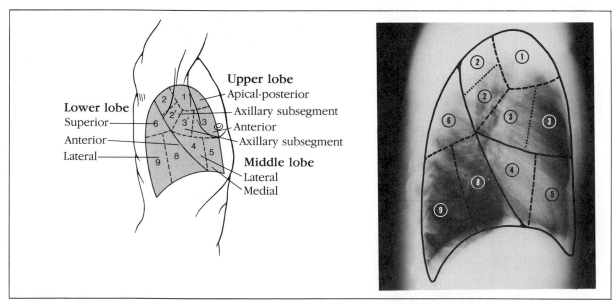

FIGURE 11-6
Segmental pulmonary anatomy (right lateral).

TABLE 11-1. Summary of the Lobes of the Lung[a]

Right Lung	Left Lung
Upper lobe	Upper lobe (superior division)
1. Apical segment (B-1)	1–2. Apical-posterior segment[c] (B-1 and
2. Posterior segment (B-3)	B-3)
2'. Axillary subsegment[b]	3. Anterior segment (B-2)
3. Anterior segment (B-2)	Lingula (inferior division)
3'. Axillary subsegment[b]	4. Superior lingular segment (B-4)
Middle lobe	5. Inferior lingular segment (B-5)
4. Lateral segment (B-4)	Lower lobe
5. Medial segment (B-5)	6. Superior segment (B-6)
Lower lobe	7–8. Anteromedial basal segment[d] (B-7
6. Superior segment (B-6)	and B-8)
7. Medial basal segment[c] (B-7)	9. Lateral basal segment (B-9)
8. Anterior basal segment (B-8)	10. Posterior basal segment (B-10)
9. Lateral basal segment (B-9)	
10. Posterior basal segment (B-10)	

[a] The Jackson and Huber nomenclature is used. The Boyden numerical system is indicated in parentheses.
[b] These axillary subsegments are listed as such because of the frequency with which they are diseased together, without the remainder of their respective segments.
[c] The medial basal segment does not present on the surface of the lung under the chest wall.
[d] The apical-posterior and anteromedial basal segments on the left are considered segments with subsequent subdivisions because they are supplied by a single segmental bronchus. In some classifications the posterior segment is referred to as (3) and the anterior segment as (2).

HISTORY

Love and a cough cannot be hidden.

LATIN PROVERB

Cough is the most common symptom of pulmonary disorders. A normal person coughs rarely, and hardly ever more than twice in a bout. Thus the complaint of cough is abnormal. Cough may also occur as a response to an inhaled irritant or aspirated material. It is caused by stimulation of afferent vagal endings and helps clear the airways of extraneous material. It occurs with focal anatomic pulmonary lesions anywhere in the respiratory system and is also frequently due to diffuse airway or parenchymal abnormality. Coughs should be characterized as productive or nonproductive of sputum, paroxysmal, brassy, loud and high-pitched, or whooplike in character.

Sputum production often accompanies cough when irritation or inflammation of any portion of the pulmonary system leads to transudation or exudation of fluids. Expectoration of sputum (phlegm) is abnormal. The tracheobronchial tree's normal secretions of 60 to 90 cc/day are swallowed. The nature and quantity of sputum should be recorded. Note the volume, color, odor, turbidity, and consistency. Some sputum is colorless, clear, and watery. Mucoid sputum is gray-white, translucent, and slimy. Globs of thicker white mucus or pus may be intermixed (mucopurulent sputum). Purulent sputum is thick and opaque; it may be green, yellow, or brown, and mixed varieties are common. Sputum may be so viscous that it sticks to the inverted specimen container.

TABLE 11-2. Some Causes of Hemoptysis

Oropharynx and nasopharynx
  Necrotizing sinusitis
  Epistaxis
  Bleeding gums
  Pharyngeal venous rupture
  Tongue (ulceration, trauma, carcinoma)
Airway (larynx, trachea, bronchi)
  Laryngeal neoplasm, tuberculosis
  Tracheitis or tracheal trauma
  Bronchitis (acute or chronic)
  Foreign body
  Bronchiectasis
  Bronchial carcinoma, adenoma
  Bronchial rupture
  Broncholithiasis
Pulmonary parenchyma
  Pneumonia
  Tuberculosis
  Fungus infections (histoplasmosis,
    coccidioidomycosis, aspergillosis, etc.)
  Other chronic infections
  Lung abscess
  Lung tumor (primary or metastatic)
  Lung trauma
  Goodpasture's syndrome
  Hemosiderosis
  Lung cysts or bulla
Pulmonary vasculature
  Pulmonary infarct
  Arteriovenous anastamosis
  Vasculitis
  Mitral stenosis
  Pulmonary edema
  Aortic aneurysm
  Anomalous vessels
  Venous obstruction

Other
  Coagulation disorders
  Parasitism (paragonimiasis, ascariasis,
    amebiasis, echinococcosis, etc.)
  Endometrial implants
  Cystic fibrosis
  Apparent (hematemesis, esophageal
    bleeding, spurious.)

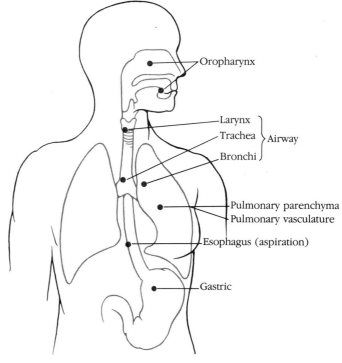

For adequate gross sputum examination the patient must save his secretions, since estimates of both the quantity and the quality are commonly very poor. Expectoration should be directly into clear plastic or glass-capped containers. The patient's course should be followed by daily measurements of volume or weight as well as the changes in the sputum character. A Gram stain of sputum should be part of the initial evaluation.

Sputum may vary in amount from a few teaspoons daily, raised predominantly in the morning, to a pint or more. Patients often are unaware of even copious sputum production if it has increased very gradually. They should be asked about it in several ways: inquire about smoker's cough, clearing throat in morning, and so forth. Morning expectoration usually implies accumulation of secretions during the night and is common to many chronic bronchopulmonary suppurative disorders. Copious sputum may be mucoid, as occurs commonly in bronchitis, or may be largely

TABLE 11-3. Distinctive Characteristics of Hemoptysis and Hematemesis[a]

Hemoptysis	Hematemesis
1. Blood coughed up	1. Blood vomited up
2. Blood may be frothy	2. Blood not frothy
3. Blood mixed with sputum	3. Blood mixed with food
4. Blood is bright red	4. Blood is dark ("coffee grounds")
5. Stools may be tarry black (melena) if enough blood is swallowed	5. Stools often tarry black
6. History of chest disease	6. History of gastrointestinal disease
7. Patient says blood from lungs[b]	7. Patient says blood from stomach
8. Hemosiderin-laden macrophages in sputum	8. No hemosiderin-laden macrophages in sputum

[a] If the amount of blood is very large, patients will often swallow some blood which may be vomited; likewise some blood may be aspirated with massive hematemesis and subsequently coughed up.
[b] Patients are sometimes remarkably perceptive in this regard and may even tell you from *which* lung the blood is coming.

purulent with superimposed infection. A large volume of purulent sputum expectorated into a glass jar ordinarily settles into four distinct layers. At the bottom is amorphous debris; a translucent layer of thin pus, mucus, and saliva is next; above this, pus globules float freely and hang suspended from the surface, which is covered with a layer of froth. Sputum of this type usually results from pulmonary destruction and suppuration and is common in lung abscess and bronchiectasis.

Note the presence of black anthracotic particles, concretions (in answer to direct questioning the patient may describe the expectoration of sand or small stones—broncholiths) casts, and foreign material.

Sniff the opened sputum jar. Most sputum is neither foul nor offensive to the patient or to the examiner. However, with certain necrotizing infections an extremely fetid odor is present, often at a considerable distance from the patient or his sputum jar.

Note specifically whether blood is present. Copious bleeding results in bright-red, frothy sputum; blood may present as small streaks on the surface or as tiny globules of darker blood intermixed with the sputum. The brighter the blood, the fresher the bleeding. Note whether the specimen is pure blood or blood mixed with pus or mucus.

Hemoptysis is frequently due to a single anatomic lesion, proximal or distal, that inflames or destroys the lung or bronchus involved (Table 11-2 outlines some causes of hemoptysis). It can occur with diffuse increase in pulmonary capillary pressure, as in cardiac disease. Blood loss into the lung can be great despite minimal external evidence of bleeding. Blood streaking of sputum commonly accompanies diffuse or localized inflammatory disorders and can be associated with paroxysmal coughing. Careful questioning and examination are required to separate hemoptysis from hematemesis (Table 11-3).

Chest pain (Table 11-4) due to pulmonary disease most often results from involvement of nerve endings in the parietal pleura, as the pulmonary parenchyma itself is insensitive. Pain can arise from major bronchial and peribronchial disease, in which case it tends to be constant, deep, and aching. Pleural pain, which varies

TABLE 11-4. Some Sources of Chest Pain

Extrathoracic
  Migraine
  Cervical arthritis
  Subdiaphragmatic disease (e.g., hepatitis, splenic infarct, pancreatitis, ulcer, gallstones)
Chest wall
  Rib fracture, neoplasm
  Intercostal muscle spasm, inflammation (Bornholm disease)
  Herpes zoster
  Costochondritis
  Thoracic vertebral pain
  Thoracic nerve disease (radiculitis)
Pleura
  Pleurisy (infectious, neoplastic, vasculitic, irritative)
Lung parenchyma
  Pneumonia ⎫
  Neoplasia ⎬ (pain uncommon with pure parenchymal lesions)
             ⎭
Lung vasculature
  Pulmonary infarction
  Pulmonary hypertension
Mediastinal structures
  Lymph nodes (pain with lymphoma, cancer)
  Esophagitis
  Aortic dissection
  Tracheobronchitis
  Pericarditis
  Myocardial pain (angina, infarct)

with respiration, is sharp and intermittent. Chest pain due to pulmonary hypertension may simulate angina pectoris. Pain may also arise from the chest wall; it is usually associated with localized tenderness.

Dyspnea is the patient's perception of shortness of breath or difficulty in breathing in an inappropriate setting, e.g., shortness of breath after running a mile ("breathlessness"), is appropriate and thus not dyspnea, while shortness of breath in a young person after walking up a flight of stairs is dyspnea. Although all symptoms require quantitation, this is essential in describing dyspnea. Each occurence of dyspnea should be recorded in relation to everyday activity, with precise details of respiratory rate and length of activity, time to recovery, and progression over time. Since dyspnea is subjective, special care is necessary in understanding the patient's description; he may complain only of fatigue or of a tightness or heaviness in the chest. The respiratory rate is almost always increased with dyspnea of an organic nature, while a normal rate associated with sighing usually indicates an anxiety state. Although the mechanisms of dyspnea are not fully defined, it appears that central mechanisms mandating regular respiratory cycles, carbon dioxide tension, pH, and reflexes originating in the lung and chest wall (that reflect the perception of inappropriate or excessive work such as a stiffened lung, a low compliance, obstructed airways, and increased resistance) play important roles.

Other symptoms of particular importance in chest disease are **hoarseness**, which may indicate damage to a laryngeal nerve by tumor or inflammation or which may be secondary to vocal cord trauma with severe coughing; **fever**, which is indicative of inflammatory or neoplastic disease; chills or a **rigor** (a shaking chill); **weight loss**; and **edema**.

A past history of pneumonia in childhood, recurrent pneumonia, or whooping cough may indicate a predisposition to respiratory tract infection, bronchiectasis, or congenital anomalies. The use of oily nose drops, poor oral hygiene, a recent dental extraction, alcoholism, or unconsciousness may predispose to aspiration pneumonia or lung abscess, or both. A history of close exposure to infectious tuberculosis, occupational exposure to certain mineral or organic dusts, travel to areas with endemic fungal infections, or inhalant allergy (e.g., hay fever) provides potentially important diagnostic information.

PHYSICAL EXAMINATION

1. Inspect for respiratory rate, rhythm, symmetry of chest and expansion.
2. Palpation for expansion (degree and symmetry), vocal fremitus, rib tenderness or deformity. Supraclavicular nodes and trachea may be done here.
3. Percuss systematically for note, borders, diaphragms.
4. Auscultate systematically for breath sounds, egophony.

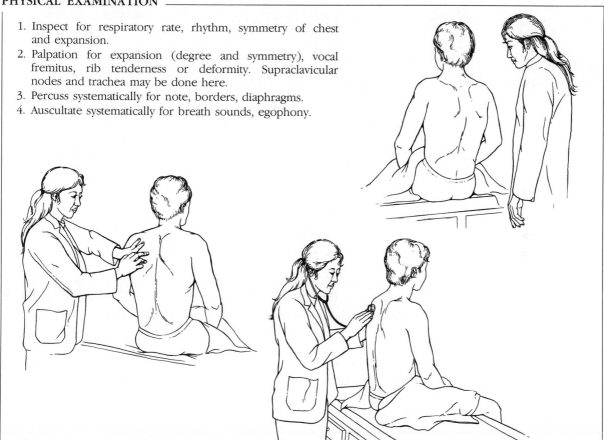

Peripneumonia and pleuritic affections, are to be thus observed: If the fever be acute, and if there be pains on either side, or in both, and if expiration be attended with pain, and the sputum expectorated be of a blond or livid color . . . the physician should proceed thus.

HIPPOCRATES
(460?–377? B.C.)

GENERAL EXAMINATION

Routine physical examination allows excellent evaluation of the ventilatory function of the respiratory tract; it permits an estimate of the volume of exchanging gas and of the rate and distribution of air flows. The other functions of the lung—that is, diffusion, perfusion, and the relation of ventilation to perfusion—cannot be well evaluated; however, the clinical findings in disease states in which these are involved are often characteristic.

Put the patient into the sitting position. If the patient is too ill to sit upright by himself, have an aide support him in the sitting position, as examination with the patient on his back or side may introduce numerous undesirable variables.

The patient is stripped to the waist; a drape is used for female patients. Sit facing the patient, but also inspect from behind, from the side, and while standing behind the patient and looking down over his shoulders at the anterior chest.

INSPECTION

Inspection has its major value in observation of abnormalities in respiration and symmetry, both of ventilation and structure, of the two sides of the thorax.

First and most important is the respiratory rate. Is it increased or decreased? Is it irregular? What is the length of inspiration? Of expiration?

The respiratory rate in the normal resting patient varies between 12 and 16 breaths per minute, although rates as high as 25 have been considered normal. Respiration is regular and quiet; the inspiratory phase lasts half again as long as the expiratory (see Chap. 5). Respirations should be counted for 30 seconds.

Is the patient in pain? Is he in respiratory distress, or is respiration noisy? Observe the chest during quiet respiration. Note the status of the skin and breasts, the muscular development, the state of nutrition, localized areas of bulging or retraction, the presence of thoracic deformities, especially if unilateral, the position of the apex impulse, scars or sinus tract openings, evidence of vascular pulsation or dilation. What are the size and shape of the chest? Pay special attention to chest contour, as it may influence other physical findings and interpretation of the chest roentgenograms. Note the angle of the costal margins at the xiphoid, the angle that the ribs make posteriorly with the vertebrae, and the slope of the ribs. Note whether the interspaces retract or bulge generally or in limited areas during ventilation. Does one area lag or flare more than another? Is respiration predominantly costal or abdominal?

After inspecting the chest in quiet breathing, ask the patient to take in a maximum breath and force it out with his mouth wide open until his lungs are completely empty (i.e., a forced vital capacity [FVC] maneuver). This should be preceded by a demonstration, and the patient should perform the maneuver two or three times to ensure maximum effort and complete emptying. The examiner should measure and record, in seconds, the time to complete this maneuver (i.e., the forced expiratory time [FET]), by listening near the mouth or with the stethoscope placed over the cervical trachea. A normal person can empty his lungs in 3 seconds or less. A prolonged FET (4 seconds or greater) provides a most sensitive and quantitative clinical measure of diffuse airways obstruction.

The hallmark of normal inspection is symmetry—both of structure and of movement. Due to the frequency of scoliosis in the normal population, however, sym-

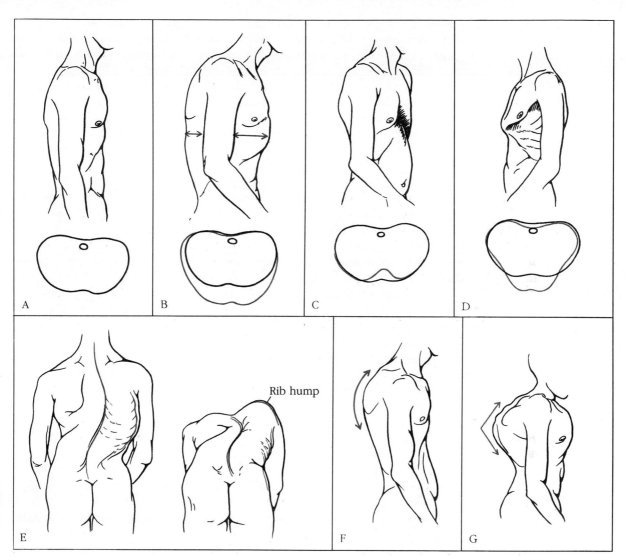

FIGURE 11-7
Chest wall contours. A. Normal. B. Barrel chest (emphysema). C. Pectus excavatum (funnel chest). D. Pectus carinatum (pigeon breast). E. Scoliosis. F. Kyphosis. G. Gibbus (extreme kyphosis).

metry is rarely perfect (Fig. 11-7). The thorax is broader from side to side than from front to back, and its shape varies with the build of the individual; it is short and broad in the stocky person, and long, flat, and narrow in the asthenic person. Minor variations from the normal structure of the thorax include a funnel-shaped depression of the lower portion of the sternum (pectus excavatum) and the reverse condition in which the sternum projects beyond the frontal plane of the abdomen (pectus carinatum, or pigeon breast). Slight thoracic kyphosis resulting from poor posture is not uncommon and is often associated with scoliosis.

Normally the interspaces between the ribs do not particularly retract or bulge during inspiration. The subcostal angle is less than 90 degrees and widens with inspiration. The ribs themselves make an angle of approximately 45 degrees with the vertebral column. Most women tend to breathe largely with their costal cage, and thoracic expansion is therefore easily noted. In most men respiration is largely diaphragmatic, and bulging of the abdomen with inspiration is seen. Inward movement of the abdomen during inspiration is paradoxical; if not voluntary it suggests severe muscle "fatigue" and may be seen with diaphragmatic paralysis. The entire rib cage moves laterally and upward with inspiration, gently rising with each breath. Ventilation is symmetric in onset and depth.

Inspection for respiratory disease requires inspection of more than the thorax. Clubbing, cyanosis, use of accessory respiratory muscles, respiratory distress, and marked sweating are important extrathoracic signs of intrathoracic disease. For example, poor veins with scarring may indicate drug addiction; peripheral thrombophlebitis may correlate with chest pain and dyspnea in pulmonary embolic disease; a rash following an intercostal nerve root distribution suggests herpes infection; a prominent bulging of the dorsal spine in a kyphotic individual, or a gibbous deformity, suggests tuberculosis; the presence of Horner's syndrome (see Chap. 8), with pain in the shoulder radiating into the arm with muscle atrophy, suggests malignancy in the lung apex; a prominent venous pattern of the chest wall may indicate vena caval obstruction; and so on.

Clubbing of the fingers is especially important (see Chap. 4). If the syndrome of pulmonary osteoarthropathy accompanies the clubbing, the periosteum over the ends of the long bones of the forearm and leg may be palpably tender. This is almost always a manifestation of carcinoma of the lung. Clubbing is commonly associated with diffuse interstitial fibrosis of the lung (idiopathic) and is almost always seen in patients with cystic fibrosis. It is not a manifestation of asthma, chronic bronchitis, or emphysema. Dilated veins may indicate compression of the venous flow within the mediastinum, and subcutaneous swellings may represent metastatic tumor nodules, abscesses, or the pointing of an empyema. Sinus tract openings or scars similarly suggest underlying infection.

Asymmetry due to localized prominence of the chest wall will occur occasionally with large tumors or large pleural effusions; in chronic conditions in which considerable scarring of the lung and pleura has occurred, localized contraction is not uncommon. Scoliosis must be eliminated as the cause of such asymmetry. A barrel-shaped appearance of the chest is common in older patients and those with emphysema. The ribs are more horizontal, and the subcostal angle is greater than 90 degrees without variation during respiration; thus, this is neither a specific nor a sensitive finding. Localized areas of diminished ventilation may reflect either local disease or the effects of severe pain with splinting on thoracic motion. Local inspiratory retraction of the intercostal spaces indicates local bronchial obstruction; generalized retractions are common in symptomatic chronic obstructive pulmonary disease, asthma, chronic bronchitis, and emphysema.

PALPATION

Palpation is the best method for the evaluation of the degree and symmetry of expansion with respiration, as well as in appreciation of the transmitted vibrations of the spoken voice. It is complementary to inspection in evaluation of respiratory ex-

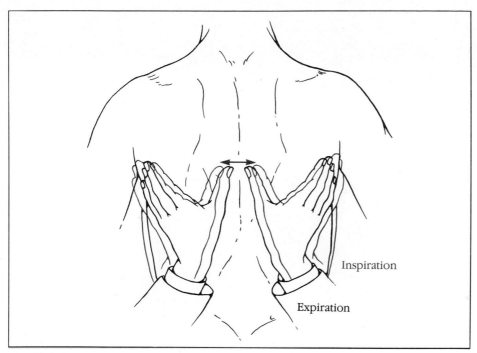

FIGURE 11-8
Palpation for expansion.

cursion. Use both hands simultaneously, and palpate symmetric areas of the thorax (Fig. 11-8). The examiner's hands must be warm. Standing behind the patient, place the hands on the lower chest with the thumbs adjacent near the spine. Tell the patient to inhale deeply, and compare the symmetry of onset and depth of inspiration. Place the hands similarly over the lower lateral chest and standing behind the patient, place them over the shoulders onto the anterior chest below the clavicles. This procedure also can be performed over the low anterior chest but is of less value there.

Costal expansion of 4 to 6 cm is considered normal. Limited costal expansion indicates diffuse obstruction or fibrosis, muscle weakness, or ankylosing spinal disease.

Palpate the chest wall and note any masses. Note the general turgor of the skin, its temperature, moistness, or the presence of edema. Note the character of the musculature. Palpate each rib, noting whether tenderness is elicited. A costal cartilage may be exquisitely tender when inflamed (Tietze's syndrome). Far from requiring severe trauma, rib fractures may occur from so ordinary a stress as heavy coughing. Firm anteroposterior compression of the chest (sternum to vertebrae) will often cause severe pain at the site of rib fracture. Note both the position of the trachea in the episternal notch relative to the midline and the distance of the trachea from the posterior surface of the sternum. This is generally ascertained most accurately by standing behind the patient and letting each index finger slide off the head of the clavicle deep into the sternal notch on either side of the intrathoracic trachea.

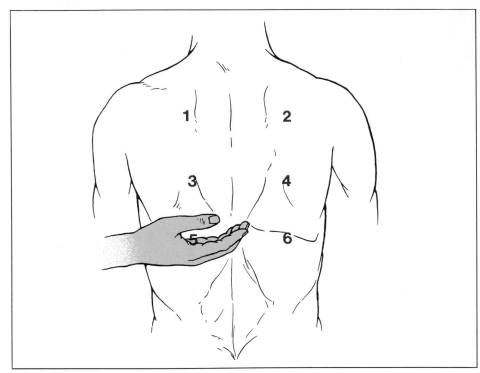

FIGURE 11-9
Evaluation of tactile fremitus.

The trachea is in the midline, admitting almost an index finger on either side at the episternal notch when palpated from behind the patient; the space between it and the sternum does not allow more than one finger at the episternal notch. The lower palpable trachea may deviate slightly to the right in older patients (see Chap. 10).

Supraclavicular lymph nodes can be sought at the same time you palpate the trachea. Nodes in this area, such as those that occur with sarcoid and neoplasia, may be brought up to the examining finger by having the patient perform the Valsalva maneuver.

With the palmar aspect of the fingers or the ulnar aspect of the hand, appreciate tactile fremitus by asking the patient to phonate (Fig. 11-9). It is standard practice to have the patient repeat "one, two, three" or "ninety-nine" to elicit fremitus; "blue moon" is also a helpful phrase. As with other chest examinations evaluate vocal fremitus over all lung segments, and note its comparative increase or decrease or its absence. It will be elicited again during auscultation, and you may wish to check your tactile findings with the auscultatory findings at this point.

Sound vibrations are best transmitted to the examiner's hand in patients with thin chest walls and deep voices. Fremitus is most prominent over areas where the bronchi are relatively close to the chest wall. It increases as the intensity of the voice increases and as its pitch drops. It is normally symmetrical except for a slightly greater intensity over the right upper lobe than over the left.

Notice if coarse vibrations associated with noisy respiration are palpable. This finding, termed *rhonchal fremitus,* implies the presence of exudate in the trachea or larger bronchial tubes, which will also produce rhonchi on auscultation. Auscultation and palpation are both necessary to differentiate rhonchal fremitus from a pleural friction rub. The pleural rub is more grating in quality and is commonly associated with pain. Palpable rhonchi are predominantly inspiratory whereas rubs involve both phases of the respiratory cycle. Ronchi may clear with cough; rubs are unaffected. Rubs are usually more localized, are heard or felt unilaterally, sound close to the ear, and are accentuated by pressure of the hand or stethoscope, features that are all absent with rhonchi.

The evaluation of tactile or vocal fremitus is at times unreliable. Take special care to compare symmetric areas of the chest, as symmetric decreases or increases in fremitus are rarely significant. Localized diminution of fremitus occurs when the transmission of the voice sound from the trachea through the vibrating lung to the examining hand or finger is interfered with by any cause. It is therefore absent in patients with an obstructed bronchus, when air or fluid in the pleural space is interposed, or when the chest wall is considerably thickened or edematous. Generalized diminution in fremitus occurs with diffuse bronchial obstruction. Localized areas of increased fremitus occur with consolidation—denser lung with a patent bronchus—and occasionally when the lung is compressed above a pleural effusion. Increased fremitus over consolidated lungs is appreciated only if the increased density of the lung extends to the pleural surface.

Remember that the intensity of fremitus and the breath sounds are influenced in the same direction by the same physical factors. They should therefore correlate at all times (e.g., diminished fremitus with diminished breath sounds, increased fremitus with loud or bronchial breathing). Minor differences in correlation, if present, are often due to technical factors of a stronger stimulus to production of breath sound or fremitus, or easier appreciation by hand or ear. The auscultatory findings are generally more reliable.

Before leaving palpation of the chest, notice if subcutaneous emphysema is present. If it is present, the fingers palpate a peculiar crackling sensation of bubbles of air underneath the skin, indicating a leak somewhere from the lung or other air-containing viscera. It is usually felt earliest in the supraclavicular area but may spread into the neck and face, over the trunk, and into the scrotum; sometimes it can be heard more easily with the stethoscope than felt. This finding may occur spontaneously or with trauma; it is usually associated with mediastinal emphysema or a pneumothorax.

PERCUSSION

The signs of hydrops of the chest on one side of the thorax, besides the general signs which I have just presented, the affected side (if it is not entirely filled with fluid) is weakened and is perceived to be less moveable on inspiration.

Moreover on percussion, there is no resonance in any part.

But if it is half filled with fluid, a greater resonance is obtained in that part which is not filled with fluid.

LEOPOLD AUENBRUGGER
(1722–1809)

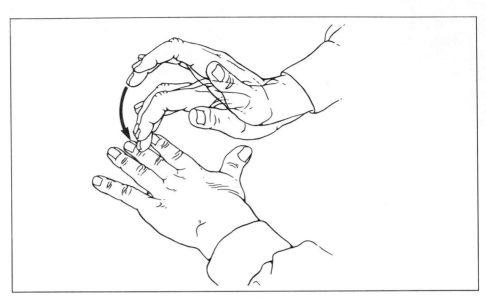

FIGURE 11-10
Mediate percussion of the chest.

Percussion has its greatest value in determining the relative amount of air and solid material in the underlying lung and in delimiting the boundaries of organs or portions of the lung that differ in structural density. Direct percussion involves tapping the chest with the middle or ring finger. It is especially valuable in percussing over the clavicle. Mediate percussion is more popular and is best learned by direct demonstration by an instructor. Figure 11-10 shows the basic method for mediate, or indirect, percussion.

Place the distal two phalanges of the middle finger of the left hand (the finger is then pleximeter) firmly against the chest wall in the intercostal spaces parallel to the ribs. Strike the distal interphalangeal joint with a quick, sharp stroke with the tip of the middle finger (which becomes the plexor) of the right hand, one or two rapid staccato blows in succession. Hold the forearm stationary and make the striking motion with the wrist. Note both the sound elicited and the sense of resistance and vibration underneath the finger. Percuss from side to side, comparing symmetrical areas of the chest. Percuss gently though firmly, making a special effort to apply equal force at all points. It will be necessary to percuss more firmly in individuals with thick chest walls, more lightly in the thin. Skillful percussion requires much practice, until the technique becomes automatic and the examiner can concentrate completely on the sounds and sensations he elicits.

Percuss the lower margins of the lungs and the width of the heart and upper mediastinum. The extent and equality of diaphragmatic excursion are well evaluated in most patients by percussion. Tell the patient to inhale deeply and hold his breath. Note the line of change in the percussion note between the resonant lung and the abdominal viscera posteriorly. Then ask the patient to exhale completely and hold his breath. The lower level of pulmonary resonance has now moved upward (Fig. 11-11). The distance between these two points represents the extent of

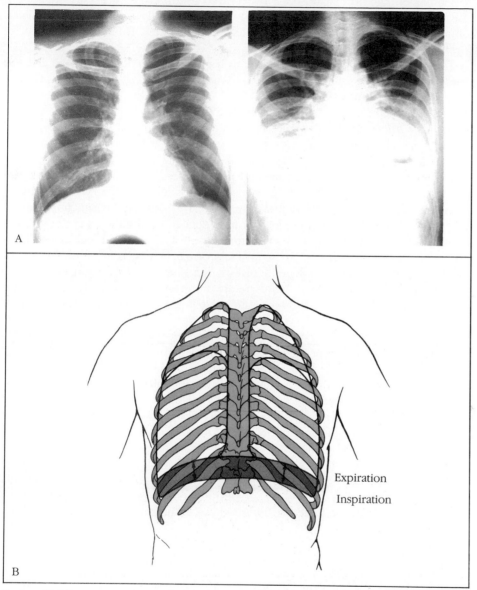

FIGURE 11-11
Normal diaphragmatic excursion. A. Full inspiration (left) and full expiration (right). B. Inspiration and expiration.

diaphragmatic excursion. The lower lung margin may vary, but in mid-inspiration it is usually at the tenth vertebra posteriorly, at the eighth rib laterally, and at the sixth cartilage anteriorly. The normal diaphragmatic excursion averages about 3 cm in women and 5 or 6 cm in men.

When the diaphragms are lower than normal or when the mediastinum is narrower than normal, hyperinflation (such as occurs with emphysema) is suggested;

when higher than normal, fibrosis or increased abdominal contents are suggested. Measured diaphragmatic excursion, when symmetrically reduced, may indicate generalized bronchial obstruction or muscular weakness. Unilateral limitation of motion implies paralysis or splinting.

The normal percussion note varies with the thickness of the chest wall and the force applied by the examiner. The clear, long, low-pitched sound elicited over the normal lung is termed *resonance.*

Dullness occurs when the air content of the underlying tissue is decreased and its solidity is increased. The sound is short, high-pitched, soft, and thudding, and lacks the vibratory quality of a resonant sound. It is heard normally over the heart and is accompanied by an increased sense of resistance in the pleximeter finger. Variations of the note intermediate between dullness and normal resonance are sometimes termed slight dullness or impaired resonance and are elicited normally over the scapulae, over thick musculature, and occasionally at the right apex. Asymmetry of apical resonance, however, is rarely elicited during the routine examination, and slight differences often require perusal of the roentgenogram to determine which side, if either, is normal or abnormal. When patients are examined while lying on the side, the dependent lung tends to have less resonance.

Flatness is absolute dullness. When no air is present in the underlying tissue the sound is very short, feeble, and high-pitched; flatness is found over the muscle of the arm or thigh.

Hyperresonance refers to a more vibrant, lower-pitched, louder, and longer sound heard normally over the lungs during full inspiration.

Tympany is difficult to describe but implies that the sound is moderately loud and fairly well sustained, with a musical quality in which a specific pitch is often noted. It is normally heard in the left upper quadrant of the abdomen over the air-filled stomach or over any hollow viscus. The pitch of tympany is variable, but it is usually high-pitched, clear, hollow, and drumlike.

The normal percussion note is resonant over all the lungs, except at the right apex, where occasionally slight dullness is detected (Fig. 11-12). Generalized hyperresonance not due to full-held inspiration may be found when the lung contains more than a normal amount of air (hyperinflation): however, unless the hyperresonance is pronounced, the considerable variations between observers, and between one observer's impressions at different times, impair the usefulness of this finding. Localized areas of hyperresonance are noted when pneumothorax is present, and occasionally over solitary bullae. Impaired resonance is difficult to evaluate but may be noted adjacent to areas of greater pathology and over lungs partially consolidated, as in diffuse bronchopneumonia. Dullness is elicited with pulmonary infiltration of almost any cause, regardless of the state of patency of the supplying bronchus, whenever the air content of the lung is partially or completely replaced by fluids or solids. When correlated with the character of the breath sounds on auscultation, and fremitus during palpation, the status of the underlying parenchyma in a dull area can be reliably predicted. Dullness also is noted when the pleurae and pleural cavity are thickened or filled with anything except air. (Rarely, air under great tension will give a dull rather than a hyperresonant note.) Extreme dullness, or flatness, is noted when no air at all underlies the pleximeter,

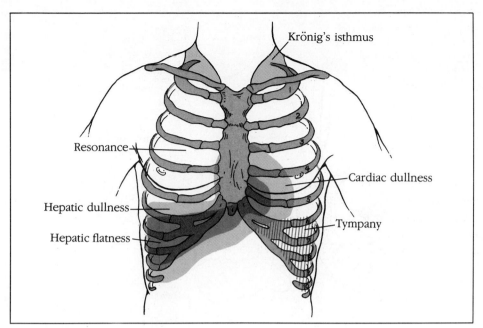

Krönig's isthmus

Resonance

Cardiac dullness

Hepatic dullness

Tympany

Hepatic flatness

FIGURE 11-12
Percussion notes over the normal chest.

as occurs, for practical purposes, only with pleural effusion. Tympany is rare over the lungs themselves. It occasionally occurs over a large pneumothorax.

AUSCULTATION

The pathognomonic signs of this disease [emphysema] are furnished by a comparison of the indications derived from percussion and mediate auscultation. The respiratory sound is inaudible over the greater part of the chest, and is very feeble in the points where it is audible: at the same time, a very clear sound is produced by percussion.

RENÉ THÉOPHILE HYACINTHE LAENNEC
(1781–1826)

Auscultation has no peer in a comparison of the state of bronchial patency of various lung divisions and in appreciation of the normal breath sounds as well as abnormal respiratory murmurs arising from diseased areas. A quiet room is essential. Use a stethoscope, preferably one fitted both with a bell and a diaphragm. Some examiners prefer one or the other—the bell is particularly helpful in very thin patients with deep intercostal spaces that do not permit the larger diaphragm to make full contact. Apply the stethoscope firmly to the chest wall and make certain that factitious sounds due to abnormal muscular movement, hair on the chest wall, and rubbing against the stethoscope do not occur. Cover systematically all portions of both lung fields posteriorly, laterally, and anteriorly, from above down, comparing areas side to side. Be certain that each bronchopulmonary segment is auscultated.

　Instruct the patient to breathe, with his mouth open, a little deeper and faster than normal; demonstrate it to him yourself. Notice especially the character of the

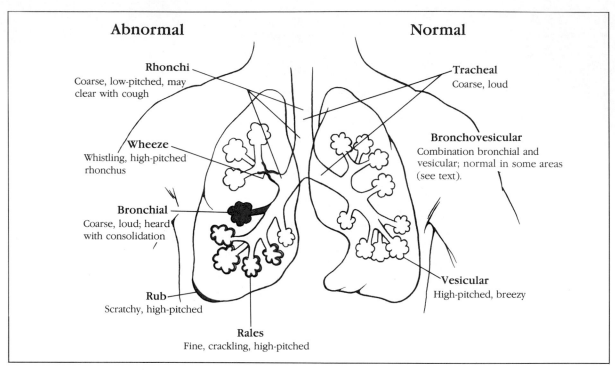

Abnormal

Normal

Rhonchi
Coarse, low-pitched, may
clear with cough

Tracheal
Coarse, loud

Wheeze
Whistling, high-pitched
rhonchus

Bronchovesicular
Combination bronchial and
vesicular; normal in some areas
(see text).

Bronchial
Coarse, loud; heard
with consolidation

Rub
Scratchy, high-pitched

Vesicular
High-pitched, breezy

Rales
Fine, crackling, high-pitched

FIGURE 11-13
Representation of normal breath sounds and abnormal sounds in the chest.

breath sounds and the presence of abnormal sounds. Notice any changes that occur during more rapid and deep respiration; in a normal person the breath sounds should increase in intensity (recruitment). Compare each area examined with the symmetric area of the opposite thorax and with other adjacent pulmonary zones. Direct the patient with instructions such as "a little deeper, please," "a little faster, please," "not quite so hard," until you are convinced that the abnormalities heard are not factitious (see Fig. 11-13). Ask him to phonate and to whisper a phrase such as "one, two, three" or "ninety-nine" and note the character of the vocal resonance perceived.

In recent years there have been renewed interest and major advances in understanding the generation of normal and abnormal breath sounds as well as adventitious sounds. This is due in large part to the availability of sophisticated sound recording equipment and the use of time-expanded wave-form analysis—an expansion of the time axis made by replaying recorded sounds from a computer memory at much slower speeds. The normal breath sounds heard at the chest wall are generated by turbulent flow in the large airways; the vibrations are transmitted through the airways and the airway walls to the chest wall. The sound is filtered, which increases the transmission of low frequencies or pitches, and attenuated. Whether a component of the sound is generated in small airways where laminar flow with its very low energy prevails is not clear. However, there is a general semi-quantitative correlation with the intensity of regional breath sounds and regional ventilation shown in 133-xenon studies.

The importance of the character of normal breath sounds is often inadequately emphasized. *Vesicular breath sounds* are breezy or swishy in character. The maximum frequency content is between 100 and 300 Hz. The inspiratory phase predominates, and the pitch is high. There is a silent pause between inspiration and expiration. Expiration is heard only as a short, fainter, lower-pitched puff less than one-quarter as long as inspiration. Vesicular breathing is normal over most of the lungs. *Bronchial breathing* is, for practical purposes, synonymous with *tracheal breathing* and is heard normally over the trachea and the main bronchi. It contains a wide band of frequencies from just audible to over 1000 Hz. In bronchial breathing, inspiration is louder and higher pitched, but the great change is in expiration, which is increased in duration so much that it actually is longer than inspiration; its pitch is high and its intensity greater. Its quality is hollow or tubular and rather harsh. *Bronchovesicular breath sounds* represent an intermediate stage; they are heard normally in the second interspaces anteriorly, in the interscapular area posteriorly, and often at the medial right apex. Inspiration is unchanged from vesicular breathing, but expiration is as loud, equal in length, and similar in pitch. Exaggerated vesicular breathing is heard normally at times in thin people and children, during exercise, and in unnecessarily loud and rapid respiration. Here the expiratory phase is more prominent than in vesicular breathing but is not of bronchovesicular character. The normal relationship of inspiration to expiration must be learned with respect to each area of the lung examined.

You must expect differences in vocal resonance due to thickness of the chest wall as well as the area to which the stethoscope is applied. Voice sounds are heard best near the trachea and major bronchi. Exaggerated voice sounds (*bronchophony*) are a normal finding over the trachea and right upper lobe posteriorly. Speech is heard only as indistinct noise.

Considerable auscultatory experience with the wide range of normal breath sounds is necessary before you can distinguish abnormal sounds with confidence. When breath sounds differ at symmetric sites of the thorax, it may be impossible to state which side is pathologic without the aid of a roentgenogram. Symmetric findings may be misleading; chronic bilateral apical tuberculosis may be present with symmetric bronchial or bronchovesicular breathing and may be misinterpreted as normal because of the symmetry. Nevertheless, comparison of one side with the other, and of the upper with the ipsilateral lower lobe, are extremely helpful maneuvers during auscultation. Factitious sounds are confusing; every student should apply the stethoscope to the hairy chest and hear the varied sounds made by hair rubbing against the stethoscope. These can be minimized by wetting the skin. In addition, apply the stethoscope to the biceps muscle while it contracts, and note the striking similarity to rales. It is for this reason that the room and the stethoscope must be warm and the patient relaxed so that involuntary muscular contractions of the chest wall will not occur and masquerade as pulmonary abnormalities.

Abnormalities of the breath sounds have great significance. What is normal in one area may be pathologic elsewhere. Bronchial and bronchovesicular breath sounds are due to increased transmission of sound through partially solidified lung, of any cause, provided the bronchus is patent. They are therefore heard with consolidation, compression, and fibrosis. Breath sounds are diminished with local or diffuse bronchial obstruction and with pleural disease. *Amphoric* and *cavernous*

TABLE 11-5. Some Causes of Wheezing

Upper airway
    Tracheal stenosis
    Laryngeal obstruction
    Laryngeal spasm
    Laryngeal edema
    Vocal cord paralysis
    Epiglottitis
Endobronchial obstruction
    Foreign body
    Bronchogenic carcinoma
    Bronchial adenoma
    Endobronchial granuloma
Endobronchial swelling, bronchospasm
    Asthma
        Allergic bronchopulmonary aspergillosis
        Toxic bronchospasm (occupational asthma)
    Anaphylaxis
    Polyarteritis nodosa
    Carcinoid
    Congestive heart failure
Loss of pulmonary architectural support
    Emphysema

breathing are terms of little practical value that refer to exaggerated forms of bronchial breathing heard over large cavities.

When bronchial breathing is heard over the upper anterior chest, the finding may be due to increased transmission through consolidated lung or merely to normal tracheal breathing due to shift in tracheal position. This distinction (which may have great importance in differential diagnosis, as the upper lobe bronchus would then be interpreted as obstructed or patent) unfortunately is often difficult to make even after correlation with the roentgenogram. Transmitted tracheal sounds rather than bronchial breath sounds are probably present if the sounds are not heard in the axilla, if they are quite harsh, without a pause between inspiratory and expiratory phases, or if an area of vesicular breathing seems to be interposed between the trachea and the abnormal breath sounds. The presence of rales, of course, strongly favors bronchial breathing.

Adventitious sounds have been divided into continuous sounds (longer than 250 msec) called *rhonchi* or *wheezes,* and discontinuous sounds (usually shorter than 10 msec) called *rales, crackles,* or *crepitations.* A single nomenclature has not yet been generally accepted. Adventitious sounds arise from abnormal airway-wall motion or intraluminal materials. *High-pitched (sibilant) rhonchi,* called wheezes, are believed to be generated by vibration of the almost touching airway walls akin to an uncoupled reed (Table 11-5). *Low-pitched (sonorous) rhonchi,* called rhonchi, usually are attributed to intraluminal content such as secretions. Crackles, rales, or crepitations are thought to be generated by the sudden release of stored energy from closed airways when they open, or from the bursting of a film of surface material as airways open, or both. Coarse rales are interrupted explosive sounds which are loud, have a low pitch, and a longer duration than fine rales. Fine rales have less amplitude, a higher pitch, and a shorter duration. Medium rales, if the term is used at all, fall in between.

Rhonchi imply disease of the trachea or larger bronchi, whereas medium and fine rales imply bronchiolar and alveolar disease. Rhonchi are usually heard earlier in inspiration than are rales. Sonorous rhonchi are low-pitched, as are coarse rales that are bubbling in quality. Both frequently clear with cough, while fine and medium rales due to inflammatory conditions are usually increased by cough.

Fine rales are short, high-pitched sounds simulated by rubbing the hair between the fingers near the ear; medium rales are louder and lower pitched. Fine moist rales may have a loud, clear consonating quality in which they sound close to the ear. The fine rales of pulmonary congestion or impaired pulmonary ventilation may disappear following a few deep breaths or coughs, but congestive rales reappear shortly thereafter. Congestive rales will move with change in position while inflammatory rales will not. Fine rales are also heard in interstitial fibrosing conditions, usually late in inspiration. The rales are usually generalized and often sound very close to the ear. Inflammatory rales may not be heard during quiet respiration but can be brought out by a special maneuver. Ask the patient to inhale, then to exhale almost completely, and then, without inspiring, to give a short barking cough. The rales are then heard in the subsequent inspiration and are called posttussive rales. The maneuver must often be demonstrated, as most individuals cough normally following inspiration. Similarly, some wheezes are elicited only by asking the patient to exhale forcibly until he empties his lungs of air.

Generalized rales and rhonchi imply conditions that affect the entire lung: bronchitis, asthma and emphysema with rhonchi, pulmonary congestion, diffuse infection, and fibrosis with moist rales. A few scattered posterior basal rales are usually heard in patients with chronic bronchitis and emphysema. Localized rales occur with localized inflammatory conditions such as tuberculosis, pneumonia, and bronchiectasis; a localized wheeze implies localized extrinsic or intrinsic bronchial obstruction, which may occur with a tumor or foreign body. Be sure that the localized or unilateral wheeze is not merely a transient localized component of generalized wheezing. A rhonchus rarely may be palpable but inaudible.

The pleural *friction rub* is a characteristic high-pitched, coarse, grating, loud sound heard close to the ear usually during both phases of respiration. It disappears when the patient holds his breath. It is pathognomonic of inflammation of the pleura. Differentiation from rhonchi is occasionally necessary.

Rarely, an extremely loud, knocking, crunching sound unlike a rub is heard over the mediastinum synchronous with cardiac action. This is *Hamman's sign,* and it occurs with mediastinal emphysema and left pneumothorax. The diagnosis is supported if subcutaneous emphysema is palpated in the neck.

Abnormal vocal resonance occurs for the same reasons as its tactile counterpart but is frequently more discriminating and reliable. The intensity of the voice sounds is decreased with pleural disease and when pulmonary ventilation is either diffusely or locally obstructed. Greater intensity and slightly increased clarity of the transmitted voice (*bronchophony*) is noted over areas of consolidation. Often a more sensitive way to define small, early, partial consolidation is to have the patient whisper while you listen with the stethoscope for distinctly heard, articulated syllables (*whispering pectoriloquy*). *Egophony* refers to a change in the quality of the spoken voice, which is louder and sounds bleating or nasal. Check for egophony by asking the patient to say "ee," which will then sound like "ay." Egophony is rarely found except over an area of compressed lung above a pleural effusion.

LABORATORY STUDIES
CHEST ROENTGENOGRAM

Careful examination of the patient is complemented by careful examination of the chest roentgenogram. Certain conditions present with abnormalities either on physical examination or roentgen examination alone; the roentgenogram always helps in the evaluation of physical findings and cannot be properly interpreted itself without correlation with them. Figures 11-14 and 11-15 show normal and abnormal chest roentgenograms, respectively.

The patient is most often examined first, and the roentgenogram is seen subsequently. Some physicians prefer to see the roentgenogram first and then the patient; it can save valuable time to identify in advance the areas that require the most meticulous examination. The sequence is immaterial as long as the patient is reexamined following study of the roentgenogram, and the roentgenogram is rechecked following careful physical examination. This procedure permits both special attention to specific areas of the patient or film and a search for unusual physical findings when indicated. To fail to elicit abnormal physical findings over an area shown subsequently by the roentgenogram to be significantly diseased is unfortunate but not rare; to fail then to reexamine carefully and to ascertain the findings is deplorable.

The roentgenogram can be a valuable aid in learning physical diagnosis. The chest examination is incomplete without inspection of the chest roentgenogram. When a roentgenographic abnormality is found, every effort should be made to obtain previous roentgenograms for comparison.

Examine the roentgenogram carefully. Be systematic, checking in order:

1. Soft tissues
2. Bones
3. Neck
4. Visible abdomen
5. Diaphragm
6. Mediastinum and heart
7. Lungs

Give special attention to areas over which physical abnormalities were elicited. If the film reveals an unsuspected abnormality, return to the patient and repeat the physical examination. Perform additional studies, such as changing the patient's position, shaking him, or checking for a tracheal tug, if the film suggests that these may be helpful. Go back and forth, if necessary, until careful correlation leads to accurate diagnosis.

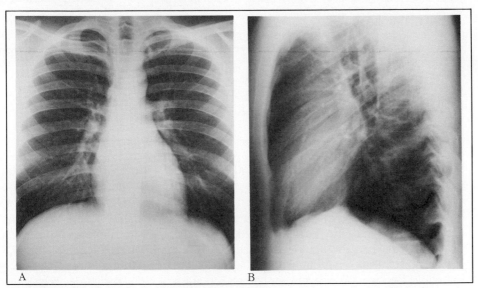

FIGURE 11-14
Normal chest roentgenograms. A. Posteroanterior. B. Lateral.

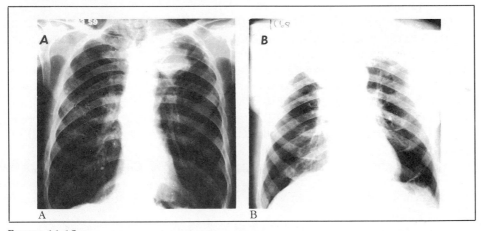

FIGURE 11-15
Abnormal chest roentgenograms. A. Elderly man with infiltration of left upper lobe with extensive calcification. Sputum had tubercle bacilli. Diagnosis: active tuberculosis. Physical findings, however, showed marked dullness and *absent breath sounds* over the left upper thorax (especially anteriorly), which suggested obstructive pneumonia secondary to bronchial obstruction; neoplasm suspected. Bronchoscopy established diagnosis of carcinoma in addition to tuberculosis. B. Elderly man with dense right upper lobe infiltration. Carcinoma suspected, yet onset of illness acute. *Breath sounds are bronchial over right upper lobe with moist rales.* Diagnosis: pneumonic consolidation without obstructing neoplasm. Abnormality cleared completely with treatment.

TABLE 11-6. Representative Normal Gas Pressures at Sea Level

Partial Pressures	Air	Alveolus	Arterial Blood	Mixed Venous Blood
PO_2	159	104	100	40
PCO_2	0.3	40	40	46
pH	—	—	7.40	7.38

ARTERIAL BLOOD GASES

It is essential to evaluate arterial blood gases—the partial pressure of oxygen (PaO_2) and of carbon dioxide ($PaCO_2$), the pH, and usually the percent saturation of hemoglobin (SaO_2)—on patients with dyspnea, tachypnea (or other respiratory rate irregularities), or significant roentgenographic abnormality (Table 11-6). Adequate oxygenation cannot be determined accurately on a clinical basis; cyanosis can be seen only when the hemoglobin saturation is markedly reduced to about 75 percent with a PaO_2 of 40 mm Hg, e.g., equal to the normal mixed venous values. The clinical estimation of hypoventilation (retention of carbon dioxide) is also unsatisfactory because the signs and symptoms are late and nonspecific.

CLASSIC FINDINGS

A single abnormal finding is rarely diagnostic; correlation with other physical abnormalities and with the chest roentgenogram is necessary before the status of the underlying lung can be determined with confidence. Dullness and absent breath sounds, for example, occur with both pleural effusion and with an obstructed lobe and often require the roentgenogram for differentiation; a small infiltrated lobe on the roentgenogram, however, may result from neoplasm or inflammatory fibrosis. Differentiation is made by the physical findings of dullness and diminished breath sounds in pleural effusion and dullness and bronchial breath sounds in an obstructed lobe.

In practice, the importance of one or another single finding may outweigh or be strengthened by others in correlative diagnosis. The following discussion describes the abnormalities that occur in various major pathologic states. Specific diseases are not emphasized.

DIFFUSE ACUTE BRONCHIAL OBSTRUCTION

The patient is in extreme respiratory distress. With laryngeal obstruction he may make crowing sounds. Bronchial obstruction gives wheezing. Respiration is rapid. The intercostal spaces retract on inspiration, and he uses accessory respiratory muscles. Fremitus is decreased, but rhonchal fremitus may be present. The percussion note is normal or hyperresonant throughout. Breath sounds are diminished in intensity, although the chest may be extremely noisy with rhonchi and coarse rales. As the obstruction *worsens,* the pitch of rhonchi increases; they become shorter in duration and less loud. With extremely severe diffuse obstruction, the chest may be almost silent even with forced expiration; this is an ominous sign. This condition may occur in patients with acute exacerbations of chronic obstructive pulmonary disease (e.g., asthma, chronic bronchitis, emphysema), bronchiolitis, or with aspiration of foreign bodies.

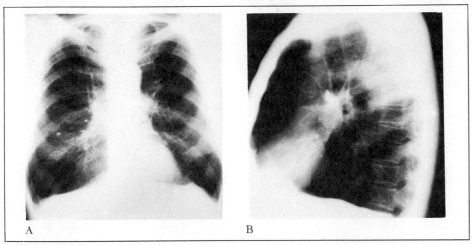

FIGURE 11-16

Roentgenograms of a man with extensive emphysema. A. Posteroanterior view. The diaphragms are flattened and the vascular markings are not uniformly distributed. B. Lateral view. The diaphragms are flattened as determined by an angle of greater than 90° between the sternum and diaphragm; and the anterior clear space—the distance between the sternum and the aorta—is greater than 3 cm (on original roentgenogram).

DIFFUSE CHRONIC BRONCHIAL OBSTRUCTION

The patient may be in no respiratory distress, although the respiratory rate may be increased. The chest may be barrel-shaped; the interspaces are wide and retract with inspiration. Fremitus is decreased, the percussion note is hyperresonant, and the breath sounds are diffusely diminished or almost inaudible. Rhonchi or rales may not be heard with quiet breathing except for a few scattered rales at the lung bases. Rhonchi may be elicited by deep breathing or the forced vital capacity (FVC) maneuver, but the breath sounds do not increase. Prolongation of the forced expiratory time (FET) may be the only evidence of airways obstruction. The diaphragms do not move well. While these findings may be elicited from time to time in any patient with chronic obstructive pulmonary disease (COPD) because of air trapping and hyperinflation, persistently decreased breath sounds in a large chest with appropriate roentgenographic findings correlate well with the presence of emphysema (Fig. 11-16).

LOCAL BRONCHIAL OBSTRUCTION

With obstruction of a large bronchus a lag may be present, the thorax may be contracted, and the trachea and mediastinal contents may be shifted toward the side of the obstruction. The shift may increase further with inspiration and decrease with expiration. Fremitus is decreased, percussion note is dull, and breath sounds are diminished or absent. No rales are heard. Bronchogenic carcinoma and, occasionally, other tumors, foreign bodies, or inflammatory stenosing lesions of the bronchi are responsible.

LOCAL PARTIAL BRONCHIAL OBSTRUCTION

It is remarkable how rarely partial bronchial obstruction manifests itself clinically. In spite of the presence of air within the parenchyma of an obstructed lobe on the

TABLE 11-7. Some Causes of Mediastinal Enlargement

Enlarged lymph nodes
  Neoplasm
    Primary
    Secondary
  Sarcoidosis
  Tuberculosis
Esophageal
  Rupture
  Achalasia
  Diverticula
Vascular
  Pericardial cyst
  Aortic aneurysm
Tumors
  Dermoids, teratomas
  Neurofibromas, sarcomas
  Goiter
  Thymoma

roentgenogram, the physical findings are often those of complete bronchial obstruction. At times, however, rales may be present, and the breath sounds may still be heard, though diminished. A localized high-pitched inspiratory or expiratory wheeze may be present; the wheeze may persist after the patient abruptly stops a forced expiration or inspiration (i.e., when breath sounds have ceased elsewhere in the lung).

COMPRESSION

An otherwise normal compressed lung above a pleural effusion may be dull or tympanic to percussion. Fremitus is increased, and breath sounds are bronchovesicular or bronchial. Egophony is elicited. The findings of pleural effusion often merge gradually with those of a normal lung without the intervening abnormality of compressed lung.

CONSOLIDATION

The patient is usually ill, depending on the underlying condition. Ventilation is usually deep and rapid. Fremitus is increased, the percussion note is dull, and the breath sounds are loud and bronchovesicular or bronchial. Fine and medium moist rales are heard that are consonating in quality. Bronchophony and pectoriloquy may be present. Consolidation occurs mainly in pulmonary infections and with large areas of pulmonary infarction.

MEDIASTINAL MASS

The patient may be either asymptomatic or quite ill; he may be unable to lie on his back. The veins may be distended if the great vessels within the mediastinum are compressed. The distance from the sternum back toward the trachea is increased if the mass is in the anterior mediastinum. The lungs may be entirely normal; however, percussion may reveal increased width of dullness anteriorly and extending laterally across the midline. Table 11-7 presents some causes of mediastinal enlargement.

TABLE 11-8. Definitions and Causes of Pleural Effusion*

I. Transudates
  A. Definition: Pleural fluid characterized by low protein content— <3 gm %—or
     pleural fluid to serum total protein ratio < 0.5; low content of lactate dehydro-
     genase enzyme (LDH) in fluid of <200 IU/L.
  B. Causes
     1. Heart disease (congestive heart failure)
     2. Renal disease (sometimes acute glomerulonephritis; most common in nephrotic
        syndrome)
     3. Malnutrition with systemic edema
     4. Severe anemia of any cause
     5. Cirrhosis of the liver
     6. Myxedema
II. Exudates
  A. Definition: Pleural fluid characterized by high protein content—>3 gm %—or
     pleural fluid to serum total protein ratio > 0.5; or high content of lactate dehydro-
     genase enzyme (LDH) in fluid of >200 IU/I.
  B. Causes
     1. Infections
        a. Bacterial
        b. Mycobacterial
        c. Viral, rickettsial
        d. Fungal
        e. Parasitic
     2. Neoplasms
        a. Primary lung
        b. Metastatic
        c. Lymphoma
        d. Mesothelioma
        e. Meigs' syndrome
     3. Pulmonary infarction, embolism
     4. Vasculitis and immune disease
     5. Pancreatic disease
     6. Drugs and toxins
        a. Allergy
        b. Toxicity
           1. Nitrofurantoin
           2. Heroin, other narcotics
           3. Asbestos
     7. Lymphatic obstruction
     8. Uremia
     9. Trauma (hemothorax)
    10. After abdominal surgery

* The divisions between transudates and exudates are not absolute. For example, long-standing heart failure may produce an exudative effusion. Specific diagnoses often require identification of an infecting organism or histologic
confirmation.

PLEURAL EFFUSION

The patient may or may not appear ill, depending on the cause of the effusion
(Table 11-8) and the rapidity with which it has developed. The affected side of the
hemithorax may bulge; ventilation may lag and be diminished. The trachea and mediastinum may be shifted to the opposite side. The percussion note is flat, fremitus
is markedly decreased or absent, and breath sounds are absent. No rales are heard.

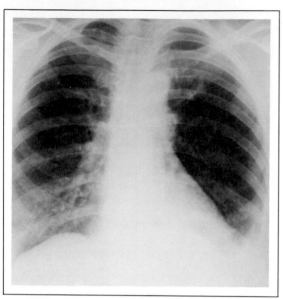

FIGURE 11-17
Pleural effusion. Note blunting of the costophrenic angle on the left. Note also the infiltrate on the right.

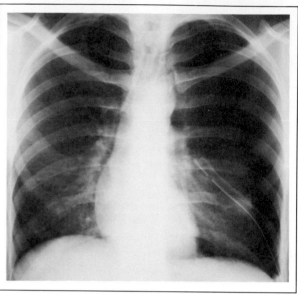

FIGURE 11-18
Chest roentgenogram showing left-sided pneumothorax.

With a moderate effusion, breath sounds may be heard underlying the effusion; physical findings of compression may be noted above it.

PLEURAL INFLAMMATION WITHOUT EFFUSION

Primary forms of this condition are rare, and physical findings of associated parenchymal pathology are often noted. Slight dullness and a pleural friction rub may be the only abnormalities elicited if the responsible adjacent inflammation is minimal, however.

PNEUMOTHORAX

Whether or not the patient is symptomatic depends on both the extent, acuteness, and rapidity of progression of the pneumothorax and on the adequacy of the remainder of the lung. Fremitus is absent, but the percussion note is hyperresonant. Breath sounds are also usually absent. When hydropneumothorax is present, a splash may sometimes be elicited by abruptly shaking the patient from side to side (a succussion splash); the dullness or flatness of the effusion shifts with change in position to a greater extent and more rapidly than in pleural effusion alone. Some causes of pneumothorax are shown in Table 11-9. A left pneumothorax is illustrated in Fig. 11-18 (note the chest tube, placed to evacuate the air from the pleural space).

PULMONARY CONGESTION

If congestion is acute and severe, the patient is in extreme distress; if congestion is partial or chronic, minimal dyspnea may be present. The respiratory rate and use of accessory musculature reflect this difference. Fremitus may be normal or slightly decreased. Associated signs of pleural effusion may be present at the base. Breath

TABLE 11-9. Some Causes of Pneumothorax

Spontaneous
  From congenital bleb
  Emphysema
  Diffuse interstitial fibrosis of lung and related vasculitides and granulomatous
    disease
  Suppurative pneumonias
  Asthma
  Neoplasm with necrosis
  Pulmonary infarction with necrosis
  Tuberculosis
  Marfan's syndrome
Traumatic
  Chest tube
  Thoracentesis or pleural biopsy (a complication)
  Rib fracture
  Stab wounds
  Complication of inserting central venous or hyperalimentation line; neck and
    supraclavicular surgery
  Mechanical ventilators
  Rapid decompression, e.g., diver's

TABLE 11-10. Correlation of Abnormal Physical Findings to Localized Disease

Disease	Tracheal Deviation[a]	Percussion	Vibration[b]	Rales
Pneumothorax	Away or N	Hyperresonant	$\downarrow$ or 0	0
Obstructed bronchus				
With atelectasis	Toward or N	Dull	$\downarrow$ or 0	0
With consolidation	N	Dull	$\downarrow$ or 0	0
Open bronchus				
With atelectasis	Toward or N	Dull	$\uparrow$	0
With consolidation	N	Dull	$\uparrow$	+
Pleural effusion	Away or N	Flat	$\downarrow$ or 0	0

N = normal; + = present; 0 = absent; $\uparrow$ = increased; $\downarrow$ = decreased. The presence of the findings will vary with
the extent of involvement.
[a] Toward or away from side of lesion.
[b] Vibration includes both fremitus and breath sounds, which vary in the same way.

sounds are of fair quality, and resonance is normal or only slightly impaired. Fine
and medium rales that do not sound close to the ear and that shift after prolonged
change of position are characteristic. With marked pulmonary edema, bubbling
coarse rales are also heard. In patients with emphysema, breath sounds may increase in intensity toward normal.

SPECIAL MANEUVERS
Compare the abnormal findings on physical and roentgenographic examination
and correlate them (Table 11-10). Recheck the physical examination carefully if any
discrepancy between physical and roentgenographic findings is noted. If the roentgenogram alone was abnormal, additional physical abnormalities may be elicited;

TABLE 11-11. Some Pulmonary Function Values*

Lung Volumes (ml)	
Vital capacity (VC)	5,000
Residual volume (RV)	1,500
Functional residual capacity (FRC)	3,500
Total lung capacity (TLC)	6,500
Ventilation	
Tidal volume (VT)	500 ml
Respiratory frequency (f)	12–16/min
Minute ventilation ($\dot{V}E$)	5,000 ml/min
Alveolar ventilation ($\dot{V}A$)	3,500 ml/min
Mechanics of Breathing	
Forced expired volume in 1 second (FEV_1)	4,100 ml
FEV_1/forced vital capacity (FVC) × 100 ($FEV_1\%$)	
% in 1 sec	83
% in 3 sec	97
Forced expired flow during middle half of forced expiratory vital capacity (FEF_{25-75})	4.6 L/sec

* For a normal 20-year-old man, 170 cm in height. Normal values are predicted according to age, sex, and height.

for example, the post-tussive inspiration may be rewarding in the demonstration of rales. If only abnormal physical findings were present, and if they persist on repeat examination, recheck the roentgenogram more carefully.

A change in the patient's position is a helpful special maneuver. It is at times difficult to distinguish the rales of inflammatory and fibrosing conditions from those of chronic pulmonary congestion. Note carefully the distribution of the rales. If they are posterior and basal, place the patient flat on his stomach and instruct him to remain stationary for at least a half hour. Recheck the examination. Congestive rales will often disappear posteriorly and appear anteriorly, whereas inflammatory rales will not be affected. Certain wheezes due to extrabronchial compression or intrabronchial polypoid lesions appear only with change in position. Dullness and absent breath sounds at one lung base may indicate either fluid or obstruction; if the patient lies on the same side for a half hour, dullness will now extend high into the axilla if free fluid is present. Obtain a roentgenogram in the lateral decubitus position to confirm the finding. The physical findings of pleural effusion change slowly with positioning; rapid change suggests combined pneumothorax and effusion. Place the patient on the contralateral side. Dullness should now be rapidly replaced with hyperresonance or tympany. A shifting linear fluid level on the roentgenogram confirms these findings. Shaking such a patient vigorously may demonstrate a succussion splash.

If a mediastinal mass is noted in the film, check for a tracheal tug. Place your fingers on the thyroid cartilage and attempt to raise it cephalad. A pulsatile resistance suggests aortic aneurysm.

If a nodular shadow connected to the hilum with broad vascular bands is seen and an arteriovenous malformation is suspected, listen over the proper anatomic area for a bruit with the patient holding his breath. Note if it increases with inspiration; it may disappear completely with a held forced expiration (Valsalva maneuver).

If the differential diagnosis between pneumothorax and a large bulla is unclear from the roentgenogram and physical examination perform the coin test. Have an aide place one coin flat against the anterior chest wall and tap it with another while you listen with the stethoscope posteriorly, or vice versa. Normally, and with bulla, you will hear only a dull thudding sound, but with pneumothorax the note will have a distinct metallic ringing quality.

CARDIOVASCULAR SYSTEM

CHAPTER 12

The heart is the root of life and causes the versatility of the spiritual faculties.
The heart influences the face and fills the pulse with blood.

HUANG TI
(2697–2597 B.C.)

The clinical examination of the cardiovascular system has been significantly modified by information made available with the advent of cardiac catheterization and advances in noninvasive techniques. A sound modern interpretation of both normal and pathologic cardiovascular phenomena requires a clear understanding of the anatomy and physiology that underlie their genesis. The unique aspect of clinical cardiovascular observation has to do with its transient nature. Phenomena pass by relatively rapidly (though recurrently) on a time axis that is constantly moving. It is understandable, then, that the cardiovascular examination presents a challenge to our perceptive ability that is unrivaled by other systems. The examiner must frequently use two or more senses simultaneously: one for identification of a finding, the other for timing purposes. This correlation of vision, touch, and sound requires patience and practice. It is, in a sense, the essence of bedside observation.

Complete evaluation of the cardiovascular system extends beyond the examination of the heart itself. It must include a careful analysis of the peripheral arterial and venous circulations. Occlusion of a coronary artery may produce alarming signs and symptoms that are easily recognized by the physician; occlusion of a deep femoral vein, on the other hand, frequently results in more subtle clinical findings that may go unnoticed but are nevertheless equally threatening to the life of the patient. In this discussion the circulatory system will be considered comprehensively.

As elsewhere in medicine, the "diagnostic negative" may be of great significance in the assessment of the circulatory system. Subtle or transient cardiovascular phenomena too often escape the casual observer. Your strategy must therefore be directed toward the conscious exclusion of certain diagnostic possibilities as you progress through a systematic evaluation. Is the arterial pulse increased? Is there an A wave? Is there a presystolic extra sound? A *No* answer to this type of inquiry is justified only if you have actively excluded the possibilities. To begin with, then, you must guard against undue preoccupation with auscultation and particularly with listening only for murmurs. This common trap most frequently awaits the inexperienced observer. Rushing for the stethoscope prematurely will certainly result in an inadequate examination. A detailed history coupled with careful preliminary observations (particularly inspection and palpation) often permits you to predict the auscultatory findings with remarkable accuracy. More importantly, when you place your stethoscope on the chest you know what you are looking for and why.

To recognize and to understand the signs of vascular disease, you must first develop an appreciation of the enormous variability of the so-called normal range. The circulatory system, perhaps more than any other, is constantly adapting to internal and external factors, with changes in cardiac rate, intravascular pressure, and stroke volume. Keep in mind that while the cardiac output may triple with heavy exercise, it may also double with excitement. If the patient is angry or fearful, if he has just smoked a cigarette or finished a large meal, if he has had to hurry to his appointment, if he is chilled or overheated, his vascular system will respond accordingly. Even the simple act of standing or of lying down on the examining table calls into play several major hemodynamic mechanisms. Thus, it is difficult for the physician to be certain of a basal or steady state at the time of examination. You must learn to recognize the physiologic variables, so as not to confuse them with signs of disease. The young conditioned athlete, the overweight businessman, and the slightly anemic young housewife must be expected to present very different patterns of blood pressure, pulse rate, and heart sounds.

Anatomy and Physiology

A sound heart is the life of the flesh.
PROVERBS 14:30

The normal relationships of the cardiac valves and the great vessels must be appreciated in order to interpret the clinical examination. As demonstrated in Figure 12-1, the mitral and tricuspid valves share a common fibrous ring, and the aortic valve also is part of this fibrous "cardiac skeleton." The projection of the normal relationship on the plain chest roentgenogram is also shown as an aid in visualizing the internal anatomy when looking at the body surface.

In normal circulation, unoxygenated blood is returned by way of the systemic veins to the right atrium and then to the right ventricle. The left atrium and left ventricle receive fully oxygenated blood from the pulmonary veins. Figure 12-2 portrays diagrammatically both the normal circulation and typical oxygen saturations and fluid pressures.

The physiology of human circulation has two very different divisions—the *systemic* and *pulmonary* (Fig. 12-3). These circuits are obviously integrally related but vary from one another in several characteristics. The pulmonary circuit is a low-pressure, low-resistance system. Although resistance vessels are found in the pulmonary circuit, they probably do not play a significant role in normal pulmonary circulation. In addition, the lung contains many potential arteriovenous shunts that, when opened, can further serve to lower pulmonary pressure. Both its distensibility and the presence of potential arteriovenous shunts allow the pulmonary circuit to permit increases in blood flow without significant increases in pressure—a property termed **capacitance**. The pulmonary circulation is therefore termed a high-capacitance circuit in the normal state. The usual pressures seen in this por-

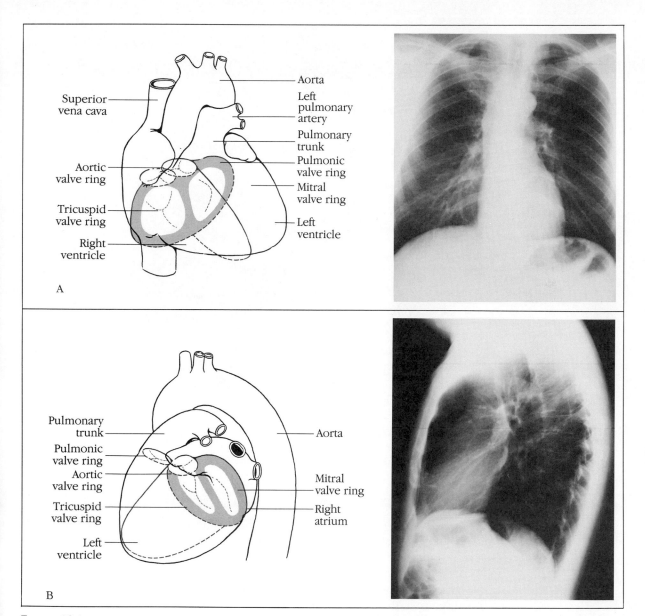

FIGURE 12-1
Normal anatomy of the heart. Anteroposterior (A) and left lateral projections (B), compared with their cardiac silhouette on chest roentgenogram.

tion of the circulation are noted in Figure 12-2.

In contrast to pulmonary circulation, the systemic circuit has been considered a high-pressure, high-resistance system. Indeed, the arterial portion of the systemic circulation does offer variable, active resistance to blood flow from the left ventri-

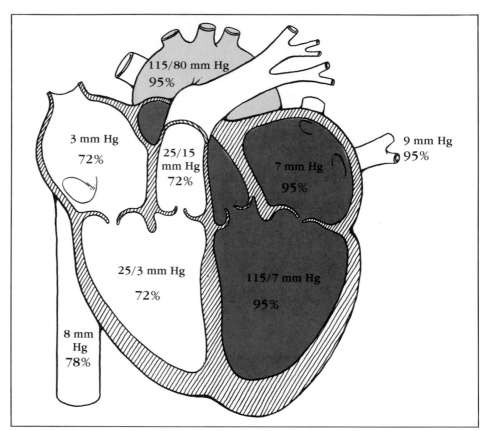

FIGURE 12-2
The normal central circulation. Oxygenated blood is depicted in red. Blood pressures (in mm Hg) and oxygen saturations (in %) are average normal values.

cle. The term **afterload** is used to refer to the strain placed on the left ventricle by this resistance to outflow. The venous portion of the systemic circulation, however, is (like the pulmonary system) a low-resistance, high-capacitance circuit. If intravascular volume is increased, the systemic veins can act as a reservoir and thereby decrease the effect of volume overload on the rest of the circulatory system. Ultimately, any major increase in intravascular volume will be reflected in increased blood return to the left heart. The volume filling the left ventricle during diastole as a result of this venous return is termed **preload** and is reflected by the left ventricular end-diastolic pressure. Examples of normal pressures in the systemic circuit are seen in Figure 12-2.

Many of the findings related to the circulatory system, which are noted in the history and physical examination in succeeding pages, result directly from these anatomic and physiologic principles. For example, evaluation of the systemic blood pressure and cutaneous perfusion will reflect with reasonable accuracy the state of systemic resistance and afterload. Observation of the venous pressure will give information related to preload and systemic capacitance vessels. The state of the pul-

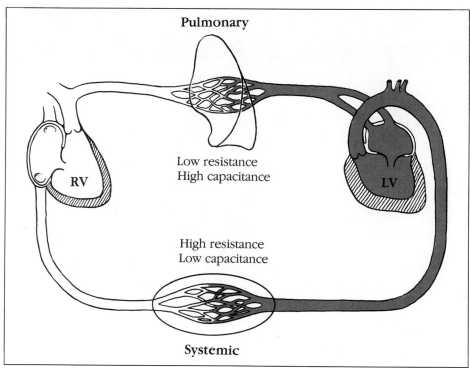

FIGURE 12-3
Normal pulmonary and systemic circuits. Oxygenated blood is shown in red.

monary vascular resistance may be suggested by findings related to the pulmonic component of the second heart sound. As you proceed through the subsequent sections, the various findings in the history and physical examination will be better understood and remembered if they are correlated with the anatomy and physiology of the circulatory system (Fig. 12-4).

History

The seat of it, and sense of strangling, and anxiety with which it is attended, may make it not improperly be called angina pectoris.

They who are afflicted with it, are seized while they are walking (more especially if it be up hill, and soon after eating), with a painful and most disagreeable sensation in the breast . . .

WILLIAM HEBERDEN
(1710–1801)

In the cardiovascular system a carefully taken, meticulously explored, and logically ordered history is highly important to correct diagnosis and therapy.

Major cardiac disease may be present in an asymptomatic patient, but far more frequently the patient's history will establish the direction of both the physical examination and special studies of cardiovascular function. In certain circumstances the history will give the diagnosis even in the face of a normal physical examination

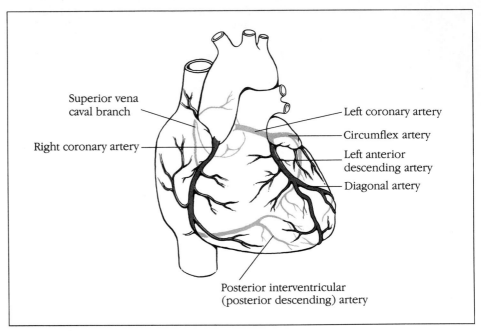

FIGURE 12-4
Anatomy of the coronary arteries.

(e.g., as frequently occurs in angina pectoris). Characteristic symptoms of cardio-vascular disease are discussed below.

DYSPNEA

Dyspnea of cardiac origin is characteristically related to effort until the advanced stages of heart disease, when it may become present even at rest. The labored respirations result from the increased work of breathing caused by decreased compliance of the lungs due to an abnormal increase in pulmonary venous pressure. Since we all experience breathlessness with heavy exertion, mild dyspnea early in the course of cardiac disability requires careful, detailed assessment. Any unexplained reduction in exercise tolerance should arouse suspicion. The patient's inability to keep up with associates of the same age is noteworthy. The level of activity that brings on the symptom must be explicitly determined and quantitated; for example, the number of flights of stairs resulting in distress. Is the complaint abnormal for the patient's age, build, and apparent physical condition? Has there been a slow progression, rapid progression, or sudden onset of the present state? How long does it take to restore the natural breathing with rest? To what extent does it interfere with daily activity? Are there associated symptoms, such as pain, palpitation, or cough? (See also Chaps. 5 and 11.)

PAROXYSMAL NOCTURNAL DYSPNEA

This describes the onset of breathlessness at night, which usually awakens the patient with an alarming smothering sensation. This invariably prompts him to assume the sitting position or to get up from bed. There may be associated wheezing and cough. It generally occurs 2 to 4 hours after lying down and infrequently occurs more than once nightly. Occasionally, non-effort-related paroxysmal dyspnea occurs during the waking hours. It is sometimes precipitated by a disturbance in cardiac rhythm with an excessively rapid or slow heart rate.

ORTHOPNEA

Dyspnea precipitated by assuming the recumbent position is referred to as orthopnea. It is a relatively late symptom and is frequently relieved or improved when the thorax is again elevated. In clinical practice, orthopnea is referred to as two-, three-, or four-pillow (or more) orthopnea, depending on the extent of elevation. It may disappear with improvement that follows therapy. It is a useful index of the patient's status.

PAIN

It is not the delicate neurotic person who is prone to angina, but the robust, the vigorous in mind and body, the keen and ambitious man, the indicator of whose engine is always at "full speed ahead."

SIR WILLIAM OSLER
(1849–1919)

Pain is an important symptom of circulatory disease. Most commonly it is a consequence of ischemia, but it may arise from the pericardium or aorta, or from elevation of the pulmonary arterial pressure.

Angina pectoris is a common manifestation of coronary artery disease and is the symptom of inadequate oxygen delivery to the myocardium. It is usually located in the retrosternal area and may radiate into the neck or into either or both arms (usually the left). It is characteristically constrictive or oppressive (from the Latin *angere,* "to strangle"), although patients will describe anginal discomfort quite variably (e.g., burning, aching, squeezing), and many will refuse to call the sensation *pain.* Factors that increase cardiac work, such as exercise, excitement, cold weather, and meals, tend to provoke angina. Anginal discomfort is not infrequently associated with transient dyspnea, diaphoresis, or nausea. The essence of the diagnosis of angina pectoris centers on distress that occurs in the substernal area, is related to effort, and is relieved within minutes by rest. Fleeting stabs or jolts of pain, or pain lasting for hours or days, is not angina pectoris. Angina pectoris is seldom restricted to the left anterior chest or inframammary region—a common site for noncardiac chest pain. While most angina results from an increase in cardiac work, spasm of a normal diseased coronary artery may also decrease myocardial oxygen delivery enough to cause ischemic pain (*variant angina*).

The observant clinician will note characteristic nonverbal suggestions of angina that will suggest further inquiry (Fig. 12-5). *Claudication* refers to ischemic pain caused by an inadequate arterial circulation to a muscle group, usually the legs (from the Latin *claudicare,* "to limp"). It is similar to angina in that it is precipitated by exercise and relieved by rest. *Pericardial* pain may be retrosternal and may mimic the pain of myocardial ischemia in many respects. It is persistent and, unlike angina, is often intensified by inspiration (pleuritic) and relieved by changes in body position, such as sitting up.

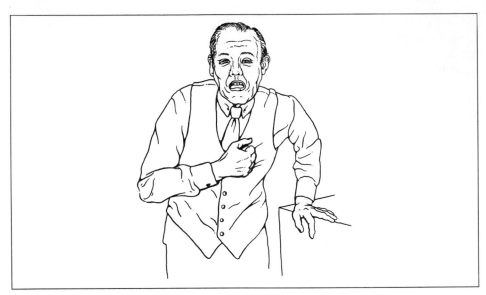

FIGURE 12-5
Levine sign. A classic nonverbal expression of angina.

PALPITATION

This is a general term that describes an awareness of the heart beat that may occur with increased stroke volume, irregularity of rhythm, tachycardia, or bradycardia. The precise identification of the underlying disturbance requires electrocardiographic confirmation. Nonetheless, a close clinical estimate may at times be possible by tapping out various cadences on the back of the hand and asking the patient to select the one that most closely simulates what he felt. Palpitation often is of no consequence, but its importance must be judged in the context of the symptoms.

COUGH

Cough, especially at night, is a common complaint with pulmonary congestion. It may be a dry hack or may produce clear, thin sputum. **Hemoptysis** may accompany cough when pulmonary venous pressures are greatly elevated, as in mitral stenosis or severe left ventricular failure (see Chap. 11). Dyspnea is usually associated with cough of cardiac origin.

SYNCOPE

Syncope of cardiac origin has two general causes: (1) inability of the heart to maintain an adequate cardiac output for a given level of activity or (2) cardiac arrhythmia resulting in sudden loss of cardiac output. Both of these mechanisms result in decreased perfusion of the central nervous system, causing loss of consciousness, occasionally seizure activity, and loss of motor control. Abnormalities that prevent the maintenance of an adequate cardiac output include left ventricular outflow obstruction (aortic stenosis, idiopathic hypertrophic subaortic stenosis [IHSS]), obstruction to flow at the mitral orifice (mitral stenosis [rare], atrial myxoma), and pulmo-

TABLE 12-1. Some Causes of Syncope

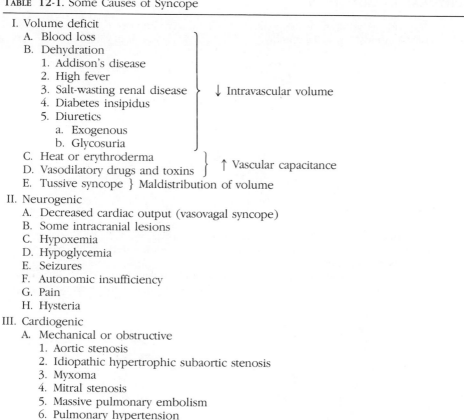

I. Volume deficit
   A. Blood loss
   B. Dehydration
      1. Addison's disease
      2. High fever
      3. Salt-wasting renal disease   ↓ Intravascular volume
      4. Diabetes insipidus
      5. Diuretics
         a. Exogenous
         b. Glycosuria
   C. Heat or erythroderma   ↑ Vascular capacitance
   D. Vasodilatory drugs and toxins
   E. Tussive syncope } Maldistribution of volume

II. Neurogenic
   A. Decreased cardiac output (vasovagal syncope)
   B. Some intracranial lesions
   C. Hypoxemia
   D. Hypoglycemia
   E. Seizures
   F. Autonomic insufficiency
   G. Pain
   H. Hysteria

III. Cardiogenic
   A. Mechanical or obstructive
      1. Aortic stenosis
      2. Idiopathic hypertrophic subaortic stenosis
      3. Myxoma
      4. Mitral stenosis
      5. Massive pulmonary embolism
      6. Pulmonary hypertension
   B. Arrhythmias

nary hypertension (severe). Syncope caused by these conditions generally occurs during physical exertion (when cardiac output cannot keep up with increased demand) and rarely happens at rest.

Either tachyarrhythmias (especially ventricular tachycardia) or bradyarrhythmias (e.g., complete heart block) can result in sufficient reduction in cerebral blood flow to cause syncope. Syncopal episodes due to arrhythmia (often termed Stokes-Adams attacks) can occur with the patient either at rest or performing activity. A history of palpitations or fatigue may also be obtained in such patients.

While syncope has many causes in association with other cardiac symptoms, including the simple faint (Table 12-1), it should alert the clinician to a limited spectrum of disorders such as those mentioned above.

PHYSICAL EXAMINATION

1. With patient sitting, note the general appearance (respiratory pattern, vital signs, color—cyanosis or pallor, fundi).

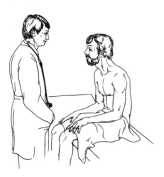

2. With patient recumbent and head elevated 30 degrees, examine the following:
   a. Upper and lower extremities (arterial pulses, venous pattern, color, nails, hair, temperature, edema).
   b. Neck (carotid pulses, jugular venous pressure, jugular venous pulse, thyroid).
   c. Precordium (inspection, direct percussion, palpation, auscultation).

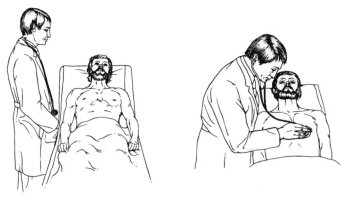

3. With patient in left decubitus position, repeat palpation and auscultation.

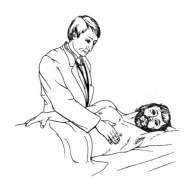

4. With patient sitting (again), repeat palpation and auscultation (precordium and neck).

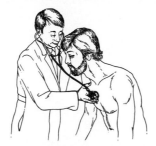

5. Perform special maneuvers (squatting, standing, Valsalva, isometric, amyl nitrite).

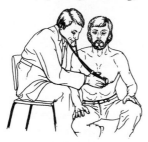

Begin with the patient sitting. Your initial observations, including examination of the fundi and lungs, have been done already in the physical examination. Then have the patient recline with arms at sides. Station yourself on the right. You may wish to retake the blood pressure. Then examine the extremities, neck, and precordium, in that order. The male patient will be disrobed to the waist. A towel is very satisfactory for draping the female chest; it can be manipulated to allow all necessary observations without causing undue embarrassment. Have adequate light and a quiet room, and eliminate all distractions as much as possible. Position the examining table or bed, which preferably has an adjustable head, at a comfortable height.

GENERAL OBSERVATION

Preliminary inspection begins during history taking (see Chaps. 3 and 4). Facies, body build, character of respiration (supine and sitting), general color, obvious pulsations, and signs of emotional tension may all be casually observed at this time.

The *face* may give clues to cardiovascular disease. In addition to the anxious expression of the patient suffering from chest pain, facial features may give clues to the discrete kind of heart disease. Patients with *mitral stenosis* may have either a malar flush or a slight cyanosis of lips and cheeks, which often is so distinctive that the valve disease can be promptly diagnosed by the experienced observer before auscultation. The protuberant eyes of Graves' disease may alert the physician to the thyrotoxic etiology of a rapid irregular heart rhythm and congestive failure. Malar telangiectasia and alopecia in a young woman with cardiac complaints requires

TABLE 12-2. Some Causes of Cyanosis

I. Central cyanosis
   A. Decreased oxygenation of blood
      1. Lung disease
      2. Arteriovenous pulmonary shunts
         a. Congenital
         b. Acquired
      3. Right-to-left intracardiac shunts
   B. Increased desaturated hemoglobin (>5 gm)
      1. Erythrocytosis
      2. Abnormal hemoglobins
II. Peripheral cyanosis (due to increased tissue oxygen extraction with slow flow)
   A. Congestive heart failure
   B. Hyperviscosity
   C. Veno-occlusive disease
   D. Hypotension
   E. Distal vasoconstriction
      1. Drugs
      2. Cold
      3. Anxiety

consideration of the myopericarditis of lupus erythematosus. The head nodding of severe aortic regurgitation should alert you to consider this diagnosis.

Cyanosis is a bluish skin color caused by a relative decrease in oxygen saturation of the cutaneous capillary blood. Normal arterial blood is about 95 percent saturated (venous blood is about 70 percent saturated). When the arterial saturation falls below 85 percent, cyanosis usually becomes manifest (unless anemia is so severe that the 5 gm of desaturated hemoglobin required to produce cyanosis in the patient are missing).

Cyanosis may be central or peripheral. *Central cyanosis* has three major causes: (1) congenital heart diseases with right-to-left shunts, (2) pulmonary arteriovenous fistulas, and (3) advanced pulmonary disease with hypoxemia. Central cyanosis is generalized and is associated with arterial oxygen desaturation. Polycythemia and clubbing are frequently present. *Peripheral cyanosis* (sometimes called acrocyanosis) is limited to the hands, feet, tip of the nose, ear lobes, and lips. It results from a critical reduction in systemic blood flow that usually is due to diminished cardiac output (heart failure shock) or obstructive peripheral arterial disease. The extremities are usually cold and mottled. Clubbing is not a consequence of these disorders alone. Light pressure will produce a sustained white print in the bluish background, which fades slowly.

Severe anxiety or pain may cause diaphoresis (sweating). Marked diaphoresis—a cold, "clammy" sweat—may be associated with an acutely decreased cardiac output, as in acute myocardial infarction. Pallor can be a component of shock as well, and is due to intense cutaneous vasoconstriction in the face of decreased cardiac output.

EXTREMITIES
GENERAL

First examine the arms and legs, paying particular attention to the hands and feet. Make your observations in the following order: (1) fingernails and toenails, (2) skin color, (3) hair distribution, (4) venous pattern, (5) presence of swelling or atrophy, and (6) obvious pulsations. Develop the habit of comparing sides. Estimate skin temperature by light, quick palpation with the tips of the fingers or with the back of the middle phalanges of the clenched fist. Compare identical sites on both sides and the gradation of temperature along the limb. The level of vascular tone in the extremities is under sympathetic control. Vasodilation results in rubor, warmth, throbbing of the distal digits, and capillary pulsations of the nailbeds, with distention of the superficial veins. Vasoconstriction results in pallor, coldness, and collapsed superficial veins. Smoking cigarettes, chilling, or apprehension may cause vasoconstriction. In the dependent position the superficial veins become distended, and the venous valves may be identified as nodular bulges; with elevation of the limb the veins collapse. These changes in caliber are at times a cause of undue concern to patients.

CLUBBING

Clubbing of the digits has been previously mentioned, in Chapter 4. Three cardiovascular causes of clubbing are cyanotic congenital heart disease, infective endocarditis, and pulmonary disease often associated with cor pulmonale.

ARTERIES

Arterial occlusion may be complete or partial; it may occur acutely or gradually. Chronic arterial insufficiency results from gradual reduction in vessel caliber, which may be due to degenerative or inflammatory processes of the vascular wall. Examination of a limb with chronic arterial insufficiency may show some or all of the following:

1. Diminished or absent pulses.
2. Audible systolic bruits, especially those extending into early diastole heard over major arteries (femoral or subclavian).
3. Reduced or absent hair peripherally (over the digits and dorsum of the hands or feet).
4. Atrophy of muscles and soft tissues.
5. Thin, shiny, taut skin.
6. Thickened nails with rough transverse ridges and longitudinal curving.
7. Mild brawny edema.
8. Coldness on palpation.
9. Intense grayish pallor on elevation of the extremity. Dependency after a minute or two of elevation produces a dusky, plum-colored rubor that develops very gradually (30 seconds to 1 minute).
10. Flat, collapsed superficial veins.
11. Delayed venous filling time. Empty the superficial veins by elevating the extremity. Prompt filling (less than 10 seconds) occurs normally with lowering.

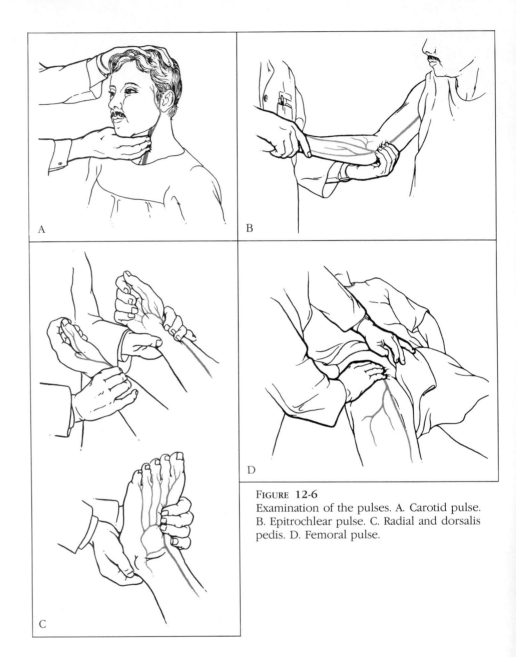

FIGURE 12-6
Examination of the pulses. A. Carotid pulse.
B. Epitrochlear pulse. C. Radial and dorsalis
pedis. D. Femoral pulse.

In examining an upper or lower extremity for suspected underlying arterial insufficiency, it is particularly important to assess the effects of exercise in order to identify early disease. Three important changes may be elicited with exercise.

1. Pallor of the skin may occur over the distal limb.
2. Arterial pulses may disappear.
3. Systolic bruits not present at rest may become apparent over the major arteries.

These important diagnostic signs may become apparent only following exercise.

Advanced arterial insufficiency shows all the above features, and in addition there may be (1) a bluish gray mottling of the skin unchanged by position, (2) early ulceration between or on the tips of the digits, (3) tenderness to pressure, (4) stocking anesthesia. These signs indicate that gangrene is imminent.

Chronic occlusion of the aortic bifurcation is associated with (1) absent femoral pulses, (2) intermittent claudication extending into the buttocks, and (3) sexual impotence. These together comprise Leriche's syndrome.

Acute arterial occlusion usually begins with agonizing pain in the affected extremity, which below the occlusion site is pale, cyanotic, and pulseless. It may also be tender and exhibit stocking anesthesia. This is a serious emergency.

Figure 12-6 illustrates several maneuvers for examining the peripheral arterial pulses. Use the three middle fingers (not simply a single finger) and vary the pressure. Occlude the vessel completely at first and release gradually. Examination of the peripheral arterial system should include auscultation over the femoral arteries, abdominal aorta, and carotid and subclavian arteries for bruits that might indicate occlusive disease.

ARTERIAL PULSE

When a patient affected by this disease [aortic regurgitation] is stripped, the arterial trunks of the head, neck, and superior extremities immediately catch the eye by their singular pulsation.

SIR DOMINIC JOHN CORRIGAN
(1802–1880)

The pulse examination is done both in assessment of vital signs (rate and rhythm, as discussed in Chap. 5) and as part of the cardiovascular examination, in which all pulses listed in the red box are examined for (1) pulse rate, (2) rhythm, (3) amplitude, (4) any special quality, and (5) elasticity of the vessel wall. Amplitude may be classified as increased, normal, diminished or absent; or a numerical system of 0 to 4+ may be used, with 2+ being normal. The following diagrammatic representation is often used in recording pulses:

		Carotid	Supraclavicular	Brachial	Radial	Aorta	Femoral	Dorsalis pedis	Posterior Tibial
Normal = 2+	(R)	2+	2+	2+	2+	0	1+	1+	1+
	(L)	2+	2+	2+	2+	0	1+	1+	1+

The ulnar and popliteal arteries are often included.

In addition to rate and regularity, the arterial pulse should be examined for its amplitude and contour. The amplitude of the pulse is largely a function of the pulse pressure, which is related to stroke volume, elasticity of the arterial circulation, and peak velocity of the ejection of blood from the left ventricle. If the stroke volume increases—as with excitement, heat, alcohol ingestion, exercise, or slowing of the heart rate—the pulse pressure widens, giving a bounding quality on palpation.

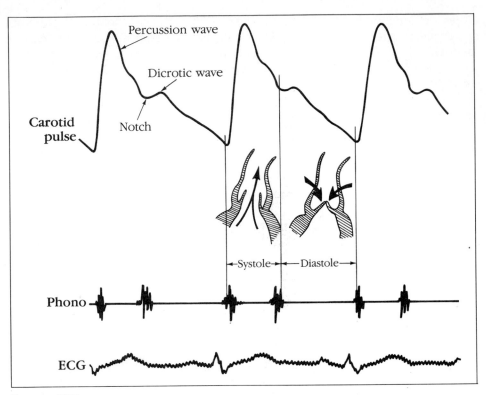

FIGURE 12-7
Normal carotid pulse. Pulse contour is shown as related to the timing of aortic valve motion, phonocardiogram, and electrocardiogram.

The amplitude of the pulse obviously contributes to its contour. However, important information about the characteristics of left ventricular ejection can be learned from assessing the rate of rise and the shape of the arterial pulse wave. Because of the distortion that occurs when the pulse wave is transmitted distally, the carotid arteries must be used for accurate evaluation of pulse contour. An excellent way of analyzing pulse contour is to correlate it with a graphic record. Figure 12-7 shows such a tracing that was recorded from a normal carotid artery. The initial percussion wave is separated from the dicrotic wave (not palpated in the normal state) by a dicrotic notch caused by aortic valve closure. A second systolic wave (tidal wave) usually follows the percussion wave but is not often palpable. The record is qualitative, but it helps the beginner to understand better what he feels. The upstroke normally takes no more than 0.10 second, and the rounded crest takes another 0.08 to 0.12 second. The brachial and femoral pulses are usually synchronous.

The *Valsalva maneuver* is a test that you can perform on yourself right at this moment. It will challenge your ability to observe and to interpret a rather complex series of physiologic variations. Close your glottis and strain down hard for several seconds while palpating your carotid or radial pulse. What happens?

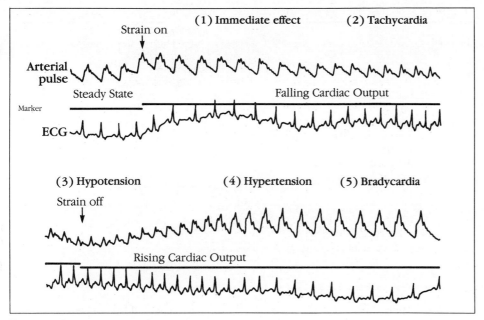

FIGURE 12-8
Normal response to Valsalva maneuver (see text).

The normal response to the Valsalva maneuver is shown in Figure 12-8. The explanation is as follows: (1) The high intrathoracic pressure decreases venous return, causing an abrupt drop in cardiac output after several seconds. (2) The normal response to the decreased output is twofold: peripheral vasoconstriction and tachycardia. (3) Despite this compensatory mechanism, the pulse pressure dwindles; that decrease causes the pulse to become feeble. (4) After release the cardiac output is suddenly restored, causing an abrupt increase in blood pressure due to the temporary increase in peripheral vascular resistance. (5) Increased blood pressure in turn triggers a reflex bradycardia (slowing), which is transient and somewhat delayed. Finally, the normal state returns. Responses (4) and (5) disappear with many forms of heart disease.

The quality of the arterial pulse may provide clues to many circulatory disorders other than peripheral vascular disease.

Water-hammer pulse (Table 12-3) is characterized by a wide pulse pressure, a low diastolic pressure, and a dicrotic notch that is absent or displaced downward on the descending limb of the tidal wave. The pulse has a collapsing, bounding quality that is reinforced by elevating the arm above the head. It is a classic sign of aortic regurgitation but is seen in other conditions in which there is a low-resistance runoff due to a leak in the arterial system—for example, patent ductus arteriosus and peripheral arteriovenous fistula. It is the basis for other peripheral signs of aortic regurgitation, including hopping carotids, pistol-shot sounds, Duroziez's sign, de Musset's sign, and others. Although interesting, these signs add little of diagnostic importance.

TABLE 12-3. Some Characteristic Arterial Pulse Wave Forms

Normal	

Water-hammer pulse
  Occurs in aortic insufficiency and other
    abnormalities associated with wide
    pulse pressure
A bounding pulse	

Anacrotic pulse (pulsus tardus) Occurs in aortic stenosis	
Bifid pulse (pulsus bisferiens) Occurs in aortic insufficiency	

Spike-and-dome pulse
  Occurs in idiopathic hyptertrophic
    subaortic stenosis	

Pulsus alternans Occurs in left ventricular failure	

Bounding pulses of lesser degree, which are characterized by a wide pulse pressure with a normal or slightly lower diastolic pressure, also occur. Fever, anemia, hepatic failure, thyrotoxicosis, and complete heart block are all capable of producing a bounding pulse. They have in common an increased stroke volume and a diminished peripheral resistance.

Weak pulse (pulsus parvus) has a normal contour but a low amplitude. It feels weak and thready. The pulse pressure is narrowed by a low stroke volume and associated peripheral vasoconstriction. It is present with low-output failures of all types. Common causes include mitral stenosis, acute myocardial infarction, shock, and constrictive pericarditis.

Anacrotic pulse (pulsus tardus) (see Table 12-3) is associated with valvular aortic stenosis. The ascending limb is delayed and the summit is broad. The pulse pressure may be narrowed. The slow rise and delayed peak can often be appreciated with careful practice.

Bifid pulse (pulsus bisferiens) (see Table 12-3) is characterized by double systolic peaks that can usually be felt with the palpating finger. Bifid pulse is found with aortic regurgitation, which may be isolated or, more frequently, may be associated with some degree of aortic stenosis.

Another type of pulse with two systolic waves is the *spike-and-dome pulse* of dynamic aortic outflow tract obstruction (IHSS, asymmetric septal hypertrophy) (see Table 12-3). This pulse is characterized by an extremely brisk initial wave (spike) followed by a rounded dome that occurs after the muscular obstruction to left ventricular outflow develops. The rounded dome is not as easily felt as the second peak of the bifid pulse of aortic regurgitation, and consequently the two waves of this pulse may be difficult to appreciate. However, the abrupt rise and fall of the spike may be a significant clue to the presence of IHSS.

The *dicrotic pulse* has two waves but only one is systolic, and the second is a very prominent dicrotic wave occurring in diastole. This pulse is best appreciated in a more peripheral artery (brachial or femoral) and is usually seen in younger patients with myocardial disease and in hypovolemic states.

In *pulsus alternans* (see Table 12-3) the regular consecutive beats are of alternating large and small amplitude. It can be detected by palpation (best appreciated in a peripheral vessel) or by use of a blood pressure cuff. Alternate systolic pressures may vary by as much as 25 mm Hg. It is an important sign of left ventricular failure.

Bigeminal pulse (bigeminy) is a coupling of two beats separated by a pause. It results most often from alternating normal and premature beats. The second beat is weak due to reduced diastolic filling time.

Pulsus paradoxus is an important sign of cardiac tamponade. It is found with tense pericardial effusions and less frequently with chronic constrictive pericarditis. The term refers to a weakening of the pulse during normal inspiration. It is really a misnomer, however, since what happens is an exaggeration of the normal (up to 10 mm Hg) inspiratory decline in systolic blood pressure. Multiple mechanisms for pulsus paradoxus have been postulated. The observed fall in systolic blood pressure with inspiration is thought to be caused by normal inspiratory augmentation of venous return to the right heart chambers in a heart with restricted capacity for diastolic filling. As a result, there is a reciprocal decrease in left ventricular filling and a fall in systolic blood pressure. Increased capacitance of the pulmonary vasculature in inspiration (with less of the right heart output entering the left ventricle from the lungs, therefore) may also play a role. Although pulsus paradoxus may be detected by palpation, it is more reliably quantitated by using the sphygmomanometer. As the pressure in the cuff is slowly reduced, the first Korotkoff sounds will appear only during expiration (upper systolic level). As one lowers the pressure, the sounds begin to occur in both inspiration and expiration (lower systolic level). A difference of greater than 10 mm Hg between these two points is abnormal. A common noncardiac cause of pulsus paradoxus is the labored respiration of the patient with obstructive pulmonary diseases (asthma, emphysema).

Abdominal bruits may be a sign of intra-abdominal disease. Because of their demonstrated common occurrence in young healthy individuals, it is important to be cautious about overinterpretation of such a bruit as an isolated finding. In the

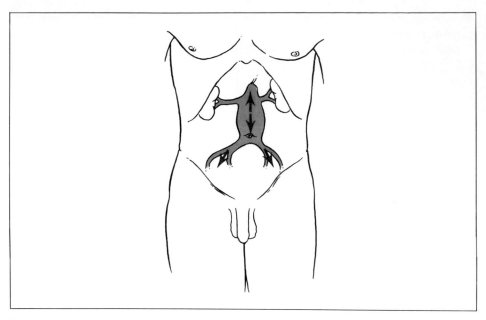

FIGURE   12-9
Abdominal aortic aneurysm. Note the radiation of the murmur, indicated by arrows.

presence of hypertension, however, a bruit heard in the epigastrium or subcostal region may be an important sign of renal artery stenosis. Abdominal bruits are best heard using the diaphragm of the stethoscope. They are commonly very soft and of medium or low pitch. Similar systolic bruits have been observed in patients with mesenteric arterial disease (abdominal angina) as well as over greatly enlarged spleens. Venous hums are at times identified over the cirrhotic liver due to torrential flow through venous collaterals. In addition, neoplasms of the pancreas, stomach, and liver may rarely produce abdominal systolic bruits due to arterial involvement or an increase in local blood flow.

There is no disease more conducive to humility than aneurysm of the aorta.
                                                            SIR WILLIAM OSLER
                                                            (1849–1919)

Aneurysm of an artery produces a pulsatile swelling along the course of the vessel. The aorta and the popliteal artery are the vessels most often involved. A systolic thrill may be felt over the aneurysm. The aorta should always be carefully palpated for the presence of an aneurysm. This is usually felt as an expansile mass in the epigastrium and midabdomen. Rupture of an aortic aneurysm is usually indicated by severe, constant back pain and is often associated with pain in one or both groins and a mass in the flank. It constitutes a serious surgical emergency and is an important consideration in any patient with an acute abdomen (see Chap. 14). If the thrill noted over such a mass is continuous, one should suspect an arteriovenous fistula.

DISORDERS OF RHYTHM

When the heart slowed down after partial recovery, I found that the jugular and liver pulses were of the ventricular form, that the presystolic murmur had disappeared, and that the heart was irregular; in other words, all evidence of auricular activity had disappeared. [*Atrial fibrillation*]

SIR JAMES MACKENZIE
(1853–1925)

The electrocardiogram is indispensable for the precise recognition and identification of arrhythmias, but much can be learned by careful examination at the bedside. Some of the common arrhythmias and their associated physical findings are listed in Table 12-4.

VEINS

That the blood in the veins therefore proceeds from inferior or more remote to superior parts, and towards the heart moving in this and not in the contrary direction, appears most obviously.

WILLIAM HARVEY
(1578–1657)

Varicose veins is the term usually applied to dilation of the superficial leg veins. *Varicose* means "dilated, swollen." The rate of blood flow through these vessels is diminished, and the intraluminal pressure is increased. There are two types of varicose veins: primary, due to an inherent weakness of the vessel wall and venous valves; and secondary, due to proximal obstruction in the vena cava, pelvic veins, or iliofemoral veins. Both the greater and lesser saphenous system may be involved. The greater saphenous vein lies superficially on the anteromedial aspect of the thigh and lower leg. It drains into the common femoral vein on the groin. The lesser saphenous vein lies superficially on the posterolateral aspect of the calf from the ankle to the popliteal space. Both saphenous veins communicate with the deep femoral venous system by means of multiple communicating or perforating veins that pierce the fascia. When the valves in the perforating veins are incompetent, the superficial saphenous varicosities may fill from the deep venous system.

Diagnosis, usually simple, is made by inspection of the dependent limb. In severe cases, pigmentation, edema, and even ulceration of the skin in the region of the medial malleolus point to significant venostasis. It is important to determine two additional facts in patients with varicose veins: Are the valves incompetent in the communicating veins between the superficial and deep systems? Are the deep veins patent?

The presence of incompetent communicating or perforating veins can be demonstrated simply. Lift the leg to empty the veins. A tourniquet is applied around the thigh with the patient in the recumbent position. When the patient assumes an erect position, the incompetent valves in the communicating veins permit the varicosities to fill rapidly from above (*Trendelenburg's test*).

Patency of the deep veins may be established by the use of the *Perthes' test*. A tourniquet is used to occlude the subcutaneous veins at knee or thigh level. This tourniquet must be at or below the lowest significant incompetent perforator. Filling of the superficial varicosities from above is prevented by the tourniquet. As the

TABLE 12-4. Some Common Arrhythmias and Their Associated Physical Findings

ECG	Jugular Venous Pulse	Arterial Pulse	Cardiac Examination
Long PR interval	Prolonged AV wave interval	No effect	Diminished intensity S_1
Short PR interval	Decreased AV wave interval	No effect	Increased intensity S_1
Left bundle-branch block	No effect	No effect	Reversed split S_2 (paradoxical split)
Right bundle-branch block	No effect	No effect	Persistently split S_2
2nd degree AV block	"Extra" A waves	Slow rate	"Extra" S_4
3rd degree AV block	Intermittent cannon A waves	Slow rate	Variable intensity S_1; intermittent S_4
Atrial fibrillation	Absent A waves	Irregularly irregular rate	Variable intensity S_1
Premature atrial contraction	Early A waves	Irregular rate	Premature cardiac cycle
Paroxysmal atrial tachycardia	Rapid venous pulsations	Rapid, often diminished	"Bouncing precordium" (loud S_1)
Premature ventricular contraction	Possible cannon A wave	Irregular	Premature cardiac cycle
Ventricular tachycardia	Intermittent cannon A waves	Rapid, usually diminished	Variable intensities, "cascade" rhythm

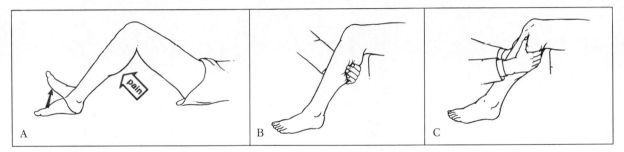

FIGURE   12-10
Examining for deep venous thrombosis. A. Homans' sign. B. Palpation of the lateral calf demonstrates muscle tenderness in the gastrocnemius. C. Palpation in the groove of the gastrocnemius demonstrates the pain or cord of phlebitis.

patient walks, the muscles exert a pumping action on the deep veins and drain the
dilated superficial varicosities. Failure of the varicosities to empty means either that
the tourniquet is placed too high and a large incompetent communicating vein permits the varices to fill, or that the deep veins have been damaged by an inflammatory process, disturbing their normal function.

Venous thrombosis may be acute (thrombophlebitis) or silent (formerly termed
phlebothrombosis), deep or superficial. Superficial thrombophlebitis produces
redness, induration, and tenderness adjacent to the involved venous segment,
which is thickened and cordlike. Diagnosis is easily made, but remember that there
may be associated deep thrombosis.

Acute inflammatory thrombosis of a major vein (deep thrombophlebitis) results
in rather striking pain, tenderness, warmth, and swelling of the involved limb. Sensation is preserved, and superficial veins may be distended. There may be considerable reflex arteriospasm, which at times may cause the extremity to become pale
and the peripheral pulses to be reduced or even absent (phlegmasia cerulea
dolens). This must be differentiated from acute arterial occlusion, which usually
occurs without swelling of the extremity.

Deep venous thrombosis involving the deep femoral and pelvic veins may be entirely asymptomatic, and fatal pulmonary embolism may occur without warning. It
is worthwhile for the physician to become "thrombosis conscious" and constantly
to watch for minor suggestive signs in his bedfast patients. These include (1) tenderness along the iliac vessels and below the inguinal ligament, along the femoral
canal, in the popliteal space, over the deep calf veins, and over the plantar veins; (2)
minimal swelling detectable only by measuring and comparing the circumference
of both calves and both thighs at several levels; (3) unexplained low-grade fever
and tachycardia; and (4) a trace of ankle edema. Homans' sign, calf pain on dorsiflexion of the foot, is also a sign of deep venous thrombosis (Fig. 12-10). With this
maneuver it is important to distinguish between calf pain and Achilles tendon pain.
The latter is common in patients who wear high heels, for example. When examining for Homans' sign it is important to flex the knee in order to reduce false positive responses. Unfortunately, the clinical diagnosis of deep venous thrombosis is
not very reliable.

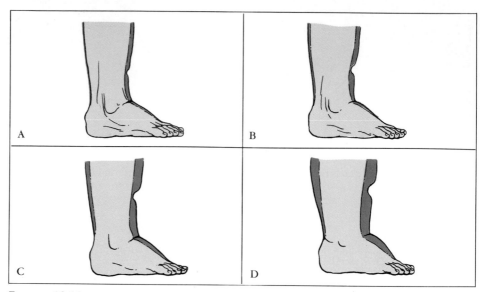

Figure 12-11
Grading of edema. A. 1+: slight pit, normal contours. B. 2+: deeper pit, fairly normal contours. C. 3+: deep pit, puffy appearance. D. 4+: deep pit, frankly swollen.

Table 12-5. Some Causes of Edema

I. Increased hydrostatic pressure in the vascular space
  A. Increased volume
    1. Congestive heart failure
    2. Renal failure
    3. Certain hormones (estrogens, corticosteroids)
    4. Certain drugs (indomethacin, sodium-rich compounds)
  B. Increased mechanical pressure (total volume normal or low)
    1. Venous thrombosis
    2. Compression of veins (tumor, scar, fibrosis, gravid uterus, etc.)
    3. Pericardial constriction
    4. Portal hypertension
    5. Prolonged standing

II. Decreased oncotic pressure in the vascular space—hypoproteinemia ($\downarrow$ albumin)
  A. Nephrotic syndrome
  B. Starvation
  C. Protein-losing enteropathy

III. Tissue or vascular damage
  A. Vasculitis
  B. Allergy
  C. Trauma
  D. Burns
  E. Ischemia
  F. Infection

IV. Other
  A. Myxedema
  B. Lymphedema

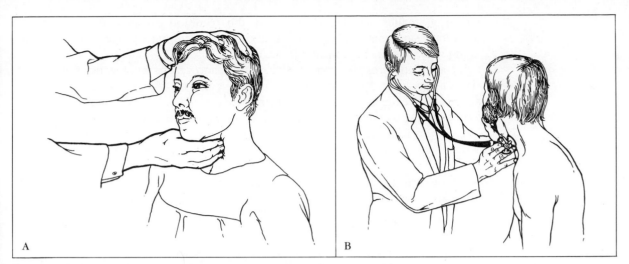

FIGURE   12-12
A. Palpation of the carotid pulse. Some examiners prefer palpating the carotid pulse with the patient in the sitting position. B. Auscultation of the carotid artery.

EDEMA

Edema has many causes. It is graded 1+ through 4+ on the basis of pitting produced by sustained, light pressure with the thumb over the medial malleolus or pretibial area. Cardiac edema is usually dependent (feet and ankles, or back and flanks if the patient is supine). It is a common though not reliable sign of congestive heart failure. Unilateral edema occurs following the occlusion of a major vein. Chronic peripheral arterial occlusion may cause mild "brawny" (nonpitting) edema.

NECK

In the assessment of cardiovascular status the physician should make four separate observations in the neck: (1) carotid pulse, (2) jugular venous pressure, (3) jugular venous pulse (wave form), and (4) venous and arterial auscultation.

CAROTID PULSE

With the patient supine, palpate each carotid medial to the sternocleidomastoid muscle just below the angle of the jaw. The three-finger method may be used, although some examiners prefer to use the thumb (Fig. 12-12A). Auscultation of the carotid arteries to detect bruits is advisable prior to carotid palpation (Fig. 12-12B).

Carotid pulsations may be striking in hyperkinetic states and particularly with aortic regurgitation (Corrigan's sign). A carotid thrill is commonly felt with aortic stenosis but may result from increased flow associated with aortic regurgitation. It also occurs with partial occlusion of the orifice of the common carotid artery. A bruit may be heard over a partially occluded carotid artery.

Diminished or absent carotid and brachial pulsations may result from a diffuse process involving the aortic arch and its major branches. This is called the aortic arch syndrome. It may be due to arteriosclerosis, aortitis, aortic aneurysm, or congenital anomalies. Isolated occlusion of the common carotid artery may cause neurologic symptoms and signs. Internal carotid pulsation may be estimated by palpating the vessel in the tonsillar fossa.

Carotid sinus pressure increases vagal tone and results in slowing of the heart rate. On occasion this response may be exaggerated, and carotid sinus pressure will result in extreme bradycardia (even cardiac standstill) or hypotension (the carotid sinus syndrome). The Valsalva maneuver, combined with carotid sinus pressure, results in more pronounced vagal tone. Carotid sinus pressure is frequently used in the diagnosis and treatment of certain arrhythmias. It is also helpful in transiently slowing the heart rate to aid in auscultation. Carotid sinus pressure should be applied cautiously (if at all) in the elderly, who are prone to have carotid artery atherosclerosis. The carotid pulse may be palpated from behind or anteriorly.

JUGULAR VENOUS PRESSURE

The first of the two sudden elevations (venous pulse) immediately precedes ventricular systole, while the second coincides nearly exactly with it; . . . in the third place and finally, a light pressure suitably applied to the lower portion of the neck can impede them or suppress them entirely, while the pulsations of the carotid persist with all their intensity.

PIERRE CARL EDOUARD POTAIN
(1825–1901)

Satisfactory examination of the neck veins requires a bed or table that will allow the patient's head and trunk to be elevated to various heights. Clothing should be removed from the neck and upper thorax, and good illumination should be available. If pillows are removed and the head is turned slightly away from the examiner (without putting a marked stretch on the neck), the neck veins can be visualized in the majority of patients. The head of the bed should be raised and lowered to bring the patient to the position where venous pulsations and the meniscus of the internal jugular vein (marking the height of the venous pressure) can be easily seen.

Maximum information can be gained only with proper technique. The thumb is placed on the opposite carotid artery for timing purposes. Occasionally, tangential lighting with a pocket flashlight is helpful. The neck veins are frequently distended with the patient supine, tending to collapse with inspiration and to refill during expiration. Light pressure over the jugular bulb causes them to distend further, and release is followed by collapse to the previous level. Because of the effects of gravity, distention usually disappears when the head of the bed is elevated to 45 degrees. This position is satisfactory for determining jugular venous pressure in the majority of instances. With severe elevation of jugular venous pressure, greater degrees of elevation of the bed may be needed.

Observe the base of the neck for venous pulsations. Four simple maneuvers should be followed in order: (1) note the general character of the pulse, which is normally diffuse and undulant; (2) observe any variation produced by respiration; (3) apply light pressure to the root of the neck, observing the effect on the pulsations; and (4) gradually elevate the head of the bed or the examining table in increments to the 45-degree level and note the overall effect. Lastly, the jugular venous pressure (JVP) is estimated by thinking of the neck veins as manometer tubes directly attached to the heart (right atrium). The internal jugular vein is more reli-

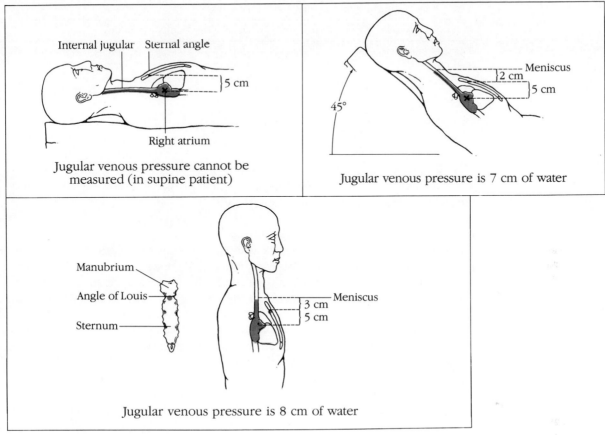

Jugular venous pressure cannot be measured (in supine patient)

Jugular venous pressure is 7 cm of water

Jugular venous pressure is 8 cm of water

FIGURE 12-13
Measuring the jugular venous pressure. The sternal angle (angle of Louis) is a bony ridge palpable between the manubrium and the body of the sternum at the level of the second intercostal space. It is always 5 cm vertically above the mid-right atrium. In any position, therefore, one may measure the distance from the sternal angle to the meniscus of the internal jugular vein and add 5 cm to obtain the jugular venous pressure.

able than the external for this purpose. Both will collapse, however, at the point at which the intraluminal pressure falls below the level of atmospheric pressure. With practice, this point can be identified, and its level above a reference point, such as the sternal angle (angle of Louis), can be estimated while the head of the bed is adjusted gradually upward. The sternal angle has been chosen for this purpose since its distance above the midpoint of the right atrium remains relatively constant (about 5 cm) in all positions (Fig. 12-13). A more direct estimate of the right atrial pressure can be achieved by using a central venous pressure catheter. Although a reasonable estimate of the jugular venous pressure in centimeters above the sternal angle can usually be achieved, a simpler scale of normal, mildly, and markedly increased will often suffice (Table 12-6).

Jugular venous pressure elevation is an important sign of congestive heart failure, although elevations of venous pressure may result from mechanical obstruction to venous inflow by intrathoracic, neoplastic, inflammatory, or vascular masses.

TABLE 12-6. Estimating the Jugular Venous Pressure

Height of Meniscus above Sternal Angle	Degree of Venous Elevation
2–4 cm	Mild
4–8 cm	Moderate
>8 cm	Severe

The presence of jugular venous hypertension may escape notice in obese or bull-necked individuals. Also, extreme venous hypertension may go unnoticed because the veins may be distended all the way to the angle of the jaw and pulsations are not seen. Pregnancy invariably increases jugular pressure. Exertion, anxiety, premenstrual increases in blood volume, and abdominal pressure (caused by corsets and binders) may produce mild elevations.

JUGULAR VENOUS PULSES (WAVE FORM)

The bedside examination of the neck veins is a noninvasive method of assessing right atrial hemodynamics. The internal jugular vein connects without valves to the right atrium and accurately displays right atrial wave form and pressure to the careful observer. Two major waves occur in the normal right atrium during each cardiac cycle (Fig. 12-14). The larger of these is the A wave, which is generated as the atrium contracts to fill the ventricle just prior to systole. As the atrium relaxes and its pressure falls, the x descent is seen while ventricular systole begins and the tricuspid valve is closed. The right atrial pressure rises as the atrium is filled from the periphery, and the V wave, which is smaller than the A wave, is generated. As the atrium empties during early diastole, a fall of the V wave or y descent is seen. (The C wave, a positive deflection on the x descent, can sometimes be recorded on pulse tracings. It probably reflects displacement of the tricuspid valve apparatus into the right atrium during ventricular systole and is of little clinical significance.)

It is important to differentiate venous from arterial pulsations. The venous pulse is diffuse and undulant and usually disappears or markedly decreases in the sitting position. Venous waves can usually be obliterated by moderate pressure at the base of the neck. Venous *pressure* decreases with inspiration, although the venous *waves* may become more prominent during inspiration. Arterial pulsations in the neck are localized and brisk and are usually best seen high and medial to the sternocleidomastoid muscle, while venous pulsations are seen lower and more laterally, either under or just behind the sternocleidomastoid muscle. Arterial pulsations are unaffected by position and do not vary with respiration, nor can they be obliterated by pressure at the base of the neck as the venous pulse can be.

To time the jugular pulse you must use two senses in order to answer the question, "Is this wave occurring before or after the first sound?" Perhaps the simplest method is to use vision and touch, observing the venous pattern while palpating the opposite carotid pulse. If the wave precedes the arterial pulsation, it must be an A wave; if it is synchronous or a little delayed, it is a V wave. A second method is to use vision and hearing. Listen to the heart while making similar observations. Exceptions to this rule are caused by the occasional rhythm disturbance which superimposes atrial and ventricular contraction.

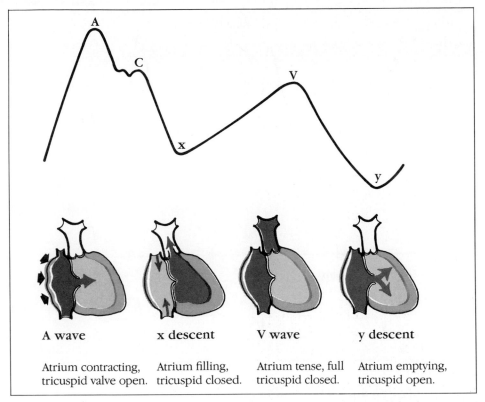

A wave | x descent | V wave | y descent

Atrium contracting, tricuspid valve open. | Atrium filling, tricuspid closed. | Atrium tense, full tricuspid closed. | Atrium emptying, tricuspid open.

FIGURE 12-14
Venous pulse. Events occurring in the right atrium are reflected in the jugular venous wave form.

Giant A waves result from very forceful right atrial contraction. They are seen with tricuspid stenosis. More commonly they result from the loss of diastolic compliance that accompanies right ventricular hypertrophy, as in pulmonary stenosis or pulmonary hypertension. Figure 12-15 shows the venous waves seen with marked pulmonary hypertension. The right atrium contracts vigorously to fill the poorly compliant right ventricle, and a large A wave is seen in the neck veins. With the onset of atrial fibrillation and the loss of the effective atrial contraction, giant A waves as well as normal A waves are no longer seen in the jugular venous pulse.

Cannon waves occur with certain arrhythmias characterized by atrioventricular dissociation (complete atrioventricular block, ventricular and nodal tachycardia, and premature ventricular beats). When atrial contraction occurs during ventricular systole, cannon waves result. The origin is the same in all these, namely, contraction of the right atrium against a closed tricuspid valve due to synchronous atrial and ventricular systole. Since the blood cannot move forward, there is striking backward regurgitation into the jugular system (Fig. 12-16).

Large V waves are transmitted to the neck with tricuspid regurgitation, which reflects abnormal right atrial filling through an incompetent tricuspid valve during

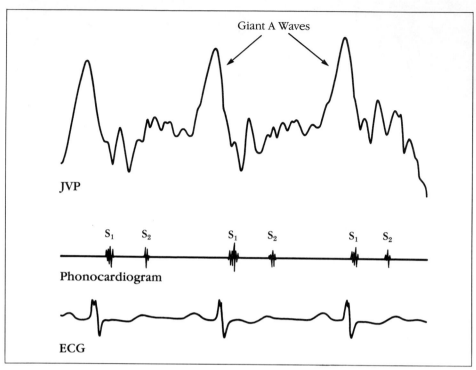

FIGURE   12-15
Giant A waves. Jugular venous pulse (JVP) tracing demonstrating giant A waves with marked pulmonary hypertension.

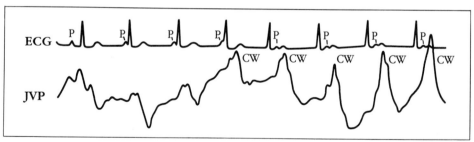

FIGURE   12-16
Cannon waves. Jugular venous pulse (JVP) tracing demonstrating cannon waves (CW). P waves on the ECG give the timing for atrial contractions.

systole. The jugular venous pulse tracing in Figure 12-17 shows V waves from a patient with rheumatic tricuspid regurgitation. Atrial fibrillation is often present with this condition. With the loss of organized atrial contractions, no A wave is seen. The large positive V wave occurs during ventricular systole (but earlier than the normal V wave) and can be timed by observation of the neck veins with simultaneous palpation of the carotid pulse or auscultation of the heart.

Sharp y descent is associated with an elevated mean pressure and is seen with chronic pericardial constriction and occasionally in acute pericardial effusion with

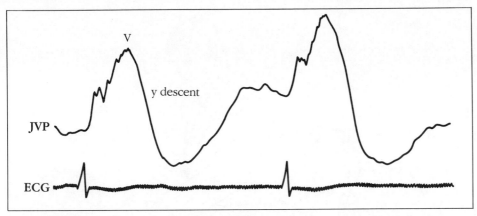

FIGURE   12-17
Large V waves. Jugular venous pulse (JVP) tracing demonstrating large V waves in a patient with rheumatic tricuspid regurgitation.

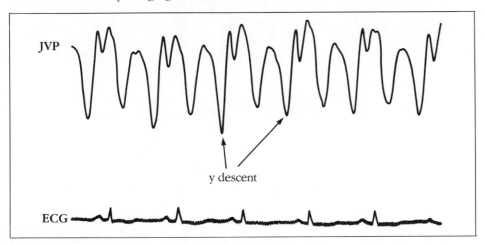

FIGURE   12-18
Sharp y descent. Jugular venous pulse (JVP) tracing demonstrating rapid y descent.

tamponade. It may be seen in severe right heart failure of any cause. In these conditions the pressure drops only briefly following tricuspid opening and remains elevated during the rest of the cardiac cycle. The sharp descents result in a characteristic **M**-shape in the jugular venous wave form (Fig. 12-18).

JUGULAR VENOUS AUSCULTATION
Venous hum refers to a phasic roaring heard in about 25 percent of normal adults (and almost always in children) at the lower border of the sternocleidomastoid muscle in the sitting position. It is accentuated in diastole and may be transmitted to the upper precordium. Hums are attenuated by compression over the jugular vein, the Valsalva maneuver, and recumbency. They are generally an innocent finding of no consequence.

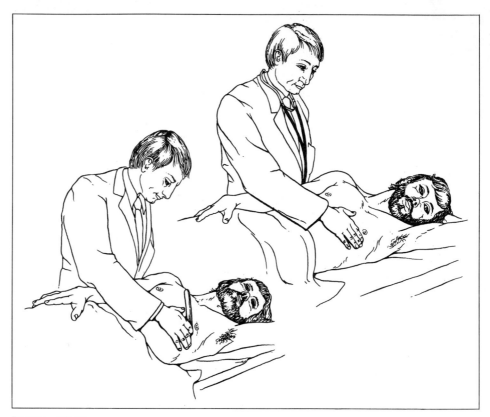

FIGURE   12-19
Palpation of the precordium. The morphology of the apical impulse can often be appreciated best in the left decubitus position. The impulse may be amplified by placing a tongue blade over the impulse.

HEART EXAMINATION

INSPECTION AND PALPATION OF THE PRECORDIUM

Move toward the foot of the bed and observe the precordium from the level of the anterior chest. The character and location of any visible cardiac impulses should be noted. Minor precordial movements can be amplified by observing during expiratory apnea. The commands "Now take in a breath, let it all out, hold it" will provide the optimal setting for detecting these pulsations. At times it may be helpful to place a tongue blade or stiff card over the precordial impulse, observing the movement of the free edge. This simply acts as a mechanical amplifier (Fig. 12-19). Now palpate the precordium carefully with the hand lightly applied, using primarily the middle and ring fingers.

Palpation of the precordium to discern movement is usually best performed using the pads of the distal and middle phalanges. Detection of thrills (palpable murmurs), however, is usually best accomplished using the sensitive area just proximal to metacarpophalangeal joints. Often, the sensation in this area is greater in one hand or the other. Trial and practice of palpation using different areas of the

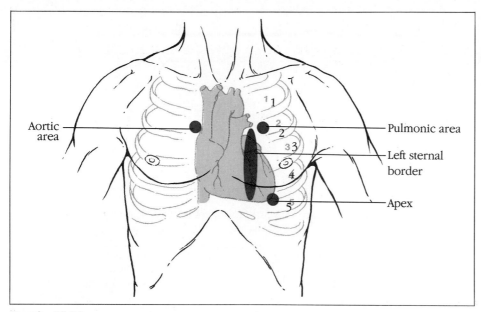

Aortic area

Pulmonic area

Left sternal border

Apex

FIGURE 12-20
Areas of routine palpation of the precordium.

hand as well as alternating hands will soon allow the examiner to determine which portion of which hand will yield the most information.

The four major areas that are explored are the apex, left sternal border, pulmonic area, and aortic area (Fig. 12-20). The apex impulse is always more forceful with the patient on his left side, which usually displaces the apex 2 to 3 cm to the left and brings it closer to the chest wall. The value of palpation lies in the estimation of heart size, ventricular hypertrophy, identification of low frequency (and sometimes inaudible) vibrations, and ectopic impulses.

What is seen and felt over the precordium varies markedly with position, phase of respiration, amount and distribution of muscle and fat, and thoracic cage configuration. In normal people the cardiac apex is usually the most lateral impulse of cardiac origin that can be felt on the chest wall. It is often referred to as the point of maximum impulse (PMI). In some patients with cardiac disease, however, the cardiac apex may not be the point of maximum impulse.

In order to appreciate the distinction between right- and left-sided events, as well as to note areas of paradoxical impulse, it is frequently helpful to palpate the precordium with two hands simultaneously. In this way, nonsynchronous movements can be distinguished from each other.

The normal apical impulse is in the fourth or fifth interspace, should not be felt in more than one interspace, usually occupies less than the first one-half of systole, and should not be felt farther to the left than halfway between the midsternal line and the lateral thoracic border. Placing the patient in the left lateral decubitus position (see Fig. 12-19) brings the cardiac apex closer to the chest wall. For purposes of auscultation and analysis of the configuration of the apical impulse, this is a useful maneuver, but assessment as to location and duration of the apical impulse

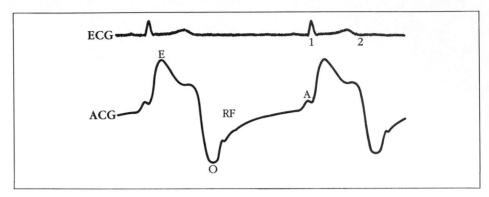

FIGURE 12-21
Normal apexcardiogram. The sharp outward movement (E) corresponds to ventricular systole and may be easily palpated at the cardiac apex. (O = end systole; RF = rapid filling.)

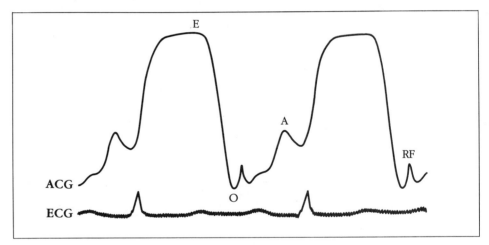

FIGURE 12-22
Apexcardiogram of left ventricular hypertrophy. Note the prolonged outward systolic motion and the exaggerated A wave, both of which are often palpable. Rapid filling (RF) in early diastole may, as here illustrated, produce a palpable impulse.

should be made with the patient supine. A graphic recording of the normal apex impulse is shown in Figure 12-21. Medial to the apical impulse one can often appreciate an inward motion that corresponds to retraction of the interventricular groove (septal retraction).

An outward systolic movement along the left sternal border is usually thought to be indicative of right ventricular pressure or volume overload; however, young, normal subjects frequently have a palpable impulse along the left sternal border, and this sign must be carefully interpreted in light of other findings. Similarly, pulmonary closure may be palpable in this group of patients without reflecting pathology.

Abnormal precordial movements are of prime diagnostic importance. They may be systolic or diastolic, outward or inward. Sustained low-frequency movements are usually visible and palpable; high-frequency vibrations are palpable only. Sustained high-frequency vibrations are called thrills, which are simply palpable murmurs. Short, high-frequency vibrations are known as shocks, which are palpable heart sounds.

Left ventricular hypertrophy produces a sustained, systolic apex impulse that may be displaced laterally and downward. A graphic record of this movement is shown in Figure 12-22. Atrial contraction in the setting of a poorly compliant, thick-walled left ventricle may result in a palpable presystolic component to the apical impulse of left ventricular hypertrophy. This presystolic distention can usually be felt with the palpating hand, especially with the patient in the left lateral decubitus position. A tongue blade held lightly over the apex will amplify this double impulse, making it easily demonstrable at the bedside without special equipment. The excursions may be timed by simultaneously listening to the heart, which usually discloses the presence of a presystolic sound or fourth heart sound in these patients. This finding is commonly associated with hypertension, aortic stenosis, and coronary disease.

Left ventricular dilatation due to heart failure also produces an abnormal, sustained apex impulse. This movement may be double for yet another reason: the effect of rapid passive filling in early diastole. An early diastolic extra sound (S_3) usually accompanies this abnormality. Advanced coronary disease, cardiomyopathies, and certain valvular diseases resulting in left ventricular failure are major causes of this abnormality. In some patients this early diastolic filling wave may be seen more easily than it can be felt or heard.

Right ventricular hypertrophy and dilatation produce similar movements that are usually more diffuse and can be felt along the left sternal edge (Fig. 12-23). The impulse of the volume- or pressure-loaded right ventricle frequently can be felt with a finger placed under the xyphoid process while the patient gently inhales. Right ventricular impulses are often single but may exhibit presystolic distention or a rapid filling wave just as the left ventricle does. The impulse of the pressure-loaded right ventricle is more sustained than the rapid outward early systolic movement found in patients with atrial septal defect (a lesion that results in selective volume overload of the right ventricle). Pulmonary artery dilatation produces a localized systolic lift in the second or third left intercostal space.

Constrictive pericarditis may produce a typical early diastolic out-thrust along the sternal border or over the midprecordium. This sometimes is associated with a short inward movement during systole. The diastolic movement is often misinterpreted as a systolic event, but when unquestionably present it is pathognomonic of this one condition. Palpate and listen at the same time!

Maneuvers that bring the heart closer to the chest wall will accentuate most of the precordial movements. Having the patient hold his breath in full expiration and/or rolling him a quarter of a turn to the left may be very helpful. Longstanding cardiac enlargement, when present during childhood, may cause a visible precordial bulge.

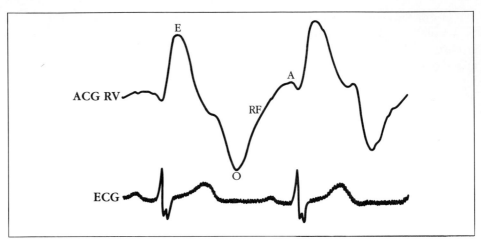

Figure 12-23
Apexcardiogram of right ventricular hypertrophy. Apexcardiogram was recorded at the left sternal border in a patient with right ventricular (RV) overload. The outward movement, which occupies only the early part of the systole, is characteristic of right ventricular volume overload. (Courtesy of the Division of Cardiology, Georgetown University Hospital.)

PERCUSSION

The methods of direct and indirect percussion described in Chapter 11 are occasionally applicable to the estimation of heart size. When the left border of cardiac dullness falls outside the midclavicular line, the heart is usually enlarged. However, as more detailed knowledge of normal and abnormal precordial movements has been accumulated, palpation has largely replaced percussion in cardiac examination. The superiority of the echocardiogram and roentgenogram for evaluation of overall heart size and chamber enlargement has relegated percussion of the heart largely to a place of historical interest.

AUSCULTATION

Immediately, on this suggestion, I rolled a quire of paper into a kind of cylinder and applied one end of it to the region of the heart and the other to my ear, and was not a little surprised and pleased to find that I could thereby perceive the action of the heart in a manner much more clear and distinct than I had ever been able to do by the immediate application of the ear.

RENÉ THÉOPHILE HYACINTHE LAËNNEC
(1781–1826)

GENERAL

Cardiac auscultation must be learned at the bedside. Diagrams, tape recordings, and phonocardiograms are of great help to the student but are no substitute for personal experience. Proficiency requires years of studied practice coupled with a clear understanding of the origin of normal and abnormal cardiac sounds. Certain frustrations are inevitable at first, but do not be disheartened.

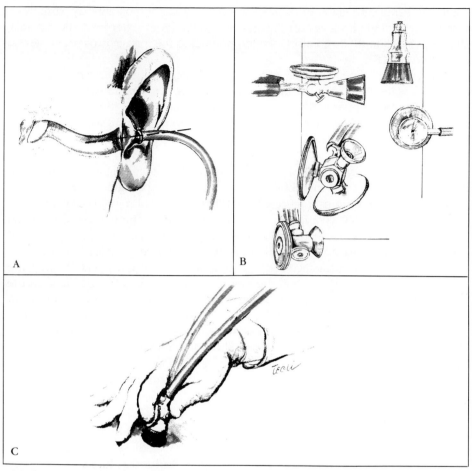

A

B

C

Figure 12-24
The stethoscope. A. Correct fit in external auditory meatus. B. Common types of stethoscope endpieces. C. Correct method for holding stethoscope endpiece, permitting variable pressure against chest wall.

STETHOSCOPE

In order for the stethoscope to function, two things have to happen. There has to be, by God, a sick man at one end of it and a doctor at the other! *The doctor has to be within thirty inches of his patient.*

Dickinson W. Richards
(1895–1973)

There is a frequently quoted saying that what you put in your ears is of less importance than what lies between them. While this is true to a great extent, a well-designed efficient stethoscope is indispensable. Several crucial factors must be considered in its selection; therefore, it is wise to try a variety of instruments before selecting your own. It will be a very close friend for a long time.

Earpieces must fit snugly. An earpiece that is too small or too tight may partially or completely occlude itself against the anterior wall of your external auditory canal. The earpieces should be comfortable and parallel to the long axis of your external auditory canal (Fig. 12-24A).

Tubing with an inner diameter of less than $1/8$ inch will attenuate high frequencies. Thick-walled tubing, particularly plastic, will reject outside noise better than the thin, flexible rubber variety. Double tubing extending all the way to the endpiece is slightly superior to the Y configuration. Tubing length should not exceed 12 to 15 inches so that the overall distance from ear to chestpiece is no greater than 21 inches.

Endpieces are of two standard types, the bell and the diaphragm. They are available in many sizes; the 1-inch bell and the $1\frac{1}{2}$-inch diaphragm are generally selected for examining adults (Figure 12-24B). The rigid diaphragm has a natural frequency of around 300 cps. It therefore acts as a filter, eliminating low-pitched sounds. High-pitched sounds, such as the second heart sound, and high-pitched murmurs are best heard with the diaphragm. The vaulted trumpet bell has been shown to have a slight advantage over the more shallow varieties. With the bell, the skin becomes the diaphragm, and the natural frequency varies depending on the amount of pressure exerted, much as the timpani player varies the pitch of his instrument by tensing the drumhead. It probably ranges from 40 cps with light pressure to 150 to 200 cps with firm pressure. When you try to detect low-pitched sounds and murmurs, therefore, the bell should be applied as lightly as possible (Figure 12-24C). Alternating firm and light pressure may aid in detecting low frequency sounds, which become more obvious "by their absence" when firmer pressure is applied.

CARDIAC SOUND

Sound intensity is objective; loudness therefore depends on both the intensity of the sound at its origin and the sensitivity of the ear. Needless to say, people vary greatly in auditory acuity, particularly at the upper and lower limits of audibility. Although the human ear at times may perceive frequencies from 20 to 16,000 cps and higher under special conditions, its maximal sensitivity is in the range of 1,000 to 2,000 cps. Figure 12-25 compares the average hearing threshold with the average intensity of cardiovascular sounds. Notice that only vibrations ranging from 25 to 600 cps achieve intensity levels that are high enough to become audible by the average listener, although the heart produces vibrations ranging from 1 to 1,000 cps.

In simple terms this means that vibrations originating in the heart with frequencies below 25 cps (and there are many) are entirely inaudible. This reinforces the importance of palpation, since with experience much information from the inaudible range can be derived by this method. Additionally, a sound of 500 cps will be perceived to be louder to the ear than one of 60 cps, even when each sound has the same intensity at the stethoscope earpiece. This means that great care must be taken to train the ear to perceive low-pitched sounds, as they are easily overlooked.

The ear adjusts itself to the intensity of sound. A loud sound causes the ear to protect itself by decreasing its receptive ability. This produces the phenomenon called "masking": if a faint sound follows a loud one, it may actually be entirely inaudible. High levels of ambient noise may also mask faint sounds and murmurs.

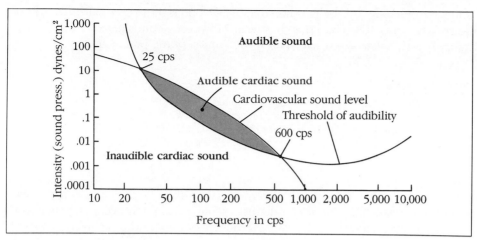

FIGURE   12-25
Ranges of audible and inaudible sound. Only a narrow range of sound generated in the heart may be heard on auscultation.

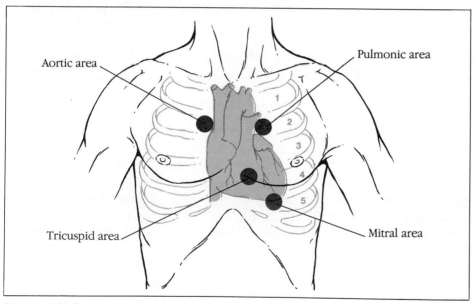

FIGURE   12-26
Areas of routine auscultation of the precordium.

TECHNIQUE OF AUSCULTATION

Four reference points are used for localization of sounds on the surface of the chest as shown in Figure 12-26. Because the pulmonic and tricuspid valves are located near the chest wall, their sounds are transmitted to auscultatory areas close by. The aortic and mitral valves, however, are situated deep in the chest, and their sounds are transmitted in the direction of blood flow to points closer to the chest wall. The mitral sounds are referred to the apex; the aortic sounds follow the ascending aorta as it curves forward and are well heard in the second right intercostal space, where the aorta is closer to the anterior chest wall. However, sounds generated at the mitral and aortic valves are usually heard over much of the precordium.

HEART SOUNDS

The gallop stroke is diastolic and is due to the beginning of sudden tension in the ventricular wall as a result of blood flow into the cavity.
It is more pronounced if the wall is not distensible . . .

PIERRE CARL EDOUARD POTAIN
(1825–1901)

GENERAL

You should clearly understand the physiologic origin of normal cardiovascular sound. Individual differences in loudness, quality, and pitch occur in patients of varying age and build. Sounds may be remarkably loud and clear in young, thin-chested patients and in patients with tachycardia due to exercise or excitement. They may be quite muffled and practically inaudible in the obese, heavy-chested individual. The heart may sound very different as the stethoscope position is changed from point to point in the same patient. This is partially due to the relative proximity of the various valves. The first sound as heard at the apex may not only become softer at the base but may also seem shorter and have a different quality due to the damping effect of the interposed soft tissues. Similarly, the second sound loses intensity and changes quality as the stethoscope is moved downward toward the apex.

The cardiac cycle is schematically represented in Figure 12-27. The sounds of greatest importance are the first and second heart sounds, which divide the cardiac cycle into systole and diastole (technically, ventricular systole and diastole). Although there is controversy concerning the origin of the first sound, it may be considered here to be related to closure of the mitral and tricuspid valves and to the related phenomena of tensing of the myocardium, atrioventricular valve (tricuspid, mitral), supporting structures (papillary muscle, chordal apparatus), as well as to changes in blood velocity. The second sound results from aortic and pulmonary valve closure. A physiologic third sound is at times audible during the period of rapid filling of the ventricles. The normal first and second heart sounds range in frequency from 60 to 200 cps. The physiologic third sound is low-pitched and usually around 40 cps or less. In Figure 12-27 these events are correlated with their corresponding systemic or left-sided pressure relationships.

TECHNIQUE OF AUSCULTATION

In order to derive the maximum benefit from cardiac auscultation, you must develop a systematic approach that is repeated in the examination of each patient. Begin by listening at the apex, but do not simply skip from one major valve area to another. Such skipping is a common mistake that results in missing much important information. Many intermediate points and satellite areas must be scrutinized as the stethoscope is moved slowly and systematically from the apex to the tricuspid area, up along the left sternal border to the pulmonic area, and thence to the aortic area. Maneuvers that bring the heart closer to the chest wall will increase the loudness of certain sounds. Two standard accessory positions should always be

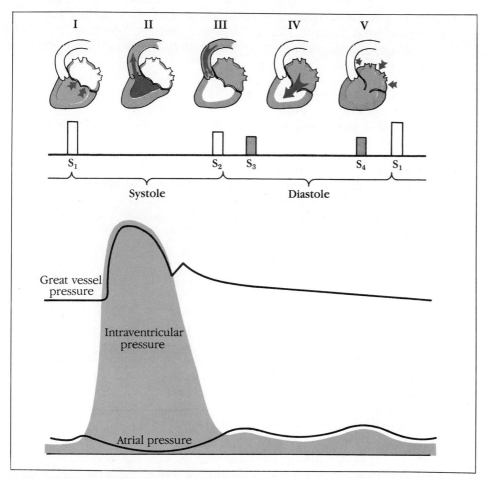

FIGURE 12-27

Heart sounds in relation to cardiac events and pulse wave forms. I. Atrioventricular valve closure corresponds in time to the first heart sound. II. Systolic ejection period begins with opening of the aortic and pulmonic valves. III. With ventricular emptying, aortic and pulmonic valve closure corresponds in time to the second heart sound (S_2). IV. With atrioventricular valve opening, the rush of blood from atria to ventricles may be associated with an early ventricular filling sound (S_3). V. Atrial contraction, causing increased ventricular filling, corresponds to tensing of the ventricular myocardium and a late ventricular filling sound (S_4).

used: the left lateral position, which usually makes louder sounds at the apex; and the sitting position, which may bring out otherwise inaudible murmurs at the base and along the left sternal border. In emphysematous patients, heart sounds, usually faint over the precordium, may be well heard over the epigastrium. Always notice the effects of position changes and of respiration on the quality of the sounds. Exercising the patient may be of great help, but it is not necessarily routine. Listening to the heart as the patient squats may also be useful in special instances.

The key to successful auscultation lies in listening to one thing at a time. It is frequently worthwhile to close your eyes and take a relaxed, comfortable position while focusing all your attention on listening. The following routine will eliminate many errors of omission:

1. **Observe and time the rate and rhythm.** Is the rate unusually fast or slow? Are there any irregularities of rhythm?
2. **Identify the first and second sounds and listen to them separately.** Is the first sound normal, accentuated, diminished? Next, listen solely to the second sound and establish its characteristics, intensity, and splitting. Compare the first and second sounds in the various valve areas.
3. **Now that the sounds are familiar, focus first on systole and then on diastole.** Listen specifically for extra sounds only (not murmurs).
4. **Listen now for the presence of murmurs—first in systole, then in diastole— scanning all major areas.** Notice the point of maximum intensity and the transmission of any murmurs heard.

At times it is difficult even for the experienced clinician to identify systole and diastole. This is particularly true with rapid heart rates in which the systolic and diastolic intervals tend to become equal in duration. Two techniques may be of value. One is to correlate the heart sounds with the apex impulse or the carotid pulse, both of which are systolic in timing. The first sound should just precede these phenomena. Because of the time required for the mechanical transmission of the pulse wave, peripheral arteries such as the radial or femoral are not suitable for timing heart sounds. The second technique is to familiarize yourself with the second sound at the base, which is invariably the loudest, and to inch the stethoscope downward toward the apex, keeping this sound clearly in your ear.

FIRST HEART SOUND

The first sound is louder, longer, and lower pitched than the second sound at the apex. Since the tricuspid component is usually not well heard at the apex, a single component first sound (mitral valve) is heard there,

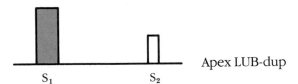

Apex LUB-dup

S_1 S_2

but because the mitral valve closes from 0.02 to 0.03 seconds before the tricuspid, splitting of the first sound is actually common normally, and is particularly well heard in the fourth left intercostal space at the left sternal border (tricuspid area).

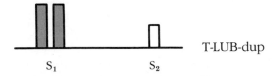

T-LUB-dup

S_1 S_2

The first heart sound is accentuated in many conditions, some of which are not abnormal. Sinus tachycardia in a healthy young person may result in a prominent first sound. Anemia, hyperthyroidism, and other disorders that result in a hyperkinetic circulation cause a similar change. The increased left atrial pressure of mitral stenosis, or a short PR interval that causes the mitral and tricuspid valves to close from a relatively open position, will also increase the intensity of the first sound.

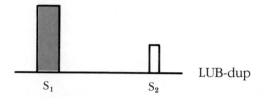

LUB-dup

Low-output states or delayed atrioventricular conduction (long PR interval) may result in a quiet first sound. Atrioventricular dissociation (complete heart block) with ventricular systole being variably related to atrial contraction, as well as atrial fibrillation with its variable diastolic filling periods, is associated with marked changes in intensity of the first sound.

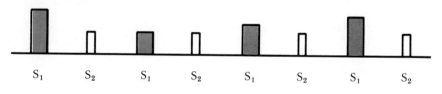

LUB-dup-LUB-dup-LUB-dup

SECOND HEART SOUND

The second sound results from combined aortic and pulmonary valve closure. It is almost always louder than the first sound at the base. The aortic component is widely transmitted to the neck and over the precordium and usually is the only component of the second sound heard at the apex.

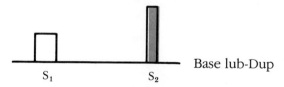

Base lub-Dup

The pulmonary component of the second sound is softer and normally is heard only along the high left sternal border. Although the second left intercostal space is called the pulmonic area, analysis of the second sound and its splitting is frequently best accomplished in the third interspace.

Respiratory variations in the timing of the two components of the second sound occur in most patients. Physiologic splitting of the second sound may be demonstrated in most normal people during inspiration. Closure of the aortic and pulmonic valves during expiration is synchronous or nearly so because right and left ventricular systole are approximately equal in duration. With inspiration, venous blood rushes into the thorax from the large systemic venous reservoirs. This increases venous return and prolongs right ventricular systole by temporarily increasing right ventricular stroke volume, with resultant delay in pulmonic valve closure. At the same time venous return to the left heart diminishes due to the increased pulmonary capacity during inspiration. This shortens left ventricular systole and permits earlier aortic closure. The two factors combine to produce transient "physiologic splitting" of the pulmonic second sound during inspiration.

Analysis of the respiratory variation of the second sound should take place during normal quiet respiration and not with forced or held inspiration or expiration. In some patients, complete fusion of the two components of the second heart sound may only occur in the sitting position.

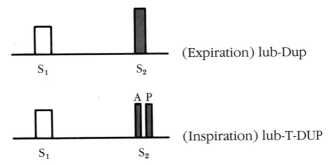

The aortic or pulmonic components of the second sound may be accentuated with elevation of the pressure in either of the respective circuits (i.e., systemic or pulmonary artery hypertension). With aortic or pulmonary stenosis they may become diminished or inaudible due to decreased mobility of the diseased cusps. Delayed pulmonic valve closure results in persistent splitting of the second sound, which may not vary at all with respiration (fixed splitting) or may vary with it in the usual manner (e.g., not fusing in expiration but widening during inspiration). Atrial septal defect with volume overload causing prolonged right ventricular ejection is the most frequent cause of fixed splitting of the second sound. Pulmonary stenosis and ventricular septal defects often cause wide splitting of the second sound with retention of normal respiratory variation. Delayed electrical activation of the right ventricle (i.e., right bundle-branch block), causes persistent splitting of the second sound with normal respiratory movements.

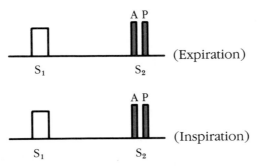

Reversed or paradoxic splitting of the second sound results from delayed left ventricular activitation (left bundle-branch block or an artificial pacemaker in the right ventricle) or prolonged emptying time of the left ventricle for mechanical reasons (aortic stenosis, marked hypertension, or poor contractility as seen in cardiomyopathy or myocardial ischemia). In paradoxic splitting, the second sound is split in expiration and "single" during inspiration, the opposite of normal respiratory variation of the second sound.

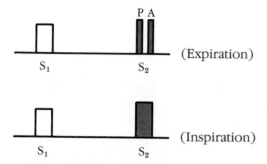

The basic cause of reversed splitting of the second sound is late aortic valve closure resulting from prolonged or delayed left ventricular ejection. Thus, in expiration right ventricular ejection is shortest and pulmonic valve closure precedes aortic valve closure. When prolonged right ventricular systole and shortened left ventricular systole occur with inspiration, the two valve sounds become superimposed. Examination for paradoxic splitting is best accomplished during normal quiet respiration or minimally exaggerated breathing with the mouth open.

EXTRA HEART SOUNDS

THIRD SOUND. Early diastolic extra sounds (S_3, ventricular gallop, or protodiastolic extra sound) occur during the period of rapid ventricular filling. They may be normal (physiologic) or abnormal (commonly heard in mitral regurgitation and ventricular failure of variable etiology).

The S_3 is low pitched and is often difficult to detect. Careful location of the cardiac apex in the left lateral decubitus position with light application of the bell of the stethoscope is imperative for detection of this sound.

The physiologic third sound is a low-pitched sound that is audible at or near the apex. It is best heard with the patient in the left decubitus position, and it frequently disappears when he sits erect. It varies in intensity with respiration, usually becoming louder with expiration. It is extremely common in children and young adults but is seldom heard in persons over 30 years of age.

In contradistinction to the physiologic S_3 of younger people the occurrence of a third heart sound at an older age is related to cardiomyopathy, ischemic heart disease, or valvular disease. Pathologic third heart sounds generally connote ventricular failure but may be seen in patients with mitral regurgitation or myocardial infarction before significant ventricular dysfunction develops.

An S_3 may arise from the right ventricle as well as the left ventricle. Right-sided third sounds tend to exhibit respiratory variation in intensity. Right ventricular S_3's occur with tricuspid regurgitation or right ventricular failure. They are usually best heard at the lower left sternal border or in the epigastrium.

PERICARDIAL KNOCK. This is a sharp sound heard in early diastole. It occurs in patients with constrictive pericarditis and is associated with the early, rapid filling phase of ventricular diastole. Its timing is earlier than a third heart sound.

OPENING SNAP. This sound, associated with rheumatic involvement of the mitral (or triscupid) valve, occurs early in ventricular diastole prior to the rapid filling phase. It results from the opening movement of the stiffened atrioventricular valve leaflets (a silent occurrence in the normal heart) and occurs earlier when atrial pressure is higher (usually connoting greater obstruction to ventricular inflow).

TUMOR PLOP. This sound, which is generated by the movement of atrial masses (most notably left atrial myxomas) into the atrioventricular orifice, also occurs in conjunction with the early rapid filling phase of the ventricles. Its characteristic quality gives rise to the term *plop*.

Each of these early diastolic sounds has a slightly different quality and timing that only repeated actual auscultatory experience will allow you to distinguish.

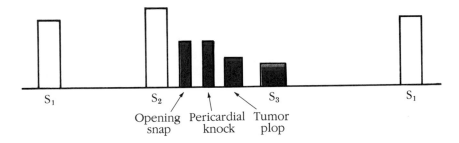

S_1 S_2 S_3 S_1

Opening Pericardial Tumor
snap   knock   plop

FOURTH SOUND. Presystolic extra sounds (S_4, atrial gallop) are dull and low-pitched. They are best heard at the apex with the patient rolled onto his left side and the bell of the stethoscope lightly applied precisely over the apex impulse. At times they are more easily felt than heard. The fourth heart sound is caused by vigorous atrial contraction in patients with decreased left ventricular compliance, which may be caused by left ventricular hypertrophy or myocardial ischemia. With pulmonary hypertension or pulmonary stenosis, a fourth heart sound originating in the right ventricle may be heard along the left sternal border. As with most right-sided auscultatory events, a right ventricular fourth sound increases with inspiration. Fourth heart sounds are so frequent over the age of 50 that their presence may not necessarily imply cardiac disease in that age group.

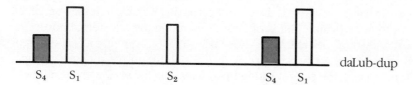

daLub-dup

GALLOPS. When an S_3 and/or an S_4 is associated with a rapid heart rate, the heart sounds assume the cadence of a galloping horse. Gallop rhythm is regarded as a sign of congestive heart failure. With more rapid rates, the third and fourth sounds are superimposed and result in a single loud prolonged "summation" gallop.

EJECTION SOUNDS. Ejection sounds occur in early systole. They may originate in either of the great vessels or their valves. They are generated by abrupt distention of a dilated great vessel during early ventricular ejection or by upward movement of stiffened deformed valve leaflets. Ejection sounds heard in congenital valvular pulmonary stenosis increase in intensity with expiration and decrease with inspiration (as opposed to most other right-sided events). The ejection sound of pulmonary hypertension is not as apt to vary with respiration. Pulmonic ejection sounds are best heard at the base and high left sternal border. Aortic ejection sounds do not vary with respiration and are heard equally well at the apex and base.

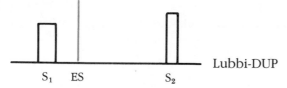

Lubbi-DUP

SYSTOLIC CLICKS. A systolic click is usually single, but two or more clicks may be heard. They are usually midsystolic, high-pitched, and sharp. They are extremely variable, changing with respiration or position or spontaneously. Clicks are heard best along the left sternal border or just inside the apex. Previously these clicks were felt to be extracardiac in origin and were regarded as benign. Now they are most often associated with prolapse of the mitral valve (or, occasionally, the tricuspid valve). Their origin is thought to be the sudden tensing of the redundant valve leaflets and chordal structures associated with the prolapse syndrome. With sitting or standing they tend to move earlier in systole, and with lying and squatting they are somewhat delayed (see Table 12-12).

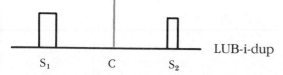

LUB-i-dup

CRUNCHES. A systolic crunch or knock (Hammon's crunch) may be heard in patients with mediastinal emphysema or a small left-sided pneumothorax. In the latter case it has been referred to as "noisy pneumothorax," frequently being audible to the patient and at times to the physician at some distance from the bedside.

RUBS. The pericardial friction rub is a sign of pericardial irritation. It may be heard anywhere over the precordium but is often loudest along the left sternal border or directly over the sternum. Sometimes it is quite loud, but frequently it is faint, high-pitched, and evanescent. Firm pressure with the diaphragm of the stethoscope, and/or auscultation with the patient sitting up and leaning forward with breath held in expiration, are maneuvers that will bring out a friction rub. Friction rubs have a superficial, scratchy, to-and-fro quality, often suggesting squeaky leather. They lag somewhat, giving the effect of being slightly out of step with the heart sounds. A fully developed friction rub has three components that correspond with the systolic, early diastolic, and presystolic phases of the cardiac cycle. One should hear at least two components before diagnosing a rub. The intensity of the rub may vary with respiration, but a true pericardial rub should be audible with respiration halted. Friction rubs may be simulated by movements of the stethoscope's end-piece on the surface of the skin, and particularly by hair.

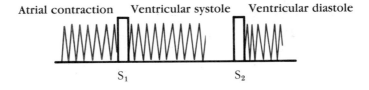

Atrial contraction   Ventricular systole   Ventricular diastole

S_1 S_2

MURMURS. Heart murmurs are immensely important in cardiac diagnosis. In order to interpret them intelligently, however, you must understand the factors that govern their production and transmission. Furthermore, you must be able to describe them in precise and appropriate terms. The phonocardiogram, though of limited diagnostic value, is helpful as a teaching tool, since it allows time for study and correlation of events that ordinarily are passing by rapidly.

Blood flow within the circulation may be laminar or turbulent. Ideally flow is silent because of its laminar character. With laminar flow through any tube, the layer of fluid adjacent to the wall is stationary while the velocity of flow increases progressively within the inner layers and is maximal at the center. As this velocity exceeds a critical level, turbulence develops and in turn produces vortices or swirls. These in turn emit high-frequency sound vibrations termed *murmurs* when heard in and around the heart and *bruits* when heard over peripheral vessels.

Production of murmurs is favored by a number of basic factors that tend to promote turbulence, including (1) lowering the viscosity of the fluid, (2) increasing the diameter of a tube, (3) changing the caliber of a tube abruptly, and (4) increasing the velocity of flow. The velocity of blood flow is vitally important in governing two important characteristics of a murmur: intensity and pitch. The intensity of a murmur is directly proportional to V^3, that is, the velocity cubed. The faster the flow, the louder the murmur. Thus, exercise, when it speeds blood flow, causes most murmurs to become louder. Pitch is also directly proportional to velocity. The faster the flow, the higher the pitch; the slower the flow, the lower the pitch. There are other causes of murmur production that are of lesser importance and will not be included here.

Transmission of murmurs also has a profound effect on both pitch and loudness. Sound intensity diminishes in direct proportion to the square of the distance that it

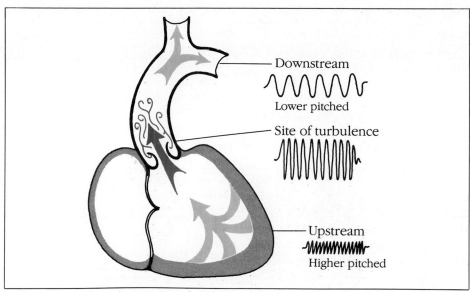

Downstream
Lower pitched

Site of turbulence

Upstream
Higher pitched

FIGURE   12-28
Differential radiation of various pitches of a murmur. Higher frequencies preferentially radiate upstream and lower frequencies preferentially radiate downstream.

must travel. Obviously the closer the murmur source to the chest wall, the louder it will sound. The natural damping effect of interposed tissues is compounded by the tendency of sound to be reflected backward at the interface between media of different densities, such as muscle, lung, bone, skin, and air. In fact, high frequencies tend to be dampened preferentially by this phenomenon; in other words, the pitch will become lower due to the effects of transmission across these interfaces. Another important factor that governs pitch is related to the transmission of a murmur within the cardiovascular system itself. As one moves backward against the stream, high frequencies tend to be preserved and lows tend to be dampened out. In moving downstream (or forward), high frequencies tend to be lost and lows tend to be preserved. This phenomenon is shown in Figure 12-28. It is not surprising, then, that many murmurs sound quite different as the stethoscope is moved over the precordium.

TYPES AND CAUSES OF MURMURS
Description of murmurs is divided into six categories: timing, location and radiation, loudness, pitch, duration, and quality. They are defined as follows:

1. **Timing:** Systolic, diastolic, continuous.
2. **Location and radiation:** Point of maximum intensity described in terms of anatomic landmarks: apex, left sternal border; left base (pulmonic area); right base (aortic area); intermediate zones by exact intercostal space. Areas to which the murmur radiates over the precordium.
3. **Loudness:** Graded on a six-point scale, described in Table 12-7.
4. **Pitch:** Low (25–150 cps); medium (150–350 cps); high (350–600 cps) (see Fig. 12-26).

TABLE 12-7. Grading of Heart Murmurs

Grade	Description
I/VI	Heard only after special maneuvers and "tuning in"
II/VI	Faint, but readily heard
III/VI	Loud, but without a thrill
IV/VI	Associated with a thrill, but stethoscope must be fully on chest to be heard
V/VI	Heard with stethoscope partly off the chest Palpable thrill
VI/VI	Heard with stethoscope entirely off the chest Palpable thrill

TABLE 12-8. Duration of Heart Murmurs

Short duration

Early systolic

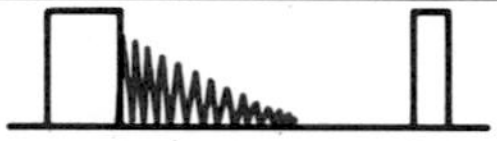

Early diastolic

Late systolic

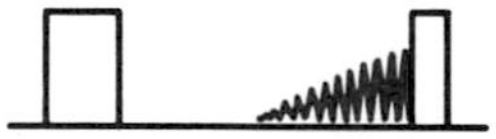

Late diastolic (presystolic)

Medium duration

Midsystolic

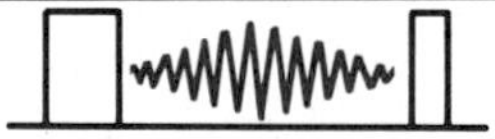

Middiastolic

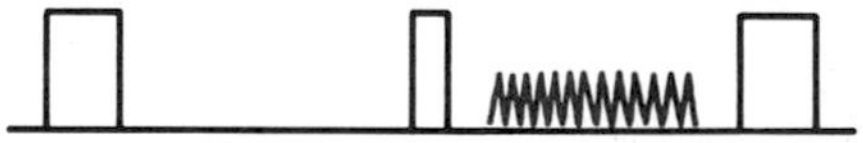

Long duration

Holosystolic

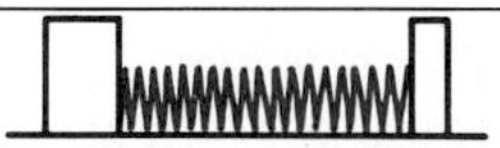

Holodiastolic

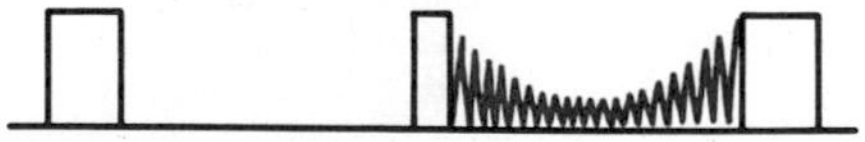

Continuous

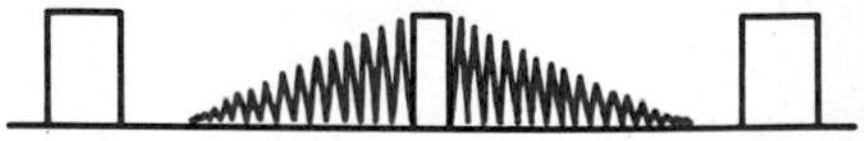

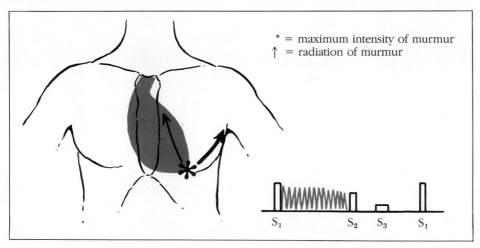

* = maximum intensity of murmur
↑ = radiation of murmur

S_1 S_2 S_3 S_1

FIGURE 12-29
Diagram of the heart sounds as it might appear in the written workup.

5. **Duration:** Classified and illustrated in Table 12-8.
6. **Quality:** Crescendo (increasing in loudness) or decrescendo (decreasing in loudness). Descriptive terms include blowing, harsh, rumbling, musical, cooing, whooping, honking, regurgitant, ejection.

On your written workup it is often useful to diagram what you hear through the stethoscope as illustrated in Figure 12-29. Note that not only duration but timing and quality (crescendo or decrescendo) are represented.

SYSTOLIC MURMURS

I found among such children, most of them quite young, a murmur of remark-able intensity, but with other characteristics which I thought unusual; what surprised me was that the murmur was almost the only sign of cardiopathy and that it was accompanied by no other physical signs (save only the purring thrill) . . . [ventricular septal defect]

HENRI ROGER
(1809–1891)

For the sake of simplicity most systolic murmurs may be grouped into one of two categories: midsystolic (often ejection) murmurs and holosystolic (regurgitant) murmurs. This subtyping of systolic murmurs correlates their quality with the underlying pathophysiologic mode of origin and eliminates errors produced by over-dependence on the geographic site of maximum intensity, which may be unreliable.

MIDSYSTOLIC MURMURS. These murmurs are usually produced by the forward outflow of blood through the pulmonary or aortic valves. Because of their hemodynamic basis, ejection murmurs have a characteristic personality in that they occur in midsystole, are medium-pitched, and rise and fall in a crescendo fashion, ending before the second sound. The four principal causes are (1) valvular or subvalvular

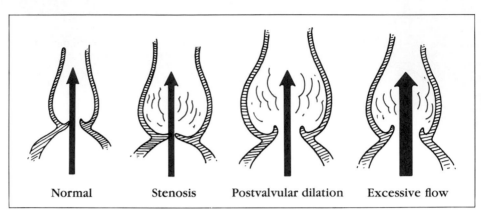

Normal   Stenosis   Postvalvular dilation   Excessive flow

FIGURE   12-30
Various mechanisms of generation of murmurs. Turbulent flow resulting from any of these mechanisms may result in cardiac sound.

stenosis; (2) high-velocity rate of ejection through the valves, which may themselves be normal (increased stroke volume); (3) dilation of the vessel beyond the valve; or (4) a combination of these factors (Fig. 12-30).

Aortic murmurs. Aortic systolic ejection murmurs occur with valvular and subvalvular stenosis (Fig. 12-31), primary dilation of the ascending aorta, and increased left ventricular stroke output. The latter may be due simply to hyperkinetic states or may be a compensatory increase in forward flow through the valve because of diastolic backflow with aortic regurgitation. Aortic systolic murmurs are usually best heard in the aortic area, but they are frequently transmitted to the entire precordium and sometimes are maximal at or inside the apex, where their pitch may seem higher or their sound musical, but they maintain their characteristic ejection quality. They are often transmitted to the carotid arteries. They may be accompanied by a thrill in the second right intercostal space. Because of an increase in stroke volume following a longer diastolic filling period, the intensity of the murmur is increased during the systole following a premature beat (postextrasystolic accentuation).

Pulmonic murmurs. Pulmonic systolic ejection murmurs occur with pulmonary valvular and subvalvular stenosis, dilation of the pulmonary artery, and increased pulmonary flow, as with atrial septal defect. They are usually best heard in the second and third intercostal spaces and may radiate to the left upper chest.

Innocent murmurs. The functional or innocent systolic murmur is commonly heard in children and young adults, especially women. It is characteristically soft, early, short, and variable (Fig. 12-32). It is usually heard best at the pulmonic area or along the left sternal border but at times is audible only at or medial to the apex. Functional murmurs vary with position and respiration and frequently have a peculiar vibratory quality. They are not associated with any structural abnormality or recognizable heart disease. The "hemic" systolic murmur commonly heard with anemia and the basal systolic murmurs frequently associated with thyrotoxicosis,

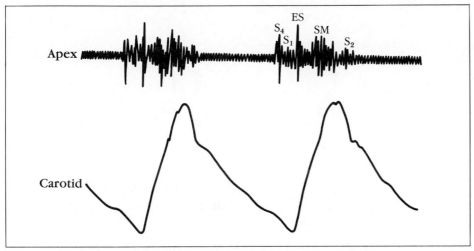

FIGURE   12-31
Systolic murmur (SM), with ejection sound (ES), generated in a patient with valvular aortic stenosis.

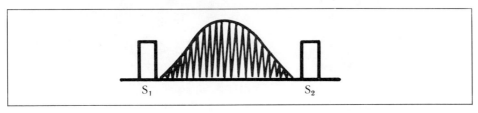

FIGURE   12-32
Representation of a functional systolic murmur.

fever, and exercise are functional murmurs, but in these instances the cardiac output is elevated.

Occasionally it may be difficult to determine whether an ejection murmur is being generated from the right or left side of the heart. This distinction may be made by having the patient perform a Valsalva maneuver. Following release, the original intensity returns within the next two or three beats when the murmur is generated at the pulmonic valve, but may take five to seven cycles to return if generated at the aortic orifice.

Subaortic murmurs. The murmur resulting from dynamic left ventricular outflow tract obstruction (IHSS, asymetric septal hypertrophy [ASH] with obstruction) has characteristics common to both mitral regurgitation and aortic stenosis (Fig. 12-33). It is usually best heard at the cardiac apex but is readily transmitted to the base (it is rarely heard well in the neck). The murmur is usually midsystolic but sometimes has a holosystolic configuration. With increases in left ventricular diastolic volume or peripheral resistance, the murmur decreases in intensity. Maneuvers that decrease left ventricular volume or peripheral resistance will enhance the intensity of the murmur. A nearly pathognomonic finding is the response of the murmur to squat-

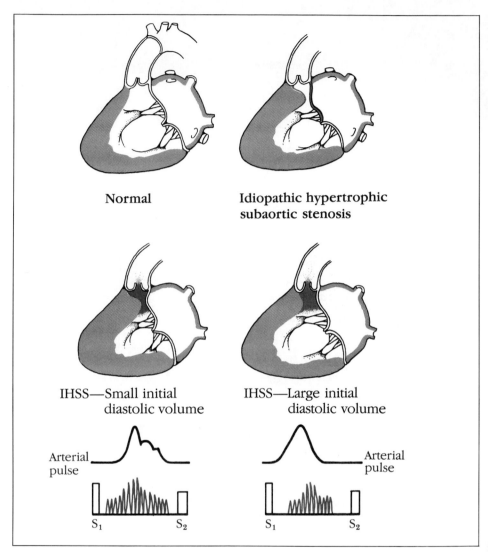

Normal   **Idiopathic hypertrophic subaortic stenosis**

IHSS—Small initial   IHSS—Large initial
  diastolic volume   diastolic volume

Arterial   Arterial
pulse   pulse

S_1 S_2 S_1 S_2

FIGURE 12-33
Idiopathic hypertrophic subaortic stenosis (IHSS). With a small diastolic volume, the obstruction of the hypertrophic septum narrows the left ventricular outflow tract to a relatively greater degree than occurs with a larger initial diastolic volume.

ting and standing—usually the murmur decreases (at least one grade) with prompt squatting (during which venous return and afterload are acutely increased) followed by an increase in intensity with standing.

HOLOSYSTOLIC MURMURS. These are produced by backflow of blood from the ventricle to the atrium through an incompetent mitral or tricuspid valve, or by flow through a ventricular septal defect. Since they are due to the escape of blood from a

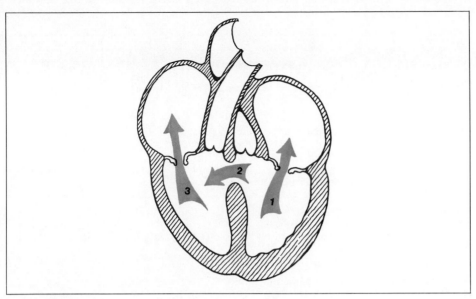

FIGURE   12-34
Mode of origin of holosystolic murmurs. 1. Mitral regurgitation. 2. Interventricular septal defect with left-to-right shunt. 3. Tricuspid regurgitation.

chamber of relatively high pressure into one of relatively low pressure, and since this pressure differential lasts throughout systole, regurgitant murmurs differ from ejection murmurs. They are longer in duration, usually holosystolic, and may engulf the first or second sound or both. They are often of constant intensity, but they may increase or decrease in late systole. They are less apt to rise and fall in intensity as an ejection murmur does. Figure 12-34 illustrates the mode of origin of holosystolic murmurs.

Mitral regurgitation usually causes a blowing holosystolic murmur. It tends to be loudest at the apex and is transmitted toward the axilla. There may be an associated thrill. The murmur of mitral regurgitation does not change in intensity during the cycle following an extrasystole.

In those cases in which mitral regurgitation has occurred precipitously, the murmur tends to decrescendo in late systole as left atrial pressure rises rapidly and decreases regurgitant flow (Fig. 12-35). When regurgitation takes place because of posterior mitral leaflet dysfunction, the anteriorly directed regurgitant stream may cause the murmur to radiate to the aortic root (the posterior wall of which is contiguous with the anterior left atrial wall).

Late systolic murmur. A murmur beginning in midsystole, often initiated by one or more systolic clicks, is characteristic of prolapse of the mitral valve (Fig. 12-36). The murmur tends to crescendo in late systole and responds in characteristic fashion to various maneuvers. When relative volume depletion occurs (as with sitting or standing), the murmur begins earlier in systole. With squatting or elevation of the legs (causing volume expansion) the murmur tends to begin later in systole. Unfor-

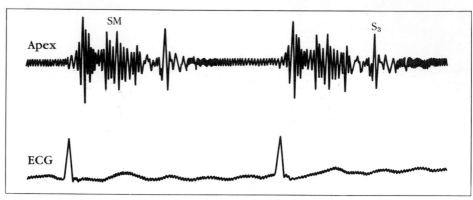

FIGURE 12-35

Decrescendo systolic murmur (SM) of acute mitral regurgitation. While caused by mitral regurgitation, the murmur tapers toward end systole as left atrial pressure rises abruptly and regurgitant flow diminishes.

TABLE 12-9. Some Causes of Systolic Murmurs

Aortic outflow obstruction
  Valvular aortic stenosis
  Subvalvular aortic stenosis
  Supravalvular aortic stenosis
Pulmonic outflow obstruction
  Valvular pulmonic stenosis
  Subvalvular (infundibular) pulmonic stenosis
Functional
  Youth
  Anemia
  Hyperthyroidism
Great vessel dilatation
  Aortic root dilatation of aging
  Idiopathic dilatation of the pulmonary arteries
Mitral regurgitation
Tricuspid regurgitation
Congenital
  Ventricular septal defect
  Atrial septal defect

---

tunately, the murmur of mitral valve prolapse is not always characteristic (see Table 12-12).

Papillary muscle dysfunction. When ischemia or myocardial infarction involves the papillary muscles or the portion of the left ventricle from which they arise, mitral regurgitation may occur as a result of a decrease in the support of the mitral valve apparatus. The resulting murmur is then said to be due to papillary muscle dysfunction. It is characteristically a nonholosystolic murmur, which may radiate to the axilla (if the anterior mitral leaflet is affected) or to the base (if the regurgitant jet is primarily due to posterior leaflet incompetence). Increases in left ventricular

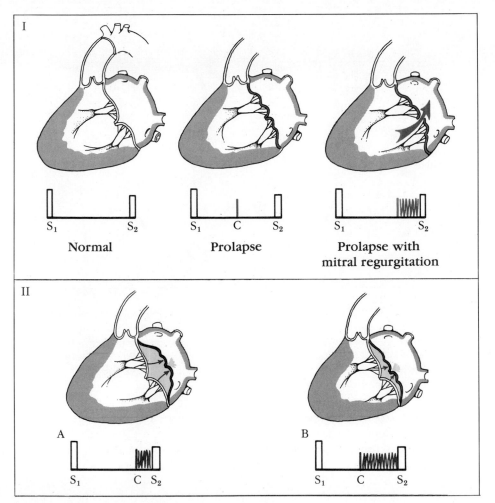

FIGURE 12-36

Spectrum of mitral valve prolapse. I. The typical findings in mitral valve prolapse. Prolapse without mitral regurgitation may result in a systolic click (C) without a murmur being heard. If mitral regurgitation is present, a late systolic murmur may be heard. II. The changes in the findings of prolapse with changes in left ventricular volume. A. Larger left ventricular volume results in a later click (C) and murmur. With increased ventricular volume more time is taken than with decreased volume for mitral leaflets to move from the position of first closure (S_1) to the point at which they are checked on their prolapse (C). B. Smaller left ventricular volume causes the click and murmur to move earlier in systole. With decreased ventricular volume less time is taken than with increased volume for mitral leaflets to move from their position of first closure (S_1) to the end of their prolapse (C). In either case, if mitral regurgitation is present, a systolic murmur follows the click.

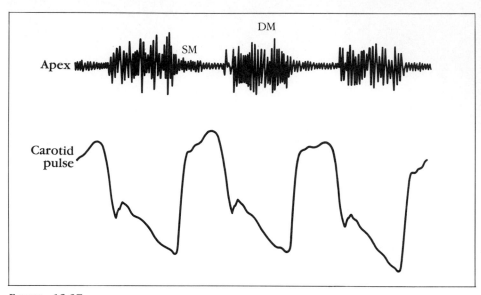

FIGURE   12-37
Diastolic murmur (DM) of aortic regurgitation. This phonocardiogram, recorded at the apex and shown with the carotid pulse tracing, also shows an early systolic murmur.

volume tend to be associated with increases in the murmur. This is thought to be due to increases in the left ventricular size with further pull of the affected leaflet from the fully closed position.

Tricuspid regurgitation. Tricuspid regurgitation causes a murmur, similar to that of mitral insufficiency, but is best heard over the tricuspid area. It can also be distinguished by the fact that it may become louder with inspiration. This quality may be accentuated by having the patient sit or stand.

Ventricular septal defect. The murmur of ventricular septal defect is heard best in the third and fourth left intercostal spaces. It frequently causes a thrill and has a loud, coarse quality that is practically pathognomonic. It tends to radiate like the spokes of a wheel about its loudest point.

DIASTOLIC MURMURS

Mitral stenosis may be concealed under a quarter of a dollar. It is the most difficult of all heart diseases to diagnose.

SIR WILLIAM OSLER
(1849–1919)

Diastolic murmurs may also be divided into two categories: early murmurs of aortic and pulmonic regurgitation, and mid- to late diastolic murmurs of mitral and tricuspid stenosis.

Aortic regurgitation results in a high-pitched murmur that begins immediately with aortic closure and diminishes progressively with diastole. Its intensity varies roughly with the size of the leak (Fig. 12-37). It is heard best along the left sternal

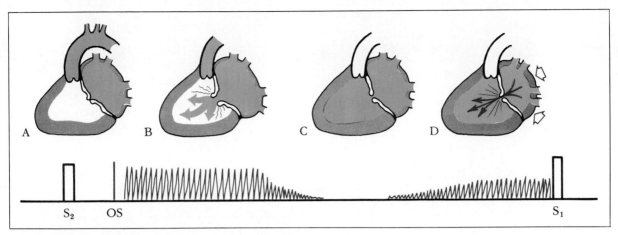

FIGURE 12-38

Hemodynamic basis for the auscultatory findings of mitral stenosis. A. Aortic valve closes; second heart sound (S_2) is generated. B. Mitral valve opens and opening snap (OS) occurs; early diastolic component is generated. C. Flow from left atrium to left ventricle diminishes, and murmur decreases in middiastole. D. Atrial systole increases flow across mitral valve, resulting in presystolic increase in intensity of murmur. Ventricular systole then causes closure of thickened mitral valve, resulting in loud first heart sound (S_1).

border with the patient sitting and holding his breath in expiration. Because of its high pitch, this murmur is best heard using the diaphragm endpiece firmly applied. A low-pitched diastolic murmur may be heard at the apex in patients with aortic regurgitation without associated mitral stenosis. This murmur, which sounds like the murmur of mitral stenosis, is referred to as an Austin Flint murmur.

Pulmonic regurgitation causes a diastolic murmur that at times cannot be distinguished from the aortic counterpart simply by auscultation alone. Its pitch, timing, quality, and location are similar, although it tends to be more localized to the pulmonic area. When pulmonic regurgitation is found in the setting of severe pulmonary arterial hypertension, the resulting sound is called a Graham Steell murmur. Congenital pulmonic regurgitation occurs with normal pressures in the pulmonary artery and results in a diastolic murmur that is low- to medium-pitched and begins at an interval after the second sound.

Mitral stenosis characteristically produces a low-pitched, localized, apical rumble. Often it can be heard only with the bell and with the patient rolled onto his left side. As is the case with the third and fourth heart sounds, the low-pitched rumble of mitral stenosis must be sought precisely over the apical impulse.

The murmur often has presystolic and early diastolic components. The early diastolic component is related to the rapid, passive filling phase. The presystolic component results from rapid flow during atrial systole and usually disappears with the onset of atrial fibrillation. The murmur of mitral stenosis may be enhanced by increasing blood flow through the valve, such as by having the patient cough or exercise.

Figure 12-38 illustrates the hemodynamic basis for the mitral diastolic murmur. The murmur is loudest in early and late diastole, at which time the pressure gradi-

TABLE 12-10. Some Causes of Diastolic Murmurs

Mitral stenosis
    Valvular disease
    Increased flow (relative)
    Left atrial myxoma
Tricuspid stenosis
    Valvular disease
    Increased flow (relative)
    Right atrial myxoma
Austin Flint
Pulmonic regurgitation
    Valvular disease
    Pulmonary hypertension (Graham Steell)
Aortic regurgitation

ent is greatest across the narrowed mitral valve. The early diastolic component is frequently initiated by a sharp click called a mitral opening snap. The opening snap can usually be heard at the apex but often is more easily discerned medial to the apex or along the left sternal border. Its separation from the second sound is related to the left atrial pressure; the higher the left atrial pressure, the closer the opening snap is to the second sound, and vice versa. This "2-OS" interval (the time between S_2 and the opening snap) may be used to estimate roughly the severity of the stenosis.

The murmur has a decrescendo quality through early and middiastole. During the latter third of diastole the gradient increases sharply due to atrial contraction, causing a presystolic accentuation of the murmur. With atrial fibrillation, effective contraction is lost, and the presystolic accentuation usually disappears. The murmur of mitral stenosis may be distinguished from the Austin Flint murmur of aortic regurgitation by altering peripheral resistance. Increases in peripheral resistance (as with isometric exercise) will increase the intensity of the Austin Flint murmur, but will decrease the intensity of the diastolic rumble of mitral stenosis. Decreases in peripheral resistance (as with amyl nitrite inhalation) have the opposite effect, decreasing the intensity of the Austin Flint murmur but enhancing the rumble of mitral stenosis.

The diastolic murmur of tricuspid stenosis is similar in timing and quality to the mitral murmur but is frequently higher pitched and localized near the tricuspid area or along the left sternal border. Inspiration usually makes it louder. A tricuspid opening snap may also occur. Some causes of diastolic murmurs are listed in Table 12-10.

CONTINUOUS MURMURS

Continuous murmurs begin in systole and continue into diastole without stopping. Although it is called continuous, such a murmur may not occupy the entire cardiac cycle. Continuous murmurs are found in those situations in which there is a flow from a high- to a lower pressure chamber that is uninterrupted by an opening or closing of cardiac valves. The prototype of a continuous murmur is the Gibson murmur of patent ductus arteriosus (Fig. 12-39). This murmur

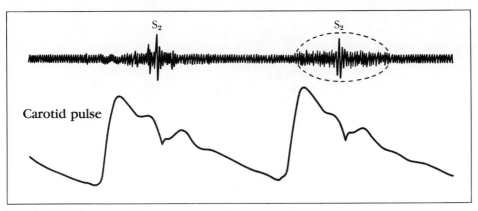

FIGURE 12-39
Continuous murmur of patent ductus arteriosus. Murmur peaks around second heart sound
(S_2).

TABLE 12-11. Some Causes of Continuous Murmurs*

Surgical or traumatic AV fistula
Patent ductus arteriosus
Pulmonary AV fistula
Coronary AV fistula
Intercostal AV fistula
Rupture of the sinus of Valsalva

* The combined murmurs of aortic stenosis and aortic regurgitation, or of mitral stenosis and mitral regurgitation,
may fill the entire cardiac cycle, but by definition they are *not* continuous murmurs. They are combinations of
separate systolic and diastolic murmurs.

begins in systole, peaks around the second sound, and then spills over into diastole, but it may not continue through to the first sound. It is heard maximally
under the left clavicle and in the pulmonic area. Other causes of continuous murmurs are listed in Table 12-11.

ENHANCING DIAGNOSTIC ACUMEN
. . . we give the name of observer to the man who applies methods of investiga-
tion, whether simple or complex, to the study of phenomena which he does not
vary and which he therefore gathers as nature offers them. We give the name ex-
perimenter to the man who applies methods of investigation, whether simple or
complex, so as to make natural phenomena vary, or so as to alter them with
some purpose or other . . .

CLAUDE BERNARD
(1813–1878)

SIMPLE MANEUVERS
Several simple bedside maneuvers that will often enhance diagnostic accuracy can
be used as adjuncts to routine cardiac examination.

ISOMETRIC (HANDGRIP) EXERCISE. Isometric exercises (simply done by having the patient squeeze tightly with both hands) results in tachycardia and increase in blood

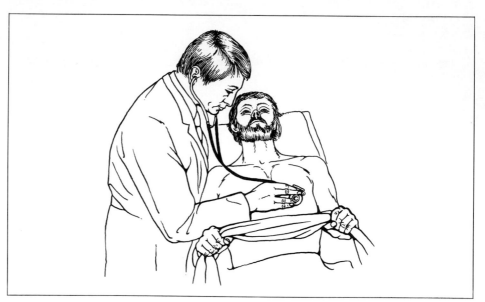

FIGURE 12-40
Isometric exercise. Patient grips towel tightly with both hands and pulls. Caution must be taken that patient does not perform the Valsalva maneuver during isometric exercise.

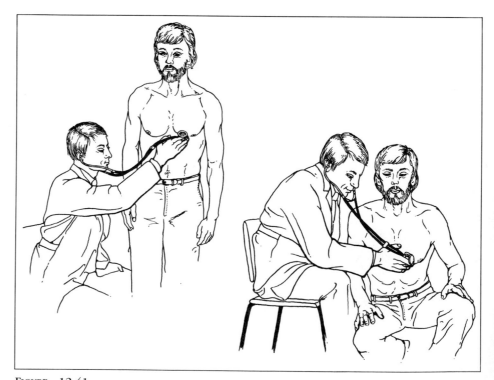

FIGURE 12-41
Prompt squatting. With the examiner auscultating from the sitting position, the patient moves quickly from standing to squatting.

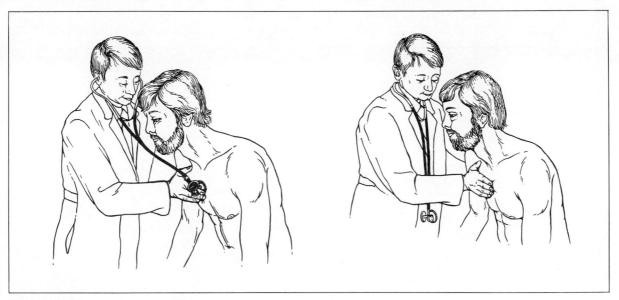

FIGURE 12-42
Palpation and auscultation with the patient in the sitting position and leaning forward. Thrills associated with aortic outflow murmurs and the diastolic murmur of aortic insufficiency may at times be appreciated only in this position.

pressure and cardiac output (Fig. 12-40). These hemodynamic alterations cause the murmurs of aortic regurgitation, mitral regurgitation, and mitral stenosis to intensify and the murmurs of left ventricular outflow obstruction to diminish.

AMYL NITRITE. The inhalation of amyl nitrite over a period of 15 to 20 seconds results in a prompt fall in mean arterial pressure with a reflex increase in heart rate, cardiac output, and stroke volume. Characteristic alterations of the auscultatory findings ensue. The lower systemic resistance produces either no change or a decrease in regurgitant murmurs (i.e., those of mitral regurgitation, aortic regurgitation, and ventricular septal defect). The increased flow causes increased intensity of outflow murmurs (i.e., aortic stenosis, pulmonic stenosis, and mitral stenosis). This intervention will help distinguish outflow from regurgitant murmurs. The murmur of organic mitral stenosis increases while the Austin Flint murmur of aortic regurgitation decreases.

PROMPT SQUATTING. Rapid squatting causes an increase in afterload and venous return (Fig. 12-41). This results in a decrease in the dynamic obstruction associated with IHSS and a resultant decrease in the systolic murmur. The murmur of valvular aortic stenosis does not change.

LEANING FORWARD. In order for the examiner to appreciate better the findings at the cardiac base, the patient should be asked to lean forward in the sitting position (Fig. 12-42). Thrills may be better palpated in this position, and soft diastolic murmurs may at times be appreciated only in this way.

TABLE 12-12. Effect of Some Physical Maneuvers on Cardiovascular Dynamics and Heart Sounds

Maneuver	Effect							
	Peripheral Resistance (Afterload)	Left Ventricular Volume (Preload)	Murmur of Aortic Stenosis	Murmur of IHSS	Murmur of Mitral Regurgitation	Click Murmur of Mitral Valve Prolapse	Murmur of Mitral Stenosis	Murmur of Aortic Insufficiency and Austin Flint
Supine with passive leg raising	— or ↑	↑	↑	↓	—	→	↑	—
Sitting or standing	↑	↓	—	↑	—	←	—	↑ or —
Prompt squatting	↑	↑	— (early) ↓ (late)	↓	↑	→	↓	↑
Isometric exercise (e.g., handgrip)	↑	↑	↓	↓	↑	→	↓	↑
Valsalva maneuver	↑	↓	↓	↑ or ↓ or —	↓	←	↓	↓
Exercise	↓	↓	↑	↑	—	←	↑	↓
Amyl nitrite	↓	↓	↑	↑	↓	←	↑	↓

↑ = increased; ↓ = decreased; — = no change; → = later in systole; ← = earlier in systole.

TABLE 12-13. Classic Physical Findings in Some Cardiac Disorders

Description	Phonocardiogram (inspiration unless noted)

MITRAL STENOSIS

Small pulse; tapping apex impulse; parasternal lift; presystolic apical thrill; accentuated S_1 and P_2; mitral opening snap; mitral diastolic rumble, with presystolic accentuation. Cold hands and feet. Atrial fibrillation (late).

DM S_1 OS   DM S_1

MITRAL REGURGITATION

Chronic, usually rheumatic

Normal or small, brisk, arterial pulse; apical systolic thrill; sustained apical lift displaced to left; normal or soft S_1, apical regurgitant systolic murmur; early diastolic extra sound (S_3). Mild forms may show murmur only.

S_1 SM S_3

Acute, severe

Usually caused by disruption of supporting structure apparatus. Varying degrees of congestive heart failure, loud S_1; harsh decrescendo systolic murmur, S_3 and S_4; right ventricular lift; increased P_2; right-sided filling sounds.

S_4 S_1 SM S_3

TABLE 12-13. (*Continued*)

Mitral valve prolapse

Normal S_1 and S_2: one or more midsystolic clicks, and/or a late systolic murmur; frequent arrhythmias; often associated with slender body habitus and minor musculoskeletal deformities.

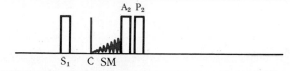

AORTIC STENOSIS

Small, slow-rising pulse; narrow pulse pressure (in severe cases); sustained apical lift displaced to the left; systolic thrill in aortic area; decreased or absent A_2; systolic ejection murmur at base and over carotids; systolic ejection sound (ES); carotid thrill. Cold hands and feet.

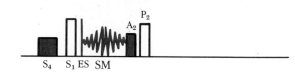

IDIOPATHIC HYPERTROPHIC SUBAORTIC STENOSIS (IHSS)

Brisk carotid pulse, often with two waves; prominent A wave in jugular venous pulse; thrill at apex or left sternal border; triple apical impulse (presystolic and two systolic waves); fourth heart sound; crescendo-decrescendo systolic murmur at apex and left sternal border.

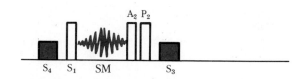

PULMONARY STENOSIS

Normal pulse; jugular A wave; parasternal lift; pulmonic thrill; pulmonary component of second sound absent or soft and delayed, causing widely split S_2; systolic ejection murmur in pulmonic area; right-sided presystolic extra sound in tricuspid area (S_4) (severe); pulmonary ejection sound (mild).

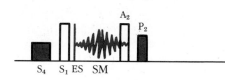

AORTIC REGURGITATION

Prominent carotid pulsations; water-hammer or bisferiens pulse. Capillary pulsations of the nail-beds; diffuse, sustained apex impulse displaced down and left; loud M_1, accentuated A_2; decrescendo diastolic murmur along left sternal border; low-pitched rumbling diastolic murmur at apex (Austin Flint).

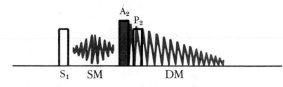

SYSTEMIC HYPERTENSION

Elevated blood pressure; carotid tortuous and usually full; hypertensive funduscopic changes; sustained double apical lift displaced to the left; normal or accentuated S_1, accentuated A_2; presystolic extra sound; aortic systolic ejection murmur.

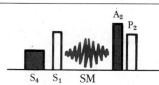

PULMONARY HYPERTERTENSION

Cyanosis (at times); small pulse; narrow pulse pressure; cold extremities; atrial fibrillation (late); giant jugular A wave; parasternal lift; systolic lift in the pulmonic area; pulmonary ejection sound; pulmonic diastolic murmur (Graham Steell); systolic ejection murmur in pulmonic area; right-sided S_3 and S_4.

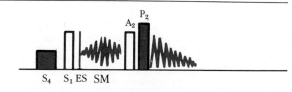

TRICUSPID STENOSIS

Small pulse; giant A wave in jugular pulse, elevated jugular pressure; quiet precordium; tricuspid diastolic murmur (DM) accentuated with inspiration (*Note:* Tricuspid stenosis is usually associated with mitral stenosis.)

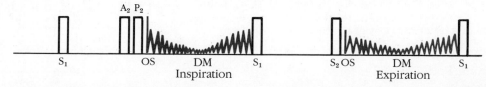

TABLE 12-13. (*Continued*)

TRICUSPID REGURGITATION

Jugular V wave; elevated venous pressure; right ventricular parasternal lift; systolic thrill at tricuspid area; tricuspid regurgitant systolic murmur louder with inspiration; atrial fibrillation; early diastolic extra sound (over right ventricle).

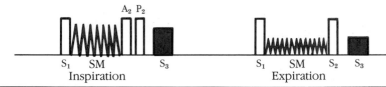

PROSTHETIC HEART VALVES

Mitral

Sharp component to first sound as valve closes; similar sound (OC) as valve opens, about 0.08 to 0.10 second after the second sound, analogous to the mitral opening snap. Characteristically no murmur is generated over such a valve.

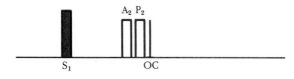

Aortic

Sharp opening component heard in the first sound; closing sound (C) heard at time of S_2; harsh systolic ejection murmur (sometimes with thrill) typically heard.

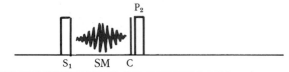

MYOCARDIAL INFARCTION

Tachycardia; pallor; small arterial pulse; narrow pulse pressure; apical late systolic bulge of ischemic myocardium; soft heart sounds; presystolic or early diastolic extra sounds; pericardial friction rub; apical systolic murmur (papillary muscle dysfunction); any of the arrhythmias.

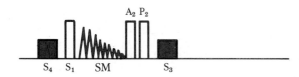

ATRIAL SEPTAL DEFECT

Normal pulse; brisk parasternal lift; lift over pulmonary artery; normal jugular pulse; systolic ejection murmur in pulmonic area; low-pitched diastolic rumble over tricuspid area (at times); persistent wide splitting of S_2.

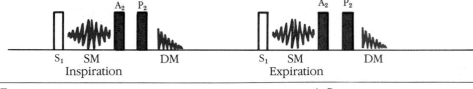

VENTRICULAR SEPTAL DEFECT

Small pulse; normal jugular pulse; parasternal lift and left ventricular apical lift; systolic thrill and loud systolic regurgitant murmur in third and fourth interspaces along left sternal border; apical diastolic rumble.

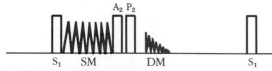

PERICARDITIS

Tachycardia; friction rub; diminished heart sounds and enlarged heart to percussion (with effusion); pulsus paradoxus; neck vein distention, narrow pulse pressure and hypotension (with tamponade).

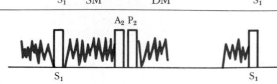

BREAST

This thy stature is like to a palm tree and thy breasts to clusters of grapes.

SONG OF SOLOMON 7:7

Careful examination of the breast should be part of every complete physical examination regardless of whether or not the patient has noted any particular signs or symptoms. Breast cancer is the most common malignancy occurring in women. It is a tumor that offers reasonable chance of a cure if it is recognized early and adequate therapy is carried out. Early detection is the key to successful treatment, and early detection of breast carcinoma is dependent on careful performance of this routine part of the physical examination.

ANATOMY

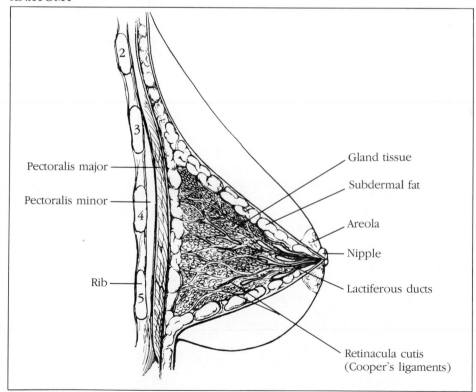

FIGURE 13-1
Cross-sectional anatomy of the breast.

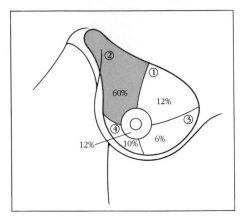

FIGURE 13-2
Clinical quadrants of the breast, with the percentage of all cancers of the breast found in each.

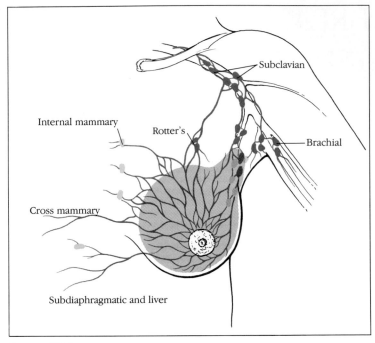

FIGURE 13-3
Nodal drainage of the breast.

HISTORY

Approximately 90 percent of breast cancers are first detected by patients themselves prior to seeking medical advice. They usually have noticed a lump or mass during bathing. Other complaints may include breast dimpling or retraction, nipple discharge, inflammation of the skin, and breast or bone pain. A family history of carcinoma of the breast in mother, maternal aunts, or sisters is a strong predisposing feature of this malignancy. To have breast-fed children is considered by some epidemiologists to lessen a woman's chance of breast cancer. Trauma to the breast probably functions more to call attention to a mass than to induce carcinomatous change.

Most breast masses are benign in origin and are associated with cyclic changes in the breast accompanying the menses. However, any mass of concern to the patient must be of equal concern to the physician. The woman complaining of such a lesion is likely to be apprehensive (with reason) about cancer and must be assured by a compassionate and thorough investigation.

PHYSICAL EXAMINATION

1. With patient sitting, inspect for asymmetry, retraction, skin change. Inspect with patient in three positions:
   a. Arms at side
   b. Arms on hips
   c. Arms overhead

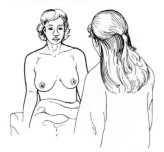 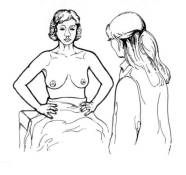 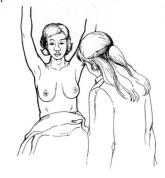

2. With patient sitting, palpate breasts with arms at side and overhead. Palpate axillary nodes.
3. With patient supine, palpate breasts and regional nodes.

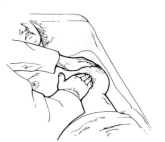

GENERAL

Complete examination of the male or female breast demands a thorough and systematic approach. Adequate exposure is important. The patient should disrobe to the waist, although the female breasts should be kept covered by a towel except during the actual examination (Fig. 13-4). The patient should be examined in both the seated position and while supine.

On the basis of a physical examination the examiner should be able to note the following diagnostic points:

1. Where is any lesion located? (Using the quadrants illustrated in Fig. 13-2, draw the lesion on your workup.)
2. Is the lesion solitary or multiple?
3. What is the consistency of the mass?
4. What is the size of the mass (in cm or mm)?
5. Is the mass tender?
6. Is the mass mobile or is it fixed to the chest wall?
7. Is the nipple displaced or retracted?
8. Is there retraction, dimpling, or erythema of the skin overlying the mass? Are there skin nodules?
9. Are there any regional lymph nodes, axillary or supraclavicular, palpable?
10. Can the lesion be transilluminated in a dark room?

The normal female breast shows considerable variation in size, shape, and consistency. In the obese patient the breast may be large and pendulous; in the slender

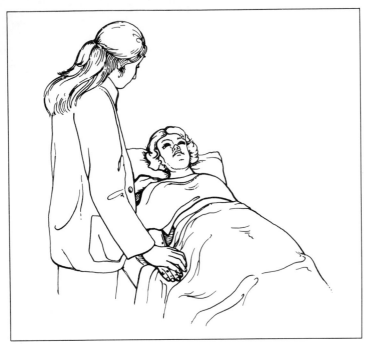

FIGURE 13-4
Woman draped for examination.

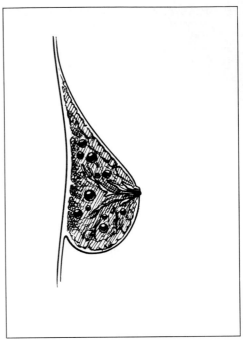

FIGURE 13-5
Chronic cystic mastitis
(also called fibrocystic disease).

person it may be thin and small. In young patients the breast tends to be firm, somewhat elastic in consistency, and cone-shaped. The borders of the breast tissue are clearly delineated, and it is possible to move the entire breast freely over the anterior chest wall. It is often very sensitive to palpation. This may be particularly marked just prior to the menstrual period. In older patients the breast develops an irregular consistency and the sharply delineated border tends to be obscured. This is particularly true after pregnancy and lactation.

The breasts tend to undergo cyclic changes that are reflected in alterations in fullness and thickness of the normal breast tissue. These changes accompany menstruation and are associated with epithelial hyperplasia and fibrosis. When such alterations are marked, one sees the clinical picture of fibrocystic breast disease (Fig. 13-5). Normal breast tissue may be characterized by a faint but distinct generalized nodularity. In some individuals this may be pronounced. This may make the recognition of a distinct tumor nodule difficult.

INSPECTION

Some degree of asymmetry is not uncommon and is usually the result of a difference in breast development. Increased size of one breast may, however, indicate the development of cyst, inflammation, or tumor. Asymmetry is most easily observed while the patient is in the sitting position.

The skin overlying the breast should be carefully observed. The edema associated with inflammatory carcinoma or the ulcerative involvement of the nipple

TABLE 13-1. Some Lesions of the Nipple

Lesion	Associations	Appearance
Inversion	Normality or, if of recent onset, malignancy	
Discharge	Blood: duct papilloma, cystic disease Milk: pregnancy, drugs, CNS disease Pus: infection	
Paget's disease	Malignancy	
Hyperpigmentation	Adrenal insufficiency	
Retention cysts	Normality	
Ulceration	Infection, neoplasm	
Inflammation	Infection, neoplasm	

seen in Paget's disease should be noted. Local areas of redness may indicate underlying inflammation and are important in the detection of early breast infection.

The nipple should be carefully examined for evidence of bleeding, discharge, retraction, or ulceration (Table 13-1).

Skin retraction is usually an indication of carcinoma, although it may result from traumatic fat necrosis. It is, however, a sign of malignancy and should be carefully searched for. The examination is best done by having the patient assume a position that will exert a pull on the suspensory ligaments of the breast. She should be examined while sitting erect and with her arms raised directly overhead. Elevating the arms should result in equal elevation of both breasts. A lesion producing shortening of the suspensory ligaments is likely to produce some retraction or deviation of the nipple. Another method of bringing out retraction is to produce contraction of the pectoral muscles, which in turn results in general traction on the breast tissue and tends to exaggerate any retraction that may be present. The patient should place the palms of both hands together and on command push the hands against each other. This may also be accomplished by placing her hands on her hips and pushing forcibly against them (Fig. 13-6A). It may be necessary to repeat these maneuvers several times so that all parts of the breasts can be adequately inspected. Another method of demonstrating retraction is to have the patient lean forward at the waist with her hands placed on the back of a chair. This demonstrates whether the breasts, as they fall away from the thorax, produce equal traction on the suspensory ligaments bilaterally. These maneuvers must be employed to detect early lesions. Obviously, with a grossly detectable lesion these steps are unnecessary (Table 13-2).

Inspection of the breasts should include careful observation of axillary and su-

TABLE 13-2. Some Visible Signs of Breast Cancer

Lesion	Cause
Peau d'orange	Lymphedema due to obstruction of lymphatic drainage by tumor

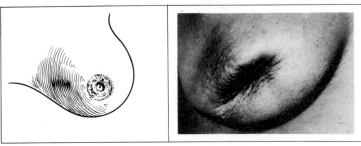

Retraction of the skin	Tumor involvement of Cooper's ligaments

TABLE 13-2. (Continued)

Increased venous pattern	Tumor obstruction of normal venous drainage

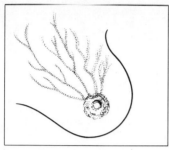

Erythema	Inflammatory tumor infiltrating skin or infection secondary to tumor

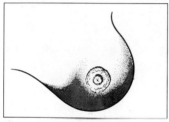

Paget's disease	Tumor originating in nipple

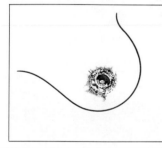 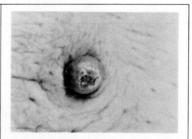

praclavicular regions for evidence of bulging, retraction, discoloration, or edema, since these are the important lymphatic drainage areas from the breasts.

PALPATION

The consistency of normal breast tissue varies widely. This variation will depend on such factors as age, obesity, stage of the menstrual cycle, and pregnancy. As experience is gained in the art of physical examination, the range of normal condition will become apparent.

Palpation of the breast is best carried out by means of a definite system of examination. Regardless of the patient's presenting complaint it is important to examine completely both breasts and their lymphatic drainage areas lest some serious lesion be overlooked. It is convenient to begin the examination in the upper lateral

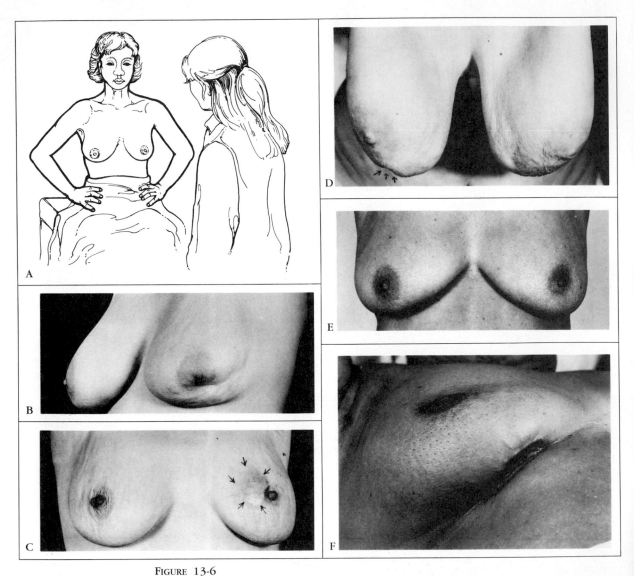

FIGURE 13-6
Some techniques of breast observation. A. Hands-on-hips technique may bring out retraction. B. Accentuation of nipple retraction and retraction of the skin, with deformity of breast contour accentuated by elevation of the arms. C. Large tumor of the medial aspect of the left breast and evidence of skin invasion as indicated by arrows. Despite its location adjacent to the nipple, there is very little evidence of nipple retraction. D. The indentation of the contour of the right breast, as indicated by arrows, is demonstrated by having the patient lean forward, thereby revealing an underlying breast tumor. E. Patient viewed from the front with both arms elevated. Both breasts are deceptively innocent. F. With the patient observed in the recumbent position, a large, ulcerative breast cancer is obvious in the costal mammary fold.

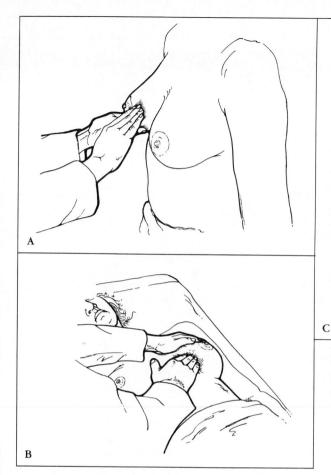

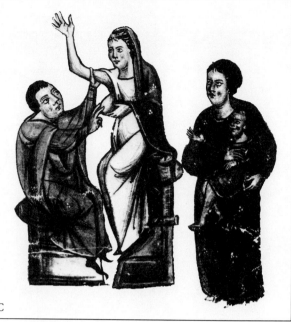

FIGURE 13-7
Technique of palpation of the breast. A. Patient seated. B. Patient supine. C. Breast palpation, from a late thirteenth century herbal.

aspect of each breast. The left breast is usually examined first, and palpation is carried out using the fingertips (Fig. 13-7). Gentle, light palpation should first be used; deeper exploration may be indicated if there is considerable breast substance. Palpation should be carried out in a clockwise direction until the entire breast has been examined. The nipple should be palpated for the presence of induration or a subareolar mass, and gentle pressure or a stripping action should be used to see whether discharge can be detected. Upon completion of examination of the left breast, the right breast is examined in a similar manner, again beginning in the upper lateral area and proceeding in a clockwise direction.

Palpation should be performed with the patient in both supine and seated positions. In both instances the breasts should be examined with the patient's arms at her side and then with her arms overhead.

The examiner should note the texture of the skin and the consistency and elasticity of the breast tissue. An increase in firmness may suggest infiltration or neoplasia. Tenderness to palpation usually indicates underlying inflammation. Malignant lesions by themselves are seldom tender but may coincide with widespread chronic cystic mastitis, in which case tenderness may be present.

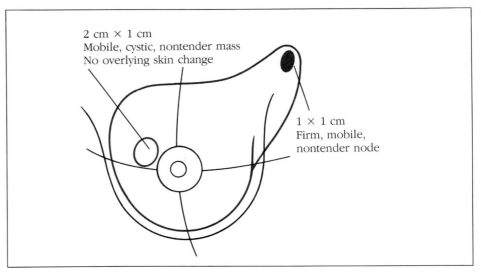

2 cm × 1 cm
Mobile, cystic, nontender mass
No overlying skin change

1 × 1 cm
Firm, mobile,
nontender node

FIGURE 13-8
Sample sketch of a cystic lesion of the left breast, such as may be recorded in the written workup.

If a mass is palpated, its size and location should be carefully recorded. This is usually done by considering the breast as the face of a clock with the nipple at the central point. The mass may be precisely located in regard to its distance from the nipple, and its size should be carefully estimated and recorded. It is often helpful to make a sketch of the area, describing the exact location and consistency (Fig. 13-8). The surface of the mass should be described, since malignant tumors may have irregular infiltrating margins while benign tumors may be sharply demarcated and smooth. The consistency of the mass may be helpful, since soft cystic lesions are more likely to be benign whereas firm and irregular masses are more likely to be malignant.

The examiner should observe whether the lesion is freely movable or is fixed in position. Benign tumors are usually movable. Inflammatory lesions may be moderately fixed; advanced malignant lesions are often fixed to other structures as they become invasive. In general, benign lesions tend to have discrete margins whereas malignancies tend to have boundaries that are difficult to define.

Both axillae should be systematically examined. This is best performed by examination with one hand while the examiner's opposite hand holds the patient's arm (Fig. 13-9). The boundaries of the axilla should be carefully palpated, and it is helpful to have the patient's arm go through a full range of motion during the examination in order to uncover any lesions that might otherwise be hidden beneath the pectoral muscle or subcutaneous fat.

The supraclavicular areas should be examined in a similar fashion; the neck should be palpated since the deep jugular nodes may be involved in metastatic spread. Since hepatic metastases are commonly found in patients with the advanced disease, the position and character of the liver edge should be noted.

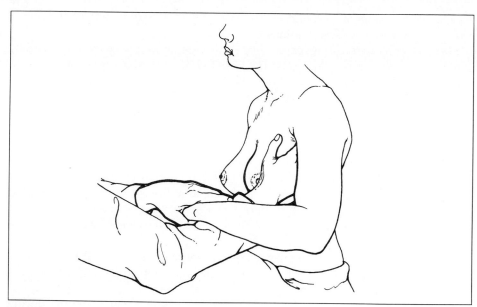

FIGURE 13-9
Technique of examination of the axilla.

If abnormalities are discovered, they are best documented in the written workup by careful description and mapping as illustrated.

Breast carcinomas are extremely variable in appearance, and a high index of suspicion is necessary if early diagnosis is to be achieved. Accurate diagnosis may only be obtained by biopsy, and this procedure should be promptly suggested if any question exists in the mind of the examiner.

Some general features of **carcinoma** include a firm or hard consistency and lack of tenderness on palpation. Lesions of moderate size shorten the supporting ligaments of the breast, producing dimpling of the skin or nipple. A bloody or purulent discharge from the nipple may occur if there is neoplastic involvement of the ducts or if the carcinoma is intraductal in origin. Advanced lesions may interfere with lymphatic drainage, producing an edematous thickening of the skin termed *peau d'orange*. Advanced carcinomas may also be associated with palpable regional lymph nodes.

Inflammatory carcinoma is a special variety of cancer characterized by infiltration in the skin that produces a red, raised margin resembling acute cellulitis. This may simulate an inflammatory lesion and be associated with pain, fever, and tenderness. This type of carcinoma is more common in premenopausal women, is sometimes seen during pregnancy, and has a bad prognostic outlook.

Intraductal papilloma is characterized by a bloody or dark discharge from the nipple. Gentle pressure in the quadrants of the breast will often permit one to identify the involved duct system. Careful palpation or stripping in this region will often result in production of the characteristic discharge.

Fibroadenoma (adenofibroma) is a nontender, firm lesion that is often multilobulated. It is most often found in young women and is difficult to differentiate from carcinoma by physical findings.

Chronic cystic mastitis is an exceedingly common breast lesion characterized by multiple nodules diffusely located in both breasts. The breast tissue is usually thickened and is often tender to palpation. The breasts frequently vary in size and degree of tenderness in association with the menstrual cycle. Occasionally the process may be fairly localized, or discrete nodules may be located in the presence of diffuse cystic changes. In either event biopsy is required for diagnosis.

Traumatic fat necrosis is a lesion that may simulate carcinoma, producing dimpling of the skin and retraction of the nipple. The consistency of the lesion is often firm, adding to the confusion. In some instances no history of trauma may be elicited. This lesion is more often encountered in large breasts containing increased amounts of fatty tissue. Absolute diagnosis can be established only by biopsy.

Paget's disease of the nipple is characterized by an excoriation or dry scaling lesion of the nipple. It may extend to involve the entire areola, tends to bleed easily on contact, and is always associated with an underlying carcinoma. It should be noted, however, that the underlying malignancy may not be palpable. Diagnosis may be achieved only by biopsy.

Mastitis is generalized inflammation of breast tissue, usually occurring during lactation. It is often associated with chills and fever. The involved breast tends to be red, edematous, and tender. Axillary lymphadenitis may occur, but fluctuation develops late or not at all. The soft, fatty nature of breast tissue tends to produce a spreading infection with little tendency to localization and abscess formation. This condition is usually associated with pyogenic infection.

Carcinoma of the male breast usually occurs as an irregular hard nodule underlying the areola. Because of the relative paucity of breast tissue, fixation to the chest wall occurs early. Metastasis is common by the time the carcinoma is detected. In general the prognosis is poor.

Gynecomastia is, by definition, a female type of breast occurring in a male patient. It is usually but not always unilateral. It must be distinguished from fatty breast occurring in a normal male. In the young patient the breast tends to assume a conical shape and be glandular in consistency, resembling the breast of a pubertal female. In elderly men the nodularity may be more irregular, and it may be difficult to rule out neoplasm. Biopsy, of course, is required under these circumstances. When gynecomastia is bilateral, it may be related to some systemic disease. For example, in patients with cirrhosis of the liver, altered metabolism of estrogens may lead to gynecomastia. Certain testicular tumors may cause gynecomastia, as may certain drugs. Other causes of gynecomastia are noted in Table 13-3. Sophisticated biochemical studies may be necessary to complete the diagnostic workup in these patients.

SELF-EXAMINATION

The technique of self-examination of the breast has been widely advocated as a means of early detection of malignant disease. Patients frequently seek advice regarding the method and frequency of its use. This brief description may be of help in advising patients on this matter.

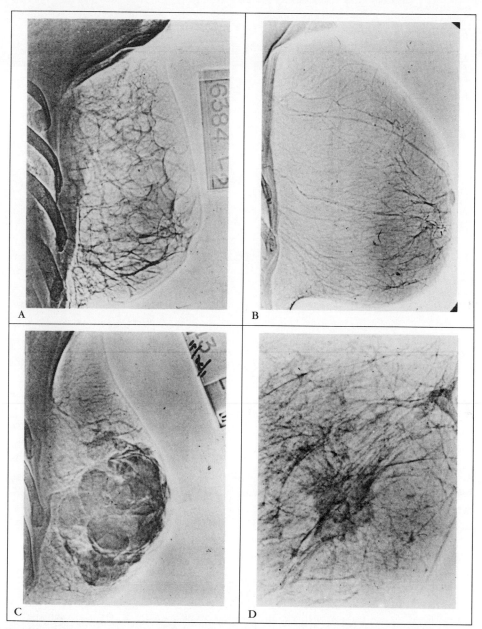

FIGURE 13-10

Xeromammography: a sensitive diagnostic study in breast disease. A. Xeromammogram of a premenopausal woman showing normal breast architecture and suspensory ligaments. B. Xeromammogram of a postmenopausal woman showing thinning and atrophy of the breast tissue and supporting structures. C. Xeromammogram of a 19-year-old woman with a firm lobulated mass within the breast. This is a typical appearance of a fibroadenoma. D. Xeromammogram of a portion of breast tissue in a postmenopausal woman with a firm but indistinct mass palpable within the left breast. The appearance is typical of scirrhous carcinoma, showing its infiltrating nature and retraction of the nipple.

TABLE 13-3. Some Causes of Gynecomastia

Physiologic
　Neonatal
　Pubertal
　Involutional
Endocrine
　Testicular failure
　Testicular tumors
　Hyperthyroidism
　Adrenocortical tumors
　Hermaphroditism
　Pituitary tumors
Liver disease
Malnutrition and renutrition
Bronchogenic carcinoma
Drugs
　Estrogens
　Chorionic gonadotropins
　Digitalis
　Phenothiazines
　Reserpine
　Aldactone

The patient should establish a regular schedule for monthly breast examination. This is ideally carried out immediately following the end of her menstrual period. An examination during the period may be unsatisfactory because of the temporary changes in consistency and tenderness that so often occur. The woman, however, may use the menstrual period as a reminder to inspect her breasts. After the menopause, monthly examination should, of course, be continued. The patient should be instructed to consult her physician immediately upon detecting a lump of any kind. The judgment and course of action should then be her physician's responsibility. She should also be warned to be alert for dimpling or puckering of the skin, retraction of either nipple, any thickening or change in consistency, or any alteration in symmetry, size, contour, or position. A discharge from the nipple may be significant. Pain, swelling, or inflammation may indicate advanced cancer, although more often they are associated with nonmalignant conditions. Having thus been advised of what to look for, she should be instructed in the following techniques:

1. **Observation.** The patient should place herself before a mirror with her arms at her sides. She should carefully examine her breasts in the mirror for symmetry, size, and shape, searching for any evidence of puckering, dimpling of the skin, or retraction of the nipple. She should then raise her arms above her head and again study her breasts in the mirror, looking for the same physical signs. She should also be alert for any evidence of fixation of the breast tissue to the chest wall. This may be displayed as she moves her arms and shoulders.

2. **Palpation.** This should be performed in the reclining position. This position permits the breasts to spread over a greater area and thins the breast tissue, making accurate palpation easier. A small pillow or folded towel should be placed beneath

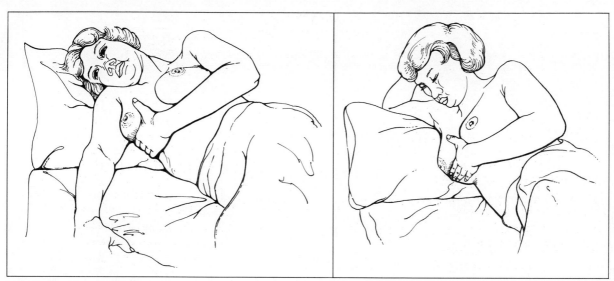

FIGURE 13-11
Self-examination of the breasts.

the shoulder on the side of the breast to be examined (Fig. 13-11). This raises that side of the body and distributes the weight of the breast tissue more evenly over the chest wall. The arm on the side to be first examined is placed at her side, and the breast is gently examined with the flat surface of the fingers of her opposite hand. The technique calls for gentle palpation of the breast tissue against the chest wall, usually beginning on the outer half of the breast, paying particular attention to the upper outer quadrant where the axillary tail of breast tissue is thickest and where most tumors occur.

She should then raise the arm above her head and thoroughly examine the inner half of the breast beginning at the sternum. When the entire breast has been carefully palpated, the pillow is placed beneath the opposite shoulder and the woman investigates the second breast in exactly the same manner.

Palpation of the breast should be thorough and unhurried. Every portion of the breast must be deliberately and carefully examined if small lesions are to be detected.

The patient should be instructed to place the greatest emphasis on the regions where most breast cancers develop, namely in the axillary tail of the breast and beneath the nipple. If the technique is to be effective, she must establish a definite habit pattern and conduct a thorough examination at monthly intervals. The method will only be effective if it is used regularly.

SECTION V
ABDOMEN AND PELVIS

Abdominal pain is one of the most common conditions which call for speedy diagnosis and treatment. Usually, though by no means always, there are other symptoms which accompany the pain, but in the majority of cases of acute abdominal disease, pain is the main symptom and complaint.

SIR ZACHARY COPE
(1881–1974)

Abdominal Examination*
1. Inspect position, general appearance, abdominal wall, flanks, and back.

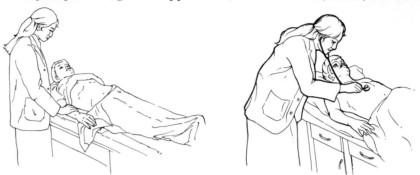

2. Auscultate abdomen for bowel sounds, rubs, hums, and bruits.
3. Percuss abdomen for organ size, masses, and tympany.

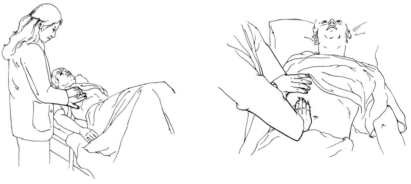

4. Palpate for tenderness, masses, and organ size.

In acute abdomen or limited physical examination proceed now to:

1. *Rectal examination* for appearance, sphincter tone, masses, and blood in stool.
2a. In men—*genitourinary examination* for hernia, testicular masses, and tenderness.
2b. In women—*pelvic examination* for tenderness, discharge, and masses.

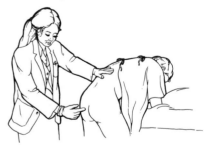

* The male genitourinary, the female pelvic, and the rectal examinations in both sexes are often done at the end of the physical examination for convenience. They are, however, logically associated with the gastrointestinal system and are an essential part of the immediate physical examination done in evaluation of an acute abdomen.

GASTROINTESTINAL SYSTEM

CHAPTER 14

A good eater must be a good man; for a good eater must have a good digestion, and good digestion depends upon a good conscience.

BENJAMIN DISRAELI, LORD BEACONSFIELD
(1804–1881)

Evaluation of the gastrointestinal system is a blend of meticulous history, careful physical examination, and judicious use of radiologic and endoscopic studies. Although proper diagnosis can frequently be obtained by history and physical, confirmation may mandate a contrast study of the bowel, selected endoscopy, or biopsy. With increased skill and experience the examiner should be able to predict confidently the findings of these special studies in the majority of circumstances.

ANATOMY

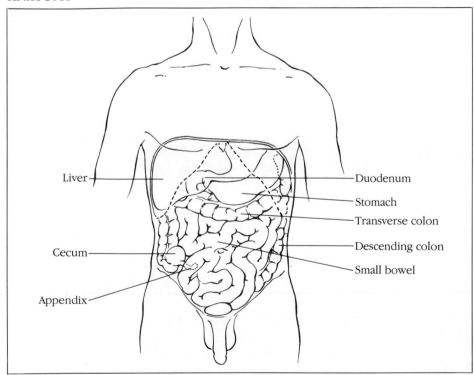

FIGURE 14-1
Schematic abdominal contents.

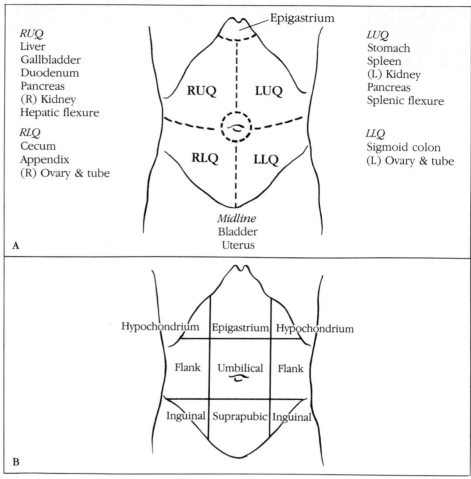

RUQ
Liver
Gallbladder
Duodenum
Pancreas
(R) Kidney
Hepatic flexure

RLQ
Cecum
Appendix
(R) Ovary & tube

Epigastrium

RUQ   LUQ

RLQ   LLQ

LUQ
Stomach
Spleen
(L) Kidney
Pancreas
Splenic flexure

LLQ
Sigmoid colon
(L) Ovary & tube

Midline
Bladder
Uterus

A

Hypochondrium Epigastrium Hypochondrium

Flank Umbilical Flank

Inguinal Suprapubic Inguinal

B

FIGURE 14-2
Superficial topography of the abdomen. A. Four-quadrant system. B. Nine-region system.

HISTORY

In the evaluation of chronic gastrointestinal complaints, a careful analysis and description of the symptoms, how they developed, the order in which they appeared and changed, are usually far more informative than the physical examination.

HOWARD M. SPIRO
(1924–   )

Gastrointestinal complaints are among the most common given by patients to their physicians.

PAIN

Pain of gastrointestinal origin varies greatly, depending on its underlying cause. The major pain mechanisms include:

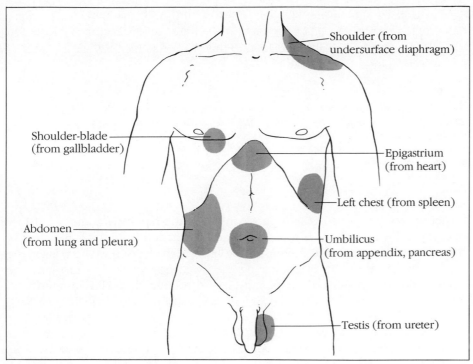

FIGURE 14-3
Common sites of referred pain.

1. Capsular stretching—as in liver congestion due to heart failure
2. Irritation of the mucosa—as in acute gastritis
3. Severe smooth muscle spasm—as in acute enterocolitis
4. Peritoneal inflammation—as in acute appendicitis
5. Direct splanchnic nerve stimulation—as in retroperitoneal extension of a neoplasm, such as carcinoma of the pancreas

The *character, duration,* and *frequency* of gastrointestinal pain are functions of their mechanism of production; the *location* and *distribution* of referred pain are related to the anatomic site of origin. *Time of occurrence* and elements that *aggravate* and *relieve* the discomfort, such as meals, defecation, and sleep, also have special significance directly related to the underlying cause.

An outline of major sites of localization of pain usually includes the following:

Esophageal: Midline retrosternal; radiation to the back at the level of the lesion
Gastric: Epigastric; radiation occasionally to back, particularly left subscapular
Duodenal: Epigastric; radiation to back, particularly right subscapular
Gallbladder: Right upper quadrant or epigastric; radiation to right subscapular or
    midback
Pancreatic: Epigastric; radiation to midback or left lumbar area
Small intestinal: Periumbilical

Appendiceal: Periumbilical, migrating later to right lower quadrant
Colonic: Hypogastrium, right or left lower quadrant, depending on site of lesion;
   sigmoid pain with possible radiation to the sacral region
Rectal: Deep pelvic localization

ACUTE ABDOMEN

It is a curious but well known fact that many who are taken with abdominal pain in the daytime endure till evening until feeling compelled to send for the doctor. It follows that important diagnoses often have to be made at night . . . when the physician, weary with the day's work, is both physically and mentally below his best.

SIR ZACHARY COPE
(1881–1974)

There is no arena of clinical diagnosis in which the rapid and complete history (and physical examination) is more dramatically urgent than in the assessment of the patient with catastrophic abdominal disease. For that reason we have taken the unconventional approach of presenting the evaluation of the patient with the "acute abdomen" prior to describing the more routine abdominal examination. You should note that the history surrounding the abdominal event is key to accurate diagnosis. Physical examination and further diagnostic studies are based on clues elicited during the carefully taken history.

The term *acute abdomen* suggests the importance and urgency which often accompanies acute intra-abdominal disease. Because of this urgency one should attempt to clarify the problem and arrive at a precise diagnosis when the patient is seen for the first time. The success of the examiner will depend on the thoroughness of his examination and his ability to pursue an orderly approach to the problem. Carelessness will be accompanied by a marked decline in accuracy. Early diagnosis is of crucial importance; the delay of even a few hours may permit peritonitis to develop or perforation of a viscus to occur. Delay also almost inevitably results in unnecessary morbidity and the likelihood of an increased mortality rate. The temptation to temporize is often strong in order to observe the course of the patient. While this may sometimes be justified, in many instances it will only result in the loss of a golden opportunity to treat surgical emergencies early and achieve superior results. It is often stated that abdominal pain that develops in a patient who has previously been well and persists for over 6 hours is caused by a condition requiring surgical attention. The practice of consistently performing a thorough examination of the acute abdomen will result in making a correct diagnosis early in the course of the disease, permitting prompt surgical treatment, if indicated.

Although the patient with acute abdominal distress is usually in pain, it is important to withhold the use of sedative or analgesic drugs until a satisfactory diagnosis has been made and one can ascertain whether surgical intervention will be required. Analgesics alter physical signs and symptoms to such an extent that accurate diagnosis often becomes impossible following their administration.

The patient who is suffering from acute, severe pain is not likely to be able to cooperate by furnishing a complete narrative history. In fact, under the urgency of the situation it may be important to depart from the routine and ask direct questions. Historical information derived from the patient himself should be supplemented whenever possible by detailed questions asked of his family and friends.

The relatives or friends who accompany the patient to the hospital should be consulted regarding significant points before they are permitted to leave.

Whenever possible, a complete and detailed history and physical examination should be performed. Under some circumstances the severity of the illness may make prompt emergency treatment imperative. Under these circumstances the diagnostic approach will require abbreviation. It is still necessary, however, to obtain sufficient information to provide an adequate working diagnosis. Shortcuts are likely to be expensive in time, accuracy, and human life. Each symptom must be carefully and thoroughly evaluated in terms of its relationship to physical findings and other symptoms.

The **patient's age** is pertinent. The occurrence of certain disease processes is often limited to certain age groups. Recognition of this factor makes it possible to improve diagnostic accuracy.

A clear **description of the disease process** is of utmost importance. The patient should be asked to fix the exact time at which the pain began and the manner of its beginning. For example, pain of gradual onset may be associated with appendicitis, while the sudden onset of acute abdominal pain, awakening the patient from sleep, may be associated with perforation of a duodenal ulcer. It should also be noted whether the onset of the pain is related to some injury or exertion, no matter how trivial. The severity of the condition may be estimated by asking whether the patient collapsed or lost consciousness at the onset of the symptoms. Severe symptoms are more likely to be associated with such intra-abdominal catastrophes as acute pancreatitis, perforated ulcer, ruptured ectopic pregnancy, or strangulation obstruction of the bowel.

The character, distribution, and mode of onset of the pain should be carefully evaluated. Even the generalized pain associated with perforated ulcer or hemorrhage from a tubal pregnancy usually begins in a specific location, later spreading and becoming generalized. With perforated duodenal ulcer, for example, pain characteristically originates in the epigastrium with severe intensity but rapidly becomes generalized. For a time the pain may be more acute in the right flank and right lower quadrant, as the irritating gastric fluid passes down the gutter on the right side of the abdomen.

Pain that arises from the small intestine is usually felt primarily in the epigastrium and periumbilical areas. This is true whether it is simple mechanical intestinal obstruction or strangulation obstruction, since the innervation of the small bowel corresponds to the distribution of the ninth through the eleventh thoracic nerves. Since the innervation of the appendix is derived from the same source, this also explains why appendicitis usually begins with onset of pain in the epigastrium, followed by radiation to the right lower quadrant as the peritoneum and the psoas muscle become secondarily involved. Pain associated with large-bowel conditions is usually referred to the hypogastrium or to the actual site of the lesion.

In addition to noting the origin of the pain, it is also significant to follow its change in **localization**. The shifting of pain from the upper abdomen to the lower abdomen may be associated with the accumulation of irritating or infected peritoneal fluid in the pelvis. This may occur with a perforated ulcer or acute pancreatitis.

The **nature of the pain** is often a help in diagnosis. Crampy, constricting pain is characteristic of biliary colic, while burning pain is more likely associated with peptic ulceration. Back pain that is severe and constant may be associated with pancreatitis. Appendicitis is usually associated with a constant aching pain, except when a fecalith is present, in which case it may be colicky in nature.

The **radiation of the pain** is often significant. This is particularly true of colic associated with obstruction of hollow viscera, for the pain radiates to the area of distribution of the nerves coming from that segment of spinal cord supplying the affected viscus. For this reason biliary colic is frequently referred to the area beneath the right scapula, and renal colic is frequently referred to the testis.

The **relationship of pain to respiration** should always be noted. With intra-abdominal sepsis, such as peritonitis or abscess, deep inspiration may cause pain. On the other hand, pleuritic pain is made worse by inspiration but often disappears when the patient holds his breath.

A complete history inquires into the possible **relationship of pain to urination.** In addition to the many urinary conditions that may produce this, peritonitis or an abscess lying adjacent to the bladder may cause pain on urination and may even be associated with hematuria.

Vomiting may be associated with the following intra-abdominal conditions: acute gastritis; irritation of the peritoneum or mesentery (e.g., vomiting may appear early in the course of peritonitis associated with appendicitis or perforated ulcer); obstruction of hollow viscera producing smooth muscle spasm (e.g., biliary or ureteral colic or intestinal obstruction may be associated with vomiting); bacterial toxins or certain tissue metabolites may have a direct central action and may produce vomiting on a reflex basis. This is often seen in cases of septic peritonitis.

It is important to note the time relationship between the onset of pain and the exact time of vomiting. With biliary-tract calculus or sudden, severe peritoneal irritation, vomiting occurs early in the course of the disease and is likely to be violent. Low small-bowel obstruction may be associated with delayed vomiting, while vomiting occurs promptly with high small-bowel lesions. With large-bowel obstruction, vomiting may be a very late feature or may not occur at all. With appendicitis the onset of pain almost always antedates vomiting by several hours.

Not all intra-abdominal emergencies are associated with vomiting. Massive intraperitoneal hemorrhage may occur in absence of vomiting, and intussusception may be deceptive because vomiting may occur late or not at all.

The physical characteristics of the vomitus should be noted. In acute gastritis the vomitus consists largely of gastric contents occasionally flecked with small amounts of blood. With intestinal obstruction the characteristics of the vomitus show considerable variation. As the condition progresses, the character changes from gastric contents to bilious material, becoming yellowish green and finally consisting of brown, feculent-smelling fluid. Feculent vomiting may occur in either dynamic or adynamic intestinal obstruction.

If the patient denies vomiting, it is worthwhile to ask him about nausea or anorexia. There is considerable variation in the ease with which people vomit, and the presence of nausea or loss of appetite may in some individuals carry the same significance as vomiting does in others.

The condition of the **bowels** and nature of the **stool** should be investigated. An estimate of the patient's normal bowel habits should be obtained as well as careful analysis of how the acute illness may cause departure from his normal routine. The presence of gross or occult blood should be noted. The combination of blood and

TABLE 14-1. Some Causes of Acute Abdominal Pain

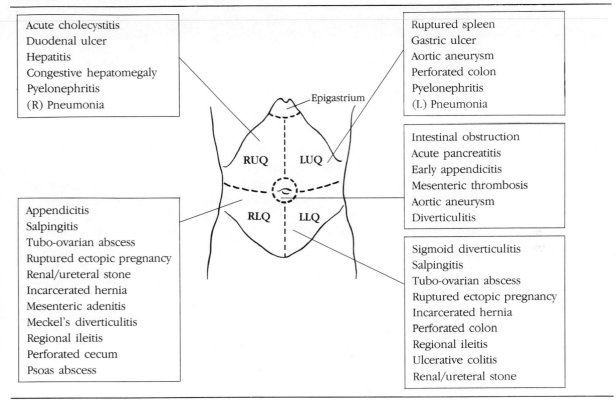

Acute cholecystitis
Duodenal ulcer
Hepatitis
Congestive hepatomegaly
Pyelonephritis
(R) Pneumonia

Ruptured spleen
Gastric ulcer
Aortic aneurysm
Perforated colon
Pyelonephritis
(L) Pneumonia

Epigastrium

RUQ   LUQ

RLQ   LLQ

Intestinal obstruction
Acute pancreatitis
Early appendicitis
Mesenteric thrombosis
Aortic aneurysm
Diverticulitis

Appendicitis
Salpingitis
Tubo-ovarian abscess
Ruptured ectopic pregnancy
Renal/ureteral stone
Incarcerated hernia
Mesenteric adenitis
Meckel's diverticulitis
Regional ileitis
Perforated cecum
Psoas abscess

Sigmoid diverticulitis
Salpingitis
Tubo-ovarian abscess
Ruptured ectopic pregnancy
Incarcerated hernia
Perforated colon
Regional ileitis
Ulcerative colitis
Renal/ureteral stone

mucus in the stool is suggestive of intussusception. Pelvic infections may alter bowel habits and produce lower abdominal pain, diarrhea, and, in some instances, tenesmus.

In women a careful **menstrual history** should be recorded, noting the characteristics of the period, including the last date of onset and the nature of the flow. Those data are necessary if one is to consider the diagnosis of threatened abortion, tubal pregnancy, and other gynecologic problems.

Vascular catastrophes, such as abdominal aortic aneurysm undergoing rupture, can produce severe pain and profound constitutional symptoms. They also require rapid diagnosis and surgical intervention.

Past history of the pain involved may be extremely valuable in making a diagnosis of such conditions as hiatus hernia, duodenal ulcer, and gastric carcinoma. The possible relationship to previous attacks of jaundice, hematemesis, melena, and so on may also contribute important information (Table 14-1).

It is obviously necessary to exclude medical diseases before deciding on the need for surgical intervention. A number of medical conditions may mimic intra-abdominal emergencies. Examples are typhoid fever, pericarditis, lower lobe pneumonia, pyelonephritis, tuberculous peritonitis, and tabes dorsalis. These possibilities emphasize the need for a thorough, objective, and systematic approach to examining entirely the patient who presents with abdominal pain.

The general rule can be laid down that the majority of severe abdominal pains which ensue in patients who have been previously fairly well, and which last as long as six hours, are caused by condition of surgical import.

SIR ZACHARY COPE
(1881–1974)

OTHER GASTROINTESTINAL SYMPTOMS

Illness isn't the only thing that spoils the appetite.

IVAN TURGENEV
(1818–1883)

The less acutely ill patient may present with a history of dysphagia, vomiting, and bowel dysfunction, which are discussed below.

Dysphagia is usually more prominent and severe with solid food than liquids. The sensation is generally localized by the patient to the approximate level of obstruction. It is an important symptom and must never be ignored. Table 14-2 presents some causes of dysphagia.

TABLE 14-2. Some Causes of Dysphagia

Mechanical obstruction of the esophagus	Dysphagia secondary to pain
Congenital stricture	Pharyngitis
Stricture due to corrosives	Laryngitis
Foreign bodies	
Carcinoma of the esophagus or stomach	
Extrinsic compression, as with aortic aneurysm	
Esophageal diverticula/pouches	
Reflux esophagitis with stricture	
Neurologic dysfunction of the esophagus	
Bulbar paralysis	
Syphilis	
Lead poisoning	
Rabies	
Tetanus	
Parkinson's disease	
Botulism	
Myasthenia gravis	
Poliomyelitis	
Achalasia of the esophagus	
Plummer-Vinson syndrome (iron deficiency anemia and esophageal webs)	
Hysteria	

Vomiting is often associated with upper gastrointestinal disorders. The patient should be questioned regarding the frequency, time of occurrence, and aggravating factors, as well as the quantity, color, odor, and taste of the vomited material.

Bowel function varies greatly among individuals. Direct observation of a stool specimen by the physician is far more accurate than a patient's description. Normal frequency of bowel action varies from several times daily to once every three to five days. Diarrhea or constipation of recent onset requires detailed description. The former is particularly important when it occurs mostly at night and suggests diabetes mellitus.

Additional gastrointestinal symptoms of importance include hematemesis, melena, anorexia, a sense of abdominal fullness, heartburn (pyrosis), regurgitation, flatulence, and belching.

There is no substitute for seeing the patient while he is having pain.

HOWARD M. SPIRO
(1924–   )

PHYSICAL EXAMINATION

1. Inspection of facial expression, respirations, position, skin (jaundice, pallor, pigmentation, etc.), nutrition, hydration, hands and nails, mouth, abdominal contour—masses, bulges, peristalsis, venous pattern
2. Auscultation for bowel sounds, rubs, bruits

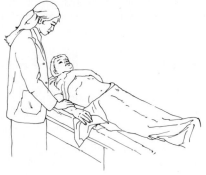 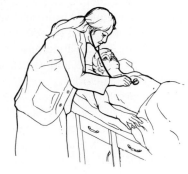

3. Palpation and percussion for tenderness, rigidity, masses, visceromegaly, rebound, fluid
4. Special maneuvers for psoas sign, obturator sign, etc. (if indicated)

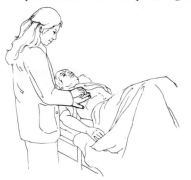 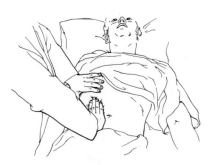

5. Rectal/vaginal examination to be considered now in acute abdominal disease

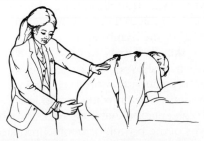

GENERAL

Jaundice is the disease that your friends diagnose.
SIR WILLIAM OSLER
(1849–1919)

As the first step in the examination of the abdomen, make sure that the patient is completely relaxed and properly positioned. His head should lie comfortably on one or two pillows, and his arms should be at his sides. The knees should be raised slightly in order to relax the abdominal musculature. Draw aside the bedclothes to make sure there is adequate exposure from the costal margin to the symphysis pubis. It is helpful to have the bed or examining table high enough to permit you to work in comfort and to have the patient close enough to the edge to permit access to the entire abdomen. Both the room and your hands should be warm, since chilling produces involuntary muscle spasm that hampers satisfactory examination. Lighting, of course, must be adequate.

A systematic plan for abdominal examination follows this sequence: inspection, ausculation, percussion, and palpation. By closely following this method the examiner may avoid omissions.

Since the gastrointestinal tract is highly sensitive to emotional state, a logical first step is to assess the patient's **face** and demeanor for signs of depression, agitation, exhaustion, hostility, and fear. A pale face with beads of perspiration may be associated with the shock accompanying acute pancreatitis or strangulation obstruction of the intestine. Pallor may be associated with massive intraperitoneal hemorrhage from a ruptured spleen or may reflect the anemia associated with acute and chronic blood loss. It should be remembered, however, that intra-abdominal catastrophes may occur without producing characteristic changes in the facies. In the late stages of many acute intra-abdominal processes, profound changes in facial expression may be accompanied by dulling of the eyes, shrinking of the tongue, and a cool skin, reflecting loss of circulating blood volume and impending failure of the circulation.

The **position** assumed by the patient is worth noting. With biliary or intestinal colic he may be unable to lie quietly; intraperitoneal hemorrhage may produce profound restlessness. This is contrasted with the patient suffering from generalized peritonitis who lies quietly with his knees drawn up to relax his abdominal muscles and relieve intra-abdominal tension.

The **respiration rate** should be noted, for a rapid rate may be associated with intrathoracic disease. Tachypnea may also be associated with generalized peritonitis, intestinal obstruction, intra-abdominal hemorrhage, or anxiety. The movement of the abdominal wall with respiration should be observed. Limitation of movement may be associated with abdominal distention, rigidity of the abdominal musculature, or limited mobility of the diaphragm.

Briefly note the state of **skin** and **nails** and the **hair distribution**. Patients with gallbladder or liver disease may show evidence of jaundice. The yellow discoloration of the sclera and skin is frequently more obvious in daylight than in artificial light, where it may pass unnoticed, even when moderately severe. Other important skin changes include (1) pigmentation that may reflect malabsorption, regional enteritis, adenomatous polyps of the bowel, or hemochromatosis; (2) xanthomas associated with biliary cirrhosis; (3) erythema nodosum from ulcerative colitis; (4) a flush suggesting carcinoid neoplasm; (5) generalized edema caused by intestinal malabsorption; and (6) spider angiomata or petechiae, palmar erythema, and hair loss, which together indicate chronic liver disease.

Outward signs of the patient's **nutritional state** indirectly reflect gastrointestinal function. Weight loss and emaciation need little emphasis here because of their obvious importance. Nail changes include (1) koilonychia (spooning) with chronic iron deficiency, and (2) clubbing with intestinal malabsorption, regional enteritis, ulcerative colitis, and hepatic cirrhosis. Dehydration may cause reduction of ocular tension, xerostomia, and persistent ridging of the skin on the dorsum of the hand when lightly pinched. Serious fluid loss frequently accompanies gastrointestinal disease.

Fever is not a constant companion of intra-abdominal disease. In the presence of shock, septicemia, acute pancreatitis, strangulating intestinal obstruction, or perforated ulcer, the temperature may be normal or subnormal at onset. A low-grade fever may accompany the early stages of acute appendicitis; higher temperatures occur with peritonitis. High fever is not often associated with the early stages of acute abdominal disease.

The **pulse rate** and its character should be carefully noted. It is true that a normal pulse does not necessarily mean a normal condition within the abdomen, although it may indicate that the patient is reacting well to his disease. It is worthwhile to follow the pulse rate at intervals, for it is likely to increase in rate as the intra-abdominal infection or hemorrhage progresses. As peritonitis advances, the pulse may show slight irregularity or be somewhat bounding. In advanced peritonitis the pulse is rapid and thready. This is a bad prognostic sign.

MOUTH

A detailed examination of the mouth is considered in Chapter 9, but it should be emphasized that inspection of the oral cavity is an important part of the gastrointestinal examination. Observe the lips, oral mucosa, teeth and gingivae, and tongue. Is salivation adequate? Although some nutritional deficiencies are reflected in the oral cavity, many nonpathologic changes may be observed. Some of these include (1) cracking of the lips due to exposure to weather and cold; (2) angular stomatitis from poorly fitting dentures; (3) mild gingivitis, a very common finding in otherwise healthy people; (4) prominent fungiform papillae, usually along the midline, giving an appearance called "geographic tongue"; and (6) normal furring or coating of the tongue, which is merely dead epithelium combined with yeast and saprophytes. The well-known "coated tongue" may be of some concern to a patient, but it is common in healthy people. Severe halitosis may occur with chronic gastroesophageal disease, particularly neoplasm (Table 14-3). Fetor hepaticus is a term describing a characteristic odor associated with severe liver failure; at times it is apparent at some distance from the patient's bed. In peptic disease of the stomach and duodenum the patient's breath often has an acid odor.

Glossitis and stomatitis often accompany deficiency states caused by chronic gastrointestinal disorders, such as sprue, with associated malabsorption and depleted body stores of iron, vitamin B_{12}, folic acid, niacin, thiamine, and riboflavin. Melanin

TABLE 14-3. Some Characteristic Mouth Odors in Disease

Name	Description	Condition
Acetone breath	Smells of acetone—sweet, like fruity chewing gum	Diabetic ketoacidosis
Fetor hepaticus	"Mousy" odor, sickly sweet	Hepatic failure
Acid breath	Acrid, acid smell	Peptic disease
Fetid breath	Sickening odor of decay	Lung abscess Esophageal diverticulum
Feculent breath	Odor like feces	Lung abscess Severe bowel obstruction
Bitter almonds	Can be detected by only some examiners (perception is genetic trait)	Cyanide toxicity
Uriniferous breath	Odor like urine	Renal failure

spots about the face and mouth are a sign of intestinal polyposis. They are frequently drab brown or dark bluish black and may be mistaken for simple freckles.

ABDOMEN

Drink a glass of wine after your soup, and you steal a ruble from the doctor.

RUSSIAN PROVERB

INSPECTION

For convenience, we divide the abdomen into topographic segments. This division permits precise localization of physical signs and symptoms and makes it possible to correlate physical signs with the anatomic location of viscera within the abdomen. A number of systems for describing topographic anatomy have been advocated, as illustrated under "Anatomy." In describing historical location or physical findings, refer to one of these systems.

As you inspect the abdomen, first observe the skin, its color, and its texture. Are there any unusual lesions, striae, or surgical scars (Fig. 14-4)?

Usually the venous pattern is barely perceptible, and the drainage of the lower two-thirds of the abdomen is downward (Fig. 14-5). Superficial abdominal veins may be dilated and tortuous because of vena caval obstruction. With portal hypertension of hepatic cirrhosis, the veins may appear to radiate from the umbilicus as a result of backflow through the collateral veins within the falciform ligament. This pattern is termed *caput medusae.*

Next, observe the general contour of the abdomen. Is it symmetrical? Is there any localized bulging or prominence? A scaphoid abdomen often accompanies cachexia; protuberance may result from gaseous distention, ascites, or neoplasm. Observe specifically for hernia.

An *umbilical hernia* protrudes through the umbilical ring. In the newborn a congenital umbilical hernia may result from improper closure of the abdominal wall; a hernia of the umbilical cord, also termed an *omphalocele,* is produced. The peritoneal sac is not covered by the skin of the abdominal wall.

True umbilical hernias are common during the first year of life. In this type the peritoneal sac is covered by skin. Increased intra-abdominal pressure due to trauma, cough, or constipation may contribute to their formation.

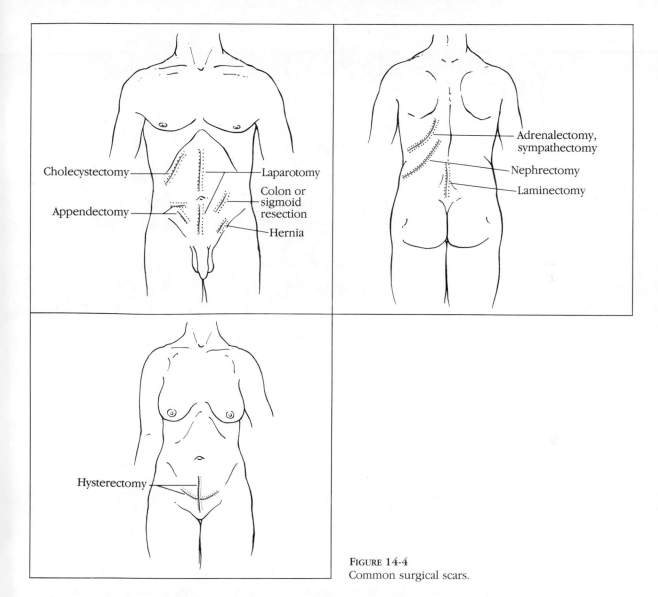

Cholecystectomy

Laparotomy

Colon or sigmoid resection

Appendectomy

Hernia

Adrenalectomy, sympathectomy

Nephrectomy

Laminectomy

Hysterectomy

FIGURE 14-4
Common surgical scars.

Umbilical hernias in adults are more common in women. Obesity, pregnancy, ascites, or congenital defect may be contributing factors. Umbilical hernias may show wide variation in size, but the neck of the sac is often small. This type of hernia usually contains omentum but may contain large or small bowel and other viscera as well. Strangulation is a frequent occurrence. Diastasis or separation of the rectus muscles is often associated.

An *epigastric hernia* occurs through a weakness in the linea alba between the xiphoid and the umbilicus, usually due to a developmental defect. Pregnancy, obesity, trauma, or constipation may be contributing factors. These hernias are most common in young adult males. The hernial sac is usually small and may contain omentum but rarely intestine. Strangulation rarely occurs.

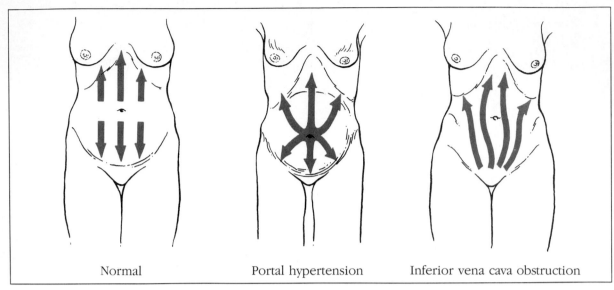

Normal   Portal hypertension   Inferior vena cava obstruction

FIGURE 14-5
Abdominal venous patterns.

Incisional hernias, as the name indicates, occur through surgical incisions. Infection, poor wound healing, faulty wound closure, postoperative vomiting, ileus, partial wound disruption, and obesity may be contributing factors. This type of hernia often reaches large size, and the intestines are usually adherent to the underside of the peritoneum. Strangulation is uncommon but may occasionally occur.

A *spigelian hernia* occurs at some point in the semilunar line at the lateral margin of the rectus muscle, usually in the lower abdomen at the linea semicircularis where the posterior rectus sheath is absent.

Is the umbilicus in the midline and normal? Instruct the patient to cough or bear down, and notice whether this produces any bulging. Does this maneuver cause any pain? Normally it does not. Note any unusual movement causing a slight protrusion with inspiration due to descent of the diaphragm. A decrease in respiratory movements of the abdomen may suggest intraperitoneal fluid, or it may be associated with acute abdominal pain, such as with peritonitis. Are there any visible peristaltic waves? With intestinal obstruction, peristaltic waves may be visible passing across the abdomen.

Finally, are there any vascular pulsations? Occasionally in the thin individual with a flat or scaphoid abdomen, the normal aortic pulsation may be evident in the epigastrium.

AUSCULTATION
Many experienced examiners will auscultate the abdomen before percussion or palpation are begun (as opposed to the classic order). In the presence of abdominal disease, percussion and palpation may cause slowing of the bowel and diminution of peristaltic sounds. Moreover, the stethoscope itself may be used, concurrent with careful auscultation, as the first instrument of light palpation. It is useful to

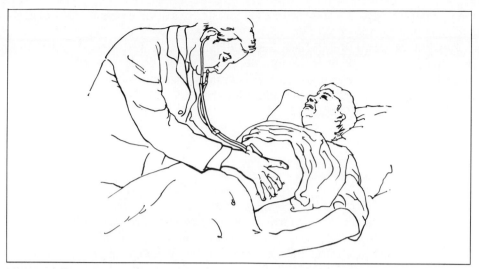

FIGURE 14-6
Checking for succussion splash.

warm the stethoscopic head (often done by simply holding it in your hand or under your armpit) before placing it on the abdomen.

Most intestinal sounds originate from the small bowel and have a high-pitched, gurgling quality, better sensed than described. Frequency of intestinal sounds varies in relation to meals, but usually five or more sounds occur each minute. The examiner should be accustomed to hearing the sounds that accompany normal peristalsis.

Abnormal bowel sounds are distinguishable only when you have developed a clear appreciation of the normal variation in peristaltic sound. Peristalsis may be increased, diminished, or absent in the presence of intra-abdominal disease. Absence of bowel sounds suggests **paralytic ileus** due to diffuse peritoneal irritation. Before bowel sounds can be said to be absent, however, it is necessary to listen for periods of at least one minute in all portions of the abdomen. Increased peristalsis will usually be audible in patients with acute intestinal obstruction. In these patients the abdomen tends to be silent between bouts of colic. As the cramps occur, the bowel sounds gradually increase in intensity, rise to a crescendo, then pass away. The patient will often complain of crampy abdominal pain that coincides with the onset of the peristaltic activity. As paralytic ileus subsides, or in the presence of chronic partial small-bowel obstruction, a variety of gurgling and tinkling sounds may be detected. These sounds are produced by peristaltic activity in dilated, fluid-filled loops of bowel. In general, no specific rhythm may be present, and it may or may not be accompanied by cramping pain.

With outlet obstruction of the stomach, a **succussion splash** is at times detectable because of the presence of fluid and gas in the distended organ. This is easily appreciated by placing the stethoscope diaphragm over the epigastrium and shaking the patient vigorously from side to side (Fig. 14-6). A characteristic sloshing and gurgling sound is readily identified. It is important to determine the interval since the previous meal, as it is possible to elicit this sign in a normal person immediately after ingestion of a large quantity of fluid.

Rubs may be heard over the liver in patients with hepatic tumor or infection, and over the spleen in splenic infarction, neoplasia, and infection. **Bruits** over these organs suggest a vascular tumor, intense extramedullary hematopoiesis (e.g., as in myelofibrosis), or arteriovenous malformation. Other vascular bruits in the abdomen are discussed in Chapter 12.

PERCUSSION AND PALPATION

Generally speaking, the looser the texture, and more tender the fibre, of animal food, the easier it is of digestion.

WILLIAM BEAUMONT
(1785–1853)

Percussion and palpation are performed together. No two physicians follow exactly the same approach, and in time you will develop your own method. Whatever it is, adhere to it strictly, for this is the surest way of avoiding damaging omissions.

Right-handed examiners nearly always prefer to approach the abdomen from the patient's right side. Since the area is sensitive and frequently ticklish, some preparation against the shock of first contact with the examining hand is helpful. Chat with the patient. Touch the patient first on the forearm, very lightly, and do not try to elicit information until he settles down. If he absolutely cannot relax, have him palpate his own epigastrium, then place your hand on top of his, and finally beneath his. Finally, ask him to withdraw his own hand. This maneuver, though rarely necessary, can be helpful with very tense patients and with children.

Keep in mind that this will be one of the most difficult parts of the routine examination. Proceed slowly: do not rush. When difficulty is encountered, have the patient breathe with his mouth open. This automatically causes some relaxation. Such suggestions as "Now, relax as if you were falling asleep" may be valuable under certain circumstances. If the bed is low, do not hesitate to kneel down beside it or sit down on the edge. The rule that prohibits sitting on the patient's bed can be violated under special circumstances if done tactfully. Finally, concentrate all your senses on the examination. In particular, watch the patient's facial expression. A slight wince or almost inaudible gasp may be of major importance as you proceed.

Consider next your objectives, which are simple and limited. You must try to determine the presence or absence of (1) tenderness (superficial or deep), (2) organ enlargement, (3) abdominal mass, (4) spasm or rigidity of the abdominal muscles, (5) ascites, or (6) exaggerated tympanites. There is no universally accepted sequence for routine abdominal examination, and you may begin in any one of the quadrants and proceed in a clockwise manner until all four have been examined.

Before beginning active palpation, ask the patient to cough. If peritoneal irritation is present, coughing will elicit a sharp twinge of pain that may then be localized to the involved area. This permits you to carry out the major portion of the abdominal examination without touching the area of maximal tenderness. You should try to begin your examination of the abdomen at the site most distant from any pain, so that the patient does not instantly tighten the abdominal musculature to protect himself, thus obscuring your examination.

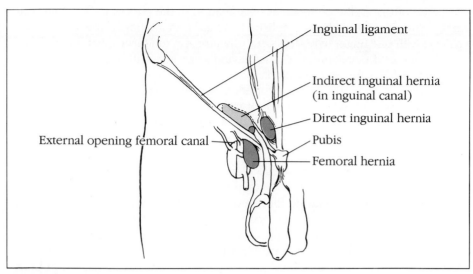

Inguinal ligament

Indirect inguinal hernia
(in inguinal canal)

Direct inguinal hernia

External opening femoral canal

Pubis

Femoral hernia

FIGURE 14-7
Common hernia sites.

Hyperesthesia should be tested for routinely. This may be done by lightly stroking the abdomen with the point of a pin, stroking the abdomen from above downward. The patient is requested to note if the pin stroke feels sharper at a given
location. Hyperesthesia suggests the presence of visceral or parietal peritoneal
irritation. It may be detected in the segmental distribution of that portion of the
spinal cord from which the affected viscus is innervated or along the distribution of
the peripheral nerves that may be involved directly by the inflammatory process.
This physical sign is helpful when present, but it should certainly not be considered
a constant finding in acute abdominal conditions, and its absence does not rule out
intra-abdominal disease.

It is important to examine the sites of possible external herniation as a routine
measure. Particular attention should be paid to the femoral canal to rule out the
presence of a small hernia or Richter's hernia. Incarcerated or strangulated hernias
are so often the cause of or associated with intra-abdominal processes that this observation should be performed without fail in all cases. The femoral artery should
be palpated during this part of the examination, since absence of its pulsations or
inequality between the two sides may suggest embolic disease or the presence of a
ruptured or dissecting aneurysm.

Test for muscular spasm of the abdominal wall. All areas of the abdomen should
be palpated to evaluate the extent of the muscular spasm present. It is helpful to ask
the patient to breathe deeply during this part of the examination, for voluntary
rectus muscular spasm will give way as the patient exhales. True muscular spasm
will not change, and the abdomen will remain rigid and tense during expiration.
Extensive rigidity involving both rectus muscles is suggestive of diffuse peritoneal
irritation. With localized or early peritonitis the spasm may be limited to a portion
of the abdomen. It is helpful to palpate both recti simultaneously in order to evaluate the extent and severity of the muscle spasm.

Palpation of the abdomen includes examination of the costovertebral angles bilaterally. This may be easily accomplished using the index finger. It is also helpful to palpate with one finger to outline gently the areas of tenderness within the abdomen. This serves the dual purpose of achieving accurate localization while producing minimal discomfort to the patient.

Light palpation is aimed primarily at eliciting minor degrees of tenderness and guarding. It is performed with the flat of the hand, not the fingertips, and sudden increases in pressure should be avoided. When changing position, remove the hand rather than drag it across the surface; the latter produces a disagreeable sensation resulting in undue muscle spasm. Such voluntary guarding may be suspected when tightness follows temporary relaxation during the first phase of expiration. It usually passes away gradually as the examination progresses.

Areas of tenderness should be localized as accurately as possible without producing undue discomfort. It may be necessary to cause additional discomfort during palpation of the abdomen. The need for this should be explained to the patient in advance so that he understands its importance.

A clear understanding of anatomic relationships and their variations is indispensable for the interpretation of tenderness of visceral origin. Sometimes, however, abdominal pain and tenderness do not actually arise from abdominal organs. This condition, referred to as parietal tenderness, is identified by having the patient, in the supine position, contract the abdominal muscles (by raising his head or feet) so as to prevent the transmission of pressure to the underlying viscera. Under these circumstances persistent tenderness on light palpation or gentle pinching probably arises in the abdominal wall itself. Similarly a mass that remains palpable under these conditions is probably situated superficially within the abdominal wall.

Percussion is of relatively limited diagnostic value, but it is a simple method of relaxing abdominal tension. Percuss the four quadrants briefly while noting the degree of resonance (Fig. 14-8 shows areas of dullness on abdominal percussion). Next, delineate the upper and lower borders of the liver in the midclavicular line. They should be no more than 10 cm apart, but liver dullness along the lower border may be partially obliterated by gas in the overlying bowel, making the overall dimension less than 10 cm. Next, outline Traube's space (the gastric air bubble) in the left upper quadrant; then, if possible, find the area of splenic dullness lateral to this, remembering that percussion has very limited value in delineating enlargement of the spleen.

Move to the suprapubic area and outline the upper border of the urinary bladder if possible. Watch carefully for evidence of tenderness while percussing. Percussible enlargement of the urinary bladder may or may not be of pathologic significance, depending on other factors. Remember always that in the premenopausal woman, an enlarged uterus may simply reflect pregnancy. A resonant note obtained in what should normally be a dull area anteriorly is suggestive evidence of free air within the peritoneal cavity. In the presence of intestinal obstruction, a gas-filled bowel may be pushed up anteriorly; in that situation percussion is of no value.

In some instances it may be possible to demonstrate the presence of shifting **dullness** by means of percussion in patients with acute abdominal disease. This test alone may be of little help, since no information is obtained regarding the charac-

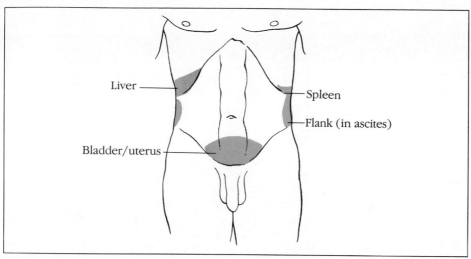

FIGURE 14-8
Areas of dullness on abdominal percussion.

ter of the fluid present, and it is seldom that this would alter the decision to operate. Needle paracentesis of the abdominal cavity may be of help in obtaining a sample of the free fluid present, permitting its culture and microscopic examination prior to laparotomy. This procedure is of little or no value in the presence of intestinal obstruction where loops of fluid-filled and gas-filled bowel predominate.

The next step in the examination consists of *deep palpation* of the abdomen in an effort to determine the size of liver, kidneys, and spleen, and to discover the presence of any abnormal intra-abdominal masses. Deep palpation requires great experience and skill. The flat of the right hand is usually used, and at times the left is placed over it for reinforcement. Pressure is very gradual and steady; special care is necessary at this point in order not to cause undue discomfort to the patient.

SPECIFIC ORGAN EXAMINATIONS

PALPATION OF THE LIVER. The bimanual technique (Fig. 14-9) is always helpful for deep palpation, particularly of the liver and kidneys. The posterior hand is placed between the twelfth rib and the iliac crest, just lateral to the paraspinous muscles. In palpating the liver, place the anterior hand firmly inward and upward in the right upper quadrant and instruct the patient to take a deep breath and hold it. You will want to release your pressure slightly at the height of inspiration, at the same time moving the fingertips gently upward toward the costal margin. When palpable, the liver edge is felt to slip over the fingertips at this moment. Proper placement of the anterior hand is important, as shown in Figure 14-9A. Horizontal placement of the hand (Fig. 14-9B) tends to force the whole liver backward, making the edge less accessible. Another common error is concerned with the level of placement of the palpating hand. Begin low, below the percussed border of dullness. Liver enlargement can be missed by palpating too close to the costal margin, so that the whole organ is beneath the hand and the edge is not palpated. At times, palpation can be better accomplished by the hooking technique (Fig. 14-9C).

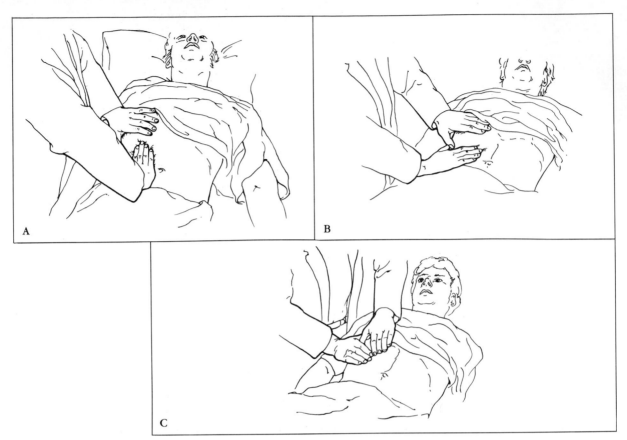

FIGURE 14-9
Palpation of the liver. A. Proper position of the hands. B. Incorrect (horizontal) positioning
(see text). C. Hooking.

The anterior hand should parallel the rectus muscle, not the costal margin. The
hooking technique is occasionally preferable. The liver edge may be normally felt,
particularly in women and children. At times the liver may extend 4 or 5 cm below
the right costal margin without actually being enlarged. Delineation of the overall
size by percussion may help to differentiate this ptosis (dropping down) from true
enlargement. Overall size in the midclavicular line is usually less than 15 cm, but
the patient's size, habitus, and pulmonary status are important considerations.

The principal causes of hepatic enlargement are congestion, cirrhosis, neoplasm,
and hepatitis. Tenderness is more likely with congestion and inflammation; irregular nodularity, with neoplasm; a very hard consistency, with cirrhosis. There are
also other causes for liver enlargement that are beyond the scope of this discussion.

The sign of inspiratory arrest (Murphy's sign) may be seen in the presence of
acute cholecystitis. This is elicited by having the patient take a deep breath while
the examiner maintains pressure against the abdominal wall in the region of the
gallbladder. As the liver descends with inspiration, the gallbladder comes in contact
with the examining hand and the patient experiences a sharp pain and inspiration
is arrested.

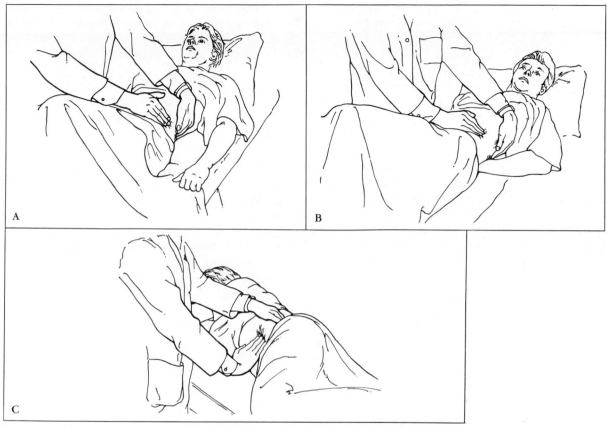

FIGURE 14-10
Palpation of the spleen. A. Positioning of examiner's hands. B. Patient's hand under his back.
C. Patient rolled to right side.

Inflammatory processes involving the liver or gallbladder may be elicited as tenderness in the right upper quadrant on fist percussion of the lower anterior chest wall. When this test is negative, one should hesitate to diagnose right upper quadrant inflammation.

SPLEEN. The spleen, though not physiologically part of the gastrointestinal system is, because of its location in the abdomen, examined here. The patient is supine, arms at side, and knees flexed slightly. Outline the area of splenic dullness as a first step. This should be done not so much to delineate the splenic size but rather to loosen the abdomen. Percussion may outline a greatly enlarged spleen, directing initial palpation to the left lower portion of the abdomen. Figure 14-10A shows the position of the examiner's hands. Note that pressure is light. Press the tips of the index and middle fingers of the right hand to a point just beneath the costal margin. Then ask the patient to turn his head to the side away from you and take a long, deep breath through his mouth. Do not move the hand as the patient inhales. The edge of an enlarged spleen will then brush against the fingers, lifting them slightly upward. As the patient exhales, probe the left upper quadrant more deeply, moving the fingertips in a slightly rotary motion. If nothing is felt, drop the hand about 1 cm and repeat. Do not dig. This will cause spasm of the muscles, making palpation difficult. Furthermore, slight splenic enlargement can be missed because the fingertips may be below the splenic edge, which will glide over the backs of the fingers.

Two special maneuvers may be helpful. First, have the patient slip his left forearm under the small of his back (Fig. 14-10B); this position will tend to thrust the spleen upward. Second, roll the patient on his right side with the right leg straight and the left knee flexed (Fig. 14-10C). The tips of the palpating fingers should be placed 1 or 2 cm below the costal margin with this maneuver. The keys to satisfactory splenic palpation are proper instructions to the patient with respect to breathing and gentleness by the examiner.

Normally the spleen is not palpable in the adult. It must be two or three times normal size before it becomes palpable.

Splenomegaly is common to many different and unrelated types of disease. It may be due to hyperplasia, congestion, or infiltrative replacement of the splenic pulp by neoplasm, myeloid elements, lipid, or amyloid.

Splenic hyperplasia occurs as a response to many systemic bacterial, parasitic, viral, or mycotic infections. Acute enlargement occurs with hematogenous dissemination of the infectious organisms as, for example, in bacterial endocarditis, septicemia, or miliary tuberculosis. Chronic enlargement of the spleen occurs with malaria, rheumatoid arthritis, and other relapsing or progressive inflammatory diseases. Splenic hyperplasia is common to many of the chronic anemias, whether due to conditioned deficiencies, hemolysis, or inherited defects in erythropoiesis. It is also the cause of splenomegaly in polycythemia vera.

Splenic congestion as a consequence of portal hypertension may be secondary to chronic hepatic disease, chronic congestive heart failure, or occlusion of the splenic or portal veins. The most common cause of congestive splenomegaly is cirrhosis of the liver.

Splenic infiltration by neoplastic cells results in the marked enlargement associated with the leukemias and lymphomas. Occasionally splenomegaly may also be produced by replacement of the splenic pulp by amyloid, lipid-filled reticuloendothelial cells (e.g., Gaucher's disease), or myeloid elements (extramedullary hematopoiesis).

A classification of splenomegaly according to the degree of enlargement is listed in Table 14-4. The designations depend on the distance (in centimeters) of the splenic edge below the left costal margin, on deep inspiration, as follows: slight enlargement, 1 to 4 cm; moderate enlargement, 4 to 8 cm; great enlargement, more than 8 cm.

If the spleen is greatly enlarged it may be missed on routine palpation. This pitfall can be avoided by (1) careful preliminary inspection during which the splenic edge may actually be visible in the abdomen with respiration, (2) preliminary percussion of the area of splenic dullness, and (3) repeated palpation at ever lower levels of the abdomen until the pelvic brim is reached. When it is suspected that the splenic capsule has been acutely distended by rapid enlargement of the spleen,

TABLE 14-4. Some Causes of Splenomegaly

Slight enlargement
Subacute bacterial endocarditis
Miliary tuberculosis
Septicemia
Rheumatoid arthritis
Syphilis
Typhoid
Brucellosis
Congestive heart failure
Acute hepatitis
Acute malaria
Pernicious anemia
Moderate enlargement
Cirrhosis of the liver
Acute leukemia
Chronic lymphocytic leukemia
Lymphoblastoma
Infectious mononucleosis
Polycythemia vera
Hemolytic anemia
Sarcoidosis
Rickets
Great enlargement
Chronic granulocytic leukemia
Chronic malaria
Congenital syphilis in the infant
Amyloidosis
Agnogenic myeloid metaplasia
Rare diseases
Gaucher's disease, Niemann-Pick disease, kala-azar, tropical eosinophilia

such as can occur in infectious mononucleosis, splenic infarction, or intrasplenic hemorrhage, great caution must be exercised lest excessive examination or manipulation lead to splenic rupture.

KIDNEYS. The kidneys are assessed as part of the abdominal examination by deep palpation below the costal margins in the supine patient, using the nonpalpating hand to lift upward from below. Since the right kidney is lower than the left, it is occasionally normally palpable, especially in very thin patients. Flank masses or tenderness in the area of the kidneys are otherwise abnormal. A full description of renal examination and associated historical and physical findings is given in Chapter 15.

URINARY BLADDER. Occasionally, a distended bladder may extend as high as the level of the umbilicus and be mistaken for a tumor. Tenderness over the bladder suggests intravesicular inflammation. As with the kidneys, a fuller description of bladder examination is presented in Chapter 15.

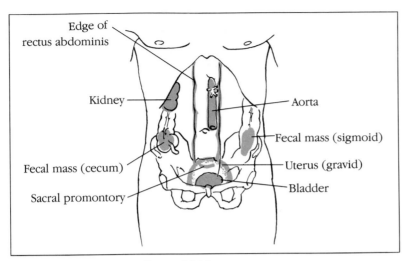

FIGURE 14-11
Some *normal* abdominal "masses."

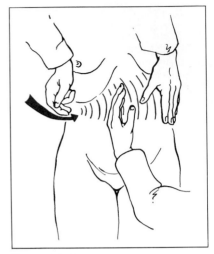

FIGURE 14-12
Demonstration of the fluid wave.

UTERUS. In women of childbearing age, a lower abdominal mass may be a gravid uterus. Full exploration of this possibility, including gynecologic examination (Chap. 16) and urine pregnancy test, must precede any radiologic studies.

OTHER FINDINGS

Normal findings on palpation and percussion are highly variable and depend largely on the degree of obesity and general body build, as well as on the patient's ability to cooperate (Fig. 14-11). The aorta is often palpable in the epigastrium and may be slightly tender. The normal aorta in the elderly, asthenic patient is easily mistaken for an aneurysm. The descending colon and cecum are commonly felt with considerable ease, particularly when they contain feces, and this normal finding may be misinterpreted as neoplasm unless roentgenographic studies are available.

Palpable masses should always be localized with respect to the previously described landmarks, and they should, if possible, be described in terms of consistency and contour. Frequently, however, they are only vaguely outlined, particularly when they are associated with tenderness or fluid or when the abdomen is obese and tense. Gastric, pancreatic, and colonic neoplasms, pancreatic cysts, and distended gallbladders may be palpable, usually at advanced stages of the disease.

Evaluation of the greatly distended abdomen is conducted by palpation and percussion. When the percussion note is high-pitched and tympanitic (drumlike), there is probably an obstruction that has produced gaseous distention of the underlying small intestine, stomach, or colon. A flat or dull percussion note suggests either the presence of fluid in the peritoneal cavity or abdominal fullness associated with ovarian cyst or obesity. The usual method for demonstrating intra-abdominal fluid requires two examiners (Fig. 14-12). The assistant places the edge of his hand on the middle of the abdomen in order to limit the transmission of the impulse by the abdominal wall. The examiner then taps one flank while palpating the opposite flank, in order to detect the transmission of a fluid wave.

A false positive sign may result if the patient is very obese or if there is a large ovarian cyst containing a sizable volume of encapsulated fluid. With ascites the distention is symmetrical and the flanks are particularly full. A tympanitic note detected in the midline, anteriorly, reflects associated gaseous distention of the bowel (the gas-containing bowel floats). The area of dullness is localized to the flanks and may be noted to shift with a change of position. In contrast, ovarian cysts may produce asymmetrical abdominal swelling; the dullness is located anteriorly with the tympanitic note in the flanks as the gas-containing bowel is displaced laterally. Shifting dullness on change of position is usually not present.

A fluid wave may not be obtained if the volume of ascites is only moderate and abdominal distention is slight. In such a case it may be possible to elicit a fluid wave if the examination is performed during the expiratory phase of a cough or during a Valsalva maneuver. This produces contraction of the abdominal muscles, reduces the volume of the abdominal cavity, and temporarily puts the ascites under enough tension to elicit a wave. This sign may be obtained in the presence of intra-abdominal cysts or fluid-filled intestines, although under these circumstances "shifting dullness" in the flanks will not be obtained.

Ascites may be associated with intra-abdominal masses, which are obscured by the presence of the fluid and therefore are difficult to palpate. Under these circumstances it is sometimes possible to detect such a mass by ballottement. This technique calls for lightly thrusting the fingers into the abdomen in the region of the suspected mass. The thrust will tend to displace the fluid, permitting the mass to bound upward, producing a characteristic tapping sensation against palpating fingers.

The recognition of masses may be made easier by repeating the abdominal examination after analgesics have been administered or the patient has been anesthetized prior to operation.

Rebound tenderness is elicited by exerting deep pressure into the abdomen in an area away from the suspected acute inflammatory process and then quickly releasing the pressure. If peritoneal irritation is present the patient experiences a twinge of pain either at the site of pressure or in the area of inflammation. This test is more reliable than cough tenderness. If the peritoneal irritation is localized to an area of inflammation, the rebound tenderness will be referred to that area. If generalized peritoneal irritation is present, rebound tenderness will be referred to the area of pressure. This test may be of particular value in obese patients. It is often accompanied by marked discomfort to the patient and should not be employed in the presence of obvious diffuse generalized peritonitis.

Intra-abdominal inflammation that secondarily involves the iliopsoas muscle may be detected by the iliopsoas test. The patient is asked to flex his thigh against the resistance of the examiner's hand. If inflammation is present in this location, contraction of the psoas muscle will be accompanied by pain. An alternative way of testing this function is to have the patient lie on the unaffected side and extend his thigh toward the affected side (Fig. 14-13). This test is not likely to be positive in the presence of subacute infection or if the abdominal wall is rigid.

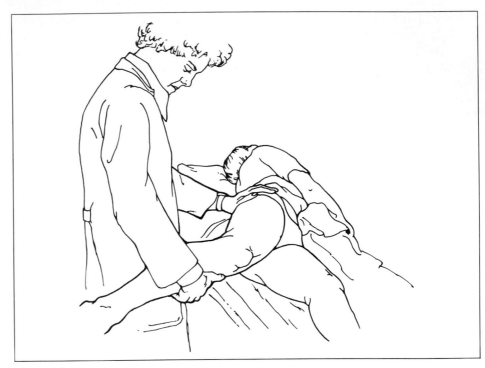

FIGURE 14-13
Psoas maneuver.

If the inflammatory process lies adjacent to the obturator internus muscle, as in the presence of pelvic abscess, lower abdominal pain may be elicited by flexing the thigh to a 90-degree angle and rotating it internally and externally. This is known as the obturator test (Fig. 14-14).

It is sometimes difficult to differentiate an acute upper abdominal process from intrathoracic disease. In this situation, deep pressure on the opposite side of the abdomen directed toward the affected side will produce pain if the basic process is intra-abdominal; however, it will not elicit pain if the disease is intrathoracic.

The chest should be examined routinely in order to rule out diaphragmatic pleurisy, lower lobe pneumonia, pericarditis, or pleural effusion. Any of these conditions may be confused with intra-abdominal disease.

No examination of the abdomen is complete without examination of the back, conveniently done just before or at the time of the rectal examination. An episode of acute abdominal pain caused by pyelonephritis may reveal itself in costovertebral angle tenderness. Ecchymoses of the flanks (Grey-Turner's sign) suggest retroperitoneal bleeding, as may occur with hemorrhagic pancreatitis. The intergluteal crease must be carefully examined for lesions. It is a favorite site for the occurrence of psoriasis. The pilonidal cyst is found overlying the sacrum and is seen as a punctate lesion just above or in the intergluteal crease which may have a tuft of hair, erythema, or both surrounding it. It can become infected, forming an abscess. The pilonidal cyst is particularly likely to occur in hirsute men.

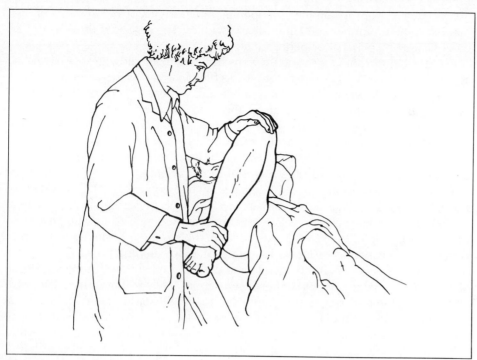

FIGURE 14-14
Obturator maneuver.

RECTUM

An important part of the examination in acute abdominal disease includes digital examination of the rectum. It is desirable in acute situations to have the patient lying on his back, permitting the rectum to be examined anteriorly, posteriorly, and on both sides with the examining finger. This maneuver may be helpful in detecting such conditions as prostatitis, seminal vesiculitis, pelvic abscess, appendicitis, and tubo-ovarian abscess. Bimanual examination of the rectum and vagina permits careful evaluation of the contents of the pelvis and the cul-de-sac. This is an important part of the examination of female patients and should be included as an integral part of all examinations of such patients with acute abdominal distress.

In any patient, it is impossible to overemphasize the importance of the rectal examination. This simple and vital procedure is too often passed by because it entails extra effort on the part of the physician and tends to be somewhat disagreeable to the patient. No gastrointestinal evaluation is complete without it.

The skin surrounding the anus should be carefully inspected for signs of inflammation or excoriation.

Local infections such as perianal and perirectal abscesses will appear as an area of swelling, with variable degrees of erythema about the anus. Local pain and tenderness are usually prominent, and the patient will usually show systemic signs of sepsis such as fever and tachycardia.

An anorectal fistula is a tract that has an external opening, often visible on inspection of the anal skin, and an internal opening into the anus or rectum. Less often it may enter the urethra or even the urinary bladder. The anorectal fistula is caused by drainage of a perianal or perirectal abscess.

External hemorrhoids are varicose veins that originate below the anorectal line and are covered by anal skin. They appear as bluish, shiny masses at the anus. They may not be visible when the patient is at rest, but will usually protrude after standing or straining at stool. If not reduced, they become edematous and may thrombose. When thrombosis occurs, local pain may be intense, and removal of the thrombus may be necessary to obtain relief. Internal hemorrhoids arise above the anorectal junction and are therefore covered by rectal mucosa. Because of their soft consistency they are not palpable by rectal examination.

The examination itself consists of digital and endoscopic study. Digital examination (described in further detail in Chaps. 15 and 16) is performed with the patient in the supine or knee-chest position, or flexed at the hips and bending over. On occasion it is helpful to examine the patient in the squatting position, for this may bring a high-lying rectal lesion within reach of the examining finger. Insertion of the examining finger should be gentle and gradual, and sufficient time should be allowed for the patient to relax after insertion has been accomplished. Excessive resistance at the anal ring is commonly due to simple spasm caused by nervousness, and this can at times be overcome by asking the patient to strain a little before palpation is begun. If there is considerable spasm and local pain due to anal pathologic changes, a local anesthetic suppository may be used to minimize discomfort.

Lesions detectable on rectal examination include anal fissure. It is a superficial linear ulcer, usually found in the posterior midline. It is tender, and patients may report pain and slight bleeding with bowel movements. The anal sphincter will usually be in spasm, and a suppository with local anesthesia may be necessary to permit examination. The fissure may be visualized directly by anoscopy.

Polyps of the rectum are a relatively common finding. They may be pedunculated or sessile, and some (villous adenomas) are so soft that they are difficult to palpate. Direct visualization and biopsy are necessary to distinguish them from rectal carcinoma. The latter lesion is usually felt as a sessile polypoid mass with nodular, raised edges and areas of ulceration. It usually has a hard consistency.

Rectal prolapse can be diagnosed by asking the patient to strain and by observing the appearance of rectal mucosa emerging from the anus. The prolapse involves the entire circumference of the bowel and may range in size from only a few centimeters to a very extensive prolapse involving a major portion of rectum.

Intraperitoneal metastases from any of several malignant sources may develop in the pelvis anterior to the rectum. These metastases may be felt as a hard, nodular area at the tip of the examining finger; this finding is referred to as a rectal shelf.

PROCTOSCOPY

Proctoscopy is a general term used for direct visualization of the terminal portion of the bowel. Anoscopy is performed with a short instrument using an external light source and is useful for seeing such lesions as fissure in ano, cryptitis, internal hemorrhoids, and the opening of a fistulous tract.

The sigmoidoscope is used for examination of the rectum and lower sigmoid. It is 25 cm in length and has a light source at its tip. It is passed to its full length and

TABLE 14-5. Examinations of the Anus, Rectum, and Large Bowel

Lesions often visible **by external examination** Dermatitis Pilonidal cyst Perianal abscess External hemorrhoids Rectal prolapse Carcinoma of the anus Anal fissures and fistulas	**Lesions (above the rectum) often demonstrable** **by barium enema** Inflammatory bowel disease Diverticula Megacolon Irritable bowel Neoplasm Polyps Strictures Ischemia Foreign bodies
Palpable lesions Cancer of the rectum Polyps Cancer of the prostate Fibroids Rectal shelf Abscess Foreign body Stricture Endometriosis (palpable during bimanual pelvic examination)	
Lesions visualized by proctoscopy Inflammation of the bowel Internal fistulous openings Cancers of the rectum and bowel Polyps Villous adenoma Internal hemorrhoids Strictures Spasm Bowel ischemia Foreign bodies Lacerations of the bowel	

the mucosa is carefully viewed as the instrument is removed. Sigmoidoscopy is helpful in the diagnosis of various types of polyps, inflammatory lesions, and rectal cancer. Biopsy can be performed easily. The bowel must be cleansed by enema in order for this examination to be conducted.

The fiberoptic colonoscope is used to study higher levels of the colon. A 60 cm model can be used to examine the rectum or sigmoid, while 100 cm models can visualize the transverse and right colon as well. Successful use of these instruments requires special endoscopic expertise and careful preparation of the patient's bowel in advance.

Radiologic studies are useful in establishing the diagnosis of various lesions above the rectum. Barium enema and air-contrast barium enema require careful preparation of the patient by laxatives and enemas if one is to visualize mucosal detail. Lesions that can be detected by barium and other studies are listed in Table 14-5.

MALE GENITOURINARY SYSTEM AND HERNIA

I have never yet examined the body of a patient dying with dropsy attended by coagulable urine, in whom some obvious derangement was not discovered in the kidneys.

RICHARD BRIGHT
(1789–1858)

Though classically recorded on the written record *before* the musculoskeletal and neurologic examinations, examination of the male and female genitalia, as well as the rectal examination, are generally done *last* in the sequence of the actual physical. These are sometimes embarrassing and uncomfortable examinations, and the understanding sympathy and deftness of the examiner will contribute considerably to the ease of the patient undergoing this sensitive but essential examination.

Examination for hernia is generally done as part of the examination of external genitalia in men; the rectal is a logical part of the internal genital examination in both men and women.

ANATOMY

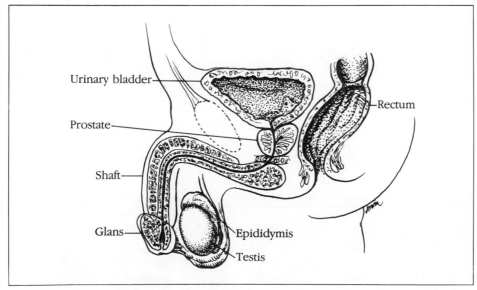

FIGURE 15-1
Cross section of male genitalia.

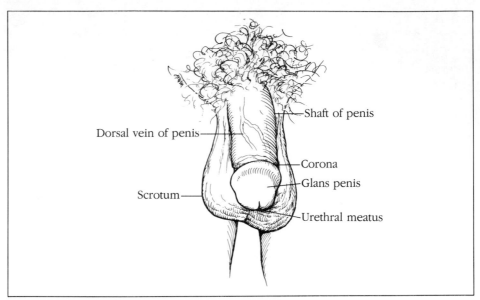

FIGURE 15-2
External male genitalia.

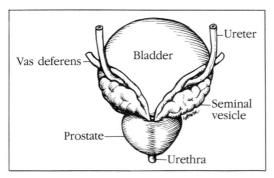

FIGURE 15-3
Prostate and seminal vesicles.

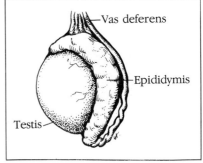

FIGURE 15-4
Testis and epididymis.

HISTORY

Pain in the testicle is met with in renal colic and in a few cases of appendicitis.

SIR ZACHARY COPE
(1881–1974)

Though difficult for many students initially, candid inquiry into excretory and sexual function is essential for their patients' well-being. If shyness or prudery allows a cancer of the prostate gland to go undetected, the price of modesty has been too high. Ask questions about the genitourinary system with the same professional objective interest you show in the rest of the history. While you should avoid embarrassing a reluctant patient, an understanding, tactful questioning will allow you to gather the necessary information.

Genitourinary symptoms may be divided into several general categories.

IRRITATIVE BLADDER AND URETHRAL SYMPTOMS

Frequency, urgency, and *dysuria* are symptoms that often occur together and are usually secondary to inflammatory disease of the bladder, the prostate, and the urethra.

Cystitis is the most common disorder of the bladder. It is far more frequent in women than in men. Infection of the bladder in men can occur, however, with obstruction (as with a large prostate gland), foreign body (such as a Foley catheter), neurologic disease affecting bladder emptying, or other predisposing states.

Acute prostatitis may result in fever, urethral discharge, and irritative bladder symptoms. *Chronic prostatitis* is usually asymptomatic.

Urethritis, not infrequently of gonococcal origin (though other organisms may cause urethral inflammation), presents with irritation and urethral discharge.

INCONTINENCE

Careful history taking will identify the type of incontinence and lead to the appropriate treatment. *Stress incontinence,* or the involuntary loss of urine caused by straining, coughing, or lifting, occurs most frequently in the multiparous woman and often is associated with cystourethrocele. This incontinence can be corrected surgically. *Urge incontinence* (precipitous micturition) is the involuntary loss of urine caused by the sudden urge to void. It may occur with inflammatory disease of the bladder and urethra but also with a neurogenic bladder with uninhibited contractions. *Dribbling incontinence* is the constant loss of urine in varying amounts with or without stress. It may be produced by a vesicovaginal fistula, ectopic ureter, or after prostatectomy when the sphincters of the bladder have been damaged. *Paradoxical incontinence,* the involuntary dribbling of urine, is due to chronic urinary retention. This may be produced either by obstruction of the urethra in the male, as in benign prostatic hypertrophy, or secondary to a neurogenic bladder, as in sensory paralytic bladder produced by tabes dorsalis (see Table 15-1).

TABLE 15-1. Some Causes of Frequency

Large Volume	Small Volume
Polydipsia	Cystitis
Renal tubular disease	Urethritis
Diuretics	Neurogenic bladder
Glycosuria	Extrinsic mass to the bladder
Diabetes insipidus	Bladder tumor
Adrenal insufficiency	Structural defects of bladder and urethra
Alcohol	(including prostatism)

PAIN

Renal pain usually is present in the costovertebral angle and may radiate anteriorly. Afferent autonomic nerves carrying sensation from the kidneys reach the spinal cord through the tenth, eleventh, and twelfth thoracic nerves. Referred pain of renal origin is therefore interpreted by the patient over the somatic distribution of these nerves in the abdominal wall. The fibers supplying the ureter enter the spinal cord from the twelfth thoracic nerve and the first three lumbar nerves. Pain referred from the ureter is distributed over the somatic distribution of the subcostal, iliohypogastric, ilioinguinal, and genitofemoral nerves, depending on the portion of the ureter that is diseased. Since both the ilioinguinal nerve and the genital branch of the genitofemoral nerves supply the scrotum, pain from the ureter often radiates into the testicle or scrotum. Renal pain may be due to pyelonephritis, calculi, perinephric abscess, tumor, glomerulonephritis, or intermittent hydronephrosis. *Vesical pain* is usually present in the suprapubic region. Pain may be severe, with bladder distention, and it may be relieved by voiding, as occurs with interstitial cystitis; or pain may be continuous when associated with urinary retention or acute cystitis. *Testicular pain* usually is due to neoplasm, infection, or local trauma, but pain may occasionally be referred to this region. *Prostatic* and *urethral pain* may be referred on occasion to the low back area.

MASS

A perceptible mass in the *renal area* is rarely noted by the patient but may occur with neoplasm. A *suprapubic mass* may signal bladder distention or neoplasm. A *scrotal mass* may be inflammatory, neoplastic, traumatic, cystic (spermatocele, hydrocele, varicocele), or a hernia.

URINARY CHANGES

CLOUDY URINE

A patient complaint of cloudy urine may suggest pus in the urine (as with infection), but is most often due simply to phosphate precipitation in an alkaline urine, a normal event.

PNEUMATURIA

Pneumaturia, usually described as "bubbles in the urine as it comes out" may develop with urinary tract infection due to gas-forming bacteria, or it may signal an enterovesical fistula caused by inflammatory or neoplastic disease of the gastrointestinal tract.

HEMATURIA

Blood in the urine must be considered to be due to neoplasm until proved otherwise. Initial or seminal hematuria is usually associated with disease of the lower urinary tract. Blood present throughout urination may come from kidneys, ureters, or bladder. Calculi, infection, trauma, and acute glomerulonephritis are frequently associated with hematuria (see Table 15-2).

NOCTURIA

Nocturia is usually a significant symptom and is seen in association with benign prostatic hypertrophy, diabetes mellitus, urinary tract infections, and with reversed diurnal rhythm such as occurs with renal and circulatory insufficiency.

GASTROINTESTINAL SYMPTOMS

Nausea, vomiting, and abdominal distention may be associated with renal or ureteral calculi. Hydronephrosis is frequently a silent lesion that may produce symptoms that suggest gallbladder disease or duodenal ulcer when the right kidney is

TABLE 15-2. Some Causes of Hematuria

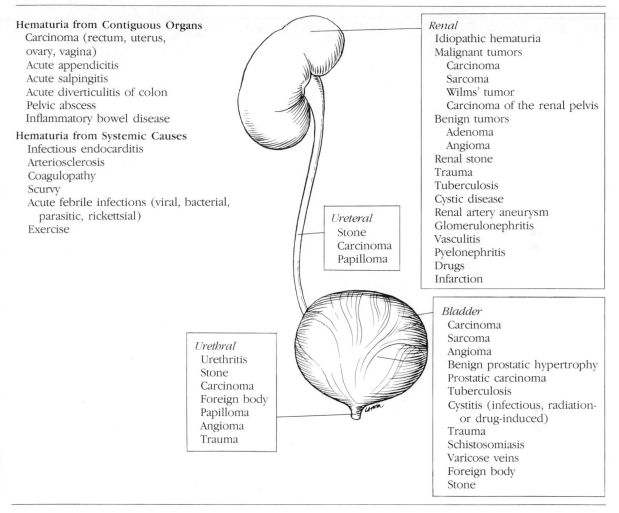

Hematuria from Contiguous Organs
  Carcinoma (rectum, uterus,
  ovary, vagina)
  Acute appendicitis
  Acute salpingitis
  Acute diverticulitis of colon
  Pelvic abscess
  Inflammatory bowel disease

Hematuria from Systemic Causes
  Infectious endocarditis
  Arteriosclerosis
  Coagulopathy
  Scurvy
  Acute febrile infections (viral, bacterial,
    parasitic, rickettsial)
  Exercise

Renal
  Idiopathic hematuria
  Malignant tumors
    Carcinoma
    Sarcoma
    Wilms' tumor
    Carcinoma of the renal pelvis
  Benign tumors
    Adenoma
    Angioma
  Renal stone
  Trauma
  Tuberculosis
  Cystic disease
  Renal artery aneurysm
  Glomerulonephritis
  Vasculitis
  Pyelonephritis
  Drugs
  Infarction

Ureteral
  Stone
  Carcinoma
  Papilloma

Urethral
  Urethritis
  Stone
  Carcinoma
  Foreign body
  Papilloma
  Angioma
  Trauma

Bladder
  Carcinoma
  Sarcoma
  Angioma
  Benign prostatic hypertrophy
  Prostatic carcinoma
  Tuberculosis
  Cystitis (infectious, radiation-
    or drug-induced)
  Trauma
  Schistosomiasis
  Varicose veins
  Foreign body
  Stone

affected, and a lesion of the colon when the left kidney is affected. The presenting symptoms of chronic renal insufficiency (azotemia) frequently are nausea and vomiting.

LOCAL LESIONS
"Sores" of the external genitalia may bring a patient to the physician. Infection (especially venereal infection) and neoplastic disease are the leading causes.

SEXUAL DYSFUNCTION
Although some men will openly admit to having sexual difficulty (or to having "lost their nature"), others will be so ashamed that they will disguise this complaint as "prostate trouble" or "fatigue," hoping that the doctor will understand and direct attention to their sexual function. Primary sexual problems include impotence, loss

TABLE 15-3. Some Clinical Features of Uremia

General	**Stomach and intestines**
Cachexia	Abdominal pain
Fatigue	Enteritis
Weakness	Ascites
Edema	**Nerves and muscles**
Vital signs	Confusion, obtundation
Tachycardia	Asterixis
Tachypnea	Paresthesias
Hypertension	Osteoporosis, pathologic fractures
Hypothermia (occasionally)	**Skin**
Head, ears, eyes, nose, throat	Easy bruising
Band keratopathy	Itching
Conjunctivitis	Hyperpigmentation
Conjunctival pallor	Pallor
Uremic breath	Uremic frost
Heart	
Pericarditis	
Congestive heart failure	
Chest	
Gynecomastia	
Pleuritis, pleural effusion	
Pneumonitis	
Dyspnea	

of libido, premature ejaculation, and loss of erection. These symptoms are sometimes psychologic in origin, although a number of common antihypertensive drugs (alpha-methyldopa, for example) and diseases (diabetes mellitus) may also induce impotence. A thorough medical and psychologic investigation is indicated for these most significant symptoms.

PROSTATISM

The symptomatic manifestations of prostatic enlargement are called, collectively, "prostatism." Symptoms produced by an enlarged prostate gland are of two major types: (1) irritative bladder symptoms as described above, and (2) obstructive symptoms characterized by a urinary stream decreased in size and force, with hesitancy and interruption of the stream during voiding. Obstructive symptoms may also be produced by a urethral stricture, a urethral valve, or a bladder neck contracture.

HYPERTENSION

Many patients will have been told that they have high blood pressure. Increased blood pressure may occur as both cause and consequence of chronic renal disease. Hypertension, therefore, calls for a careful historical and physical assessment of the urinary system.

UREMIA

The symptoms (and signs) which may occur in uremia are given in Table 15-3.

PHYSICAL EXAMINATION ────────────────

1. Palpate kidneys and urinary bladder as part of abdominal examination.

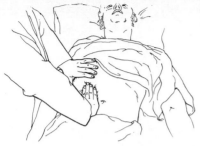 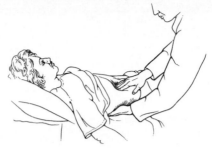

2. Inspect external genitalia: hair distribution, scrotum, and penis.
3. Palpate regional nodes, penis, testes, and epididymis.
4. Check for hernia bilaterally.

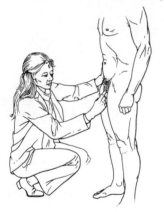 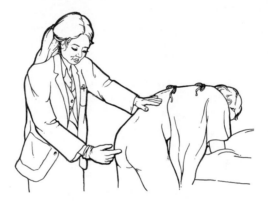

5. Consider doing rectal examination now if not done as part of gastrointestinal examination: sphincter tone, prostate, ampulla, stool for occult blood.

The examination of the urine is the most essential part of the physical examination of any patient with Bright's disease.

THOMAS ADDIS
(1881–1949)

KIDNEYS, URETERS, AND URINARY BLADDER

The upper urinary tract is assessed as part of the abdominal examination. The patient is supine with knees slightly raised. Begin by scrutinizing the upper abdomen for obvious symmetry or bulging, particularly in the flanks. Close observation during the patient's deep inspiration and expiration may give important clues as to the site of pathologic change.

KIDNEYS

In palpating the **renal areas**, place one hand posteriorly beneath the costal margin and press directly upward (Fig. 15-5). The other hand palpates for the kidney and is placed below the costal margin at about the midclavicular line. The patient is then

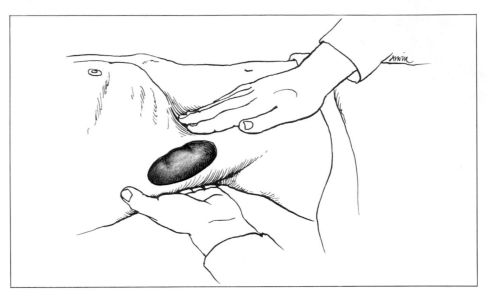

FIGURE 15-5
Palpation of the kidney.

asked to take a deep breath, a maneuver that depresses the diaphragm and pushes the kidney downward. As the patient inhales, the hand is pressed inward and upward toward the costal margin. The technique is similar to that used for palpation of the liver and spleen except that the hand is gradually pressed more deeply into the abdomen. The right kidney is palpated from the right side, while the left kidney is examined by reaching across the abdomen or preferably by moving around the patient to his left side. When pathology is suspected, it may be valuable to have the patient lie on his side. The uppermost kidney tends to fall downward and medially in this position, making it somewhat more accessible to palpation.

Percussion is not used routinely, but it may be valuable at times in generally outlining masses in the renal areas that are unusually large. Auscultation is valuable for detecting bruits that may originate in the renal arteries. It is carried out over the costovertebral angles posteriorly and in both upper quadrants of the abdomen. Auscultation is particularly important in the hypertensive patient, since renal-vascular disease causing an elevated blood pressure may be surgically remediable. Transillumination is a particularly valuable technique in children. The room is darkened and the light source is pressed into the costovertebral angle posteriorly. A hydronephrosis will transmit light; a solid tumor will not.

Since the right kidney normally is somewhat lower than the left, it is occasionally palpable, particularly in asthenic patients.

The usual causes of renal enlargement are infection, tumor, hydronephrosis, and polycystic kidneys. (In dramatic circumstances of polycystic disease, the palpating hand may detect a crepitant—"crackling"—sensation over the kidney as the multiple cysts are compressed.) Masses in the area of the kidney may also be due to bowel lesions (tumors, abscesses), retroperitoneal tumor, gallbladder, or spleen.

The examiner should look also for possible tenderness originating in and around the kidney. Renal pain is elicited by pressure at the costovertebral angle—

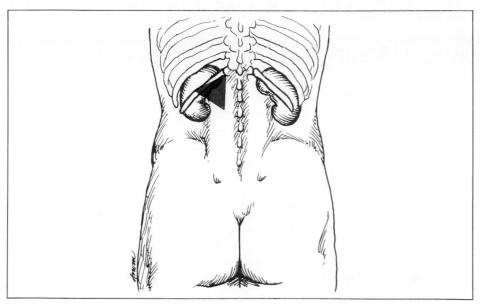

FIGURE 15-6
Costovertebral angle.

the angle formed by the junction of the twelfth rib and the paraspinous muscles (Fig. 15-6). In this region the kidney is nearest to the skin surface, and deep pressure by the examiner's fingers may elicit pain due to intrinsic renal parenchymal disease. Costovertebral angle pain must be differentiated from pain produced by muscular spasm. Muscle pain can be demonstrated by deep palpation directly over the back muscles that lie medial to the costovertebral angle.

Acute pyelonephritis usually produces fever, and the patient may be extremely ill. There is tenderness to deep palpation or percussion in the costovertebral angle, and the entire flank region may be tender. When the peritoneum overlying the kidneys is affected by the inflammatory reaction, signs of peritonitis are present, with abdominal distention, muscle spasm, rebound tenderness, and hypoactive bowel sounds.

Perinephric abscess may be associated with a low-grade or septic elevation in temperature. There usually is exquisite tenderness on the affected side, and frequently a bulging mass may be felt in the flank. Scoliosis of the spine with the concavity pointed toward the affected side occurs because of irritation of the psoas major and quadratus lumborum muscles. The diaphragm is elevated and somewhat fixed on the affected side; because of inflammatory reaction, basilar rales may be present. Edema of the skin may occur over the abscess.

Hydronephrosis (or pyohydronephrosis) occurs when there is obstruction to the flow of urine from the intrarenal collecting system. Obstructive uropathy, regardless of its location, produces an increase in the hydrostatic pressure within the renal collecting system. In general, the higher in the urinary tract the lesion is located, the greater the effect on the kidneys. Initially there is hypertrophy of the musculature of the renal pelvis, but as the obstruction persists or progresses, decompensation and dilation occur. The resultant enlarged kidney may be palpated

TABLE 15-4. Renal Stones

Type of Stone and Incidence	Causes	X-Ray Appearance

Calcium oxalate
Calcium phosphate
Calcium oxalate and phosphate } (74%)
	Hypercalciuria
	  Most common cause—idiopathic hyper-
	    calciuria
	  Common cause—primary hyperpara-
	    thyroidism
	  Rarer causes
	    Renal tubular acidosis
	    Vitamin D excess
	    Vitamin A excess
	    Calcium carbonate excess
	    Sarcoidosis
	    Hyperthyroidism
	    Paget's disease of bone
	    Prolonged immobilization
		Radiopaque

	Hyperoxaluria
	  Most common cause—small bowel disease,
	    malabsorption
	  Uncommon causes
	    Genetic hyperoxaluria
	    Vitamin B_6 deficiency
	    Ethylene glycol (antifreeze ingestion)
	    Vitamin C excess
	    Dietary excess of oxalate (rhubarb, spinach)
	    Methoxyfluorine anesthesia
		Radiopaque

Magnesium-ammonium phosphate (15%)	Recurrent urinary tract infection with urea splitters giving decreased urinary pH	Radiopaque

Uric acid stone (8%)	Excess uric acid excretion
	  Idiopathic
	  Associated with gout
	  Associated with myeloproliferative disease
		Radiolucent

Cystine, xanthine (3%)	Genetic—rare	

on bimanual examination. In small children, transillumination of the renal areas may help to differentiate cystic mass from solid tumor. As the back pressure increases, the hydronephrotic process progresses; the renal blood supply is compromised, producing ischemia. Eventually the renal parenchyma is destroyed, leaving a thin-walled cystic mass.

Benign tumor of the kidney is rare and usually is too small to be palpated.

The *embryoma* (Wilms' tumor) is malignant. It usually occurs in children under the age of 5 years. The presenting sign often is a palpable mass in one or both renal areas. Renal cell carcinoma (hypernephroma), the most common renal malignant neoplasm, may produce a palpable mass in the flank. Extension of the tumor into the renal vein and inferior vena cava will produce dilated veins in the abdominal wall. The left spermatic vein empties into the left renal vein and may be obstructed by a tumor growing into the renal vein. This obstruction produces a varicocele on the left side of the scrotum that does not decompress when the patient is supine.

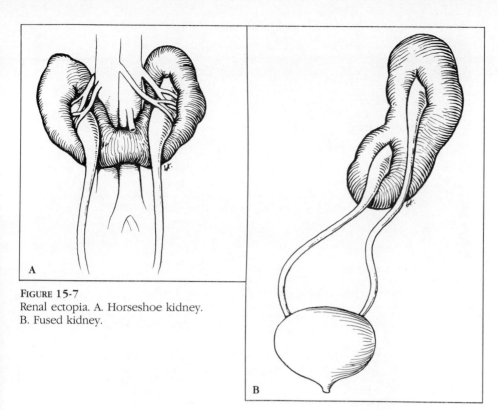

FIGURE 15-7
Renal ectopia. A. Horseshoe kidney.
B. Fused kidney.

*Gout produces calculus in the kidney. . . . The patient has frequently to enter-
tain the painful speculation as to whether gout or stone be the worst disease.*

THOMAS SYDENHAM
(1624–1689)

Renal stone disease is very common and can present with excruciating pain
(renal colic) in the back, flank, or radiating to testis, thigh, or penis. On physical
examination, marked costovertebral angle tenderness may be present, especially if
there is an associated pyelonephritis. Acute renal colic frequently produces abdominal distention and either hypoactive or absent bowel sounds. A history of predisposition to stone should be sought (Table 15-4) when the diagnosis is suspected,
and a urine analysis (which often shows microscopic blood) and abdominal film
(showing calcium stones) should be obtained.

Renal ectopia will produce a palpable mass in the lower part of the abdomen
(Fig. 15-7). In crossed renal ectopia, both kidneys are on the same side and are
often fused, giving rise to a rather large mass that suggests neoplasm. A *horseshoe
kidney* is produced by the fusion of the lower pole of each kidney, producing an
isthmus of renal tissue across the midline, which may be palpable in a thin patient.
Polycystic kidneys are usually bilateral and contain multiple cysts. As the cysts enlarge, palpable masses are produced in the renal areas. Unless infected, the renal
masses are usually not tender. In this progressive genetic disease, renal failure ultimately occurs.

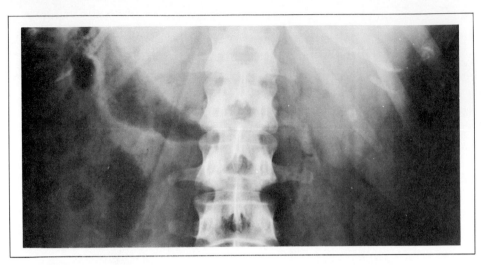

FIGURE 15-8
Nephrolithiasis on plain film (radiopaque stone).

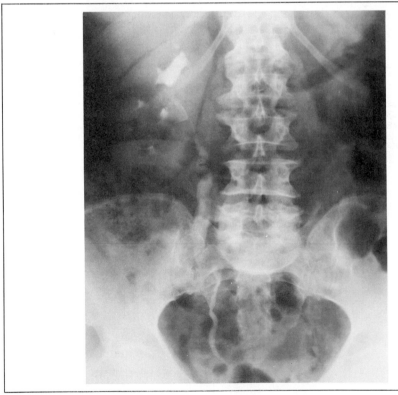

FIGURE 15-9
Nephrolithiasis on intravenous pyelography with hydroureter (radiolucent stone).

URETERS

The ureters are not accessible to physical examination. Ureteral obstructions and strictures, however, may produce hydronephrosis on the involved side. Ureteral obstruction may result from stones as they pass from the kidney. The stones commonly are arrested in their passage at the three narrowest areas of the renal-ureteral-vesicular pathway: the ureteropelvic junction, the pelvic brim where the ureter crosses the iliac vessels, and the ureteral-vesical junction. The passage of the stone, or its arrest in the ureter, may be associated with the violent pain and other findings described as renal colic.

Ureteral stricture may occur congenitally or as a result of inflammation, fibrosis, surgical accident, or tumor in the retroperitoneum.

URINARY BLADDER

The **bladder** is examined by inspection, percussion, and palpation. When distended it produces a bulging mass in the lower part of the abdomen over which dullness may be elicited by percussion. At times this dullness may extend up as far as the umbilicus. The region of the symphysis should be carefully palpated. Bladder pain is usually elicited by direct palpation over the suprapubic area. Bimanual examination may be performed at the time of rectal examination with the man in the lithotomy position; the examiner places one finger in the rectum pressing upward, the opposite hand on the lower abdominal wall (Fig. 15-10). The best results are obtained with the patient under anesthesia. In women, the bladder is easily palpated bimanually at the time of pelvic examination.

The empty bladder is not accessible to physical examination, but when distended with urine it can be mistaken for a lower abdominal tumor unless this possibility is kept in mind. On bimanual examination the empty bladder feels much like a thick-walled, collapsed balloon. It is not tender and is freely movable, with no lateral extensions or palpable discrete masses.

Cystitis, which occurs particularly in women, is the most common disorder of the bladder. Tenderness is often elicited by palpation over the suprapubic region (Table 15-5). Obstruction below the bladder may be due to vesicle neck contraction, hypertrophy of the prostate, or hypertrophy of the urethral valves. Chronic obstruction causes trabeculation, cellules, and diverticula of the bladder. As residual urine increases, bladder capacity may increase, producing a decompensated bladder. The bladder may then be palpable in the suprapubic region as a midline mass. When large diverticula occur, these may also be palpated. *Tumors* and *calculi* of the bladder are common, particularly in men, but usually produce no physical findings unless the lesions are large.

In those cases where there is a sandy sediment in the urine, there is calculus in the bladder or kidneys.

HIPPOCRATES
(460?–377? B.C.)

A *neurogenic bladder* is one in which neurologic disease leads to bladder dysfunction. Physical findings may be pathognomonic of the various types of neurogenic bladder (Fig. 15-11).

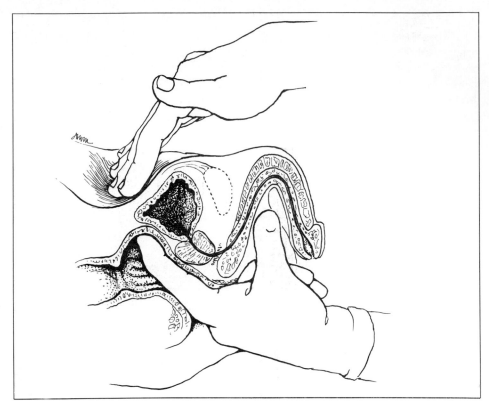

FIGURE 15-10
Bimanual palpation of the urinary bladder.

TABLE 15-5. Some Causes of Cystitis

In women
Short urethra
Postcoital ("honeymoon") cystitis
Recent urinary catheterization
Incomplete emptying of the bladder
Obstruction (prostatic disease)
Cystocele
Neurogenic bladder
Urethritis
Pyelonephritis
Intravesicular disease
Foreign body
Stone
Tumor
Parasites
Some systemic immunosuppressive diseases (e.g., diabetes mellitus)
Radiation to bladder
Drugs and chemicals

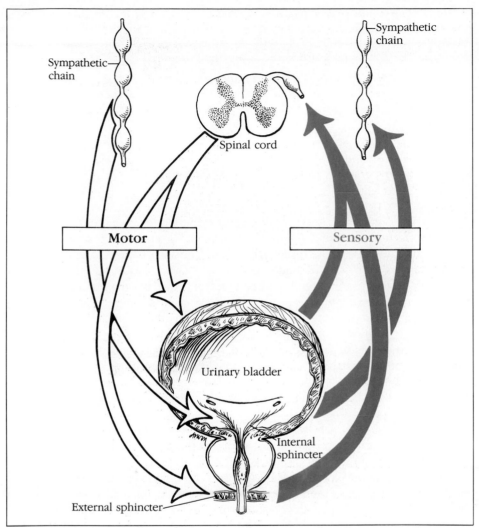

FIGURE 15-11
Simplified scheme of the neurologic control of the bladder. Both sensory and motor components of normal bladder function depend on autonomic and somatic neurologic integrity.

1. *Sensory paralytic bladder* is produced by a lesion on the sensory side of the reflex arch as in tabes dorsalis. There is no bulbocavernosus reflex, and saddle anesthesia is present. When the bladder becomes decompensated, a suprapubic mass may be palpated.

2. *Motor paralytic bladder* results from a lesion affecting the motor side of the reflex arch, as in poliomyelitis. There is no bulbocavernosus reflex, but saddle anesthesia is absent. The patient is unable to initiate micturition, and a large distended bladder is palpable in the suprapubic region.

3. *Autonomous neurogenic bladder* is produced by a lesion affecting sacral segments 2, 3, and 4, such as occurs in myelomeningocele or myelodysplasia. There is no bulbocavernosus reflex, and saddle anesthesia is present. Urine can be forced from the bladder by pressure in the suprapubic region.

4. *Reflex neurogenic bladder* due to a transverse myelitis of the spinal cord, as in trauma, characteristically produces a hyperactive bulbocavernosus reflex and saddle anesthesia. Associated neurologic findings due to the paraplegia facilitate this diagnosis.

5. *Uninhibited neurogenic bladder* is seen in normal infants before myelinization of the spinal cord and after cerebrovascular accidents. The bulbocavernosus reflex is normal or hyperactive, and there is no saddle anesthesia.

External Genitalia

In the normal uncircumcised man the foreskin should be easily retractable. At the time of retraction the external meatus is examined by separating it with the thumbs placed on either side of the distal glans penis. The shaft is then carefully palpated while searching for areas of tenderness or induration, and the urethra is milked downward to express any secretions present. Congenital anomalies of the penis are uncommon. *Balanoposthitis* is seen in uncircumcised men, because of recurrent infection of the prepuce and glans penis. There is erythema, local discomfort, and sometimes a purulent discharge. *Phimosis* occurs when it is impossible to retract the prepuce and is usually secondary to recurrent balanoposthitis (Fig. 15-12). There may be local signs of infection. *Paraphimosis* results when the prepuce is retracted behind the glans penis and cannot be returned to its normal position. Impairment of local circulation to the glans in this circumstance may lead to edema and, if not relieved, gangrene.

Stenosis of the external urethral meatus produces a serious obstructive lesion. There is often meatal ulceration and crusting. *Hypospadias* may be discovered on close inspection of the ventral surface of the penis. Its classification is dependent on the location of the external urethral meatus. An associated chordee is produced by fibrosis in the area of the malformed urethra, producing a downward curvature of the penis on erection. *Epispadias,* in which the urethra opens in the dorsum of the penis, is less common than hypospadias and is often associated with exstrophy of the bladder. Urinary incontinence is often an associated finding. Urethritis produces a few abnormal physical findings. The urethra may be tender to palpation, and often there is a purulent urethral discharge.

The *primary lesion of syphilis,* which appears 2 to 4 weeks after infected sexual contact, is a painless ulcer with indurated borders and a relatively clear base. Palpable inguinal lymph nodes are often present. *Lymphopathia venereum* begins with a small penile lesion that may be papular or vesicular. Painful enlarged inguinal lymph nodes called buboes may ulcerate and drain. *Granuloma inguinale* results in a painful superficial ulceration that is erythematous and velvety in appearance.

Herpes progenitalis, a viral infection, produces multiple superficial vesicles on the foreskin or glans. This should be distinguished from *condylomata acuminatum* (venereal wart), a variant of the ordinary wart that may occur anywhere on the skin.

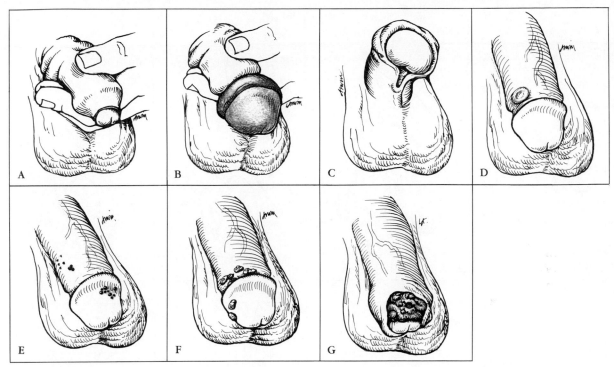

FIGURE 15-12
Some lesions of the penis. A. Phimosis. B. Paraphimosis. C. Hypospadias. D. Syphilitic chancre. E. Herpes progenitalis. F. Condylomata acuminata. G. Epidermoid carcinoma.

Epidermoid carcinoma is usually found in uncircumcised men as a painless ulceration that fails to heal. Growth frequently begins beneath the prepuce. Palpable lymph nodes may indicate metastatic extension of the neoplasm.

The skin of the scrotum is inspected, and each testis is palpated between the thumb and the first two fingers. The comma-shaped structure bulging on the posterolateral surace of each testis is the epididymis, and it is palpated in the same manner. The spermatic cord extends upward from the epididymis to the external ring. The vas deferens can be easily palpated between the thumb and index finger as a small solid cord, using the opposite hand to exert gentle downward traction on the testis.

Normally no masses or areas of tenderness are palpable along the shaft of the penis. The testes lie freely in the scrotum. In the average man they are 3 or 4 cm by 2.5 cm in size, being correspondingly smaller in boys. The epididymis and vas deferens are discretely palpable but not tender. Transillumination is a commonly employed technique for examining the scrotal contents. It is performed in a darkened room. Normally the testes are not translucent.

Acute epididymitis results in a painful mass in the scrotum (Fig. 15-13). Initially it may be possible to distinguish the enlarged tender epididymis from the testis, but later the testis and epididymis become an inseparable mass. The spermatic cord is often thickened and indurated. *Chronic epididymitis* results from recurrent bouts

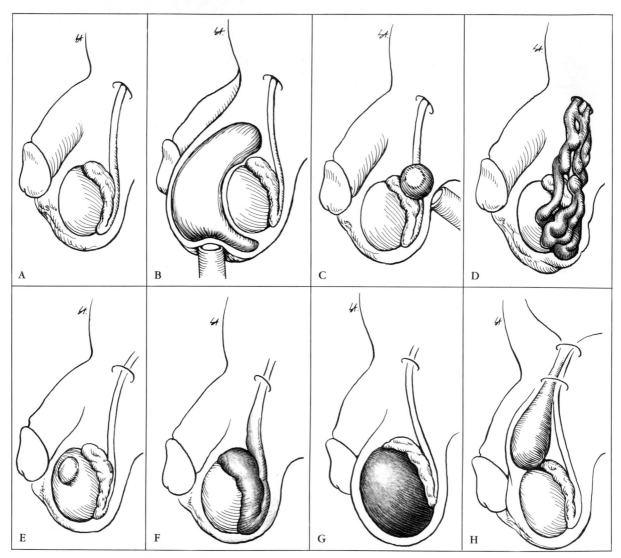

FIGURE 15-13
Some scrotal lesions. A. Normal. B. Hydrocele. C. Spermatocele. D. Varicocele. E. Testicular tumor. F. Epididymitis. G. Orchitis. H. Hernia.

of epididymitis. The epididymis is enlarged and indurated. Tuberculous epididymitis may mimic acute and chronic epididymitis. The vas deferens often contains a group of enlargements that resembles a string of beads, giving rise to the term *beading of the vas deferens.*

Acute orchitis may occur from any infectious disease process but most often is associated with mumps parotitis. The testis is enlarged and painful, and the overlying scrotal skin is erythematous.

A *testicular tumor* usually results in an enlarged testis that is not translucent. Any painless nodular area in the testis must be regarded as a tumor. *Hydroceles* may

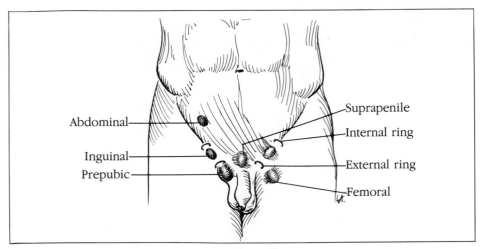

FIGURE 15-14
Common sites of testicular ectopia and cryptorchidism.

develop secondary to tumors; when the testis cannot be palpated because of a hydrocele, aspiration of the fluid will facilitate palpation. Simple hydroceles are common. They transmit light readily.

Torsion of the spermatic cord occurs spontaneously, most often in prepubertal boys, resulting in acute ischemia to the distal parts of the epididymis and testis. Examination of the scrotum reveals a painful mass that is usually elevated. In this condition, elevating the testis may increase the pain, in contradistinction to epididymitis, in which elevation of the testis will somewhat relieve the pain.

When no testis is palpable in the scrotum, it may be *ectopic*. In this case the testis has not descended normally but has been arrested along the normal path of descent (*cryptorchidism*) (Fig. 15-14). Displaced testes are not only sterile, if correction is not accomplished by the fifth or sixth year of life, but have increased potential for malignant change.

HERNIA

Abdominal hernias have in common a sac lined with peritoneum that protrudes through some defect in the abdominal wall. The contents of inguinal and femoral hernias are variable. Omentum, small bowel, large bowel, or bladder may be encountered within the hernial sac (Fig. 15-15).

Examination of the inguinal canal is not difficult (Fig. 15-16). The examining finger is inserted in the lower part of the scrotum, and the scrotum is inverted so that the finger passes along the inguinal canal to palpate the external ring. When performed slowly and carefully this examination causes minimum discomfort to the patient. The examining finger should always identify the following normal structures: the extent of the os pubis, the spermatic cord as it lies within the inguinal canal, the size and perimeter of the external inguinal ring, and the area of Hesselbach's triangle medial to the deep epigastric vessels.

The indirect inguinal hernial sac emerges through the internal ring, traverses the inguinal canal with the contents of the cord, and appears at the external ring. If it

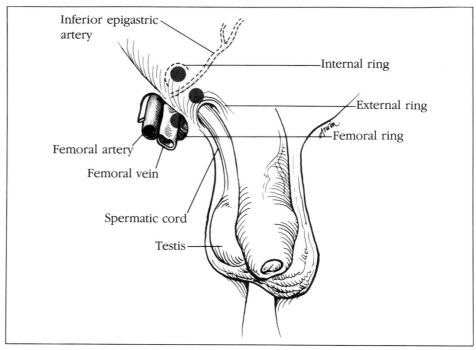

FIGURE 15-15
Common sites of hernias.

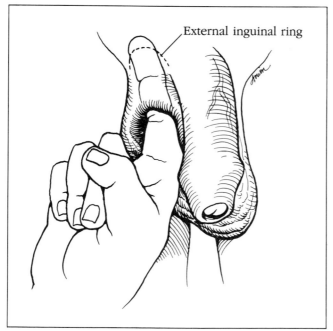

FIGURE 15-16
Technique of examination for inguinal hernia.

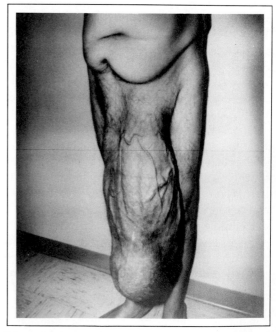

FIGURE 15-17
Massive inguinal hernia.

extends into the scrotum it is termed a scrotal hernia. The neck of the indirect hernial sac lies lateral to the deep epigastric artery.

Indirect hernias are the most common inguinal hernias. They are thought to be congenital and may result from failure of the processus vaginalis to obliterate. Hernias in children and young adults are usually of the indirect type. Hernias limited to the inguinal canal are termed incomplete, while those that emerge from the external ring are complete. In the female a complete hernia may enter the labium majus as a labial hernia.

The direct inguinal hernial sac protrudes through Hesselbach's triangle medial to the deep epigastric artery and appears at the external ring without passing through the inguinal canal. It is apparent, therefore, that the direct hernial sac does not lie in close relationship with the spermatic cord. *Direct hernias* usually result from weakness of the fascia transversalis in the region of Hesselbach's triangle and present as a rounded swelling. They are almost always reducible and rarely enter the scrotum. Most direct hernias occur in individuals over 40 years of age.

On physical examination the external ring may sometimes appear to be enlarged. Relaxation of the external ring, however, is insufficient evidence on which to make a diagnosis of indirect inguinal hernia. If the examining finger encounters a mass in the inguinal canal, the presumptive diagnosis of hernia may be made. This may be confirmed by palpating an impulse in the external ring when the patient coughs. The differentiation between an indirect inguinal and a direct inguinal hernia should not be difficult. If the hernia can be completely reduced, the examining finger may be inserted into the external inguinal ring, and when the patient coughs the leading edge of the hernia may be palpated with the tip of the finger. On the other hand, if the finger is inserted into Hesselbach's triangle, the sac of an indirect hernia will be felt striking the side of the finger.

It may sometimes be difficult to establish the diagnosis of inguinal hernia in a woman. It should be possible to identify the inguinal ligament and os pubis and from these anatomic points to locate the external inguinal ring. If a sac is palpated when the patient coughs, the diagnosis of inguinal hernia may be made. It may help to place the palmar surface of the hand over the area of the internal inguinal ring in an effort to feel an impulse with cough. It is occasionally possible to see a small indirect inguinal hernia as a bulge that appears on coughing. Examination in both standing and supine positions may help to bring these points out.

Examination of the femoral region is more difficult than is the study of the inguinal area. The external opening of the femoral canal may be located anatomically just medial to the femoral artery and deep to the inguinal ligament. A simple precept to remember in examining the patient's right femoral area is that when the examiner's right index finger is placed on the patient's right femoral artery, the middle finger will overlie the femoral vein and the ring finger will overlie the femoral canal. A swelling lying within the femoral canal that transmits an impulse on coughing may be diagnosed as a *femoral hernia*. It must be distinguished from psoas abscess, lymphadenitis, and saphenous varix.

Femoral hernia is the most common hernia in women, and the points raised in the above discussion of examination of the femoral region are applicable in examining the female patient as well.

As a general rule, the incidence of strangulation is high in femoral hernias. Consequently, early operation is desirable.

A *sliding hernia* is a special type that deserves mention. The large bowel (or bladder) slips retroperitoneally between the leaves of its mesentery to herniate or protrude through the defect in the abdominal wall. On the right side the cecum may be the presenting part, while on the left the presenting part may be the sigmoid colon. In either event it is important to recognize this entity, since the wall of the bowel or bladder rather than a peritoneal sac makes up the leading edge of the hernia. Failure to make the proper diagnosis may lead the surgeon to open the bowel accidentally, thinking he is incising a hernial sac. It is often difficult to reduce a sliding hernia, and irreducibility should raise the examiner's suspicions as to this possibility.

When a hernia can no longer be reduced and the contents of the hernial sac cannot be returned to the peritoneal cavity, it is said to be *incarcerated.* If the blood supply to the viscera lying within the hernial sac has been cut off, it is said to be a *strangulated hernia.* It is often difficult and sometimes impossible to tell with certainty whether a hernia is simply incarcerated or whether it is strangulated. It is reasonable to attempt to reduce an incarcerated hernia if the incarceration is recent and one can be certain that the contents are completely viable. Strangulated hernias usually show local signs of inflammation, although this is not invariable. When inflammatory signs are present it is unwise to attempt vigorous reduction lest strangulated bowel be returned to the peritoneal cavity.

If it is decided to attempt nonoperative reduction of an incarcerated hernia, this should be performed with the patient in the recumbent position. This may be accomplished by exerting constant gentle pressure over the sac. The patient will often be experienced in reducing the hernia himself and may be able to accomplish this with ease. In difficult cases it may be necessary to lower the head of the bed, flex the leg on the affected side to relax the abdominal muscles, and attempt to gently guide the contents of the hernial sac through the inguinal ring. If local pain and tenderness are present, presumptive diagnosis of strangulation may be made and operative reduction and repair of the hernia is the procedure of choice. It should be noted that it is sometimes possible to reduce the entire hernia, together with the internal ring, into the abdominal cavity without actually freeing the contents of the hernial sac from the constricting internal ring. Under these circumstances, continued pain or tenderness in the region indicates the need for urgent surgical attention.

Large femoral hernias may be difficult to diagnose correctly because of their tendency to leave the abdominal cavity by way of the femoral canal and then be directed upward to overlie the inguinal ligament. They may be differentiated from inguinal hernias, however, if it is remembered that the sac of the femoral hernia lies lateral to and below the level of the symphysis pubis, while the sac of the inguinal hernia lies medial to it and above.

It is sometimes difficult to detect early strangulation in femoral hernias, since such local signs as pain or tenderness may be minimal. The femoral canal is the most likely site for the development of a *Richter's hernia.* The systemic signs of strangulation—such as tachypnea, leukocytosis, and fever—should invariably lead

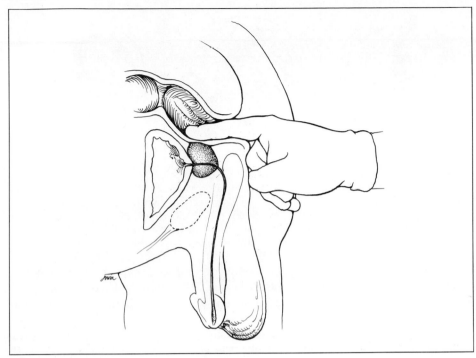

FIGURE 15-18
Examination of the prostate.

one to inspect this area with great care. The localized gangrene of the bowel wall without intestinal obstruction may lead to perforation and abscess formation just below the inguinal ligament. This should be differentiated from psoas abscess and femoral lymphadenitis.

Hydrocele of the canal of Nuck may occur in women. In the course of embryologic development, the round ligament leaves the retroperitoneal area to traverse the inguinal canal and insert itself on the labium majus. A processus vaginalis of peritoneum descends with the round ligament, and if the process is incompletely fused and obliterated, a hydrocele may result. A hydrocele may lie anywhere between the internal inguinal ring and the labium majus. Hydrocele of the canal of Nuck may be difficult to demonstrate but is characterized by its cystic, irreducible, translucent appearance.

Occasionally a patient will have indirect and direct hernias simultaneously. These are termed *saddlebag hernias.*

PROSTATE GLAND
As explained previously, the prostate is assessed during rectal examination. The technique of digital examination of the rectum is considered in Chapter 14. The prostate gland is best examined while the patient is standing and bending over the examining table (Fig. 15-18) or, when he is unable to stand or is in bed, in the Sim's position. Ample lubrication of the examining finger and perianal region facilitates

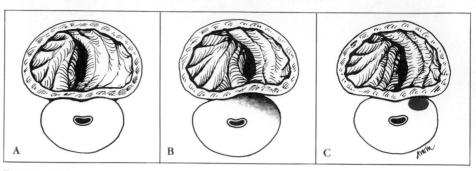

FIGURE 15-19

Diagnosis of some prostatic lesions. A. Normal. An approximately 2.5-cm, firm, smooth, heart-shaped gland. The medial sulcus can be felt as a depression between the two lateral lobes. B. Inflammatory nodule. The area of inflammation is raised above the surface of the gland, with induration decreasing at the periphery of the nodule. C. Cancerous nodule. The cancer is not raised. There is an abrupt demarcation of induration at the periphery of the lesion.

the procedure. The index finger is introduced pointing toward the umbilicus, as this approximates the direction of the anal canal. The patient is asked to bear down slightly, which helps to relax the anal sphincter, and with gentle pressure the finger is easily introduced into the anal canal.

The muscle tone of the anal sphincter is estimated and the bulbocavernosus reflex is tested. The patient is asked to relax the sphincter as much as possible, and the glans penis is squeezed with the opposite hand. Normally this produces involuntary contraction of the anal sphincter. Voluntary contraction may produce a false positive test. The presence of a bulbocavernosus reflex signifies an intact reflex arc in the region of the sacral cord, which also innervates the urinary bladder.

The prostate gland is examined by gentle palpation of the anterior wall of the rectum. The upper limits, lateral margins, and medial sulcus should be outlined. Each lobe is carefully palpated while the examiner searches for areas of irregularity or enlargement. The region of the seminal vesicles extends upward and laterally along the upper margin of the prostate gland.

Normally the sphincter tone is good, and the bulbocavernosus reflex is present. The prostate varies greatly in size, usually increasing with age. It is smooth and rubbery in consistency and normally not tender. The lateral borders are usually well defined (Fig. 15-19). The seminal vesicles are normally not palpable.

Acute prostatitis results in fever, urethral discharge, and an exceedingly tender, enlarged prostate gland on rectal examination. An abscess may develop and can be demonstrated as a fluctuant mass in the prostate gland. The seminal vesicles often are involved in inflammatory reaction and may be dilated and extremely tender. *Chronic prostatitis* is usually asymptomatic. At times rectal examination shows the prostate to be boggy or irregular. Areas of fibrous tissue may be palpated, thus simulating neoplasm. *Prostatic calculi* are seldom of clinical importance. They may often be palpated at rectal examination and mistaken for carcinoma.

Benign prostatic hypertrophy is extremely common in men over 50 years of age. The prostate is of variable size. Small glands may be as obstructive as the large glands because it is the intraurethral protrusion that produces obstruction, not extraurethral enlargement. The gland is usually symmetric and has a smooth, rubbery consistency. The medial sulcus can be identified, and the lateral borders are well defined.

Carcinoma of the prostate occurs in approximately 20 percent of men over 60 years of age. The initial lesion usually involves the posterior lobe and is readily palpable at rectal examination. The early lesion feels like a small nodule on the posterior surface of the gland. Similar nodules can also be caused by calculi, chronic infection, or benign adenoma. More advanced malignant lesions usually are stony hard, irregular, and painless on palpation.

FEMALE GENITOURINARY SYSTEM

CHAPTER 16

There is only one way to be born and a thousand ways to die.

SERBIAN PROVERB

The objective of this portion of the physical examination is to assure normality or to diagnose abnormalities of the reproductive organs of the woman. More specifically the objective is to determine the size, shape, and mobility of the reproductive organs and to locate any source of intrapelvic pain and evidence of inflammation, discharge, or structural abnormality in the genitalia.

In view of this objective, it is well for the student to acquire the habit of referring to the procedure as a pelvic examination rather than as a vaginal examination. The latter, of course, implies an examination only of the vagina itself rather than of the entire pelvic contents.

The pelvic examination is an essential part of the total evaluation of female patients. Although there is a natural reluctance on the part of both patient and physician about this portion of the physical examination, such reluctance must not interfere with prompt and thorough evaluation of the pelvic area. A physical examination in which the pelvic examination is deferred is as incomplete as one in which the cardiac examination is deferred.

ANATOMY

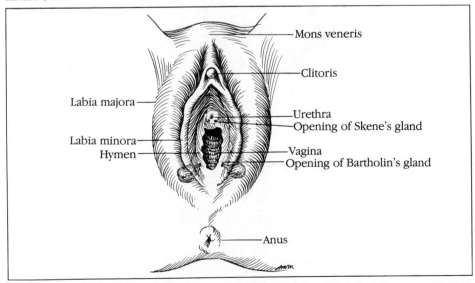

Mons veneris

Clitoris

Labia majora

Urethra
Opening of Skene's gland

Labia minora
Hymen

Vagina
Opening of Bartholin's gland

Anus

FIGURE 16-1
External female genitalia.

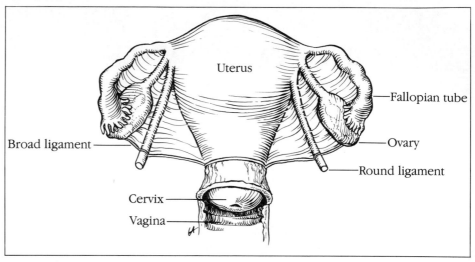

FIGURE 16-2
Internal female genitalia.

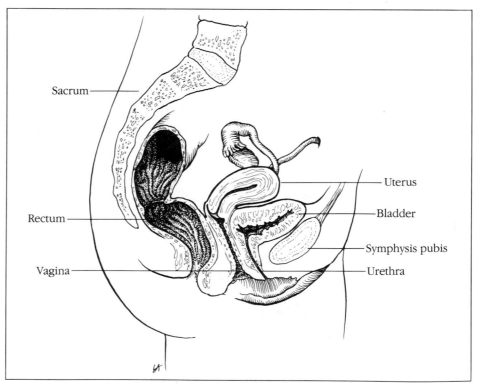

FIGURE 16-3
Cross-sectional anatomy of the female pelvis.

HISTORY

No one who is not female can be in a position to make accurate statements about women.

OTTO WEININGER
(1880–1903)

Gynecologic symptoms may point to local disease (infections, tumors) or signal systemic disorders (menstrual irregularities with thyroid disease and the vulvo-vaginitis of diabetes, for example). Moreover, gynecologic disorders may be associated with generalized symptoms resulting from a primary pelvic disease.

Menstrual symptoms are common. Specific inquiry should always be directed to the following:

1. Age at onset
2. Amount of discharge per period
3. Duration of period
4. Interval between periods
5. Character of menstrual discharge
6. Menstrual symptoms—especially pain
7. Intermenstrual period.

Endocrine disorders may precipitate an early menarche (onset of first period) or delay puberty and menstruation. A delay in sexual maturation may occur with any debilitating disease (starvation, inflammatory bowel disease, juvenile arthritis) around the time of puberty.

The amount of menstrual blood lost at each period varies from woman to woman. In an individual woman, however, marked decrease or increase in flow may be the hallmark of systemic (especially endocrine) or local (e.g., tumor) disease (Table 16-1).

TABLE 16-1. Some Causes of Excessive Menstrual Bleeding

Endocrine
    Puberty (anovulatory)
    Maturity (anovulatory, progesterone deficient)
    Menopause
    Hypothyroidism

Genital
    Fibromyoma
    Chronic salpingo-oophoritis
    Endometriosis
    Malignancy of the uterus
    Acute infectious systemic disease

Vascular
    Chronic right heart failure
    Arteriosclerosis

Hematologic
    Coagulation defects
    Leukemia

A normal flow can last anywhere from 2 to 6 days. However, this is extremely variable. Similarly the interval between periods—a traditional 25 to 28 days—is not fixed, even in individual women. However, marked variations in interval may also suggest gynecologic disease.

Menstrual blood is generally dark and is normally without clots. With excessive menstrual bleeding, however, the menstrual flow may be redder and clots may form.

Menstrual pain (*dysmenorrhea*) is not always abnormal. It may begin a day or two before flow and continue well into the menstrual period. Some women are so afflicted that they must take to their beds for the duration of their period. Constitutional, psychologic, and local factors may all produce dysmenorrhea.

Bleeding between periods (spotting) may occur as the menopause approaches but is also a cardinal signal of gynecologic malignancy. It should be thoroughly investigated.

The date of the last menstrual period should be ascertained, particularly since delay—while potentially due to a variety of emotional, structural, or metabolic upsets—may also be due to pregnancy. Other symptoms of pregnancy include weight gain, morning sickness, and breast swelling and tenderness.

Vaginal discharge worries many women. Leukorrhea, a white discharge, may suggest bacterial, fungal, or parasitic infection. The duration, character, odor, and irritation caused by the discharge should be recorded in the history.

Gastrointestinal symptoms may be the hallmark of gynecologic disease or pregnancy. Nausea and vomiting may hint at pregnancy. Loss of appetite, weight loss, constipation, and abdominal pain and distention can be symptomatic of gynecologic malignancy.

Urinary symptoms, as discussed in Chapter 15, may be associated with vaginal or uterine disease as well as disorders primary to the urinary system.

Sexual dysfunction and *infertility* in women are serious complaints that may require extensive evaluation, beginning with a careful and complete history and physical and including pelvic examination.

PHYSICAL EXAMINATION

1. Abdominal examination (see Chap. 14).
2. Inspection of external genitalia, including Bartholin's and Skene's glands and urethra.
3. Speculum examination, including appropriate cultures and Papanicolaou smear.
4. Bimanual examination of internal genitalia.
5. Rectovaginal examination.

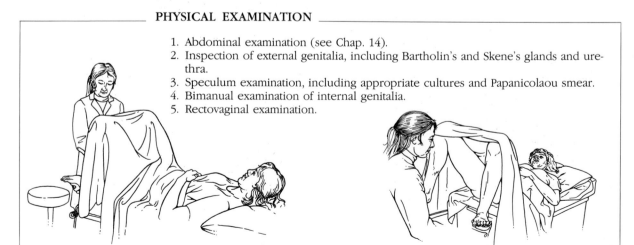

Rupture of a tubal gestation is one of the causes of sudden death in young women who have previously been in perfect health.

SIR ZACHARY COPE
(1881–1974)

GENERAL

To understand the importance of acquiring competence in this particular aspect of physical diagnosis, one should consider two questions: (1) Who should have such an examination? and (2) who should carry out the examination?

First, of course, all hospitalized women should have the benefit of careful pelvic examination. In addition, any woman coming to the physician because of pelvic complaints (or with the request for routine prophylactic pelvic checkup) should be examined, as well as women with systemic complaints of any kind. The old axiom "If the nature of the story is such that the physician palpates a woman's abdomen, then he is obligated to examine her pelvis" is, if anything, too restrictive.

There is often a great reluctance on the part of physicians (and parents) to examine the very young. This attitude can be very detrimental. In a recently reported series of cases of ovarian malignancy, those patients who were teen-aged or younger had a significantly worsened prognosis, chiefly because of the much greater amount of time lost through postponement of the examination necessary to make a correct diagnosis. Actually, gentle rectal examination in even very young girls can yield a great deal of helpful information; and if there is any suspicion of a pelvic lesion, examination under light anesthesia should be carried out. Youth does not convey an immunity to pelvic disease, and the physician should not deny his patients the best possible care simply because they are young. In general, if a mother thinks the problem is serious enough to bring her daughter to the doctor, the doctor should consider the complaints to be serious enough to examine the patient.

Second, who should carry out the examination? Pelvic examination of the female patient is a specialized gynecologic procedure only in the sense that auscultation of the heart is a specialized procedure reserved for the cardiologist. In other words, any physician who retains among his basic skills the ability to percuss the cardiac border or listen to the heart sounds should also retain the ability to use the vaginal speculum and carry out careful bimanual pelvic examination.

In either instance—for either the noncardiologist or the nongynecologist—the purpose of such examinations is to identify those patients who should be referred for specialized diagnosis and treatment. Such referral is also an obligation when the examination has been unsatisfactory or incomplete. Thus, to reassure a woman that "everything is all right" when both ovaries have not been clearly felt could be signing her death warrant. All physicians—internists, surgeons, pediatricians, as well as gynecologists—should perform pelvic examination on their patients. If the examination is inadequate or the results are inconclusive, careful referral, not bland reassurance, is required.

None of us consider our reproductive organs in the same sense that we regard other parts of our anatomy. Thus, the embarrassment that some women anticipate in relation to this type of examination may cause them to postpone it. Similarly, in their personal hygiene, some women will often fail to inspect or palpate lesions that, on other parts of the body, they would examine minutely. As a physician, therefore, one must proceed with this embarrassment clearly in mind and do one's best to place the patient at ease. This has practical as well as humane aspects—the more relaxed the patient, the more easily the examination will be accomplished. Patient cooperation is essential, and an undue tightening of the abdominal muscles or the levator ani sling can effectively bar the physician from accomplishing the objective of this examination.

It should be remembered that the pelvic examination, if done by a male physician, should never be performed without a female nurse or aide present.

The examination is best conducted in a room designed and equipped for that specific purpose. Ideally, separate toilet and dressing facilities should be part of the room. A curtained cubicle is no substitute for four walls and a solid door.

The patient should empty her bladder and rectum immediately before the examination and should disrobe completely.

Draping the patient is important. The most satisfactory draping is a square sheet. The patient holds one corner over her xiphoid, the corners adjacent to this are placed one over each knee, and the fourth corner hangs between her legs and over her perineum. Draping in this manner minimizes embarrassment to the woman while permitting adequate exposure for the examination.

The routine nature of the office ritual helps put the patient at ease. The relative impersonality of the physician's behavior and the manner of arranging the draped sheet all heighten the reassuring effect. In elevating the corner of the sheet which hangs over the perineum and tucking it under the sheet on her abdomen, one is well advised to be looking not at her perineum but directly into her eyes, and to be commenting on something far afield from the complaints of the moment.

The perineum is as tender and sensitive as any area examined in the course of physical diagnosis. The doctor who hurts a patient instantly makes her an opponent rather than an ally in the job of accomplishing a satisfactory examination.

Anyone—man or woman—placed in the lithotomy position and then touched abruptly on the perineum will experience the anal sphincter reflex. The external anal sphincter (and portions of the levator ani) will involuntarily contract, creating a barrier to a comfortable examination. Accordingly the examiner's initial contact with the perineum should be at some distance from the labia and should be firm but gentle.

All the tender areas of the introitus are anterior (clitoris, labia minora, and urethral meatus), and insertion of the intravaginal fingers should be posterior, with adequate lubrication. Jamming or shoving motions should be avoided. Although subsequent portions of the examination are inevitably somewhat uncomfortable, the entire initiation of the procedure can be such that optimum patient comfort (and hence patient cooperation) is achieved and maintained.

EXTERNAL GENITALIA

Inspection precedes palpation here as in other realms of physical examination. However, the inspection can be brief and unembarrassing to the patient. One is seeking superficial skin lesions of the groin and perineum, evidence of erythema on the labia, and signs of an abnormal vaginal discharge.

Palpation also can be effected briefly and can yield evidence of the strength of the pelvic floor, the presence of Bartholin's cysts (Fig. 16-4), or the presence of pus in Skene's glands. Evaluate the general strength of perineal support by asking the

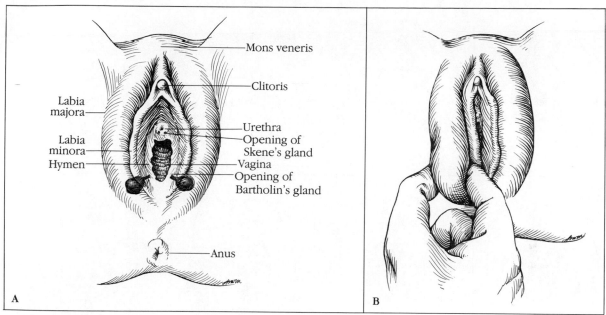

Labels (left, top to bottom): Labia majora, Labia minora, Hymen

Labels (center/right, top to bottom): Mons veneris, Clitoris, Urethra, Opening of Skene's gland, Vagina, Opening of Bartholin's gland, Anus

A　　　　　　　B

FIGURE 16-4
A. Bartholin's glands. B. Technique of palpation of Bartholin's glands.

patient to bear down and then observing any ballooning that may develop anteriorly (cystocele) and posteriorly (rectocele) (Fig. 16-5). The perineal body may be assayed by depressing the posterior fourchette with two fingers of the gloved hand and testing the general resistance. The presence of pus in Skene's glands can be determined by gently stripping these areas upward and watching for the appearance of purulent material at the urethral meatus.

With the exception of instances in which you must pause for an unexpected finding (e.g., vulvar or labial lesions), the inspection and palpation of the external genitalia can be expertly completed in 1 to 2 minutes.

SALINE DROP

Before introduction of the intravaginal fingers, it is well to obtain material for microscopic examination. This is achieved by inserting a saline-moistened swab into the vagina to collect a specimen and then placing the swab in a small test tube containing 1 ml or at most 2 ml of physiologic saline solution. It is advantageous to keep the solution slightly warm, perhaps by having the attendant hold the test tube in her clenched fist. The examination of this specimen as simply a drop on a regular slide, without stain or fixation of any kind, will yield considerable information. The value of the procedure—as is true of so many diagnostic tests—is usually in direct proportion to the frequency with which the physician carries it out.

Under most circumstances the principal cellular element noted will be the vaginal epithelial cells. The bacterial content will be largely Döderlein's bacillus and *Escherichia coli.* A significant number of leukocytes imply inflammation, and a significant number of erythrocytes indicate a bleeding lesion. The *Trichomonas vaginalis* parasite is recognized by its flagellate motion; *Candida albicans,* by its

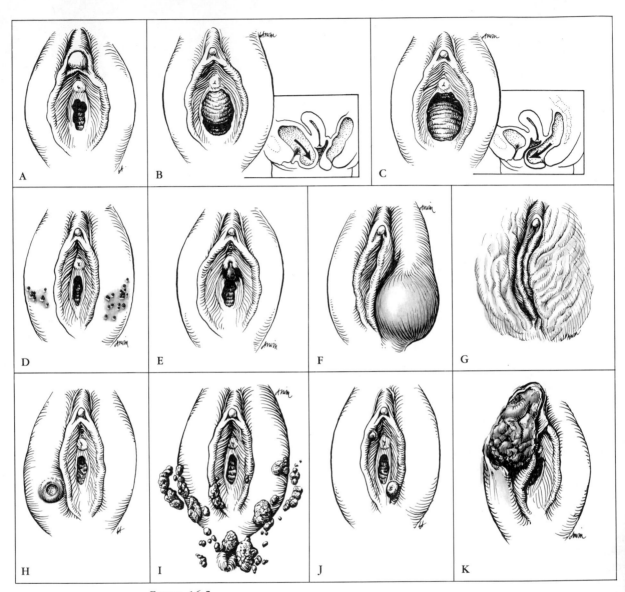

FIGURE 16-5
Some lesions of the external female genitalia. A. Clitoral enlargement. B. Cystocele.
C. Rectocele. D. Herpes of vulva. E. Urethral caruncle. F. Bartholin's gland cyst. G. Labial
varicosities. H. Syphilitic chancre. I. Condylomata acuminata. J. Hidradenoma of vulva.
K. Carcinoma of vulva.

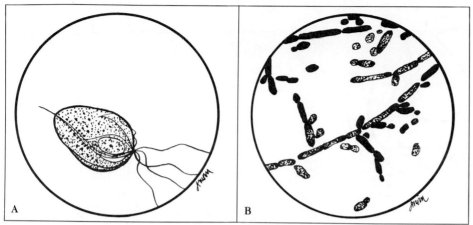

FIGURE 16-6
Saline drop. A. *Trichomonas vaginalis.* B. *Candida albicans.*

configuration (Fig. 16-6). For the few moments spent in examining this preparation, its diagnostic value is great.

SPECULUM EXAMINATION

Inspection of the cervix and upper vagina precedes internal palpation and is accomplished by means of the vaginal speculum. This is perhaps the most valuable single diagnostic instrument in gynecology, and the student is well advised to spend a few moments learning its simple mechanism.

The Graves or duck-billed speculum is made up of two blades. The posterior blade is fixed and the anterior is movable. The two blades are held together by a thumbscrew on the handle that can be loosened to separate the blades. The thumbscrew should always be tightly fastened and the blades in close approximation when the speculum is in ordinary use, or the chances of pinching the labia are increased.

The anterior blade is hinged and carries the thumbpiece on the side, which permits it to be elevated, separating the two blades when the speculum is assembled. The thumbscrew here should be all the way back, permitting the blades to be in close approximation on introduction of the speculum into the vagina.

In order to avoid interference with cytologic studies and to minimize discomfort, the speculum should have no lubrication other than warm water. It is best held with the handle grasped loosely and the blades firmly held between the index and middle fingers. On introduction of the speculum, the pressure should be largely against the posterior fourchette and the blades should be oblique. If the flat surfaces of the blades are horizontal, the introitus is often overly stretched; if the blades are vertical, the suburethral area can be hurt.

As soon as the broad portions of the blades have passed the introitus, the speculum is rotated so that the blades are horizontal, and the handle is elevated so that the speculum is advancing at a 45-degree angle toward the examining table. The blades should not be separated until the speculum is fully inserted. As the thumb presses the lateral thumbpiece to elevate the top blade, the hand should lift on the

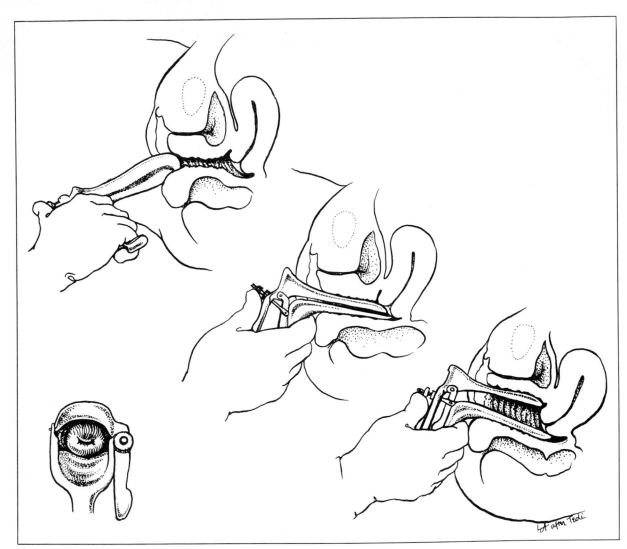

FIGURE 16-7
Insertion of the vaginal speculum (see text).

handle to lower the fixed posterior blade. In this way the two blades move away from each other, and the cervix and vaginal walls are exposed (Figure 16-7).

Inspect the vaginal wall and cervix carefully under a good light (see Table 16-2 and Figs. 16-8 and 16-9).

SPECIAL TESTS

CULTURES

In any population of sexually active women, it may be wise to obtain a sample of vaginal secretions for gonorrhea cultures. Women with *Neisseria gonorrhea* vaginitis, cervicitis, or proctitis need *not* have *any* symptoms.

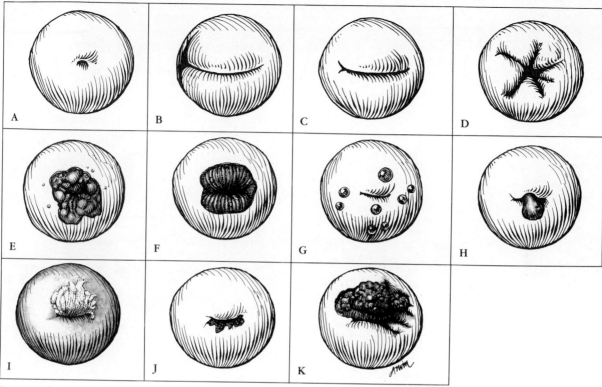

FIGURE 16-8
Some cervical lesions. A. Virgin. B. Parous. C. Minor tear. D. Stellate tear. E. Erosion.
F. Eversion. G. Cysts. H. Polyp. I. Leukoplakia. J. Early cancer. K. Advanced cancer.

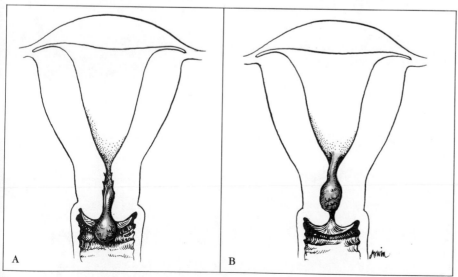

FIGURE 16-9
Cervical polyps. A. Exocervical. B. Endocervical.

TABLE 16-2. Some Vaginal Lesions

Lesion	History	Physical Signs	Appearance
Bacterial vaginitis (*Hemophilus,* gonococcus)	Leukorrhea, yellow discharge; dyspareunia, burning discharge	Vaginal wall inflammation Cervix inflamed; pooled pus from os cervix	
Senile vaginitis	Postmenopausal bleeding, discharge, itching, burning, dyspareunia	Friable mucosa small, shrunken introitus; small cervix	
Candida vaginitis	Discharge (thin to purulent); irritation and redness of vulva	Mucosal redness Whitish or grayish patches	
Trichomonas vaginitis	Leukorrhea, soreness, burning, itching	"Strawberry" punctate erosions of cervix and mucosa Foamy pus pooled in fornix	

TABLE 16-2 (*Continued*)

Lesion	History	Physical Signs	Appearance
Gartner's duct cyst	If large, possible bulging from vaginal outlet	Cyst on anterolateral vaginal wall	

PAPANICOLAOU SMEAR

There are many ways to obtain the cells for cytodiagnosis. Perhaps the most important single requirement is to obtain an adequate representation of the endocervical sample. The procedure described here is the Fast technique, which is designed to combine samples from the posterior vaginal pool and from the cervical canal and cervical face. Since this test is for the identification of epithelial lesions, the specimen should be obtained before the upper vagina and cervical face are wiped off.

The slide and the bottle of ether-alcohol fixative should be labeled and prepared in advance to facilitate prompt fixing after spreading the cellular specimen. By using the handle of the Ayres spatula or a similar spatula, a thick sample of cells from the posterior cul-de-sac is obtained and placed on the slide at the frosted end. The spatula is immediately reversed, the longer arm of the tip is placed in the cervi-

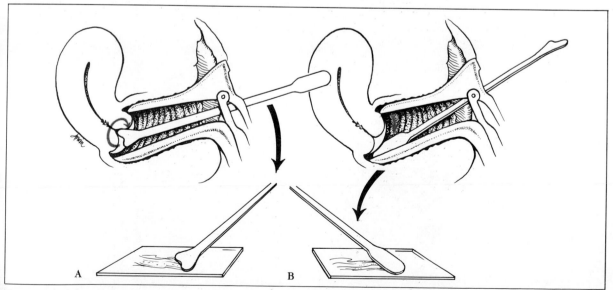

FIGURE 16-10
Technique of the Papanicolaou smear. A. Cervical scraping. B. Vaginal pool sampling.

TABLE 16-3. Classification of Cervical Carcinoma

Stage	Extent
0	Carcinoma in situ (preinvasive)

Stage	Extent
I	Carcinoma is confined to cervix

II	Carcinoma extends beyond cervix but has not yet reached pelvic wall It may involve vagina but not lower third

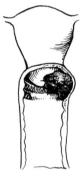

III	Carcinoma has reached pelvic wall, involves lower third of vagina, or is associated with lymph node metastases on pelvic wall

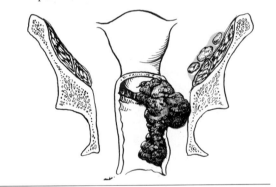

IV	Carcinoma involves bladder or rectum or has extended outside true pelvis (e.g., metastases to vulva, abdomen, lungs, bones, distant nodes)

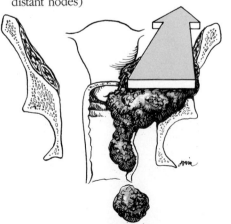

cal os, and the blade is rotated a full circle. This portion of the sample is spread the length of the slide, catching and distributing some of the original cul-de-sac specimen. Then, with the tip of the spatula the entire specimen is spread evenly and the slide dropped immediately into the ether-alcohol.

A Papanicolaou ("Pap") smear should be part of the routine pelvic examination in every woman. The frequency with which a Pap smear is taken is determined by the patient's sexual activity, family history, use of contraceptive drugs, past cytologic diagnoses, and other considerations.

CERVICAL BIOPSY

The cervix is insensitive to cutting, and a liberal biopsy can be taken without discomfort to the patient. Various punch biopsy forceps are available that will obtain samples from the cervical face and endocervix without distortion.

It should be remembered that cervical cytology has not replaced the biopsy. Cytologic study has its greatest value for the normal-appearing cervix, as an aid in screening, and in raising the examiner's index of suspicion. Where there is an evident lesion, the examiner's suspicion should already have been alerted and a biopsy should be taken. A negative cytologic report in the presence of a lesion does not remove the need for biopsy. Table 16-3 presents the classification of cervical carcinoma.

BIMANUAL PELVIC EXAMINATION

After the specimens are obtained and the speculum removed, bimanual pelvic examination is carried out. The age-old debate as to whether the intrapelvic examination should be done with the right or the left hand is fruitless. The point is to achieve the stated objectives of the pelvic examination without concern about which hand is used. Indeed, it is often useful to change the intrapelvic hand, since the adnexal regions can often be felt best with the hand of the same side (for example, right hand for right adnexal region).

In general, the abdominal hand brings the pelvic structures within reach of the intravaginal fingers for palpation. It is well to remember that the area that can be covered depends largely on the position of the abdominal hand. The beginner tends to place the abdominal hand too close to the pubic bone, and he should be encouraged to move it at least three-quarters of the way toward the umbilicus (Fig. 16-11).

The examining fingers should be well lubricated and gently inserted over the posterior fourchette. It is often most comfortable to rest one foot on a low stool, with the elbow of the intrapelvic hand resting on the knee.

CERVIX

The cervix will be most easily palpated, and as a general rule it points the opposite way from the fundus. If the cervix points posteriorly, the fundus of the uterus will usually be found anteriorly; if the cervix is in the axis of the vagina, the fundus will more often be retroverted and found in the cul-de-sac (Fig. 16-12). Motion of the cervix should not produce pain. However, it is just as well not to ask a direct question on this score since most patients will answer in the affirmative simply on the basis that the entire examination is uncomfortable. The pain one is seeking (as in

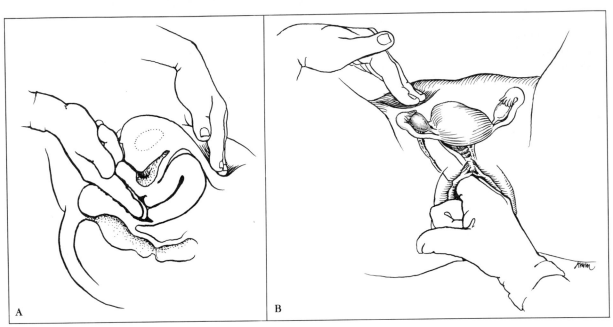

FIGURE 16-11
Technique of bimanual pelvic examination. A. Lateral view. B. Perineal view.

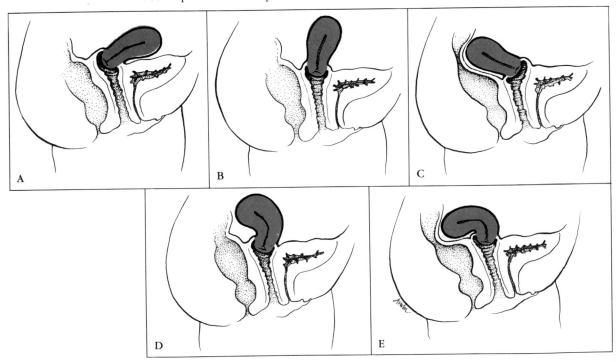

FIGURE 16-12
Some malpositions of the uterus. A. Normal position. B. Slight retroversion. C. Marked retroversion. D. Slight retroflexion. E. Marked retroflexion.

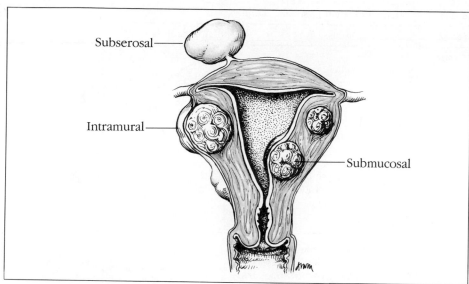

FIGURE 16-13
Uterine fibroids (myomata). These are truly benign smooth muscle tumors and are the most common of pelvic tumors.

ectopic pregnancy or adnexal inflammation) is severe enough that the patient will usually indicate its presence without questioning.

UTERUS

The body of the uterus is then held between the examining hands, and its size, contour, and mobility are determined. Irregularities in its surface (as with myomata) can usually be determined with ease (Fig. 16-13). The cul-de-sac area should also be examined for bulging, tenderness, and masses. A uterine mass always requires further investigation, but x-rays should not be ordered until you are certain that your patient is not pregnant.

The broad ligament structures beside the uterus do not generally yield palpable findings. The vaginal fingers go posteriorly under the broad ligament, and the abdominal fingers beside the uterus approach them so that the tissues of the broad ligament and the fallopian tube can be run between the fingers from bottom to top. In a normal patient no masses should be encountered.

OVARIES

The intravaginal fingers now move downward and backward again at the lateral wall, the abdominal hand moves over just inside the anterior superior spine of the ileum, and the same process is repeated. Here the examiner should encounter the ovary, and size, shape, and mobility can be determined. (Tables 16-4 and 16-5 describe some important ovarian lesions.) The gonads of women are as sensitive to pressure as the gonads of men; again, direct questions on this score are meaningless, and gentleness is imperative.

TABLE 16-4. Benign Ovarian Cysts and Tumors*

Lesion	Discussion	Appearance
Cystic Non-neoplastic	Follicle, lutein cysts, etc.—functional retention cysts arising in follicles or corpora lutea Usually no symptoms, but may undergo spontaneous rupture, bleeding, torsion Also includes inflammatory and endometrial cysts	 *Follicle cyst*
Neoplastic	Pseudomucinous, serous, and dermoid cysts May grow to huge size	 *Dermoid cysts (containing hair, teeth)*
Solid	Fibroma (of fibrous muscle tissue), Brenner tumor of epithelial cells (rarely malignant)	 *Solid mass, though cystic degeneration may occur*

* On physical examination, all tumors may be felt as abdominal or pelvic masses, depending on size.

TABLE 16-5. Clinical Manifestations of Ovarian Tumors

Benign	Malignant
1. May be totally asymptomatic	1. May be totally asymptomatic
2. Rupture or hemorrhage may mimic an acute abdomen	2. Necrosis or rupture may mimic acute abdomen
3. May undergo torsion, with or without infarction	3. Torsion is rare
4. Infection is rare	4. Symptoms of vague abdominal distress, bladder and bowel irritability 2° pressure
5. Symptoms and signs are those of intra-pelvic or intra-abdominal mass	5. Abdominal swelling
	6. Irregular vaginal bleeding
	7. May cause ascites, weight loss, intestinal obstruction, metastatic disease

RECTOVAGINAL EXAMINATION

The examination is completed by rectovaginal abdominal palpation (Fig. 16-14). Entry into the rectum is facilitated by liberal use of lubrication and having the patient bear down. The middle finger is gently inserted in the rectum and the index finger in the vagina. This immediately gives much greater access to the adnexal regions and the posterior surface of the broad ligament and also reveals the presence or absence of rectal lesions.

Hard, fixed nodules in ureterosacral ligaments, cul-de-sac, or rectovaginal septum may represent *endometriosis*—the deposition of functional endometrial tissue

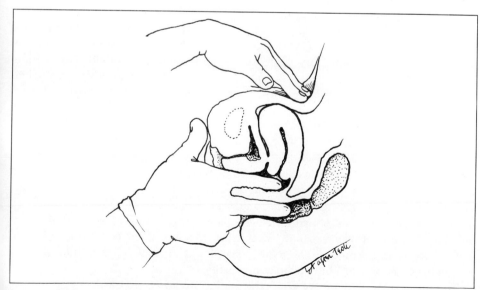

FIGURE 16-14
Technique of rectovaginal examination.

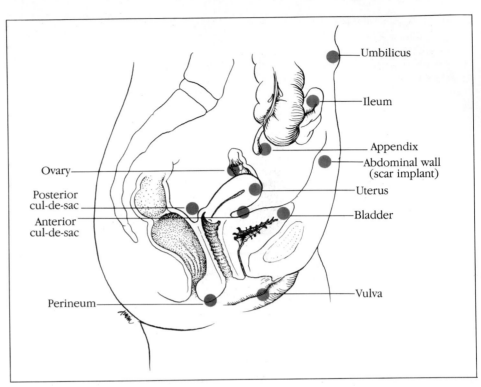

FIGURE 16-15
Some sites of endometrial implants.

in areas outside the uterus (Fig. 16-15). Multiple sites usually are involved. The patient is commonly a young, nulliparous woman with dysmenorrhea, infertility, dyspareunia, bowel dysfunction (including rectal bleeding), hematuria (if the bladder is involved), or other symptoms, depending on the site of implantation of the endometrium, which goes through cyclic menstrual proliferation and bleeding much as does endouterine tissue. Almost one-fifth of patients with endometriosis will have no symptoms at all.

INFECTIONS OF THE FEMALE GENITALIA

The label "pelvic inflammatory disease" has been used to the detriment of patients as a diagnostic term for pelvic pain of unknown etiology. Its use should be limited to the occurrence of pelvic peritonitis as a result of an infection involving the uterus, tubes, or ovaries, caused by pathogenic organisms (Fig. 16-16).

The clinical diagnosis of acute pelvic inflammatory disease has an accuracy of less than 75 percent. The remainder of the individuals with the commonly accepted clinical signs and symptoms of acute pelvic infection have either other surgical problems or no discernible pelvic abnormalities.

The increasing incidence of gonorrheal infection combined with recognition of asymptomatic male carriers of gonorrhea requires that physicians be knowledgeable of the symptomatology and clinical findings of pelvic infections in women.

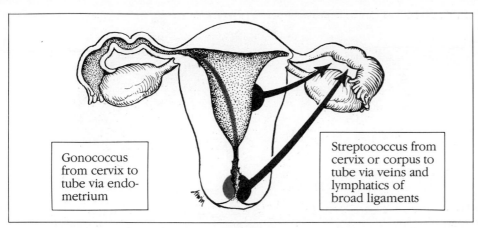

Gonococcus from cervix to tube via endo-metrium

Streptococcus from cervix or corpus to tube via veins and lymphatics of broad ligaments

FIGURE 16-16
Routes of pelvic infection.

Patients with pelvic peritonitis present with a complaint of lower abdominal pelvic pain that is associated with a fever ranging from 100°F to 104°F. They frequently date the onset of symptoms to immediately following the last menstrual period. Usually patients are without gastrointestinal complaints, and their appetites are usually not impaired.

Positive physical findings are limited to the lower abdomen and pelvis. On abdominal examination the lower abdomen and suprapubic areas are tender, with the suggestion or presence of rebound. Intestinal sounds are most commonly active. On pelvic examination there may or may not be a vaginal discharge. There is a history of a malodorous discharge before the last menstrual flow. Bimanual examination will demonstrate bilateral adnexal and uterine tenderness. This tenderness will be accompanied by guarding, and one frequently will be unable to delineate the adnexal structures clearly. Moderate-size ovarian or tubal masses may be missed. Rectal examination is mandatory because it allows demonstration of the presence of posterior pelvic masses characteristic of tubo-ovarian or pelvic abscesses.

Unfortunately the outlined physical findings may be the result of a variety of clinical entities. Such findings are observed in appendicitis associated with perforation, or an inflamed appendix that is adherent to pelvic viscera. Other gastrointestinal inflammatory states may also result in pelvic peritonitis. These include the uncommon Meckel's diverticulum and diverticulitis. Leaking ovarian cysts or twisting either of ovarian tumor or adnexa may result in similar complaints. Benign uterine tumors such as degenerating myomata can also cause similar physical findings.

The patient's history may be of assistance in suggesting an exposure to gonorrheal infection (Fig. 16-17). In such cases the collection of cervical cultures may demonstrate the gonococcus without difficulty, and the patient may respond rapidly to antibiotics such as penicillin. The duration of the clinical course is frequently related to the number of pelvic examinations, which should be minimized.

RECURRENT PELVIC INFECTION
The continued destruction of ovarian and tubal architecture as a result of recurrent

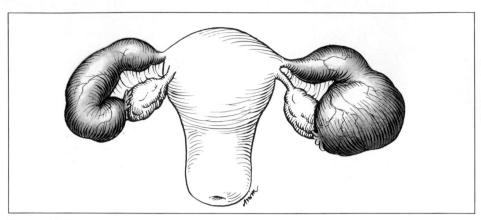

FIGURE 16-17
Chronic pelvic gonorrheal infection.

and inadequately treated infections may result in the evolution of tubo-ovarian abscesses or ovarian abscesses. The major problem with such abscesses is rupture with intraperitoneal leakage of their contents. This syndrome is associated with inordinate mortality if operative intervention is not prompt. Those patients who have intraperitoneal leakage develop progressive peritonitis with disappearance of intestinal function and development of ileus associated with nausea and vomiting. Their heightened temperature and tachycardia do not respond to antibiotic therapy. On pelvic examination, pelvic masses will be found in at least 50 percent of the cases. These patients often require immediate exploration and cannot be treated in a nonsurgical manner.

PREGNANCY

At the moment of child-birth, every woman has the same aura in isolation, as though she were abandoned, alone.

BORIS PASTERNAK
(1890–1960)

DIAGNOSIS OF PREGNANCY

The most prominent changes in the pelvis during early pregnancy revolve around the vascular congestion that takes place. The cervix softens and the uterus grows slightly larger and softer. Subsequently cyanosis of the upper vaginal tissues and of the cervix becomes prominent (Chadwick's sign).

The initial enlargement of the uterus is not usually symmetrical but is more pronounced on one horn, apparently the side of conception. Subsequently globularity of the uterus becomes evident, in contrast to the anteroposterior flattening normally present. A softened area 2 or 3 cm in diameter appears on the anterior wall (Ladin's sign).

There is also fullness and congestion of the breasts and increased prominence of the superficial veins.

DIAGNOSIS OF PREVIOUS PREGNANCY

The nipples and areolae retain the brown color acquired during pregnancy and do not resume the former pink color. The linea alba remains brown. The cervical os never resumes the round and symmetrical configuration but will be irregular and slightly enlarged. The perineum may show a loss of tone, or there may be scarring of the posterior fourchette (episiotomy).

EXAMINATION OF THE ABDOMEN DURING PREGNANCY

It is contrary to nature for children to come into the world with feet first.

PLINY THE ELDER
(23–79)

The initial prenatal visit calls for a complete examination and an estimation of the capacity of the pelvis. Subsequent examinations in the average case call only for a brief interval history and a limited examination. The patient's weight and blood pressure should be obtained, and the urine should be examined for albumin and sugar.

Abdominal examination should be performed on every visit. The height of the fundus of the uterus above the pubic bone should be measured to estimate continued and appropriate uterine growth. The uterus first rises above the symphysis pubis at about the third month. Thereafter, the number of centimeters divided by four equals the months of pregnancy. This rule is only approximate, but marked deviations from it suggest the possibility of twins or hydramnios if the measurement is great, or of fetal abnormality or death if the fundal height fails to increase.

Palpation of the fetus within the uterus usually begins about the fifth month with an attempt to locate the fetal head by grasping it above the pubic bone with the thumb and middle finger. If the pole of the fetus in this area gives the impression of being pointed rather than firm and rounded, the head should be sought in the fundus, with both hands placed flat on the abdomen and parallel to the uterine axis. The back of the fetus can also be located with the hands flat on either side and the fingers parallel to the uterus. The fetal small parts feel knobby and irregular in comparison with the back, on which the hand can be fitted flat.

SECTION VI

NEUROMUSCULAR SYSTEM

The main object of all science is the freedom and happiness of man.

THOMAS JEFFERSON
(1743–1826)

1. Patient sitting
   a. General inspection
   b. Cranial nerve testing (may be done as part of head examination
      —see Section III)

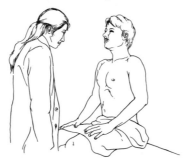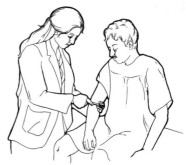

   c. Motor function upper extremities including reflexes
   d. Joint examination—neck and upper extremities
   e. Cerebellar testing (begin)

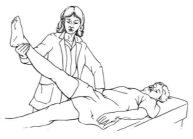

2. Patient recumbent
   a. Motor function lower extremities
   b. Joint examination—lower extremities
   c. Reflexes
   d. Sensory examination
   e. Cerebellar testing (finish)

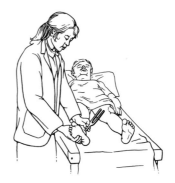

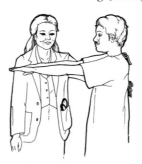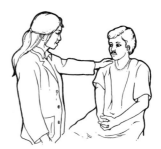

3. Patient standing—posture, station, gait, deformities, Romberg test
4. Patient sitting again—mental status, reflexes

MUSCULOSKELETAL SYSTEM

No muscle uses its power in pushing but always in drawing to itself the parts that are joined to it.

LEONARDO DA VINCI
(1452–1519)

Trauma, arthritis, degenerative change, congenital and acquired deformities, and general aches and pains are prevalent complaints in the American population. The increasing emphasis on sports and fitness have led to a burgeoning number of orthopedic injuries.

The musculoskeletal examination of an individual who has not been acutely injured differs greatly from the examination of an acutely injured patient. For example, the active and passive range of motion of the cervical spine should be determined when the patient shows symptoms of a nontraumatic disorder of the neck and upper extremity. However, this determination is not performed in an individual who has been acutely injured until the mechanical stability of the cervical spine has been demonstrated by roentgenogram. The importance of this distinction cannot be overemphasized.

The physical examination of an adult differs in some respects from the physical examination of a child and especially from that of an infant. The method detailed here is that used for the examination of an adult.

ANATOMY

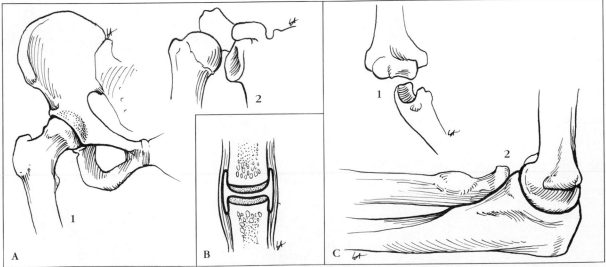

FIGURE 17-1
Types of joints. A. Ball-and-socket: hip (1), shoulder (2). B. Synovial. C. Hinge: elbow disarticulated (1), elbow articulated (2).

TABLE 17-1. Innervation of the Muscles of the Extremities

Upper Limb Muscles	Nerve	C2	C3	C4	C5	C6	C7	C8	T1
Sternocleidomastoid; trapezius	Spinal accessory	X	X	X					
Diaphragm	Phrenic		X	X	X				
Deltoid	Axillary				X				
Supraspinatus	Suprascapular				X				
Infraspinatus	Inferior scapular				X	X			
Teres minor	Axillary				X	X			
Subscapularis; teres major	Subscapular				X	X			
Serratus anterior	Long thoracic				X	X	X		
Rhomboideus	Dorsal scapular				X				
Clavicular pectoralis major	Anterior thoracic				X	X	X		
Biceps; brachialis	Musculocutaneous				X	X			
Brachioradialis	Radial				X	X			
Latissimus dorsi	Thoracodorsal					X	X	X	
Sternopectoralis major	Anterior thoracic					X	X	X	X
Flexor carpi radialis; pronator teres	Median					X			
Extensor carpi radialis, longus & brevis; extensor digitorum communis; extensor indicis proprius; extensor carpi ulnaris; extensor pollicis, longus & brevis; abductor pollicis longus; triceps	Radial					X	X	X	
Flexor digitorum sublimis	Median						X	X	X
Flexor digitorum profundis	Volar interosseous; ulnar							X	X
Flexor carpi ulnaris	Ulnar							X	
Pronator quadratus	Volar interosseous							X	X
Dorsal interosseous; volar interosseous	Ulnar							X	
Lumbricals; flexor pollicis brevis	Median; ulnar							X	X
Adductor pollicis brevis; opponens	Ulnar							X	X
Biceps tendon reflex	Musculocutaneous				X	X			
Extensor pollicis tendon reflex	Radial						X		
Triceps tendon reflex	Radial						X	X	

Lower Limb Muscles		Nerve	L1	L2	L3	L4	L5	S1	S2	S4	S5
Hip flexion	Iliopsoas; sartorius; rectus femoris; tensor fasciae latae	Lumbar plexus; femoral; superior gluteal; obturator		X	X	X	X	X			
Hip adduction	Adductor major; adductor brevis; adductor longus	Obturator		X	X	X					
Knee extension	Quadratus femoris	Femoral			X	X					
Hip abduction	Gluteus medias; gluteus minimus; tensor fascia femoris	Superior gluteal				X	X	X			
Foot inversion & dorsiflexion	Tibialis anterior	Peroneal				X	X				
Toe extension	Extensor digitorum, longus & brevis	Peroneal				X	X	X			
Great toe extension	Extensor hallucis, longus & brevis	Peroneal					X	X			
Foot eversion	Peroneus, longus & brevis	Peroneal					X	X			
Foot inversion & plantar flexion	Tibialis posterior	Tibial					X	X			
Toe flexion	Flexor digitorum, longus & brevis	Tibial					X	X			
Great toe flexion	Flexor hallucis longus	Tibial					X	X	X		
Hip extension	Gluteus maximus	Inferior gluteal					X	X	X		
Knee flexion	Biceps femoris; semimembranous; semitendinosis	Peroneal; tibial					X	X	X		
Foot plantar flexion	Gastrocnemius; soleus	Tibial						X	X		
	Cremasteric reflex	Genital-femoral	X								
	Patellar tendon reflex	Femoral			X	X					
	Achilles tendon reflex	Tibial						X	X		
	Anal reflex	Pudendal								X	

HISTORY

Some men ('gainst Raine) doe carry in their backs
Prognosticating Aching Almanacks;
Some by a painefull elbow, hip or knee
Will shrewdly guesse, what weather's like to be.

JOHN TAYLOR ("The Water Poet")
(1580–1653)

Pain, deformity, and **limitation of function** are the major symptoms of musculo-skeletal abnormality. Limitation of function in itself may be due to pain associated with movement, to bone or joint instability, or to the restriction of joint motion. The joint restriction in turn may be due to muscle weakness from neurologic disease or trauma, muscle contractures from previous injury or disease, bony fusion, or a mechanical block by bone fragments or torn cartilage within the joint.

Pain is a broad and significant symptom. It is important to note its characteristic location and relation to the patient's activity. The pain of bone erosion caused by tumor or aneurysm is usually described as deep, constant, and boring. It is apt to be more noticeable and more intense at night, and it may not be relieved by rest or position.

The pain of degenerative arthritis and muscle disorders is an aching type that is often accentuated by activity and lessened by rest. The discomfort may be increased by certain positions or motions. For instance, the pain resulting from degenerative changes in the cervical spine is often accentuated by maintaining the neck in extension. Subjective paresthesias that do not follow a dermatome distribution are often noted by the patient with degenerative changes involving the cervical or lumbar spine. These paresthesias are often described as a "sandy" feeling or as if the foot (or arm) were "going to sleep."

The pain of fracture and infection of bone is severe and throbbing and is increased by any motion of the part. Acute nerve compression causes a sharp, severe pain radiating along the distribution of the nerve. It is often associated with weakness of muscles supplied by the nerve and sensory changes over the area supplied by it.

Referred pain is that perceived by the patient in an anatomic location removed from the site of the lesion. Pain resulting from a disorder of the hip is often first noted by the patient in the anterior and lateral aspect of the thigh, or in the knee. Pain from a shoulder lesion may be felt at the insertion of the deltoid muscle on the lateral aspect of the proximal portion of humerus. Pain from the lower cervical spine is often referred to the interscapular region of the back, along the vertebral aspect of the scapula, or to the tips of the shoulders and lateral aspects of the arms.

PHYSICAL EXAMINATION

1. Inspect posture and gait. Look for obvious deformities and inflammation of joints, muscles, and bones.

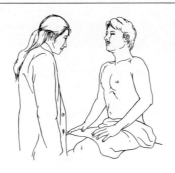

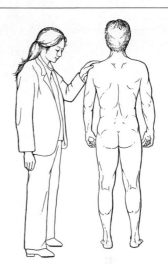

2. Inspect, palpate, and do range of motion* for the following:

   Cervical spine
   Thoracic spine
   Lumbar spine
   Shoulder
   Elbow
   Wrist
   Hand
   Hip
   Knee
   Ankle
   Foot

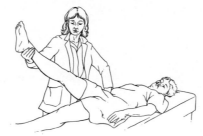

3. Inspect, palpate, and do strength testing of muscle groups as you follow the sequence of joint examination in (2).

   * Emphasis, of course, is on those joints to which history or gross inspection casts suspicion of disease.

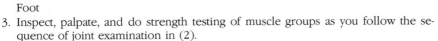

Science is the father of knowledge, but opinion breeds ignorance.

HIPPOCRATES
(460?–377? B.C.)

GENERAL

POSTURE AND GAIT

Begin the examination by observing posture and gait as the patient enters the examining area. Gait is divided into two broad phases—stance and swing. The stance phase includes heel-strike (as the heel strikes the ground), midstance (as the body weight is transferred from the heel to the ball of the foot), and push-off (as the heel leaves the ground). The swing phase includes acceleration, swing-through (as the foot travels ahead of the opposite foot), and deceleration (as the foot slows in preparation for heel-strike). Observe each phase and note any awkwardness or change in rhythm. For example, a patient with a painful callus on the ball of the foot will not bear weight normally on that part of the foot during midstance and push-off.

Abnormalities in gait may be caused by

1. Mechanical or structural abnormalities
2. Pain (antalgic gaits—Table 17-2)
3. Muscle disease
4. Neurologic disease
5. Psychiatric disease

TABLE 17-2. Some Causes of Antalgic Gait

Bone disease
  Fracture
  Infection (osteomyelitis)
  Tumor
  Avascular necrosis (if in childhood, often called by eponym)
    Femoral head (Perthes' disease, Legg-Calvé's disease)
    Tibial tubercle (Osgood-Schlatter's disease)
    Tarsal navicular (Köhler's disease)
Muscle disease
  Traumatic rupture, contusion
  Cramp secondary to fatigue, strain, malposition
  Inflammatory myositis
Vascular disease
  Claudication of arterial insufficiency
  Thrombophlebitis
Joint disease
  Traumatic arthritis
  Infectious arthritis
  Immune arthritis (rheumatoid, lupus, vasculitis of other sorts)
  Crystalline arthritis (gout, pseudogout)
  Hemarthrosis (hemophilia, scurvy)
  Bursitis
Neurologic disease
  Lumbar spine disease with nerve irritation or compression
  Pelvic masses involving sacral roots
Other
  Foot trauma (including blisters, ingrown toenails)
  Foreign bodies of the foot
  Corns, bunions

Look for gross deformities, areas of swelling, and areas of discoloration. The presence of ecchymoses suggests previous trauma. A red swollen area that is warm and tender to palpation suggests inflammation. If such an area is about a joint and is associated with fluid within the joint, acute synovitides such as rheumatoid arthritis, gouty arthritis, or infectious arthritis are suspected. If such an area is over the diaphyseal region of an extremity, infectious lesion of the underlying bone or soft tissues or noninfectious inflammatory lesion (e.g., thrombophlebitis) is suspected.

EXAMINATION OF A JOINT

Observe the joint and note any gross deformity and swelling. Swelling within a joint may represent either fluid or thickened synovial tissue. In the former, a fluid wave can be demonstrated; in the latter, the firm and somewhat boggy tissue can be palpated and no fluid wave is noted unless, of course, excessive fluid is also present. Palpate about the joint for masses and for points of tenderness that may indicate a torn ligament, an area of osteoarthritis or synovitis, or the torn attachment of a meniscus. Determine the active and passive range of motion of the joints, comparing those on opposite sides. Palpate the joint during active and passive motion to detect crepitation. Test the ligaments that help stabilize the joint and the muscles.

EXAMINATION OF A MUSCLE

. . . and at the same time as the sparks were obtained, there were produced wonderfully strong contractions in each muscle of the joints just as if an animal in tetanus had been used.

LUIGI GALVANI
(1737–1798)

In the examination of a muscle or a muscle group, ascertain the status of the muscle fibers as well as the nerves that supply them. Inspect the muscle for gross hypertro-

TABLE 17-3. Testing for Muscle Strength

100%	5	N	(normal)	Complete range of motion against gravity with full resistance
75	4	G	(good)	Complete range of motion against gravity with some resistance
50	3	F	(fair)	Complete range of motion against gravity
25	2	P	(poor)	Complete range of motion with gravity eliminated
10	1	T	(trace)	Evidence of slight contractility No joint motion
0	0	0	(zero)	No evidence of contractility

TABLE 17-4. Some Causes of Muscle Atrophy

Old age

Generalized wasting diseases
  Malignancy
  Tuberculosis or other chronic infections
  Starvation
  Thyrotoxicosis
  Diabetes mellitus
  Cushing's disease
  Addison's disease

Disuse atrophy (affects unused muscle mass locally)
  Fractured bone
  Casting or immobilization
  Painful or ankylosing joint disease
  Hysterical paralysis

Lower motor neuron lesions with flaccid paralysis
  Spine
    Disc disease
    Syringomyelia
    Cord tumor
    Poliomyelitis
    Amyotrophic lateral sclerosis
  Spinal root
    Disc disease
    Tumor entrapment
    Radiculitis due to meningitis
  Peripheral nerves
    Infective mononeuropathy or polyneuropathy
    Toxic mononeuropathy or polyneuropathy
    Vasculitic mononeuropathy or polyneuropathy
    Trauma

TABLE 17-5. Some Causes of Muscle Weakness (Myopathies)

Congenital
  Muscular dystrophies: limb-girdle,
    facioscapulohumeral, Duchenne,
    distal, myotonic, etc.
  Glycogen storage diseases: Pompe's,
    McArdle's, etc.
  Inherited spinal muscular atrophies,
    myositis ossificans
  Huntington's chorea
	Hypomagnesemia
	Hypoglycemia
	Myasthenia gravis
	Diabetes mellitus
	Cushing's disease
	Addison's disease
	Hyperparathyroidism
	Hyperaldosteronism
	Acromegaly
	Malnutrition

Infectious
  Virus: influenza
  Bacteria: tuberculosis, pyogens,
    syphilis, actinomycosis
  Parasite: trichinosis, toxoplasmosis,
    trypanosomiasis
	Vascular insufficiency
	Immune/idiopathic
	  Scleroderma
	  Systemic lupus erythematosus
	  Polyarteritis nodosa

Toxic
  Alcohol
  Heavy metals: mercury, lead, arsenic
  Corticosteroids
  Organophosphates
  Drugs: vincristine, Adriamycin, heroin,
    chloroquine, etc.
  Botulism
	Rheumatoid arthritis
	  Polymyalgia rheumatica
	  Sarcoidosis
	  Polymyositis/dermatomyositis
	Traumatic
	  Exercise
	  Injury
	  Seizure

Metabolic
  Hyperthyroidism
  Hypothyroidism
  Hypokalemia
  Hypophosphatemia
  Hypocalcemia
	Neoplastic
	  Carcinomatous myopathy
	  Eaton-Lambert syndrome
	  Carcinoid myopathy

phy or atrophy and for fasciculations, which are isolated contractions of a portion of the fibers. Look for areas of muscle spasm that can be easily palpated and often are accentuated as the joint they span is moved passively. Areas of muscle spasm are tender to palpation. Measure the circumference of an extremity at a given point above and below the patella or above and below the olecranon and compare this measurement with that of the opposite side. Test the strength of the muscle according to the criteria given in Table 17-3. Note the consistency of the muscle to palpation and the presence of tenderness over the muscle or its tendon. The spinal segments and the peripheral nerves that generally innervate major muscle groups of the extremities are listed in Table 17-1.

EXAMINATION OF A BONE

Observe the soft tissues covering a bone for obvious deformity, such as bowing, angulation, and tumor. Palpate the bone for areas of tenderness and for masses (Table 17-6). Tenderness of a bone suggests underlying tumor, inflammation, or the sequelae of trauma. This impression is strengthened when percussion of the bone at a site distant from the site of tenderness produces pain, not at the site of percussion but at the point of tenderness to palpation. Test the gross structural in-

TABLE 17-6. Some Causes of Bony Masses or Swelling

Trauma	Tumor
Heterotopic bone; myositis ossificans	Osteoma
Fracture callus	Chondroma
Fracture	Fibrocystic disease
Infection	Giant cell tumor
Osteomyelitis	Angioma/angiosarcoma
Tuberculosis	Osteogenic sarcoma
Syphilis	Periosteal fibrosarcoma
Typhoid periostitis	Ewing's sarcoma
Metabolic disease	Metastatic tumor to bone
Rickets	Myeloma
Scurvy	Neurofibroma
Acromegaly	
Paget's disease	

tegrity of a bone by noting its ability to resist a deforming force. Lack of resistance suggests a fracture or the result of a fracture (pseudoarthrosis).

SPECIFIC EXAMINATIONS

CERVICAL SPINE

In the cervical part of the spine evaluate the vertebrae, the articulations between them (the facet joints posteriorly and the intervertebral discs anteriorly), and the structures that are totally or partially contained within these bone structures (the spinal cord, the cervical nerve roots, and the vertebral artery).

Inspect the spine for gross deformities and visible muscle spasm. Among the possible deformities are absence of the normal cervical lordosis, or abnormal shortness of the neck, which may be associated with congenital malformation of the cervical vertebrae. Determine the active and passive range of motion of the cervical spine in flexion, extension, lateral bending, and rotation (Fig. 17-2). *Do not* perform this maneuver on patients with severe rheumatoid arthritis or those who have sustained recent neck injury, as serious damage to the spinal cord may result. Transient giddiness or even unconsciousness that is induced by a particular head or neck position suggests temporary occlusion of a vertebral artery within the neck. This diagnosis may be suspected on physical examination but must be confirmed by arteriography.

Palpate the tips of the spinous processes for general alignment and for points of tenderness. Palpate the cervical muscles—which include the posterior paraspinal muscle group, the trapezius muscle, the sternocleidomastoid muscle, and the scalene muscles—for tenderness and muscle spasm. Decreased motion of the cervical spine associated with points of tenderness to palpation over the spinous processes is commonly seen in tumors and infections of the cervical vertebrae, as well as in degenerative, prolapsed, and herniated cervical intervertebral discs. Palpate the cervical spine anteriorly, with the palpating finger passing medial to the carotid vessels and lateral to the trachea and esophagus. Tenderness is noted in the presence of disc lesions, infections, and certain tumors.

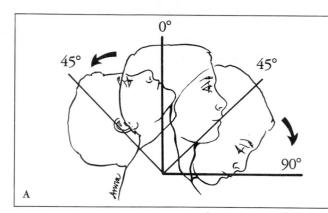

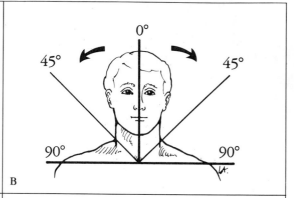

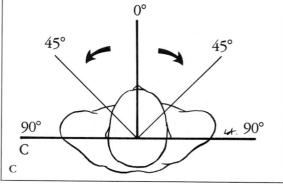

FIGURE 17-2
Passive range of motion of the cervical spine. A. Anteroposterior motion. B. Lateral motion. C. Rotation.

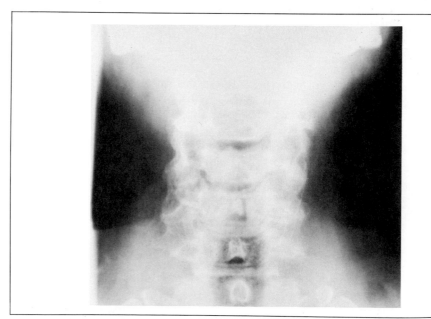

FIGURE 17-3
Roentgenogram showing osteoarthritis of the cervical spine.

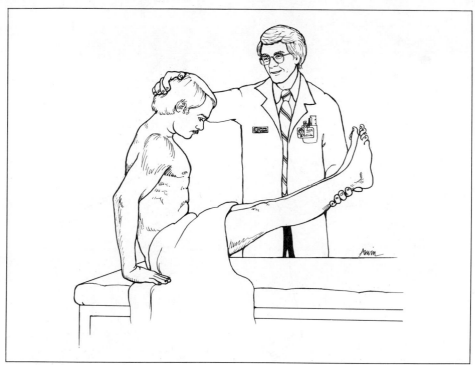

FIGURE 17-4
Lhermitte's sign.

Maintain the neck in extension by having the patient look at the ceiling for 60 seconds. This test will produce discomfort in the base of the neck, the interscapular region of the back, or the lateral aspect of the shoulders or arms when there are degenerative changes involving either the cervical intervertebral discs (anteriorly) or the facet joints (posteriorly). Vertically compress the extended cervical spine by pressing on the head. This will intensify discomfort in the same areas in the presence of degenerative, prolapsed, or herniated intervertebral discs.

Increase in the symptoms on vertical compression of the extended cervical spine with the head tilted to the side indicates degenerative changes in the facet joints or the uncovertebral articulations (so-called joints of Luschka). Test for *Lhermitte's sign,* with the patient sitting, by flexing the neck and the hips simultaneously with the knees in full extension (Fig. 17-4). Sharp pain that radiates down the spine and into the upper or lower extremities suggests irritation of the spinal dura either by tumor or by a protruded cervical disc.

Examine the *thoracic outlet* routinely as part of the examination of the cervical spine. Palpate the supraclavicular fossae for muscle spasm, vascular thrills, masses, and points of tenderness. Perform the *Adson maneuver* with the patient sitting with the forearms in supination and resting on the thighs (Fig. 17-5). Palpate the radial pulse on the side to be tested. Instruct the patient to extend the neck and turn the chin to the side to be tested. The transient disappearance of the radial pulse during inspiration signifies temporary occlusion of the subclavian artery as the anterior

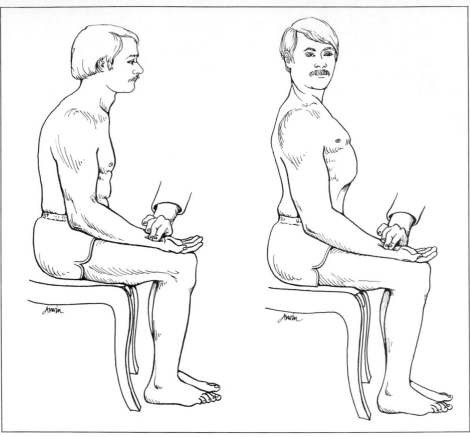

FIGURE 17-5
Adson maneuver.

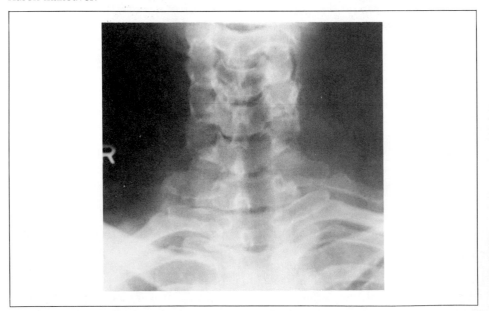

FIGURE 17-6
Roentgenogram showing cervical rib.

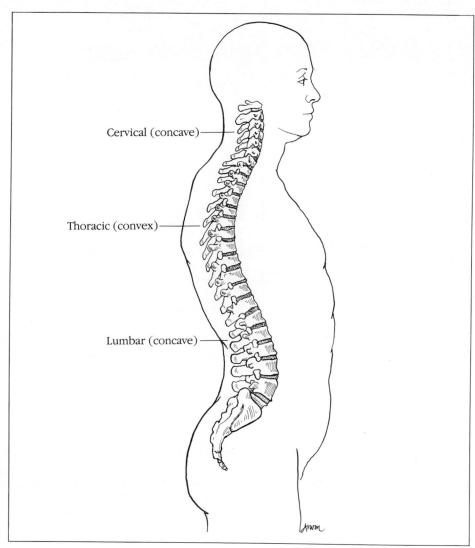

Cervical (concave)

Thoracic (convex)

Lumbar (concave)

FIGURE 17-7
Normal spinal contours.

scalene muscle is tensed (by extension of the neck and rotation of the skull) while the "floor" of the thoracic outlet rises during inspiration. This may be due to the presence of a cervical rib, for example (Fig. 17-6). Compression of the brachial plexus in the supraclavicular fossa is suggested by intensification of pain and paresthesia in the arm as the Adson maneuver is performed, by tenderness to palpation over the brachial plexus, and by neurologic changes in arm and hand (particularly a decrease in the ability to appreciate light touch over the fourth and fifth fingers of the hand). These signs may be intensified as the shoulder is abducted and externally rotated. Measure the circumference of the upper arm and forearm and compare the measurements with those of the opposite arm. Test muscle strength, sensory modalities, and deep tendon reflexes in the upper extremity.

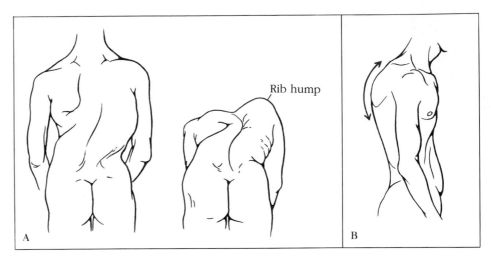

FIGURE 17-8
Deformities of the thoracic spine. A. Scoliosis. B. Kyphosis.

THORACIC SPINE

Palpate the tips of the spinous processes for general alignment and points of tenderness. Test the motion of the thoracic spine during flexion, extension, and lateral bending and observe the symmetry of the ribs. Small rotational deformities of the thoracic spine that produce asymmetry of the rib cage are best appreciated by inspecting the flexed thoracic spine and rib cage from the rear (Fig. 17-8).

LUMBAR SPINE

Note the contour of the lumbar spine with the patient standing. A lumbar lordosis is normally present; its absence suggests a spinal abnormality. Palpate the paraspinal muscles for tenderness and spasm; palpate the tips of the spinous processes, noting their general alignment and any points of tenderness that may be present. Carefully differentiate spinal tenderness from flank tenderness, which would indicate an abnormality in the retroperitoneal space. When a spondylolisthesis is present, anterior displacement of the superior spinal segment produces a "step" deformity in which the spinous processes of the superior (cephalad) segment can be palpated anterior to those of the inferior (caudal) segment. Test the range of lumbar motion in flexion, extension, lateral bending and rotation (Fig. 17-9). Limitation of flexion exerted by tightness of the hamstring muscles in the posterior aspect of the thigh is

TABLE 17-7. Signs of Disc Disease of the Lumbar Spine

Diminished or obliterated lumbar lordosis
Decreased flexion of spine
Painful extension of spine
Asymmetrical limitation in straight-leg raising
Percussion tenderness over affected disc
Atrophic change in muscle mass of affected leg (occasionally seen)
Neurologic defect of lower extremity, depending on level of the lesion

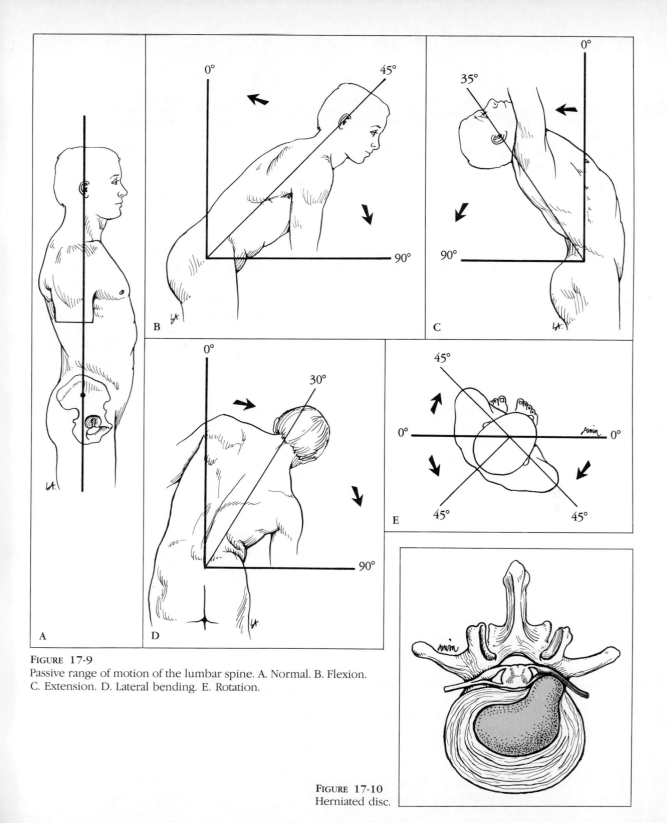

FIGURE 17-9
Passive range of motion of the lumbar spine. A. Normal. B. Flexion.
C. Extension. D. Lateral bending. E. Rotation.

FIGURE 17-10
Herniated disc.

TABLE 17-8. Localization of Ruptured Disc of the Lumbar Spine

Disc	Pain	Paresthesias	Weakness	Atrophy	Reflexes
L_3–L_4 (3–5%)	Anterior thigh	Anteromedian thigh	Quadriceps	Thigh	Decreased or absent knee jerk
L_4–L_5 (45%)	Posterior thigh, calf, top of foot	Medial dorsal foot, great toe	Anterior tibialis, dorsiflexors, toes	Lower leg	Normal or slightly increased knee jerk, slightly decreased ankle jerk
L_5–S_1 (50%)	Posterior thigh, calf, ankle	Lateral dorsal foot, small toe	Calf, plantar flexors, toes	Calf	Decreased or absent ankle jerk

associated with spondylolisthesis and less commonly with tumors, arachnoiditis, and herniated intervertebral discs in the lumbar and lower thoracic regions (Fig. 17-10).

Perform the straight-leg-raising test with the patient lying supine on the examining table. Flex the hip with the knee in full extension by raising the foot (Fig. 17-11). A sharp pain traveling from the lower back or buttock down the posterior aspect of the leg indicates irritation of the sciatic nerve or its roots of origin within the spine (Table 17-9). In the absence of such irritation, this maneuver may be limited by muscle tightness at the back of the thigh but not by sharp pain.

As part of the complete physical evaluation you will, of course, perform a rectal examination, a brief evaluation of the urinary tract, an examination of the abdomen, and an evaluation of the femoral pulses. Prostatic disease in men, pelvic abnormalities in women, and diseases of the kidneys and ureters may produce discomfort in the lower back. Occlusion of the distal aorta or of the hypogastric arteries, as well as an abdominal aortic aneurysm, may produce pain in the lower back or in the buttocks.

Tenderness to palpation over the lumbar spinous processes associated with limited motion of the spine may indicate disc lesions, osteoarthritis, spondylolisthesis, tumor, or infection. Laxity of the sacroiliac joints may be detected by palpation while the patient, standing erect, lifts first one knee and then the other ("marching in place"). A click can be felt if subluxation of the sacroiliac joint occurs. With the patient supine, stress the articulation between the fifth lumbar vertebra and the sacrum by acutely flexing the patient's hips and knees. Resultant pain in the lower back suggests a mechanical abnormality at the lumbosacral articulation. Tilting the pelvis in this position by rocking the knees to the left and right causes pain when abnormalities of the sacroiliac joint are present.

Measure the leg length from the anterosuperior spine to the medial malleolus. Measure the circumference of the thigh and calf and compare the measurements with those of the opposite leg. Test muscle power of the dorsiflexors and plantar flexors of the foot and ankle by having the patient support the body weight on the toes and on the heels. Test deep tendon reflexes at the knee and ankle and the sensory modalities of light touch, pain, and position sense.

SHOULDER

Inspect the shoulder anteriorly and posteriorly and look for loss of normal contour and muscle atrophy. Three major muscles are easily visible about the shoulder: (1)

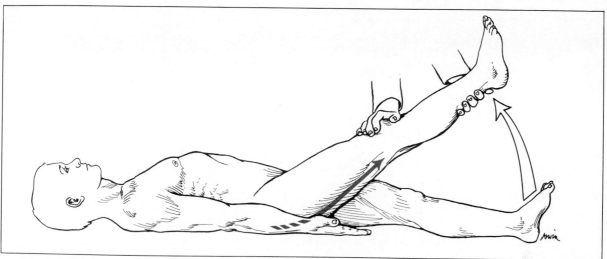

FIGURE 17-11
Straight-leg-raising test.

TABLE 17-9. Some Causes of Sciatica

Nerve root compression	**Inflammatory disease of the nerve**
In the spinal cord	Toxins
Protruded disc	Alcohol
Tumor	Heavy metals
Abscess	Diabetes mellitus
In the intervertebral foramen	Syphilis
Arthritis of the spine	**Direct trauma to the nerve**
Vertebral collapse	
Tumor of the nerve in the foramen	
Extruded disc	
Inflammatory synovitis of the facet joint	
(Marie-Strümpell arthritis)	
In the pelvis or buttocks	
Intrapelvic tumor	
Intrapelvic or gluteal abscess	

deltoid (which covers the shoulder anteriorly, laterally, and posteriorly), (2) supraspinatus, and (3) infraspinatus, the last two of which originate on the posterior border of the scapula above and below the scapular spine. Visible atrophy of the deltoid muscle follows disuse, injury to the axillary nerve, and diseases of the nervous system, such as poliomyelitis. Visible atrophy of the supraspinatus and infraspinatus muscles is seen following nerve injury, diseases of the nervous system, tears of the insertion of these muscles into the rotator cuff of the shoulder, and calcific tendinitis involving that portion of the rotator cuff that represents their insertion. Determine function of the anterior serratus muscle by having the patient push with both hands against a wall. The medial border of the scapula is not held firmly against the chest wall but is displaced posteriorly ("wings") when weakness of the anterior

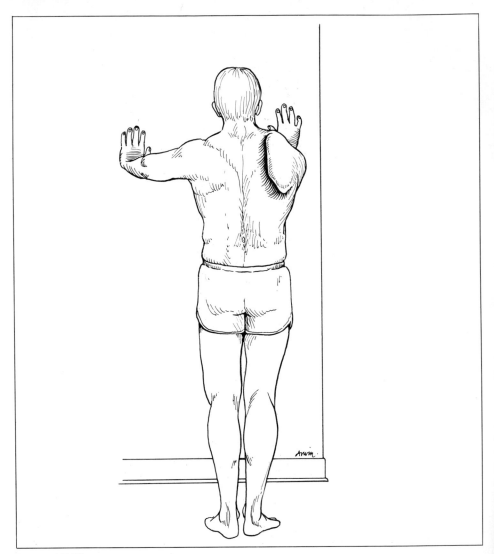

FIGURE 17-12
Winging of the scapula in injury of the nerve to the anterior serratus muscle.

serratus muscle is present (Fig. 17-12). Weakness of this muscle frequently follows injury to the long thoracic nerve of Bell either in the neck or in the axilla.

Note the bony contour of the shoulder and the position of the humeral head. Flattening of the lateral portion of the shoulder is seen when the humeral head is not in its proper position but is displaced, as in a subcoracoid dislocation of the shoulder. Prominence of the distal end of the clavicle indicates a dislocation of the acromioclavicular joint or a tumor of the distal end of the clavicle.

Carefully palpate the structures about the shoulder, particularly the rotator cuff, for points of tenderness. The rotator cuff of the shoulder represents the insertion of the subscapularis, supraspinatus, infraspinatus, and teres minor muscles into the proximal humerus. Tenderness to palpation of a segment of the rotator cuff indi-

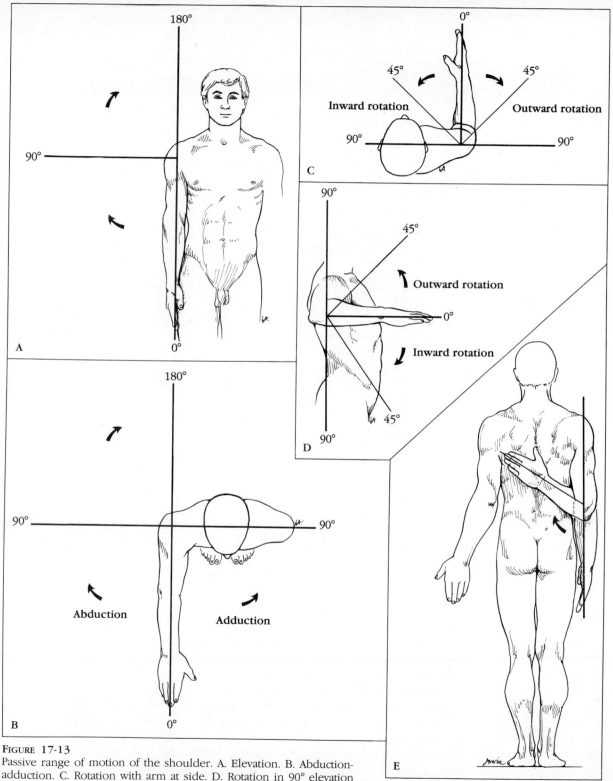

FIGURE 17-13
Passive range of motion of the shoulder. A. Elevation. B. Abduction-adduction. C. Rotation with arm at side. D. Rotation in 90° elevation and 90° abduction. E. Internal rotation posteriorly.

TABLE 17-10. Some Causes of Shoulder Pain

Originating in the shoulder
  Trauma
  Arthritis
  Bursitis
  Myositis
  Neuritis (brachial plexus)
  Tendinitis (calcific tendinitis)
Originating outside the shoulder (referred pain)
  Cardiac ischemia or infarction
  Pleuritis
  Lung tumor
  Pneumothorax
  Gastric or duodenal disease
  Gallbladder or liver disease
  Pancreatic disease
  Subdiaphragmatic irritation (fluid, pus)
  Neurologic disease of cervical spine

cates a rotator cuff tear or calcific tendinitis. Diffuse tenderness over the entire cuff suggests pericapsulitis (frozen shoulder) or synovitis of the joint. Tenderness over the long head of the biceps tendon as it lies in the bicipital groove between the greater and lesser tuberosities of the humerus suggests tendinitis of the biceps tendon. This diagnosis is further suggested if shoulder pain is accentuated when the forearm is flexed and supinated against resistance.

Determine active and passive motion of the shoulder and compare with the opposite side (Fig. 17-13). If passive motion of the shoulder is normal but active motion is limited, a tear of the rotator cuff or muscle weakness about the shoulder should be suspected. If active and passive motion are both limited to an equal degree, contractures, arthritis, or a mechanical block (such as calcific tendinitis) should be suspected. Determine sensation over the lateral portion of the shoulder, which is supplied by the axillary nerve.

Before putting through vigorous maneuvers the patient who gives shoulder pain as a major complaint, ascertain by careful history and physical examination of other systems that the shoulder pain is not referred from the heart or abdomen (see Table 17-10).

ELBOW

Note the contour and the carrying angle of the elbow. The carrying angle is the angle formed by the upper and lower arm when the elbow is observed from the front with the forearm in full extension and supination (Fig. 17-14). Change in this angle may be seen following damage to the elbow from trauma, rheumatoid arthritis, or osteoarthritis. Determine the relationship between the olecranon and the medial lateral epicondyles, which form a triangle. Note points of tenderness and the presence of palpable effusion of synovitis within the joint. Palpate the head of the radius and the tissue just anterior to it for points of tenderness as the forearm is supinated and pronated.

Tenderness lateral or anterior to the radial head may indicate lateral epicondylitis ("tennis elbow") and may be accentuated as the patient pronates the forearm

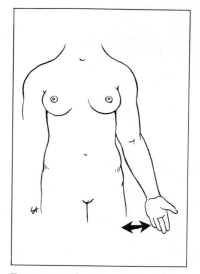

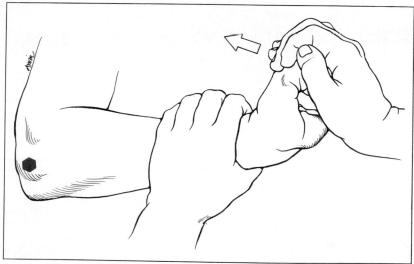

FIGURE 17-14
Normal carrying angle of the elbow.

FIGURE 17-15
Cozen's test. Dorsiflexion of the wrist against resistance causes pain in the area of the lateral epicondyle in epicondylitis (tennis elbow).

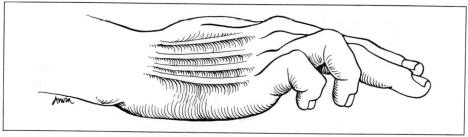

FIGURE 17-16
Position of fourth and fifth fingers and atrophy of hand muscles in ulnar nerve palsy.

and extends the wrist against resistance (Fig. 17-15). Palpate the ulnar nerve in the groove in the posterior aspect of the medial condyle of the humerus. Localized tenderness over the ulnar nerve at this spot suggests irritation of the nerve, which frequently follows fractures about the elbow. It may be associated with pain and paresthesia in the fourth and fifth fingers and weakness of those muscles in the hand supplied by the ulnar nerve (adductor pollicis, third and fourth lumbricales, and interossei) (Fig. 17-16). Test the active and passive ranges of motion of the elbow in flexion, extension, supination, and pronation and compare with the opposite side (Fig. 17-17). Palpate the subcutaneous surfaces of the proximal ulna for nodules that are often found with rheumatoid arthritis, even when rheumatoid involvement of the elbow is not present (Fig. 17-18).

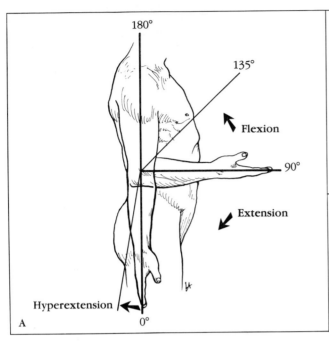

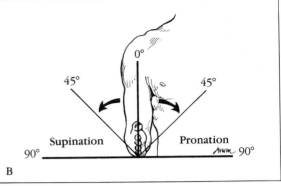

FIGURE 17-17
Passive range of motion of the elbow. A. Flexion and extension. B. Forearm (elbow and wrist).

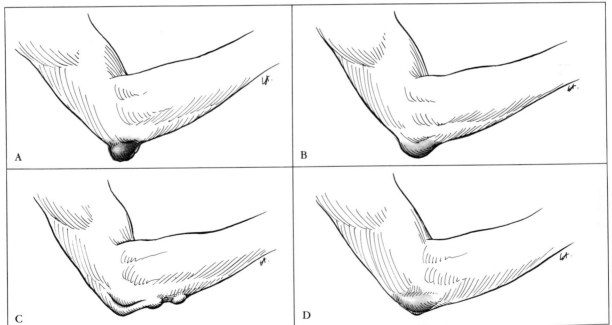

FIGURE 17-18
Some lesions of the elbow. A. Gouty tophus is deposited over the olecranon. Elbow may be inflamed, tender, and firm to palpation and may drain chalky material. B. Bursa may be inflamed or swollen or both. Bursitis may be caused by trauma, infection (staphylococcus), or rheumatoid arthritis. Elbow is tender and boggy. C. Rheumatoid nodules are firm, nontender nodules at pressure points on the ulna. D. The arthritic elbow has fluid or boggy synovium in the groove between the epicondyle and olecranon. Elbow is inflamed, tender, and swollen.

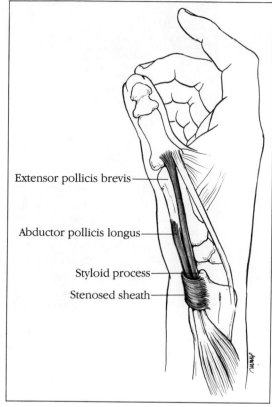

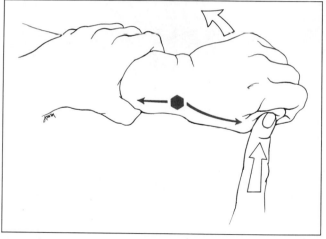

FIGURE 17-20
Finkelstein's test. The patient makes a fist enclosing the thumb. Pressure on the fist into ulnar deviation induces pain in the radial styloid process that may radiate to the thumb or toward the elbow.

FIGURE 17-19
De Quervain's disease. This condition occurs only in adults, generally women. In chronic circumstances a small swelling may be felt just proximal to the styloid process. Fine crepitus may also be present.

WRIST

Observe the contour of the wrist and note any fullness about the joint. Palpate the bony and tendinous structures about the wrist for tenderness and nodularity. Tenderness over the anatomic snuffbox in the lateral aspect of the wrist may be associated with abnormality of the navicular or greater multangular bones. Tenderness over the lateral aspect of the distal radius suggests inflammation of the tendon sheaths of the extensor pollicis brevis and the abductor pollicis longus, *de Quervain's disease* (Fig. 17-19). The diagnosis is confirmed when a tender nodule can be felt within one or both of the tendons over the lateral aspect of the distal radius and when a positive Finkelstein's test is noted. Perform *Finkelstein's test* (Fig. 17-20) by moving the wrist rapidly into ulnar deviation as the patient holds the thumb flexed in the palm. The test result is positive if it induces sudden pain that extends to the thumb or toward the elbow.

Compression of the median nerve at the wrist causes tenderness over the nerve, loss of normal sensation in the portion of the hand supplied by this nerve—the flexor surfaces of the thumb, the index and middle fingers, and the lateral half of the ring finger—and weakness of those muscles of the thumb supplied by the me-

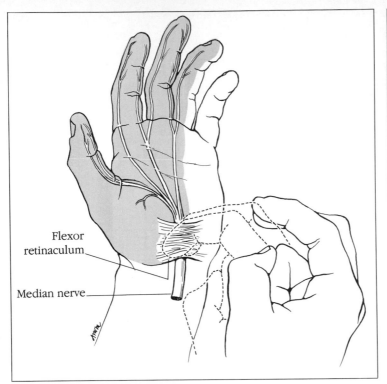

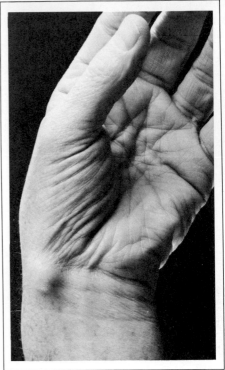

FIGURE 17-21
Tinel's sign. Strike the median nerve in the wrist as it passes through the carpal tunnel. A tingling sensation radiating from the wrist to the hand is a positive indication.

FIGURE 17-22
Ganglion of the wrist.

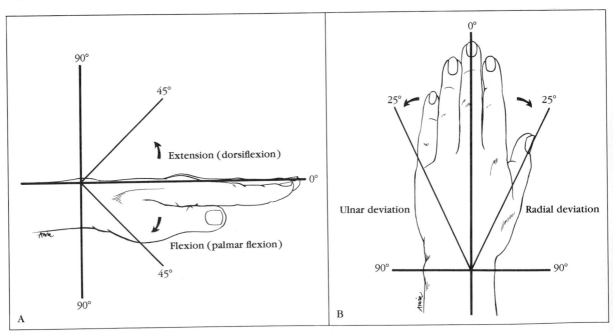

FIGURE 17-23
Passive range of motion of the wrist. A. Flexion and extension. B. Lateral deviation.

TABLE 17-11. Some Causes of the Carpal Tunnel Syndrome

Idiopathic
Synovitis of the wrist or flexor tendons
Ganglion of the wrist
Acromegaly
Hypothyroidism
Pregnancy
Fracture about the wrist

dian nerve, i.e., carpal tunnel syndrome (some causes of which are presented in Table 17-11). In addition, percussion over the median nerve at the wrist will produce pain or tingling radiating distally into the hand—a positive *Tinel's sign* (Fig. 17-21).

A *ganglion* is the result of myxomatous degeneration of a portion of connective tissue in a joint capsule. The cystlike swelling may occur on ankle, foot, or finger, but is more common on the wrist (Fig. 17-22). The swelling is not inflamed but may be slightly tender.

The wrist may also be the site of arthritis (rheumatoid, infective, gouty) and trauma.

HAND

Inspect the hand for deformities. Test active and passive ranges of motion of the fingers for evidence of nerve injury, tendon rupture, muscle fibrosis, joint contracture, or arthritis. Test the function of each muscle to the fingers and wrist. The pres-

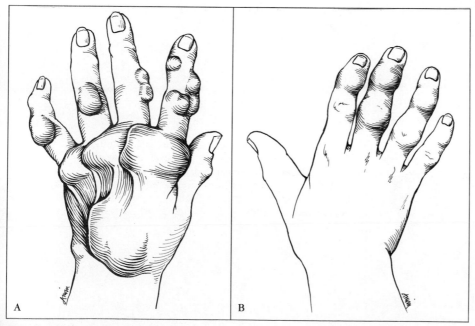

FIGURE 17-24
A. Rheumatoid arthritis. B. Osteoarthritis.

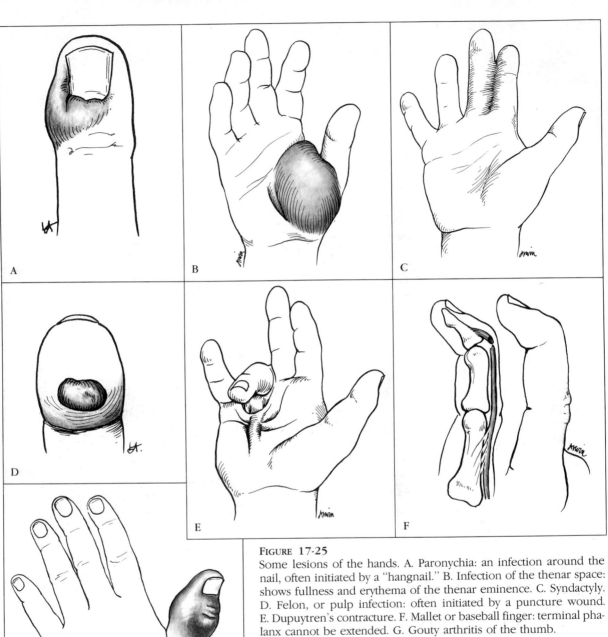

FIGURE 17-25

Some lesions of the hands. A. Paronychia: an infection around the nail, often initiated by a "hangnail." B. Infection of the thenar space: shows fullness and erythema of the thenar eminence. C. Syndactyly. D. Felon, or pulp infection: often initiated by a puncture wound. E. Dupuytren's contracture. F. Mallet or baseball finger: terminal phalanx cannot be extended. G. Gouty arthritis of the thumb.

TABLE 17-12. Some Differential Diagnostic Aids to Distinguish Rheumatoid from Degenerative Arthritis

Features	Rheumatoid Arthritis	Osteoarthritis
Age at onset	Younger, but may occur at any age	Older (40+ years)
Onset	May be explosive or gradual	Generally insidious
Systemic symptoms (fever, malaise)	Present	Absent
Joint involvement	Often symmetrical, progressive	Localized, affects the most active joints
Inflammation	Common	Less common
Effusion	Common	Uncommon
Subcutaneous nodules	May be present	Absent
Activity	Increases pain in active joint	Ameliorates pain in active joint
Extra-articular involvement	May be present	Absent
Sedimentation rate	Increased	Often normal
X-ray changes	Erosion	Hypertrophy

ence of nodules within the palm, associated with firm fibrous bands that limit extension of the fingers suggests *Dupuytren's contracture.* A palpable nodule within a flexor tendon overlying a metacarpophalangeal joint, associated with a palpable click as the finger is flexed or extended, suggests a *trigger finger* in which a nodular enlargement of a flexor tendon snaps into or out of the fibrous tunnel through which it passes.

Nodules along the distal interphalangeal joints (*Heberden's nodes*) occur in degenerative osteoarthritis. These nodules must be distinguished from the *tophi* of chronic gout. Carpal, proximal, and middle interphalangeal joint deformity, swelling, and erythema—all of which symmetrically involve both hands—are characteristic of rheumatoid arthritis (Table 17-12 and Fig. 17-24). Figure 17-25 illustrates some common lesions of the hand.

HIP

Examination of the hip begins with the initial evaluation of the patient's gait. Leg-length inequality, muscle weakness, habit patterns, fusion, contractures, and pain-producing lesions of the hip, knee, ankle, and foot all may produce abnormalities of gait. Fairly specific for abnormality of the hip, however, is the *Trendelenburg gait,* which is marked by a fall of the pelvis, rather than the normal rise, on the side opposite the involved hip when it is weight bearing (Fig. 17-26). This indicates weakness of the abductor muscles due to intrinsic muscle disease, lack of normal innervation of the muscle, or an unstable hip joint. In the antalgic ("antipain") gait of hip disease, the patient attempts to minimize the force borne through the hip by leaning over the involved hip as weight is borne through it. This moves the body's center of gravity toward the hip joint, decreasing the force exerted on the hip and thus decreasing the discomfort.

Palpate the hip anteriorly for points of tenderness and fullness within the joint. The location of the femoral head is approximately 1 inch distal and 1 inch lateral to

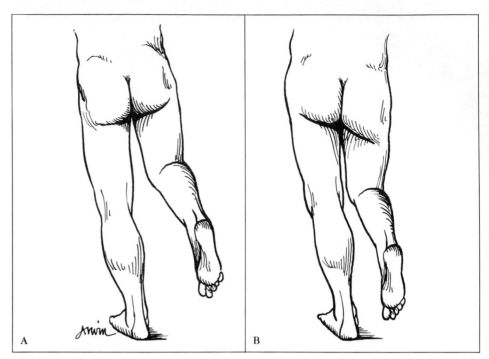

FIGURE 17-26
Trendelenburg's sign. A. Normal. The right side of the pelvis rises when weight is borne on the left leg. B. Positive Trendelenburg's sign of the left hip. The right side of the pelvis falls when weight is borne on the left leg.

the point at which the femoral artery crosses the inguinal ligament. In addition, palpate the greater trochanter laterally and the ischial tuberosity posteriorly. Inflamed bursae in either of these locations may account for pain in the hip region. Although more than 18 bursae have been described about the hip, only four of these are commonly clinically affected. When the iliopectineal bursa is inflamed, tenderness may be present over the anterior hip at about the midpoint of the inguinal ligament. Pain will occur on extension, internal rotation, or adduction of the hip and may radiate down the front of the leg.

Patients with ischiogluteal bursitis have great tenderness over the ischial tuberosity. It develops in those whose jobs require long periods of sitting on hard surfaces (*weaver's bottom*).

Deep trochanteric bursitis may present as pain on any movement of the hip, radiating down the back of the thigh. There is tenderness over the greater trochanter.

Superficial trochanteric bursitis presents as pain and swelling over the bursa, without pain on motion of the hip. Test the range of motion of the hip in flexion, extension, abduction, adduction, and rotation (Fig. 17-27). Test for flexion contracture of the hip by maximally flexing the opposite hip with the patient supine on the examining table. In this maneuver the pelvis is flexed on the lumbar spine, and any lumbar lordosis present is eliminated (Fig. 17-28). If a flexion contracture is present, the involved thigh will flex. The angle that the involved thigh forms with the

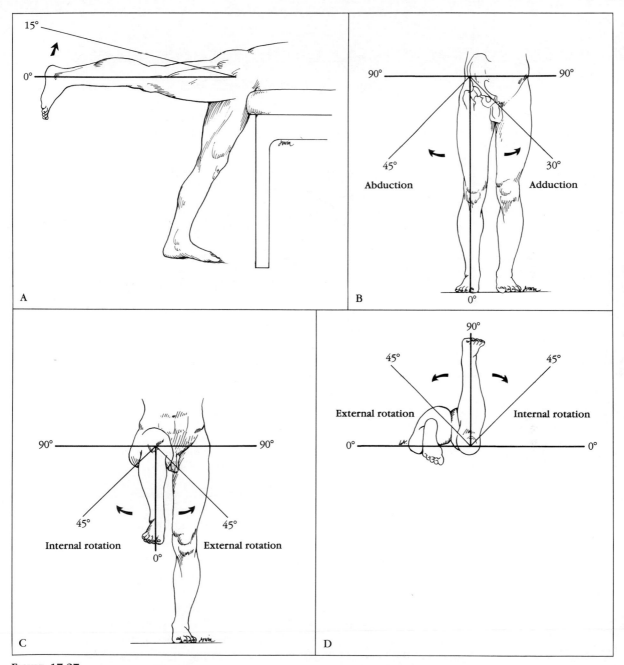

FIGURE 17-27
Passive range of motion of the hip. A. Extension. B. Lateral motion. C. Rotation in flexion.
D. Rotation in extension (prone).

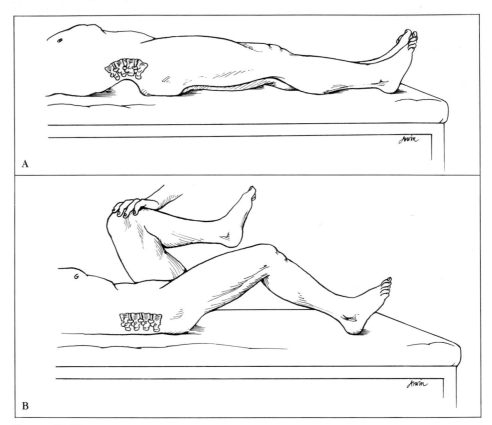

FIGURE 17-28
Thomas test. A. With the patient supine a flexion contracture of the hip may be masked by lordosis of the lumbar spine. B. When the lumbar lordosis is eliminated by maximally flexing the left hip, the angle that the right thigh makes with the examining table designates the degree of flexion contracture in the right hip.

surface of the examining table indicates the degree of contracture (Thomas test). Determine the strength of the flexor, extensor, abductor, and adductor muscle groups by having the patient move the thigh against the resistance of the examiner's hand.

KNEE

Inspect the knee for joint swelling and gross deformity, and the thigh for atrophy of the quadriceps muscle group, which may indicate a significant knee abnormality.

Test for excessive fluid within the knee joint by pressing the patella against the femur with the knee in full extension and gently tapping one side of the joint while feeling for a fluid wave on the other side of the joint. In addition, note whether ballottement of the patella is possible (Fig. 17-29). Palpate about the joint line, about the circumference of the patella, over the attachments of the medial and lateral collateral ligaments, over the anserine bursa (on the medial posterior aspect of the proximal tibia about 1 inch distal to the joint line), and in the popliteal fossa. When tenderness is noted over the medial or lateral joint line, a torn meniscus is

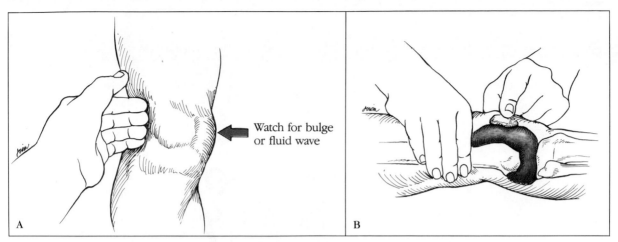

FIGURE 17-29
Testing for fluid in the knee joint. A. The bulge sign. B. The patellar tap will suggest fluid in the knee as the patella clicks against the femur. With greater amounts of knee fluid, the patella will be ballotable.

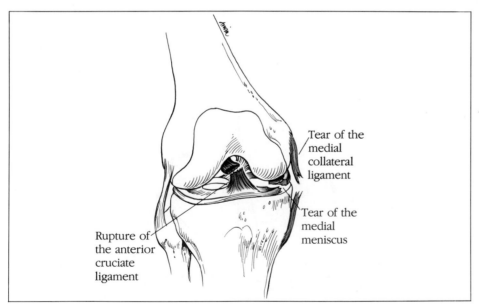

FIGURE 17-30
Three common severe injuries of the knee.

suspected (Fig. 17-30). Tenderness about the patella suggests osteoarthritis or chondromalacia. The diagnosis is confirmed if crepitation and pain are elicited when the patella is moved medially, laterally, proximally, and distally while it is firmly pressed against the underlying femur. Tenderness over the medial or lateral collateral ligament suggests a tear of the ligament or an inflamed bursa between the ligament and the bone. Tenderness over the prepatellar bursa or in the popliteal fossa suggests symptomatic bursitis in these regions (Fig. 17-31).

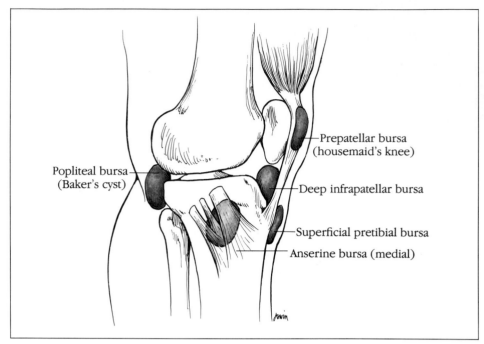

FIGURE 17-31
Common sites of bursitis in the knee.

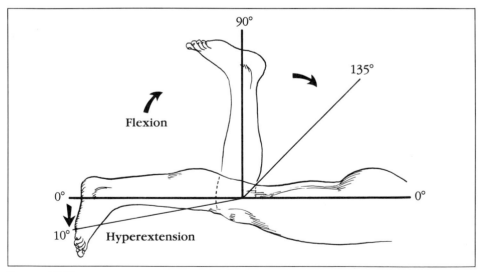

FIGURE 17-32
Passive range of motion of the knee.

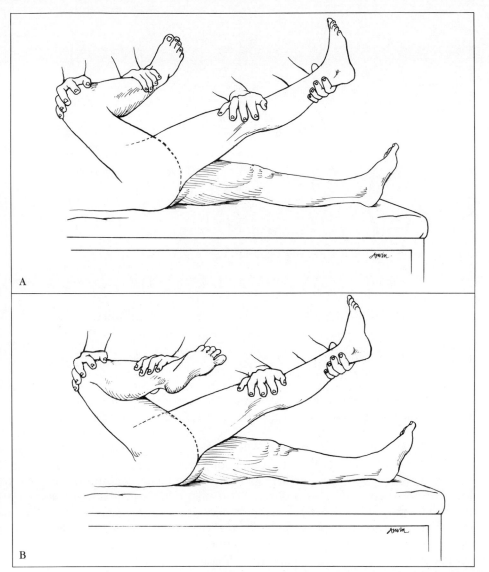

FIGURE 17-33
McMurray maneuver. A. Extension in internal rotation. A palpable or audible snap suggests a lesion in the lateral meniscus. B. Extension in external rotation. A palpable or audible snap suggests a lesion in the medial meniscus.

Determine the range of motion and compare with the opposite side. Full extension and at least 120 degrees of flexion from full extension are normally present (Fig. 17-32). Palpable crepitation within the knee joint during flexion and extension suggests a mechanical incongruity of the joint that may be the result of arthritic changes, a tear of the medial or lateral meniscus, or a loose fragment of cartilage or bone within the joint. Locking of the joint during flexion or extension definitely

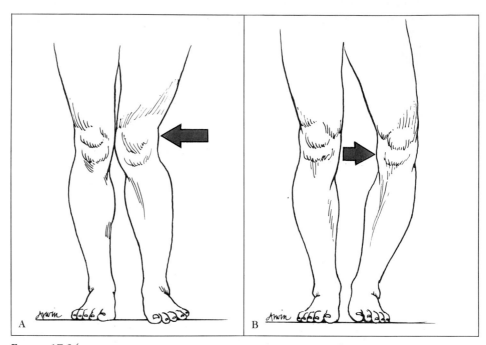

FIGURE 17-34
Forced valgus and varus. A. Forced valgus suggests instability of the medial collateral ligament. B. Forced varus suggests instability of the lateral collateral ligament.

signifies a mechanical block within the joint, most commonly a torn meniscus or a bone fragment. A mechanical block preventing full extension, or a contracture of the posterior capsule, is suggested when the knee cannot be fully extended passively. Test for a positive spring sign, which indicates a mechanical block with the consistency of cartilage, by maximally extending the knee passively and then forcibly extending the knee further. The joint will extend and then quickly snap back into flexion when the sign is positive. A torn meniscus is further suggested by a positive McMurray sign. To perform the *McMurray maneuver* (Fig. 17-33), flex the knee fully with the patient recumbent, steadying the knee with one hand, and slowly extend the knee while holding the tibia in internal rotation. A palpable or audible snap associated with momentary discomfort as the knee is extended suggests a tear in that portion of the lateral meniscus that was between the femoral condyle and the tibial plateau when the snap occurred. This test is repeated with the tibia held in external rotation, which tests the posterior aspect of the medial meniscus. This test is generally not positive when the tear involves the anterior one-third of either meniscus.

Test the integrity of the medial collateral ligament by attempting to force the knee into valgus (knock-knee) deformity with the knee in full extension. If more than 5 to 10 degrees of deformity can be produced, instability of the medial collateral ligament is suspected. Test the lateral collateral ligament by attempting to force the knee into varus (bowleg) deformity with the knee in full extension (Fig. 17-34). Again, if more than 5 to 10 degrees of deformity can be produced, instability of the

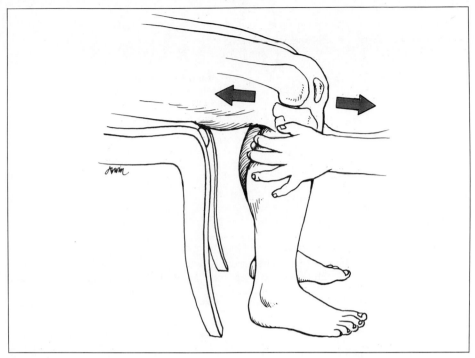

FIGURE 17-35
Drawer sign.

ligament is suspected. Test the cruciate ligaments with the patient sitting with the knees flexed to 90 degrees. If the tibia can be pulled anteriorly from under the femur (a positive drawer sign), laxity of the anterior cruciate ligament is present (Fig. 17-35). If the tibia can be pushed posteriorly under the femur, laxity of the posterior cruciate ligament is present.

ANKLE
Inspect the ankle for gross deformity or swelling and palpate for points of tenderness or fullness within the joint. Tenderness over the medial or lateral malleolus suggests previous injury to these bony structures. Tenderness distal to the tip of the medial or lateral malleoli but over the medial or lateral ligaments of the ankle suggests previous injury to these ligaments. Tenderness just anterior to the Achilles tendon at its insertion into the calcaneus suggests an inflamed bursa, often noted in patients with rheumatoid arthritis. Tenderness over the posterior tibial tendon as it lies just posterior to the medial malleolus or tenderness over the peroneal tendons just behind the lateral malleolus suggests inflammation of these structures. Occasionally tenovaginitis of the posterior tibial tendon or the peroneal tendons, similar to de Quervain's disease of the wrist, is seen. In such cases tenderness is present over the tendon at the point of the constriction posterior to the malleolus. Passive motion of the foot will intensify the discomfort, and a palpable nodule may be present within the tendon itself.

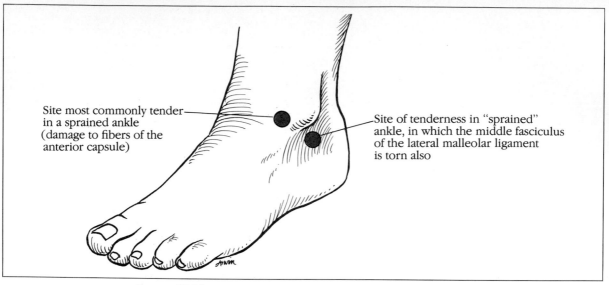

Site most commonly tender in a sprained ankle (damage to fibers of the anterior capsule)

Site of tenderness in "sprained" ankle, in which the middle fasciculus of the lateral malleolar ligament is torn also

FIGURE 17-36

Sprained ankle. A *sprain* implies that no fracture has occurred but that the ligaments of the ankle have been stretched, with but a few fibers torn. In more severe injury the term *ligament rupture* should be used.

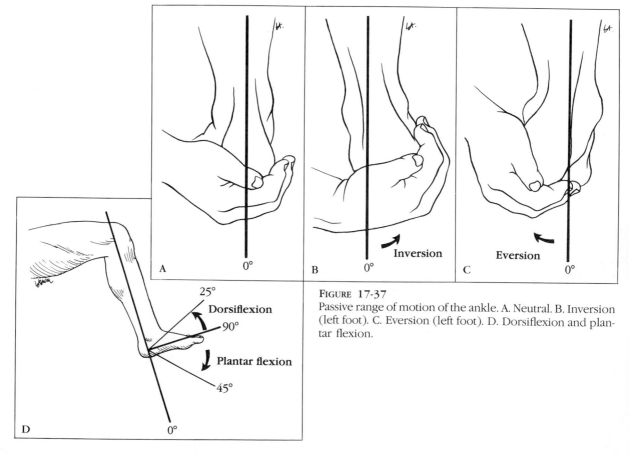

A — 0°

B — Inversion — 0°

C — Eversion — 0°

D

25° Dorsiflexion — 90°

Plantar flexion — 45° — 0°

FIGURE 17-37

Passive range of motion of the ankle. A. Neutral. B. Inversion (left foot). C. Eversion (left foot). D. Dorsiflexion and plantar flexion.

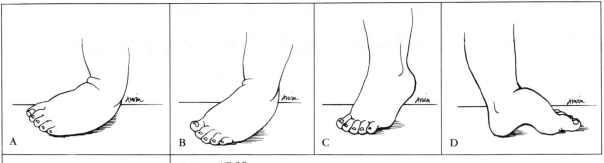

FIGURE 17-38
Some lesions of the foot. A. Varus (forefoot inverted in relation to the heel). B. Equinovarus (plantar flexed and inverted). C. Equinus (plantar flexed). D. Pes cavus (hollowing of instep). E. Pes planus (flatfeet—congenital or acquired).

Test the active and passive motions of the ankle joint (Fig. 17-37). At least 10 degrees of plantar flexion and 15 degrees of dorsiflexion should be present. Test the stability of the joint, particularly in inversion and eversion. Normal ankle motion is dorsiflexion and plantar flexion. If tilting of the talus can be demonstrated as the ankle is forced into eversion, instability of the medial collateral ligament is present.

Determine the strength of the muscles crossing the ankle joint by having the patient support body weight first on the heel and then on the ball of the foot.

FOOT
Inspect the foot for obvious deformities and swelling. Observe the heel from the rear. The axis of the heel is normally a continuation of the long axis of the lower leg. If the heel is tilted toward the midline of the body, the heel is in varus—a deformity frequently associated with clubfoot and cavus foot (Fig. 17-38). If the axis is tilted away from the midline, the heel is in valgus—a deformity associated with flatfeet. A bony prominence just anterior to and below the medial malleolus suggests the presence of an accessory navicular bone, which may be associated with flatfeet and which makes proper shoefitting difficult. A swelling over the medial aspect of the metatarsophalangeal joint of the great toe is termed a bunion and may be associated with a medial deviation of more than 15 degrees when compared with the lateral four metatarsals (metatarsus primus varus), or with lateral deviation of the great toe (hallux valgus). Inspect the toes for abnormalities such as claw-toe, in which the proximal interphalangeal joint is acutely flexed while the metacarpophalangeal joint remains in neutral position. Inspect the sole of the foot for the presence of calluses over the metatarsal heads (Fig. 17-39). Observe the state of nutrition of the tissues of the foot by palpating the skin, noting the presence or absence of hair on the dorsum of the toes, and palpating the dorsalis pedis and posterior tibial pulses.

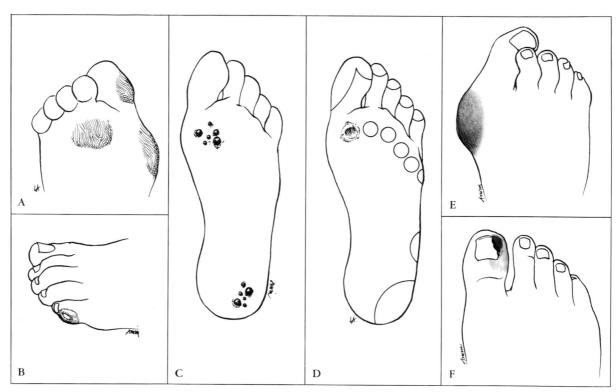

FIGURE 17-39

Some other lesions of the foot. A. Callosity: hard protective layer of skin over stress site. B. Hard corn: highly compressed keratotic cells with central white core. C. Plantar warts: a viral infection giving a dark pearl on the skin of the sole; very painful. D. Neurotrophic ulcers: painless perforations seen in peripheral neuropathies. Most common sites are outlined. E. Hallux valgus with bunion: proximal phalanx in valgus, often congenital. A bunion is an inflamed bursa over a hallux valgus. F. Ingrown toenail.

Test inversion and eversion of the foot by rocking the heel medially and laterally while stabilizing the lower leg, rotating the foot by supinating and pronating the metatarsals as a unit while stabilizing the heel, and flexing and extending the toes. Test the individual muscles by having the patient perform the appropriate movements against the resistance of the examiner's hand.

Palpate for points of tenderness indicating inflammation of bursae or joints. Diffuse tenderness over the calcaneus itself is often associated with early rheumatoid arthritis or with Reiter's syndrome. Inflammation detected in any of the joints of the foot may be caused by septic arthritis, rheumatoid arthritis, osteoarthritis, or gout. Tenderness to palpation over the metatarsal heads on the ball of the foot indicates metatarsalgia; tenderness between the metatarsal heads on the dorsum of the foot suggests interdigital neuroma. The latter possibility is strengthened if a sensory abnormality can be demonstrated on the opposing surfaces of the contiguous toes supplied by the involved interdigital nerve, and if medial to lateral compression of the forefoot induces metatarsal pain that radiates into the involved toes.

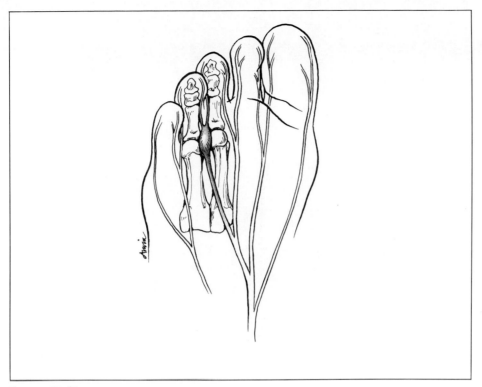

FIGURE 17-40
Plantar neuroma just above the division of the plantar nerve into its terminal branches.

A lancinating pain in the toes and metatarsal tenderness, especially in women, suggests a neuroma just above the division of the plantar nerve into its terminal branches (Fig. 17-40).

NERVOUS SYSTEM   CHAPTER 18

From the brain, and from the brain only, arise our pleasures, joys, laughter and jests, as well as our sorrows, pains, griefs and tears.

HIPPOCRATES
(460?–377? B.C.)

Examination of the nervous system has a reputation for being complicated to perform and difficult to interpret. This reputation is only partially deserved. The examination is time-consuming only while one is acquiring proficiency. With repetition, interest increases, and the speed with which an adequate neurologic examination can be done also increases. A screening neurologic examination can be accomplished in 15 minutes. That time can be cut down further if various parts are assimilated into the general physical examination.

ANATOMY

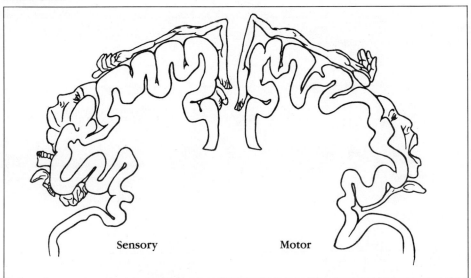

Sensory   Motor

FIGURE 18-1
The cortical topography of neurologic function: Sensory homunculus (sensory cortex); motor homunculus (area 4, or anterior central gyrus).

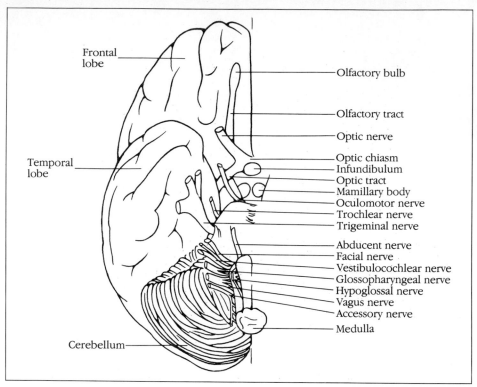

FIGURE 18-2
Brain stem with cranial nerves.

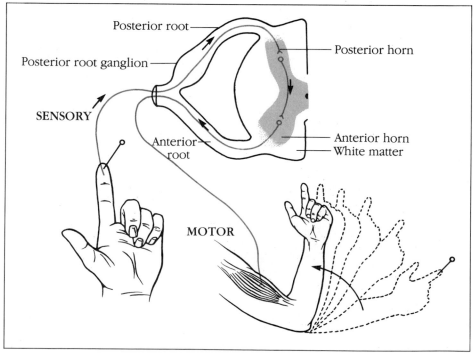

FIGURE 18-3
Cord with sensory and motor tracts.

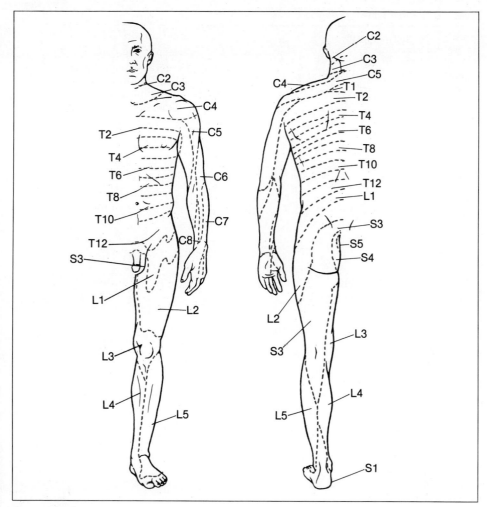

FIGURE 18-4
Dermatomes.

HISTORY

The Brain —is wider than the Sky —
For —put them side by side —
The one the other will contain
With ease —and You —beside —
                    EMILY DICKINSON
                    (1830–1886)

Patients with neurologic symptoms are often highly anxious about them, fearing that they represent brain tumor or impending stroke. Moreover, neurologic impairment—because it can affect memory, perception, or speech—may make the history difficult to obtain. It is essential, therefore, that the greatest patience and care be exerted to obtain the best history from the patient, his friends, or relatives.

TABLE 18-1. Some Causes of Coma

Cerebral vascular accidents
  Cerebral infarction
  Cerebral hemorrhage
  Cerebral embolism with infarction
  Subarachnoid hemorrhage

Cerebral trauma
  Concussion
  Cerebral contusion
  Subdural hematoma
  Epidural hematoma

Drugs and toxins
  Alcohol
  Narcotics
  Barbiturates
  Insulin
  Aspirin
  Carbon monoxide
  Heavy metals (lead, arsenic)
  Other sedatives and drugs

Endogenous toxins or states
  Diabetic coma
  Uremia
  Hepatic failure
  Hypoxemia
  Hypoglycemia
  Myxedema
  Hypothermia
  Hypercalcemia
  Hyponatremia
  Adrenal insufficiency
  Avitaminosis
    (B_{12}, thiamine)
  Profound anemia
  Heat stroke

Infections
  Severe systemic sepsis
  Central nervous system infections

Brain tumors

Postepileptic coma

Cerebral hypoperfusion
  Carotid thrombosis
  Arrhythmias
  Stokes-Adams disease
  Severe congestive heart failure

Psychiatric "coma"
  Hysteria
  Schizophrenia

Other
  Akinetic mutism
  Locked-in syndrome

Often such "personality traits" as suspicion, euphoria, and moodiness may be significant clues to neurologic disease and should be explored in questioning.

The following symptoms in the neurologic review are particularly important and require elaboration:

Changes in consciousness. The state of awareness of the patient may vary from mild drowsiness to unresponsive coma. Coma may be transient or permanent; there are many causes of coma, some of which are presented in Table 18-1.

Disturbances of vision may be due to drugs or eye disease, but organic lesions of the central nervous system may present with a history of visual field loss (stroke, brain tumor), double vision (multiple sclerosis, trauma, basilar artery insufficiency, chronic basilar meningitis, tumor), flashing lights (migraine, occipital lobe lesions), visual hallucinosis (temporal lobe lesions, drugs), and transient blindness (vascular lesions, migraine).

Disturbances of smell and taste suggest a focal lesion of the olfactory nerves.

Fits, seizures, or convulsions are important symptoms. Their prodrome (if any), the situation in which they occurred, focal components of the convulsion, and a minute description of the convulsion itself from a witness (if possible) should all be ascertained.

Vomiting may characterize central nervous system disease, especially if it is unaccompanied by nausea and is projectile in its force. Vomiting may also occur with migraine, with cerebellar and vestibular disease, and with neurosis.

Difficulty with bladder and bowel control, as well as **sexual dysfunction**, may signal spinal cord or autonomic dysfunction. Other autonomic symptoms include abnormal patterns of sweating, flushing, and palpitations.

Disturbance of gait should be categorized as due to motor weakness or incoordination or due to sensory dysfunction (does the patient know where his feet are?).

Disturbance of speech may be noted by the physician as the history is given or may be the patient's major complaint. Try to discern if the difficulty is one of articulation (*dysarthria*) or of word command (*aphasia*). Are there associated difficulties with chewing or swallowing?

Abnormal motor movements may have seriously disturbed the patient's ability to function. Is there a tremor?

Numbness usually indicates peripheral nerve or spinal cord (posterior column) involvement but may also be due to sensory pathway interruption in the brain stem, thalamus, or parietal cortex.

Weakness may result from abnormalities of the muscle, myoneural junction, or nerve, or of the corticospinal tract in the spinal cord, brainstem, internal capsule, or motor cortex. Involvement of other central pathways connecting to this main motor system also produces weakness.

Dizziness usually means one of three things: vertigo, imbalance, or faintness. *Vertigo* is caused by dysfunction of the inner ear balance mechanisms or the vestibular portion of the acoustic nerve or its central connections. *Imbalance* may result from peripheral nerve, posterior column, cerebellar, or main motor pathway involvement.

Fainting or loss of consciousness results from loss of function of the brain due to loss of blood supply, inadequate nutrition (oxygen, glucose), imbalance of nutrients, abnormal cerebral electrical discharge (epilepsy), or cerebral destruction due to any cause.

Pain is due to distortion, transection, or irritation of pain endings and pain fibers of peripheral nerves or of the central pain pathways (spinothalamic tracts) in the spinal cord, brain stem, or thalamus.

Headache is caused by distortion of or traction on blood vessels or the meninges or other covering structures of the brain, or by pressure, distortion, traction, or displacement of almost any extracerebral structure in the head, including the skull, paranasal sinuses, scalp, and posterior suboccipital muscles of the neck.

Defective memory or thinking. Difficulty with these two cerebral functions may result from lesion in almost any area of the brain, although a specific memory defect may result from small lesions in the hypothalamic-thalamic-temporal lobe structures (see Table 18-2).

TABLE 18-2. Some Causes of a Chronic Dementia* (*not* in order of frequency)

Dementias associated with systemic disorders	**Dementias associated with other neurologic signs**
Avitaminosis (B_{12}, thiamine)	Huntington's chorea
Hypothyroidism	Slow virus disease (e.g., Jakob-Creutzfeldt)
Hypercorticosteroidism	Demyelinating disorders (e.g., Schilder's disease)
Dementias associated with some cancers	Lipid storage diseases (e.g., Tay-Sachs)
Hepatolenticular degeneration (Wilson's disease)	Myoclonic epilepsy
Syphilis	Parkinson's disease
Chronic alcoholism and/or drug use	Hereditary ataxias
Porphyria	Cerebral atherosclerosis (multiple stroke syndrome)
Dementias in which dementia may occur as the sole evidence of disease	Brain tumor
	Brain trauma (multiple, old)
Senile and presenile dementias	Low-pressure hydrocephalus
Some brain tumors of the frontal lobes or central structures	

* *Dementia:* A clinical state characterized by failing memory and loss of other intellectual functions due to chronic, progressive degenerative disease of the brain.

PHYSICAL EXAMINATION

1. Assay mental status (history, recent and remote memory, judgment, affect).
2. Auscultate and palpate the head and the carotids in the neck.

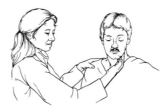 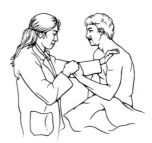

3. Test cranial nerves II—XII (cranial nerve I not generally tested in routine examinations).
4. Test motor function (abnormal movements, muscle mass and tone, strength, reflexes).
5. Test cerebellar function (finger to nose, heel to shin, rapid fine and alternating movements).

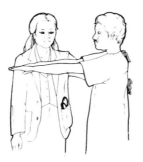 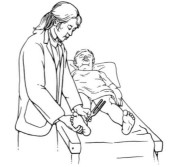

6. Test station and gait (Romberg test included).
7. Test sensation (temperature, superficial pain, vibration, light touch, deep pain).

*The auditory nerves were atrophied. . . . The convolutions of the brain, which
was rather soft and edematous, seemed to be twice as deep and twice as numerous as normal.*

Report of autopsy on Ludwig van Beethoven
JOHANN WAGNER
(1800?–1833)

GENERAL

Some observers prefer to examine the nervous system by regions rather than by
systems; that is, the legs are examined as to motor, sensory, reflex, and cerebellar
responses, and then the arms are examined, and so forth. This approach has advan-
tages but probably should be left to those with considerable experience. It is not
necessary to do the examination in the order listed here, however. It is often better
to examine first the part or function complained of by the patient and then return
to the established routine.

The examiner should have available a reflex hammer, tuning forks (128 and 256
cps), an ophthalmoscope, a small flashlight, tongue blades, sharp pins, and cotton
or a camel's-hair brush. A stethoscope and otoscope are also often required.

MENTAL STATUS

You will have obtained considerable information about your patient's recent and
remote memory, affect (mood), judgment, basic intelligence, and alertness during
the history and physical examination already done. Take care not to confuse cultural difference or deafness with poor cognition, language difficulty with stupidity,
and aphasia with dementia. An awareness of your patient's socioeconomic and educational levels will help you in your analysis of his cognitive function. Specific questions may be used to discern orientation in those who appear confused: what date
is it? (orientation to time); what hospital is this? (orientation to place); what is my
name, and who am I? (orientation to person).

Memory may be tested by asking your patient to recite U.S. presidents, starting
with the incumbent, back as far as he can remember. Record in your physical examination the most distant president the patient could name, such as "presidents back
to Truman." A better test of recent memory is for you to give the patient the names
of three objects (for example, "doll," "book," "dog") with instructions to remember them and to repeat them back to you when you ask for them in 5 minutes. Then
don't forget to ask for them when the 5 minutes are up! Ask the patient what he ate
at his last meal.

The ability to do *calculations* is often tested by "serial sevens." Ask the patient to
subtract seven from one-hundred (93), then seven from that (86), and seven from
that (79), and so on, as far as the patient can go. Both the accuracy of the computa-
tions and the number to which the patient can go are recorded.*

The capacity for *abstract thought* is addressed by asking your patient to interpret
proverbs; for example, "What is the meaning of the old saying 'People who live in
glass houses shouldn't throw stones'?" Concrete interpretations, such as "The glass
will break if they do," suggest organic cognitive dysfunction or psychosis.

---

* An easy way to do serial sevens is to subtract ten and add three to each successive number.

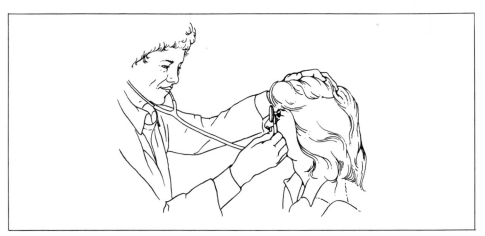

FIGURE 18-5
Auscultation of the eye.

An idea of the capacity to exercise *judgment* may be obtained by presenting the patient with specific situations and asking them what they would do: "If you found a stamped, addressed envelope lying on the ground next to a mailbox, what would you do?"

Affect, or mood, is best appreciated by observation over the course of the entire history and physical examination. If the patient is depressed, is it appropriate to the situation? Is he inappropriately lighthearted in the face of devastating illness? Does the patient show lability of mood, switching from happiness to tears without reasonable restraint? Is there a significant emotional component to his speech, or is the affect inappropriately "flat"? Record your subjective impressions in the physical examination.

In all these questions, exercise tact and gentleness. Many patients with impaired mentation are very frightened by their perceived loss of ability and will have erected defenses to its discovery. In breaking through those defenses the physician may become threatening to them. Patients who lack formal education may interpret your probing as an attempt to belittle their intelligence. If you meet with a hostile or disturbed response during mental status testing, back off for a while and, if you can, come back to it later.

EXAMINATION OF THE HEAD AND NECK

Palpate the common carotid arteries in the neck and the temporal arteries just in front of the ears. Palpate both radial arteries at the wrist, noting both strength and simultaneousness of impulse.

With the bell of the stethoscope listen for a bruit over each eyeball after asking the patient to close both eyes. Place the bell over one eyeball firmly and ask the patient to open the other eye and look steadily at an object (Fig. 18-5). Listen also for a bruit over both carotid arteries high in the neck at the angle of the jaw and in each supraclavicular space. If a bruit is heard in either of the latter two spaces, compare blood pressure in the arms.

The carotid pulses are usually equal and normal, and when absent or markedly

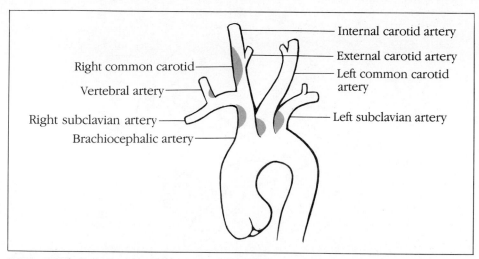

FIGURE 18-6
Frequent sites of atherosclerosis in the aortic arch. Eighty percent of lesions are at the bifurcation of the common carotids. Obstruction may also occur at the take-off of the great vessels from the aorta, at the origin of the vertebral artery, or at the origin of the subclavian arteries. Subclavian occlusion may (rarely) produce the "subclavian steal."

decreased may suggest an occlusion. However, complete or partial occlusion can take place in the presence of what is apparently a normally palpable carotid artery. If the common carotid artery in the neck gives a full pulse, but the pulse in the temporal artery on the same side is decreased or absent, there is presumptive evidence of occlusion of the external carotid. Retinal artery pressure testing and Doppler ultrasound mappings give a more reliable clue as to the patency of the internal and common carotid systems than does simple palpation. The ophthalmodynamometer may also be used to determine the blood pressure in the temporal artery. The subclavian, brachial, and radial pulses and also the dorsalis pedis, posterior tibial, and femoral pulses, if absent or definitely decreased, may give hints of occlusion of the main branches of the aorta, and this may be helpful in neurologic diagnosis.

Auscultation of the skull may reveal a bruit on the side of increased or decreased blood flow through a carotid or vertebral artery. Increased flow may be due to occlusion on the opposite side or to an arteriovenous anomaly or tumor on the same side. A bruit due to decreased flow occurs with partial or complete occlusion on the same or opposite side, or even in the absence of vascular disease.

A bruit in the supraclavicular space may indicate partial or complete occlusion of the subclavian artery with possible production of the "subclavian steal" syndrome. With this syndrome there may be also a decrease in the blood pressure in the affected arm and a delay in the radial pulse on the same side. Proximal obstruction in the subclavian artery decreases the pressure in that artery at the point of origin of the vertebral artery (Fig. 18-6); this condition may result in an actual reversal of flow in the vertebral artery, with blood draining from the basilar artery into the arm as it is exercised.

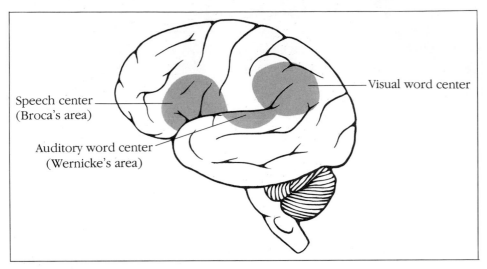

FIGURE 18-7
Some centers of language in the brain. Left cerebral hemisphere (dominant in right-handed individuals). In actuality, the centers shown overlap.

SUPPLENESS OF THE NECK

The most easily tested of the meningeal signs is that for *nuchal rigidity* (stiff neck). Ask the patient to relax, and then with both hands flex his neck on his chest. If nuchal rigidity is present, there will be resistance and pain. *Brudzinski's sign* is flexion of the hips when the head is flexed in this manner. Test for *Kernig's sign* by flexing the hip on the trunk, allowing the knee to flex at the same time. When the hip is flexed to 90 degrees, extend the knee. In the presence of meningeal irritation there will be resistance, pain, and sometimes a tendency toward flexion of the neck.

APHASIA

In most cases it is not necessary to do detailed testing for aphasia. A good idea of the patient's ability to express himself and to understand what is said to him can be gained in the course of the initial history. If aphasia is suspected, simple tests can be done. Ask the patient to name objects as you point to them, such as thumb, nose, ear, eye, watch, watch crystal, tie, and colors in the tie. Auditory receptive aphasia can be tested by asking the patient to perform such commands as "Touch your finger to your nose" or "Touch your left first finger to your right ear" and by having the patient do so without any demonstration by the examiner. Testing to determine the patient's ability to read can be done by asking the patient to perform written instructions, such as "Touch your finger to your nose." The patient's ability to recognize printed words and simple objects can be tested even in the presence of a marked expressive aphasia by printing the names of simple objects, such as key, pencil, and coin, on a piece of paper and by placing the objects next to the paper. The patient quickly understands that he is to match the printed word with the object.

A normal patient will of course demonstrate no dysarthria or aphasia. It is important to know the handedness of the patient, although if this cannot be ascertained it is usually safe to assume that the left cerebral hemisphere is dominant (Fig. 18-7). (About 98 percent of all people, including at least half of those who are left-handed, have left-hemisphere dominance.) Involvement of the dominant hemispheres by any type of disease often produces aphasia or dysphasia (partial aphasia).

In the common cerebral infarct in either hemisphere there will be some short-lived dysarthric slurring of speech. It should not be confused with aphasia. The ataxia of speech of cerebellar disturbances and multiple sclerosis is also to be differentiated from dysarthria and aphasia. Lesions of the brain stem or bilateral cerebral lesions produce a bulbar or pseudobulbar speech that is similar to the dysarthria produced by a lesion of one hemisphere but is more marked and more likely to persist. The significance of abnormalities found on testing for aphasia is a confused and complicated subject and will be discussed only briefly. If the patient's aphasia is mainly expressive and the word flow is diminished (nonfluent), his lesion is likely to be in the front half of the dominant hemisphere; if the aphasia is receptive, the lesion is on the back half. If the aphasia is mixed and the word flow is good (fluent) but inaccurate, as it usually is, the lesion may include frontal, parietal, or temporal lobes or may be deep in the hemisphere.

EXAMINATION OF THE CRANIAL NERVES

A large part of the cranial nerve examination is commonly done at the time of examination of the head, eyes, ears, nose, throat, and neck (see Chaps. 8–10, Sec. III).

I: OLFACTORY

Ask the patient to identify, with his eyes closed, any common nonirritating odor, such as coffee, tobacco, vanilla, turpentine, or cloves. Each nostril is tested separately. If these scents are not readily available, items at the bedside, such as oranges, flowers, and cigarettes, may be used. Normally the patient should be able to approximately identify familiar odors. Care must be taken here to differentiate between inability to smell the substance and inability to identify it properly. Many patients smell the substance correctly but are unable to name it. For this reason very familiar odors are probably best. Loss of the ability to smell (anosmia) is abnormal but does not usually indicate disease of the nervous system and is therefore of little localizing value. Local nasal disorders are far more common as a cause of loss of smell.

The most common neurologic causes of anosmia are head injuries and tumors, especially meningiomas of the olfactory groove. The ability to smell commonly decreases with advancing age.

II: OPTIC

Examination of the optic nerve is divided into three major subdivisions: (1) vision, (2) visual fields, and (3) funduscopic.

Visual acuity is best tested with standardized charts or with small pocket-size testing cards. If these are not available, the examiner can use any printed material and compare his own visual ability (assuming he knows his own acuity) with the patient's. Because we are interested in lesions of the retina and optic pathways and not in errors of refraction, the patient should be tested with his glasses on. Test each eye separately. If the acuity is so diminished that the patient cannot read even large print, ask him to count extended fingers at various distances. If even this is impossible, test his ability to see moving objects or to distinguish light from dark. Visual acuity, with correction, should be 20/20. In youth, the visual acuity is usually better than this, and in fact an acuity of 20/20 in the young can represent some loss of vision.

Check the *visual fields* by the confrontation method. Ask the patient to cover one eye and with his other eye look straight into your eyes. Slowly bring from behind the patient one constantly moving finger (wiggling), held 12 to 18 inches from his head. A small test object such as a cotton applicator may be used. As the test object is moved forward, the patient will let you know when he first sees it. All four quadrants should be tested at 45-degree angles from the horizontal and the vertical. Each eye must be tested separately, but most field defects of central nervous system origin can be found with both of the patient's eyes open. Finer testing can be done with small test objects and screens made for the purpose. Many scotomas cannot be found without such special equipment. Extinction, or suppression, is tested by wiggling a finger first in one half of the field, then repeating on the opposite side with a finger on the other hand. Then both fingers are moved simultaneously. The patient is asked the same question each time that one or both fingers are moved: "On which side do you see the finger wiggle?" Normally the visual fields are full, without any obvious blind spots, and there is no extinction; that is, both fingers are seen to wiggle simultaneously.

The *optic fundi* should be examined with the ophthalmoscope. The presence of a sharp disc outline and of pulsations of the veins in the discs is of particular interest from a neurologic standpoint, since these findings indicate a normal intracranial pressure. The two most common funduscopic abnormalities of concern during neurologic testing are swelling or edema of the optic disc and optic atrophy. Papilledema first appears as a loss of distinctness of the disc margins that progresses until all evidence of margin disappears. It then may become raised above the surrounding retina, and the edema may spread into the retina. One should be careful not to attach significance to minimal indistinctness of the disc margins along the nasal or medial aspect of the disc, since this is often normal. Optic atrophy is usually manifested by a combination of pallor of the lateral aspect of the disc and a lack of normal vascularity in that area.

The most common gross visual field defect of neurologic importance is that of a homonymous hemianopia, in which, for instance, the right visual field is lost in the right and left eyes. This would indicate that the left optic tract or visual radiation is diseased somewhere between the optic chiasm and the left visual cortex. A homonymous quadrantanopic defect usually indicates disease involving the visual radiations as they pass through the parietal or temporal lobes. An upper quadrantanopic defect usually indicates involvement of the visual radiations in the opposite temporal lobe, and a lower quarter field defect indicates involvement of the opposite parietal lobe. Bitemporal field defects or involvement of the lateral half of the visual field in each eye indicates a lesion in the center of the optic chiasm interrupting the fibers as they cross from one optic nerve to the opposite tract. The most common lesion causing this defect is a tumor of the pituitary gland.

A fuller discussion and illustration of the optic examination and its relationship to neurologic evaluation is provided in Chapter 8.

III, IV, AND VI: OCULOMOTOR, TROCHLEAR, AND ABDUCENS

These nerves supply the muscles of eye movement and are tested as a unit. Each eye is tested separately and then both together. Ask the patient to follow an object such as a fingertip, keeping his head motionless. Move the object laterally from side to side, and then vertically up and down when lateral gaze is reached. Test elevation and depression with the eyes in the midposition also. Pause for a moment at each end point and inspect for nystagmus and weakness of eye muscle. The test object is then brought from a distance of 3 or 4 feet to within an inch of the patient's nose. In this way both convergence and the normal pupillary constriction to convergence are tested.

Paralysis of cranial nerve III results in a dilated pupil, external deviation of the eyeball, and ptosis of the upper lid. Cranial nerves IV and VI carry no parasympathetic fibers, and their paralysis results only in weakness of the appropriate muscles. The eye is deviated inward with *paralysis of cranial nerve VI* (lateral rectus muscle weakness). Sixth-nerve weakness has only moderate localizing value because it may result from increased intracranial pressure regardless of cause, especially in children. *Paralysis of cranial nerve IV* is not quite so easy to detect and is rare. There is weakness of internal rotation of the eyeball and of gaze downward and inward. The patient may tilt his head so that the eye with the paralyzed superior oblique muscle is elevated somewhat above the plane of the normal eye. This is done to bring the horizontal axes parallel and thus prevent diplopia (see Chap. 8).

The eyes are inspected for *ptosis,* and any difference in the width of the palpebral fissures is noted. Check the *pupillary response to light.* The light is directed into one eye, watching for pupillary constriction in the eye being tested (direct light reflex) and in the other eye (consensual light reflex). At rest, depending on the amount of light in the examining room, the pupils are normally equal and about 2 to 3 mm in diameter. They react quickly to light both directly and consensually and also to convergence.

Anisocoria (unequal pupils) may be caused by a variety of abnormalities, including a sympathetic paralysis (Horner's syndrome), syphilis (Argyll Robertson pupil), diabetes, multiple sclerosis, and trauma or disease of the iris. Anisocoria may also be congenital and have no pathologic significance. If both pupils are markedly larger or smaller than normal, inquiry should be made into the use of drugs, especially stimulants such as *d*-amphetamine or eye drops for ocular disease such as glaucoma.

A unilateral dilated pupil often occurs with increased intracranial pressure, and in this case it is an early sign of cranial nerve III weakness. The dilated pupil is usually on the side of the lesion causing the increased pressure. The *Argyll Robertson pupil* is usually smaller than normal and reacts to convergence but not to light. *Adie's pupil* is usually found in young women with decreased or absent tendon reflexes; the pupil is larger than normal and reacts only slowly to light. (Table 8-8 describes abnormal pupils).

When the eyes are moved to the limit of lateral gaze in any direction, there normally may be minimal *nystagmus.* There should be *no* nystagmus on elevation and depression of the eyes, even at the extremes.

Nystagmus often gives a definite clue as to location and even type of neurologic

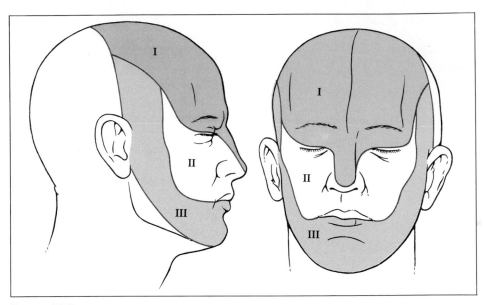

Figure 18-8
Three sensory divisions of the trigeminal nerve: ophthalmic (I), maxillary (II), and mandibular (III).

disease present. Of special importance is the *dissociated nystagmus* with lesions of the medial longitudinal fasciculus. In this type of nystagmus the eye on the side to which the gaze is directed participates strongly with a horizontal nystagmus, whereas the opposite eye will show less nystagmus but will show some weakness of internal rotation. Multiple sclerosis is the most common cause of this type of nystagmus.

Nystagmus is common in acute and chronic conditions of the cerebellum and brain stem, in which case it is usually more pronounced on looking toward the side of the lesion. There also may be a minimal to moderate nystagmus with strictly cerebral lesions, in which case it is usually more evident in looking away from the side of the lesion.

V: TRIGEMINAL

The areas supplied by the three divisions of the trigeminal nerve (Fig. 18-8) are tested for their sensitivity to light touch (cotton), pinprick, and temperature. If a medullary or upper cervical cord lesion is suspected, it is important to test pain, temperature, and touch on the face; with a lesion involving the descending tract of the trigeminal nerve, touch may be intact with absence of pain and temperature. In such lesions, the loss of pain and temperature sensation extends exactly to the midline. It may, however, involve only the first, second, or third divisions of the trigeminal nerve because of the arrangement of these divisions in the descending tract. For this reason it is important to test all three divisions.

The corneal reflex is important and can be tested by carefully placing a fine, elongated wisp of the cotton on the cornea while the patient is looking away from the

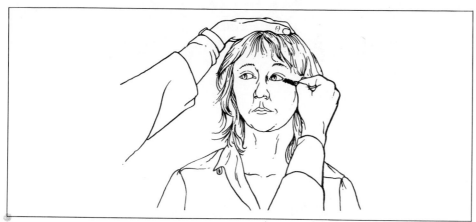

FIGURE 18-9
Testing the corneal reflex.

approaching cotton (Fig. 18-9). *Both eyes should blink quickly with this stimu-lation.* Each eye is tested separately.

The corneal reflex may be diminished unilaterally from either a peripheral or a central lesion. A decreased corneal reflex may be an early clue to a peripheral le-sion of cranial nerve V. At times the corneal reflex may be consciously suppressed and thus may be decreased or absent in stoical persons or in conversion reactions. It is not difficult to differentiate the absence of a corneal reflex due to a lesion of a fifth nerve from that caused by a seventh-nerve paralysis (weakness of the face).

The masseter and temporalis muscles should be palpated with the patient clenching his jaws. Deviation of the jaw on opening the mouth should be assessed. Test also the strength of the jaw on lateral movement. Check the strength of jaw closure by asking the patient to grip a tongue blade with his teeth on each side while you try to extract the blade. Normally all of these modalities are intact and muscle strength is good.

With the usual type of cerebral infarct there may be some decrease in sensation on the opposite side of the face, but this usually does not extend exactly to the midline. There is usually no appreciable weakness of the masseter and pterygoid muscles on the side opposite a "central" (cerebral) lesion.

VII: FACIAL

The facial nerve is tested by asking the patient to show his teeth and smile, to show strong closure of the eyes against resistance, to elevate his eyebrows, and to con-tract the platysma (Table 18-3). Each of these maneuvers may be first shown to the patient by movements of your own.

All facial movements should be equal bilaterally. Some individuals, however, ha-bitually talk and smile more out of one side of their mouth than the other. These habit patterns must be kept in mind while looking for possible evidence of weak-ness.

In a "central" (*upper motor neuron*) weakness of the face, such as is typically seen with the usual cerebral infarct, there is moderate to marked weakness of the

TABLE 18-3. Right Facial Weakness

Central (Upper Motor Neuron)	Maneuver	Peripheral (Lower Motor Neuron)

I. Face at rest

Loss of nasolabial fold on right

Corner of mouth droops on right

To a limited degree, widening palpebral fissure on right

Loss of nasolabial fold on right

Corner of mouth droops on right

Widening palpebral fissure on right

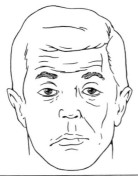 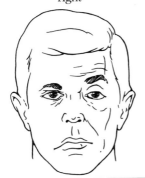

II. Elevation of eyebrows

Patient can elevate both eyebrows

Unable to elevate eyebrow on right

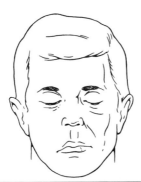 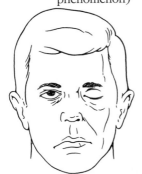

III. Closing eyes

Patient can close both eyes

Right eye does not close and eyeball turns up (Bell's phenomenon)

TABLE 18-3. (Continued)

Central (Upper Motor Neuron)	Maneuver	Peripheral (Lower Motor Neuron)
	IV. Emotion	
Smile symmetrical		Smile asymmetrical

opposite lower facial muscles, including the platysma, the orbicularis oris, and sometimes the lower part of the orbicularis oculi. With a small lesion there may be only minimal drooping of the opposite corner of the mouth at rest and some weakness of that corner of the mouth on voluntary movement. The patient, however, will be able to close his eye and wrinkle his forehead on the side opposite the cerebral lesion fairly strongly. With weakness of the face due to a lesion of the seventh-nerve nucleus or of the nerve itself (peripheral facial paralysis, *lower motor neuron disease,* Bell's palsy) there is weakness of all parts of the face on the side of the lesion. The patient will be unable to wrinkle his forehead, close his eye, or show his teeth.

Weakness of one side of the mouth, even though minimal, may be an important clue in determining whether the lesion responsible for the accompanying weakness of an arm (or an arm and a leg) on the same side is in the spinal cord, the brain stem, or the cerebrum. If the lesion is in the spinal cord, there should be no weakness of the face. If it is in the pons, the facial weakness will be on the side opposite that of the affected arm and the leg. If the lesion is above the brain stem, weakness of the face, arm, and leg will be all on the same side.

Test *taste* with sugar or salt. Place a few grains on half of the anterior two-thirds of the protruded tongue and instruct the patient to keep his tongue out until he tastes the substance. At times it helps to have him point to the word *sweet* or *salt* written on a piece of paper rather than to withdraw his tongue and state what he has tasted. Each side of the tongue should be tasted separately.

VIII: AUDITORY

The two divisions of the auditory nerve—the cochlear and the vestibular—are tested separately. The patient's ability to hear a watch tick or a whispered voice at a definite distance from each ear may be all that is necessary to test. Hearing may also be tested with a tuning fork of 256 or more cycles per second. Normally the patient's hearing should be equal in both ears, and air conduction should be about twice the duration of bone conduction.

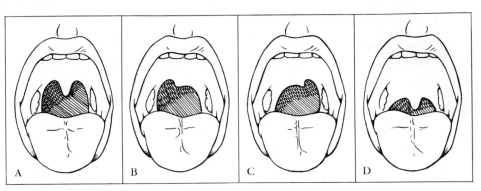

FIGURE 18-10
Tests of uvular deviation (cranial nerves IX and X). A. Normal. B. Left IX and X palsy. C. Right IX and X palsy. D. Bulbar palsy.

A lessening of the time of air conduction with preservation of bone conduction indicates that there is *conductive* (middle ear or external ear) deafness. If both air conduction and bone conduction are reduced, the deafness is *perceptive* (nerve) or mixed. With unilateral nerve deafness the patient will hear the tuning fork when it is placed on the midline of the skull (Weber's test) in his good ear, whereas if the defect is in the middle ear or external ear the patient will hear it in his deaf ear (often much to his surprise). Lesions central to the cochlear nuclei do not cause unilateral deafness; therefore, unilateral perceptive deafness indicates a lesion of the cochlear nuclei (rare), cranial nerve VIII, or the end-organ (cochlea). To differentiate between these it is sometimes helpful to test the vestibular portion of cranial nerve VIII. The vestibular function will be preserved if deafness is caused by a lesion of the cochlear nuclei but may be lost in lesions of the nerve or end-organ.

Tests of hearing are described in detail and illustrated in Chapter 9.

IX AND X: GLOSSOPHARYNGEAL AND VAGUS

These two complex cranial nerves are tested together and, in fact, are rather simple to evaluate. Note the quality of the patient's voice and his ability to swallow. Ask him to open his mouth and say "ah." Observe the position of the soft palate and uvula at rest and with phonation (Fig. 18-10). Check the gag reflex with a tongue blade by touching each side of the posterior pharyngeal wall separately. Taste on the posterior one-third of the tongue can be examined when an abnormality is suspected.

Normally the uvula and palate rise in the midline with phonation. It is important to test this function with the patient's head in the midline and not turned to either side.

If there is unilateral paralysis of cranial nerves IX and X, the palate will deviate to the unparalyzed side during phonation. The distance between the soft palate and the posterior pharyngeal wall will be less on the paralyzed side. The arch of the palate at rest on the paralyzed side will tend to droop lower than on the normal side. The sensory component of the gag reflex is mediated by cranial nerve IX and the motor by X. However, paralysis of cranial nerve IX alone is difficult to detect, since sometimes there may be no apparent sensory loss in the pharynx. If there is any doubt about the presence of a vagus paralysis, the vocal cords should be visualized to see whether or not there is unilateral or bilateral weakness.

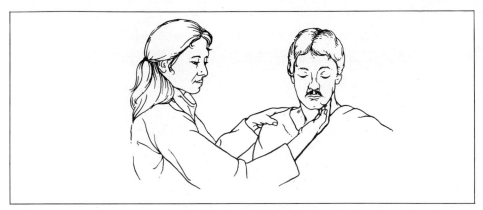

FIGURE 18-11
Testing the strength of the sternocleidomastoid muscle (cranial nerve XI).

Marked palatal and vocal cord paralysis on the same side indicates a lower motor neuron lesion. However, some patients will show moderate and temporary palatal weakness of the side opposite a large upper motor neuron lesion such as that caused by a large cerebral infarct. Marked unilateral paralysis of the palate, pharynx, and vocal cords without evidence of long sensory or motor pathway involvement nearly always indicates that the lesion is not within the brain stem (affecting the nucleus ambiguus) but involves the cranial nerves IX and X after they have left the medulla. Bilateral weakness can result from lesions of the upper motor neurons (bilaterally), giving a pseudobulbar palsy, or from involvement of the nuclei in the medulla, the nerves, or the muscles, giving a bulbar palsy.

XI: SPINAL ACCESSORY

Ask the patient to turn his head to one side against the examiner's hand on that side. Meanwhile palpate the opposite sternocleidomastoid muscle (Fig 18-11). Palpate the trapezius muscle and test the strength of the patient's "shrug" while you press down on the shoulders with both hands. Make sure that there are no fasciculations present. Normally the strength of the sternocleidomastoid and trapezius muscles is equal bilaterally.

If unilateral weakness and atrophy of the trapezius and sternocleidomastoid muscles occur, one can be certain that the responsible lesion is outside the brain stem, since the nerve has its origin in the upper cervical cord. Marked bilateral weakness and atrophy of these muscles are often found in primary muscle disease, such as muscular dystrophy.

XII: HYPOGLOSSAL

Ask the patient to protrude his tongue in the midline, and observe any deviation or atrophy. If atrophy is suspected, the tongue may be palpated. Another test for weakness or deviation of the tongue is to ask the patient to stick his tongue into his cheek while the examiner presses against the bulging cheek. Unilateral tongue weakness is manifested by a deviation of the protruded tongue toward the weak side and often by atrophy and fasciculations on the affected side. When the tongue is lying in the mouth, however, it will be pulled toward the strong side (Fig. 18-12). The reason for this pull is that the sets of tongue muscles in action when the tongue

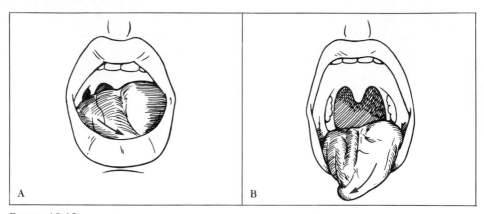

FIGURE 18-12
Hypoglossal nerve (cranial nerve XII). A. Right XII paralysis, tongue at rest. B. Right XII paralysis, tongue protruding.

is protruded are different from those sets in action when the tongue is resting in the mouth.

It is important to check the tongue carefully for fasciculations; they may be the earliest sign of lower motor neuron disease affecting the hypoglossal nerve nuclei. Normally a few small tremulous movements are seen in the tongue. These movements should not be confused with the continuous "wormy" movements (fasciculations) over the entire tongue seen in amyotrophic lateral sclerosis. Occasionally, as with the palate and pharynx, there may be temporary unilateral weakness of the tongue on the side opposite a large acute upper motor neuron lesion. Associated with this weakness may be a transient dysarthria; both usually clear within a few days. With a bilateral upper motor neuron lesion there may be anarthria and inability to protrude the tongue beyond the lips.

EXAMINATION OF THE MOTOR SYSTEM

INSPECTION

Observe the patient's musculature for abnormal movements, either large (capable of moving a joint) or small (within the belly of the muscle itself). *Fasciculations* may be emphasized by strong contraction of the suspected muscle before examination and by tapping the muscle with the reflex hammer. Since the presence of fasciculations is important in the diagnosis of diseases of the anterior horn cells, inspection should be careful and thorough.

Atrophy (Fig. 18-13) and *hypertrophy* may give important clues in the diagnosis of muscle disease. If atrophy is present or if a progressive disease that might cause atrophy is suspected, the circumference of the muscle should be measured bilaterally; record the point at which the measurement is taken. The limbs of the normal individual at rest do not demonstrate any movement either of the joints or in the body of the muscles themselves except for an occasional rare and random fasciculation. A concept of normal muscle bulk is gained only by experience. Great variation is normally present among persons of different ages, sexes, and occupations. Chronic illness in itself may produce generalized wasting of the muscles.

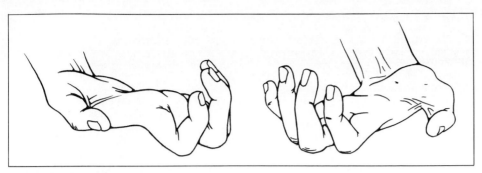

FIGURE 18-13
Hand muscle atrophy.

Abnormal movements should be carefully observed and described (Table 18-4). The abnormal movement of parkinsonism is a *resting* (nonintention) *tremor* (4 to 5 per second) that is usually more evident in the hands but is also found in the arms, head, face, tongue, and legs. It may be associated with rigidity or increased tone of the muscles and thus may produce the typical *cogwheel effect,* which is a rhythmic increase and decrease in tone superimposed on passive movements produced by the examiner. The *essential* (familial or senile) *tremor* is not present at rest but is more pronounced with sustained posture or with movement. It is not associated with any alteration in tone and is more likely to involve the head than is the tremor of parkinsonism. The *intention tremor* characteristic of such diseases as multiple sclerosis is usually combined with some degree of ataxia and is brought out with purposeful movement such as the finger-to-nose test.

Choreic movements are irregular, involuntary, spontaneous movements usually involving more than one joint. They are purposeless but may not appear so at first glance. They are most easily characterized as being similar to the "fidgets" or normal restlessness seen in children. They involve any extremity, the face, the mouth, and the tongue. They are not associated with an increase in tone. *Athetoid movements* are characteristically slow, writhing movements involving mainly the proximal parts of the extremities and also the trunk and face. They are often associated with other neurologic abnormalities found in cerebral palsy.

STRENGTH

In testing the strength of all appropriate muscle groups, pay particular attention to the relative strength of the two sides and the differences between proximal and distal groups. Special attention should be paid to any area that the patient considers weak. It is not necessary to do a complete detailed muscle examination on every patient, especially if he does not complain of weakness. A screening examination would logically include testing the strength of dorsiflexion and plantar flexion of the feet, extension of the wrist, and flexion and extension of the forearm and shoulders. Strength can be graded from 0 to 5. A system of grading by percentage of the normal may also be used (Table 18-5).

The strength of different individuals varies greatly. The handgrip normal for a society matron would certainly not be considered normal for a farmer. The difference in strength between the nondominant and dominant sides of the body is

TABLE 18-4. Some Causes of Abnormal Movements

Tremor Type	Characteristics	Seen In
Simple tremor		
Essential, familial, or senile tremor	Not present at rest, except in head	With a family history: Fatigue Advanced age Stimulants Fever Alcohol Thyroid excess
Parkinsonism (resting tremor)	Present in hands at complete rest Associated with rigidity, decreased associative movements, small steppage gait, masked face	Parkinsonism of all types
Cerebellar tremor	Worse with motion and associated with cerebellar signs	Multiple sclerosis Wilson's disease Hereditary ataxia
Chorea	Jerky, irregular, sudden movements; intermittent fidgeting (some tremors of simple tremor may be very choreiform at times)	Acute rheumatic fever (Sydenham's chorea) Huntington's chorea
Athetosis	Upper limbs predominate Slow, sinuous, writhing movements	Congenital athetosis Cerebral palsy Torsion dystonia
Myoclonus	Sudden jerks of single muscles or muscle groups	Epilepsy Encephalitis Hyponatremia Hyperosmolar state Some degenerative CNS diseases
Tetanic spasms	Sustained contractions of single muscles or muscle groups	Tetanus Strychnine poisoning Tetany Spasticity

usually very minimal and should not be used as an explanation for unilateral weakness.

It is important to test both distal and proximal muscle groups in both the upper and lower extremities. In some muscle diseases, such as muscular dystrophy, there may be marked weakness of the shoulder and hip girdle musculature and surprising strength of the hands and feet. If weakness is present, detailed tests of all muscle groups are indicated to determine the extent, distribution, and degree of weakness. Much diagnostic information can be obtained in this way.

The muscular weakness of myasthenia gravis will characteristically be accentuated by repetitive or continuous use of the muscles (arms held over the head, eyes fixed upward in a steady gaze, or hands clenched in a continuous grip).

TABLE 18-5. Grading of Muscle Strength

Grade	Percentage	Criteria
0		No movement of the muscle
1 (trace)	0–5	Trace movement Cannot move the joint
2 (poor)	5–20	Minimal movement
3 (fair)	20–50	Can move the joint against gravity
4 (good)	50–90	Good power but not normal
5 (normal)	90–100	Normal strength

Strength testing before and after a trial dose of edrophonium is the most certain method of identifying this disease.

Feigned muscle weakness may fool the most sophisticated observer. It is said that a tendency to "give way" in a jerky fashion is characteristic of nonorganic muscular weakness, but some tendency toward giving way may be found in certain definitely organic diseases.

MUSCLE TONE

Check muscle tone by both fast and slow flexion and extension at the elbows, wrists, shoulders, knees, and ankles. Ask the patient to relax as much as possible during this examination. In healthy cooperative adults the muscles are normally somewhat hypotonic. The normal patient should be able to relax his extremities sufficiently so that the examiner can easily test for tone. In older or senile patients or in patients with decreased intelligence, there is sometimes marked difficulty in producing the necessary relaxation of the extremities. The patient tries to cooperate and voluntarily moves the arm in the same manner as the examiner, thus defeating the examiner's purpose. In a few people it may be impossible to assess tone adequately for this reason.

Muscle tone is normally decreased in diseases of the anterior horn cells and peripheral nerves and in uncomplicated diseases of the cerebellum. An increase in tone is found in upper motor neuron diseases (pyramidal tract), in which case it is characterized as *spasticity*. Spasticity is the most common abnormality of tone and is classically of the clasp-knife type. The tone varies from normal as one rapidly extends or flexes the joint to a marked increase when full flexion or extension is approached. With continued pressure the muscle then gradually gives way.

On the other hand, *rigidity,* which characterizes the extrapyramidal group of diseases such as parkinsonism, is characterized by an increase of tone that is present throughout the full range of motion of the joint, producing steady resistance to the examiner's superimposed movement. In addition there may be a "cogwheeling," as mentioned above.

A tendency to slowed relaxation of the muscles is characteristic of such diseases as hypothyroidism, myotonia, and myotonic dystrophy. It is most evident in patients with myotonia. It may be demonstrated by percussion of affected muscles, such as the quadriceps, the forearm groups, or the thenar muscles, with the reflex hammer. The percussed muscle will contract and then relax at a rate several times slower than normal.

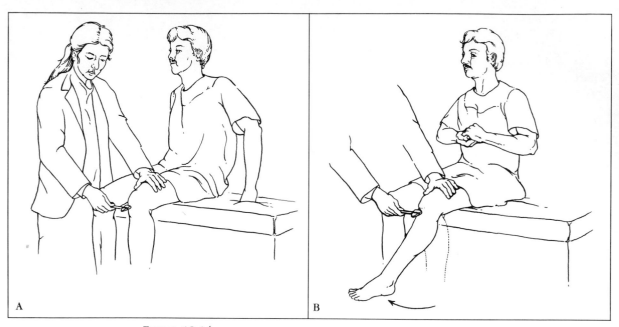

FIGURE 18-14
Reinforcement of the patellar reflex. A. Patient at rest. B. Patient pulls against his own fingers just as tendon is struck.

REFLEXES

Check the biceps, triceps, radial periosteal, patellar, and Achilles reflexes in all patients. The tendon (or bone) is struck directly and smartly with the reflex hammer. The limb to be tested should be relaxed and in a flexed or semiflexed position. The biceps reflex is best tested by tapping the examiner's finger or thumb, which has been placed over the patient's tendon.

In normal young adults reflexes may be minimal or apparently absent and may be elicited only by asking the patient to "reinforce" by pulling with one hand against the other at the time the tendon is tapped (Fig. 18-14). A reflex is not considered truly absent until there is proof that it cannot be elicited by this maneuver. In certain patients the reflexes may be extremely active, but sustained *clonus* (persistent involuntary flexion and extension of the joint under extension or flexion pressure) is never present in the absence of central nervous system disease.

It is good to develop the habit of charting all the reflexes completely. This is easily done by drawing the figure of a man, labeling the sides right and left, and placing the state of the reflex represented by 0 through 4+ at the appropriate joint. An abbreviated chart may also be used for this purpose. Reflexes may be represented as follows: 0, absent; 1+, decreased; 2+, normal; 3+, hyperactive; 4+, hyperactive with clonus. These methods are illustrated in Figure 18-15.

Reflex asymmetry has more pathologic significance than the absolute activity of the reflex. That is, 3+ hyperreflexia bilaterally in the knee jerks may occur as a result of anxiety, for example, and is less diagnostic of neurologic abnormality than a 3+ reflex in the right knee with 2+ in the left. The reflex examination is one of

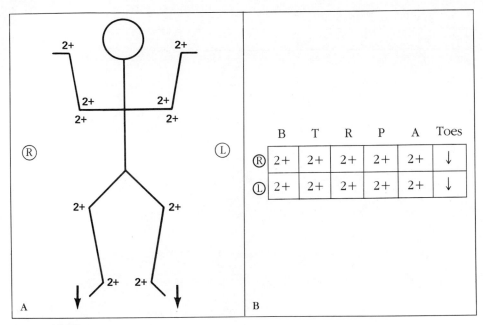

FIGURE 18-15
Recording the reflexes. One may record the deep tendon reflexes by drawing them on a stick figure (A) or may record them graphically (B) in the written physical. The examiner should always designate the normal on his or her scale.

the most important parts of the neurologic examination because abnormalities in this sphere are difficult to feign and thus represent an objective assessment of the patient's neurologic status. Anything that interferes with the anterior horn cell, the sensory or the motor part of the reflex arc, the motor end-plate, or the muscle may eliminate or decrease the reflex. On the other hand, a pathologic increase in reflexes almost invariably represents disease of the upper motor neuron or pyramidal tract. The lesion, of course, can by anywhere from the cerebral cortex to just above the appropriate anterior horn cell. Any isolated reflex change, either increase or decrease, requires special consideration by the examiner.

It is important to memorize a few reflex arc levels that are helpful in determining the level of spinal cord lesions (see Table 18-6).

PATHOLOGIC REFLEXES. The pathologic reflexes are extremely important and should be carefully looked for. There are two basic pathologic reflexes—the *Babinski* and its variants, and the *Hoffmann* and its variants.

The *Babinski reflex* is tested by stroking the sole of the foot with a pointed instrument from the heel, along the lateral edge of the foot, and then across the ball of the foot medially. The *Chaddock reflex* is elicited by stroking the lateral edge of the foot from the heel to the toes just above the sole. The *Oppenheim reflex* is elicited by firmly pressing down on the shin with the knuckles from the knee to the ankle. The *Gordon reflex* is tested by squeezing the calf firmly. Normally, after infancy, there is no extensor response of the foot and toes to any of these maneuvers.

TABLE 18-6. Reflex Examination

Name	Technique	Reflex Arc Level
Biceps		C 5–6
Triceps		C 6–7–8
Radial periosteal		C 5–6

TABLE 18-6. (Continued)

Name	Technique	Reflex Arc Level
Patellar		L 2–3–4

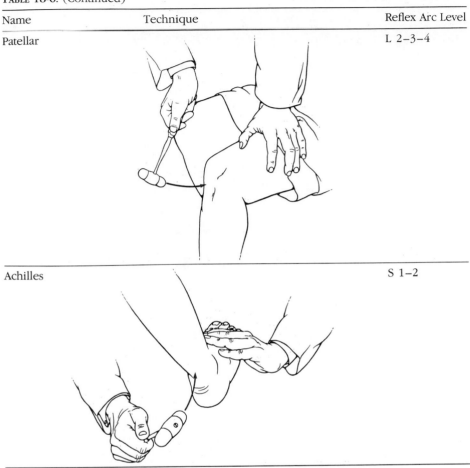

| Achilles | | S 1–2 |

Therefore, the presence of these reflexes is an unequivocal sign of disease of the pyramidal tract (Table 18-7).

With extensive pyramidal tract disease there may be some withdrawal of the entire leg with flexion at the ankle, knee, and hip.

There are several sources of difficulty in interpreting the Babinski response. At times the response may be equivocal with perhaps only fleeting dorsiflexion of the large toe and no fanning of the other toes. There may be no response to plantar stimulation at all; when this occurs, it is usually significant if there is a difference in the responses of the two feet. Another source of difficulty is the tendency of some patients voluntarily to withdraw their lower extremity when the sole of the foot is stimulated. Often this can be overcome by simply asking them not to withdraw. Some Babinski responses are strongly abnormal, with withdrawal of the entire lower extremity, and yet are stated to be equivocal because the examiner incor-

TABLE 18-7. Reflex Examination in Pyramidal Tract Disease

Reflex	Technique	Illustration
Babinski	Firmly hold the knee or ankle to prevent withdrawal Stroke the **lateral** sole of the foot with a blunt point (a key is good for this); the stroke must not be painful A Babinski sign (extensor plantar response) is dorsiflexion of the great toe with fanning of the other toes	
Chaddock	Stroke with a blunt point around the side of the foot, from external malleolus to the small toe In a positive test, there is dorsiflexion of the great toe	
Oppenheim	Firmly press down on the shin and run the thumb and the knuckles along the anterior medial tibia toward the foot In a positive test, there is dorsiflexion of the great toe	

TABLE 18-7. (Continued)

Reflex	Technique	Illustration
Gordon	Firmly squeeze the calf The great toe dorsiflexes in a positive test	

rectly thinks that the withdrawal is voluntary and not part of the reflex. It is only with experience that the examiner learns to differentiate between these two types of withdrawals.

The Babinski response is one of the most reliable signs in neurology and should be tested for in all patients. A Babinski sign, from a semantic point of view is either present or absent, not positive or negative.

The *Hoffmann reflex* is tested by quickly extending or flexing the last joint of the middle finger. While suspending the limp hand by its middle finger, quickly flip the tip of the finger upward or downward (Fig. 18-16). Normally there is very little if any response to this maneuver, but a flexion response of the thumb and fingers is not an unequivocal sign of pyramidal tract disease. It should be equated more with the tendon reflexes and is only significant when markedly exaggerated or unilaterally present.

Clonus is tested by quickly flexing or extending a joint and maintaining the tension (Fig. 18-17).

SUPERFICIAL SKIN REFLEXES. The main superficial reflexes are the abdominal and cremasteric reflexes. The *abdominal reflex* in men and women is elicited by stroking with a firm or slightly irritating object (such as a somewhat sharp stick) over all four quadrants of the abdomen. The stroke can be directed either toward or away from or at right angles to the umbilicus. Normally the umbilicus moves toward the stimulus. The *cremasteric reflex* in men is elicited by stroking along the internal aspect of the upper thigh. A normal response results in an upward movement of the testicle on the side stimulated due to involuntary contraction of the cremaster muscle (Fig. 18-18).

Both of these reflexes are normally present in the young, relaxed patient, but their absence is common and may be due to a variety of causes. Diseases of either the upper or the lower motor neurons will eliminate the superficial reflexes. In

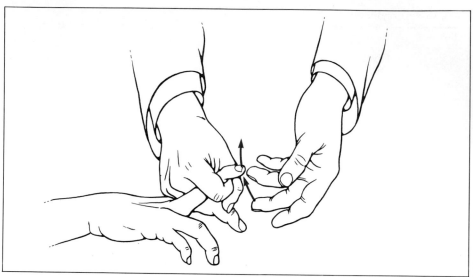

FIGURE 18-16
Hoffmann reflex.

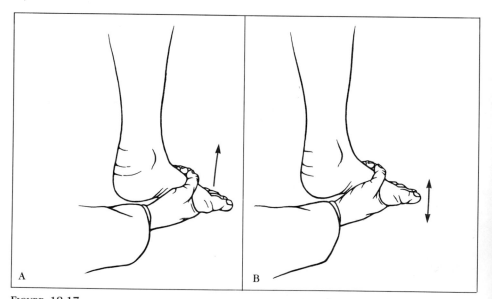

FIGURE 18-17
Testing for clonus at the ankle. A. Grasp and quickly dorsiflex the foot. B. Holding the foot in dorsiflexion, you will feel the rhythmic contractions ("beats") in your hand.

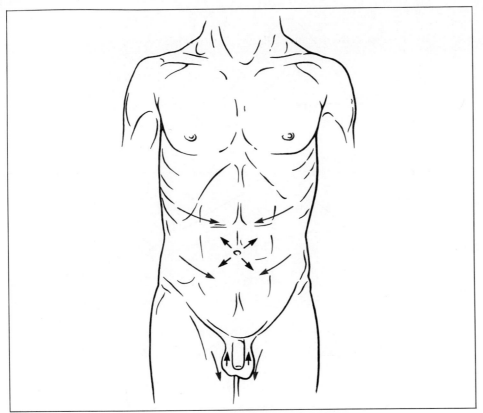

FIGURE 18-18
Abdominal and cremasteric reflexes. Sites of testing for these superficial reflexes are indicated by red arrows. Reflex response is indicated by black arrows.

addition the superficial reflexes may be difficult to elicit in the tense, obese, pregnant, or uncooperative patient. Although they have been said to be of special significance when absent, they are not usually of diagnostic importance. Unilateral absence or absence of either the upper or lower abdominals may be of significance and may be helpful in ascertaining the "sidedness" of a lesion, or the level of a lesion in the spinal cord. In this regard it is important to remember that the upper abdominals are innervated by segments T7 through T9 and the lower by T9 through T11.

CEREBELLAR FUNCTION
Coordination and the ability to perform skilled and rapid alternating movements in the upper and lower extremities are tests of cerebellar function.

UPPER EXTREMITIES. The patient is asked to supinate and pronate his hand alternately as rapidly as possible on each side. He should be able to perform rapid alternating movements nearly as well with his nondominant as with his dominant hand. Direct him to touch the index finger of his outstretched arm to the tip of his nose slowly, with his eyes closed (finger-to-nose test). The ability to perform rapid fine move-

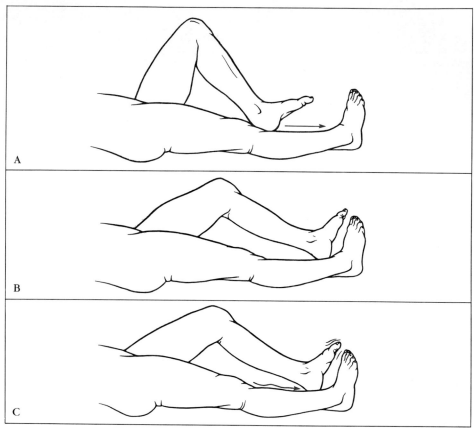

FIGURE 18-19
Heel-to-knee-to-toe test. A. Beginning the test. B. Normal result: The heel runs smoothly and straight down the shin. C. Abnormal result: The heel is ataxic and jerky and may even fall off the shin.

ments of the fingers, such as touching the tip of the index finger to the thumb, can also be assessed.

LOWER EXTREMITIES. Ask the patient to tap his foot against the floor as rapidly as possible, then direct him to touch one heel to the opposite knee and run it slowly down his shin to the big toe (heel-to-knee-to-toe test) (Fig.18-19).

Normally the patient is able to perform these maneuvers without any wavering, tremor, or ataxia. The heel-to-knee-to-toe test should show no falling off of the heel from the shin. The patient should be able to tap the floor quickly with either foot.

Many things may interfere with cerebellar testing or may give false cerebellar signs. Among these are sensory loss, especially loss of proprioception. In addition pyramidal tract disease may give slowness in cerebellar testing; marked weakness of lower motor neuron or peripheral nerve origin may also show this slowness. A combination of these defects may produce cerebellarlike signs that make it difficult to determine whether or not the ataxia is really of cerebellar origin. Certainly one

TABLE 18-8. Some Causes of Ataxia

Generalized weakness or fatigue of any cause

Drugs and toxins
  Alcohol
  Sedative-hypnotics
  Phenytoin (Dilantin)
  Narcotics

Sensory defects
  Posterior column disease
    Vitamin B_{12} deficiency
    Tabes dorsalis (syphilis)
    Diabetes
  Peripheral neuropathy (if severe)
    Diabetes
    Alcoholism
    Guillain-Barré syndrome
    Vasculitis (rare)
    Porphyria
    Carcinomatous neuropathy
    Nutritional disorders
  Multiple sclerosis of the cord
  Lesions of the thalamus, internal capsule, sensory cortex

Cerebellar lesions
  Multiple sclerosis
  Alcoholism
  Vascular events
    Thrombosis
    Bleeding
  Hereditary ataxia
  Tumor

Hysteria

should be careful to do adequate sensory testing on any patient with apparent cerebellar disease to determine whether or not proprioception is intact.

Disease of one cerebellar hemisphere produces signs on the same side of the
body. That fact is important to remember when attempting to localize a lesion because the thalamic, pontine, and occasionally frontal lobe lesions of the opposite
side may produce ataxia similar to that from involvement of the cerebellum itself.
Since some diseases are characterized by the production of cerebellar signs that
are more prominent in the distal or the proximal parts of the extremities, it is important to state the exact nature and location of the tremor or ataxia. In addition,
since ataxia may be drug-induced and therefore transitory, it may be necessary to
test the patient more than once. Some causes of ataxia are presented in Table 18-8.

STATION AND GAIT
Ask the patient to walk as normally as possible for some distance. Notice his general
posture, the size of his steps, the lateral distance between his feet as he places them
on the ground, the amount of associated arm swinging present, and his balance
while walking. Test his ability to start and stop on command. Sometimes walking
will be normal but running impossible. If walking balance is to be tested further,

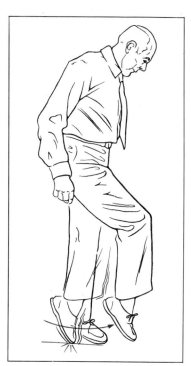

FIGURE 18-20
Steppage or footdrop gait. To avoid dragging his toes against the ground, (since he cannot dorsiflex the foot), the patient lifts his knee high and slaps the foot to the ground on advancing.

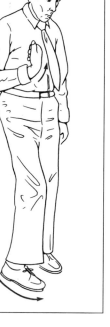

FIGURE 18-21
Hemiplegic (hemiparetic) gait. The arm is carried across the trunk, adducted at the shoulder. The forearm is rotated; the arm is flexed at elbow and wrist and the hand at the metacarpophalangeal joints. The leg is extended at the hip and knee. The patient either swings his affected leg outward in a circle (circumduction) or pushes it ahead of him.

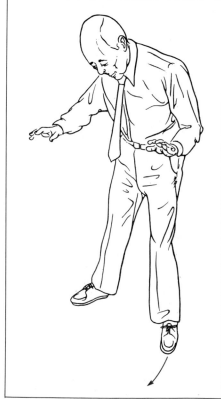

FIGURE 18-22
Ataxic gait. In *cerebellar ataxia* the patient has poor balance and a broad base; therefore he lurches, staggers, and exaggerates all movements. In *sensory ataxia* the patient has a broadbased gait and, since he cannot feel his feet, slaps them against the ground and looks down at them as he walks. In both types of ataxias the gait is irregular, jerky, and weaving.

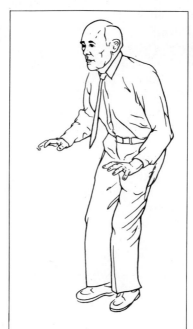

FIGURE 18-23
Parkinsonism. The head, trunk, and knees are flexed; the arms are held rather stiffly with poor associative movement. The gait is shuffling or characterized at times by short, rapid steps (marche à petits pas). The patient may lean forward and walk progressively faster, seemingly unable to stop himself (festination).

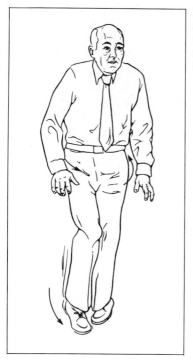

FIGURE 18-24
Scissors gait. Spasticity of thigh adduction, seen in spastic paraplegics, draws the knees together. The legs are advanced (with great effort) by swinging the hips.

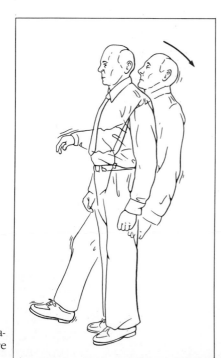

FIGURE 18-25
Positive indication of Romberg's sign. The patient falls backward only when his eyes are closed.

the patient can be asked to walk a straight line, putting one heel directly in front of the toes of the other foot. This is called *tandem walking*.

Abnormalities in gait should be described as closely as possible. A difference in length of stride between the feet should be mentioned. Any tendency toward dragging of the toes and high lifting of the knees due to weakness of the dorsiflexors of the feet (*footdrop gait* of peroneal palsy or multiple neuritus) (Fig. 18-20) should also be commented on. The *hemiplegic gait* (Fig. 18-21) with circumduction of the affected leg, weakness of dorsiflexion of the foot, and some tendency toward flexion at the knee on the affected side is a classic characteristic of corticospinal tract damage. Similarly the wide-based *ataxic gait* (drunken gait) (Fig. 18-22) is the classic gait of cerebellar dysfunction. Also diagnostic is the typical *gait of parkinsonism* (Fig. 18-23), with small shuffling steps, lack of normal arm swing, flexion of the trunk, and a tendency to increase the speed and fall forward. The dancing gait of advanced *Huntington's chorea* is distinctive, as are the wormlike, athetoid movements of the limbs and trunk in athetosis. Congenital spasticity (Little's disease) produces a *scissors gait* (Fig. 18-24), with a tendency toward internal rotation of both legs and scraping together of the semiflexed knees as the patient drags them forward. The typical gait of *tabes dorsalis* is characterized by ataxia, foot slapping, and a tendency for the patient to watch his feet (since he does not know where they are) when he walks.

The patient's standing balance is tested for *Romberg's sign* by asking him to stand with his feet together, first with his eyes open and then with his eyes closed. The examiner should be ready to catch the patient, as there is often a tendency to fall when eyes are closed. Finer tests of balance include standing on one foot and hopping or jumping on one foot.

Indications of Romberg's sign are positive only when the patient falls backward with his eyes closed and his feet together and *does not fall with his eyes open* (Fig. 18-25). In falling, knees do not flex, and arms are thrown forward in an attempt to right oneself. This is said to be diagnostic of posterior column disease but may also be found in unilateral or bilateral weakness, cerebellar disease, or disease of the peripheral nerves.

SENSORY EXAMINATION

GENERAL

The sensory examination is difficult to perform well and interpret correctly. It is subject to great variation, depending on the experience and skill of the examiner and the cooperation and emotional balance of the patient. It is of primary importance, however, and can give clues to a diagnosis that can be obtained in no other way. Sensory testing is usually done with the patient's eyes closed.

VIBRATION, MOTION, AND POSITION (POSTERIOR COLUMN SENSES)

With a 128-cycle tuning fork, test the duration of vibration perceived on a bony prominence in all four extremities. Use the lateral malleolus on each ankle and the first knuckle of each hand. The tuning fork should be struck with the same strength and held with the same degree of firmness against each prominence. In this way a fairly good quantitive estimate of vibratory sense can be obtained (Fig. 18-26). Next, grasp one toe or finger of each of the four extremities, move it up and down, and

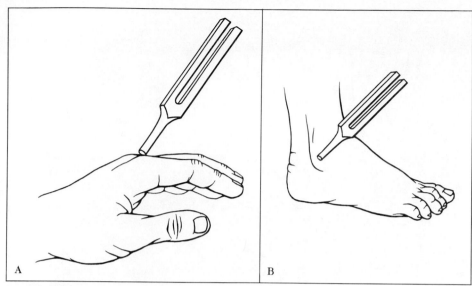

FIGURE 18-26
Testing for vibration sense. A. Upper extremity. B. Lower extremity.

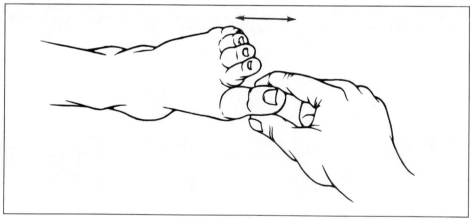

FIGURE 18-27
Testing for position sense in the lower extremity.

ask the patient to identify the digit with his eyes closed (Fig. 18-27). After moving the digit up and down repeatedly, leave it in the upward or downward position and ask him to identify its direction. Ideally the digit should be grasped by the sides rather than the top and bottom, but that hold is not always feasible. The vibratory sense is the best and most easily assessed posterior column function and therefore should be tested in all patients. Position and motor sense are usually not decreased until vibratory sense is markedly diminished or lost.

In addition to giving an index to posterior column function, vibratory sense may also be used to determine the level of a spinal cord lesion. Simply "walk" up the body with a tuning fork, going from bony prominence to bony prominence until

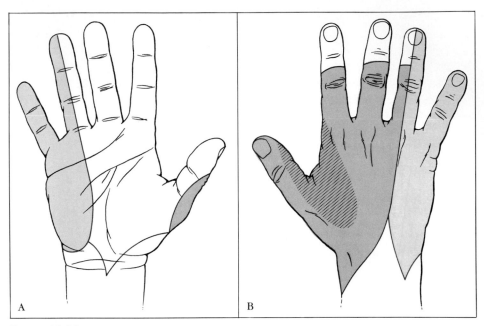

FIGURE 18-28
Sensory change on the hand with peripheral nerve injury. A. Palm. B. Dorsum. Cross-hatching indicates area of "pure" radial nerve supply, the only area of sensory loss in some patients with radial nerve loss. Ulnar area is pink; median, white; radial, shaded.

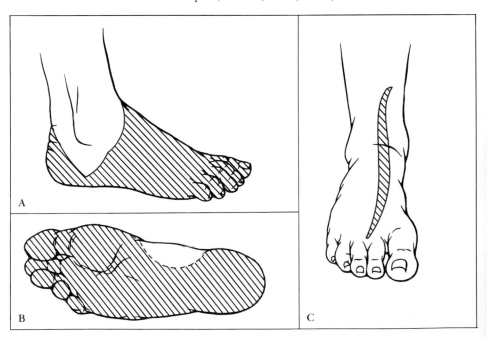

FIGURE 18-29
Sensory change on the foot with peripheral neuropathy. A. Sciatic nerve. B. Tibial nerve. C. Common peroneal nerve.

vibration is felt by the patient. The level of sensory perception in the bones corresponds well to that of the skin over them. If vibratory sense is intact, it is usually not necessary to test motion and position sense. If vibratory sense is decreased or absent, motion and position sense should be tested. If motion and position sense are absent in the toes, for instance, they should then be tested at progressively higher levels. Some diseases are characterized by posterior column sensory loss (posterolateral sclerosis) and will show marked loss of vibratory and motion and position senses.

PAIN AND TEMPERATURE

Pinprick testing may be more often misleading than helpful. Temperature sensation can be tested with any cool or warm object. The tines of the examiner's tuning fork or the metal handle of the reflex hammer will often serve well enough. Temperature testing, which gives the same information, often serves better than the pinprick test to check the spinothalamic system because it does not produce withdrawal. The sensations of both pain and temperature need not be routinely tested inasmuch as they travel the same pathway. If temperature testing shows abnormality, you may outline the areas of definite loss with the pin (Figs. 18-28 and 18-29).

Pinprick sensation is tricky to test, and one may easily obtain abnormal responses in a normal person. Such difficulties are partly due to the natural variations in the pressure put on the pin and the sensitivity of different areas of the skin. Some patients, especially the neurotic and some highly intelligent, careful individuals, may report pinprick decrease that is not significant. In this case the examiner is wise to go to some other part of the examination and then return later so as not to emphasize the "abnormality" that he has found. Another error in examining with a pin occurs when testing one side of the body against the other. The second or last side tested will often apparently be more sensitive to the pinprick. In this case the examiner should reverse the order of the sides tested.

Pinprick testing is the most common way of determining the sensory "level" caused by a spinal cord lesion. There is usually an area of increased response to the pin at the level of the lesion, normal response above the level, and decreased response below.

Deep pain sensation may be assessed by firmly pinching the Achilles tendon or the thenar eminence. Squeezing the nipple or testicle is a barbaric method of deep pain testing, in our opinion.

FINE SENSORY MODALITIES

Fine sensory modalities include touch, two-point tactile sensation, stereognosis, graphesthesia, and extinction. Test for *light touch* with a wisp of cotton on the hairy surfaces of the body. Include the trunk and all four extremities, and test one side against the other. Normally a very light wisp of cotton can be felt only on the hairy surfaces, and the movement of one hair can usually be perceived. However, very light touch that does not indent the nonhairy skin, such as the palms or soles, frequently cannot be perceived.

Two-point tactile discrimination is tested with two dull points. Ask the patient to close his eyes; then simultaneously touch two places on the same extremity. Compare one side of the body to the other. The threshold at which the patient feels two distinct points, or conversely at which he feels them as one, is recorded. Two-point

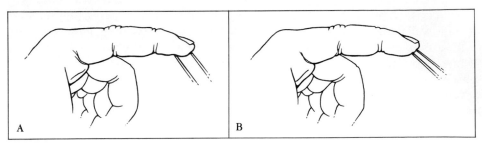

FIGURE 18-30
Two-point discrimination. A. The patient perceives the touch of two wooden sticks at 33 mm apart as two distinct stimuli. B. When the sticks are less than 3 mm apart, the touch is felt as though one stick were being used.

discrimination is usually tested on the tips of the fingers. The threshold on the tip of the index finger on a normal person is about 3 mm, that is, the points are 3 mm apart or less when they are perceived as one (Fig. 18-30).

Stereognosis is tested in the hands. Ask the patient to close his eyes and identify objects placed in his hands by moving them around and feeling them with his fingers. Any convenient objects, such as coins and keys, can be used. A normal person can differentiate between a penny, nickel, quarter, and half dollar.

Test *graphesthesia* by drawing numerals on various parts of the patient's skin and asking him to identify them. The size of the identifiable numeral will naturally vary with the area.

Extinction (*suppression*) can be tested by the method of double simultaneous stimulation. Have the patient close his eyes, and touch him, for example, on the back of the hand. Ask him where he was touched. Touch him then on the identical spot on the other side of his body and repeat the question. The third time, touch him in both places simultaneously and with equal pressure. Suppression is normally not present, and the patient feels both sides. If extinction is present, it is usually significant.

Since motion, position, and vibratory senses have already been checked to test the function of the posterior columns, most of the finer modalities do not need to be tested in the usual patient. However, they are useful in evaluating parietal cortex function and should be tested when disease is suspected in that region. If a patient demonstrates extinction or suppression, he will feel the stimulus only on his "good" side, which will be opposite his normal parietal lobe.

Since these finer sensory modalities travel in the posterior columns of the spinal cord, they also may be useful in the analysis of hysterical (conversion reaction) sensory loss. Some patients with hysterical sensory loss have loss of vibration but good stereognosis. The reverse of this may also occasionally be true.

Before stating that a patient has astereognosis, one should be careful to determine that there is no more obvious sensory loss in the extremity. If there is a definite sensory loss in the extremity and stereognosis is also decreased, the loss would better be called stereoanesthesia and does not necessarily indicate parietal cortex dysfunction.

CONVERSION REACTION

Although many neurotic patients may present with neurologic complaints of functional origin, the diagnosis of hysteria or conversion reaction on the basis of findings on the neurologic examination is dangerous. It is true that a stocking or glove anesthesia, a sensory defect extending exactly to the midline, a sensory defect with changing borders, paralysis of the legs or of half the body, "giving way" on strength testing, and other "hysterical" neurologic findings can be and sometimes are nonorganic, but they are also found in bona fide neurologic disease. A stocking or glove sensory loss is also found in peripheral neuritis; a hemisensory defect to the midline is found in several types of lesions of the brain stem and spinal cord; and normally there is some variability in the borders of most true sensory defects. The organic causes of paraplegia are many, and anyone with such a defect, if it is recent, will naturally demonstrate some anxiety and perhaps appear hysterical. The same is true of a hemiparesis. Giving way on strength testing may be found when testing patients with true weaknesses. One must be wary of making an easy diagnosis of hysteria. Many a spinal cord tumor has delivered its fatal blow while the physician was investigating the psyche. Such confusion is as great an error as treating a patient for organic disease when there is none.

SECTION VII
SPECIAL EXAMINATIONS

Christopher Robin
Had wheezles
And sneezles,
They bundled him
Into
His bed.
They gave him what goes
With a cold in the nose,
And some more for a cold
In the head.
They wondered
If wheezles
Could turn
Into measles,
If sneezles
Would turn
Into mumps;
They examined his chest
For a rash,
And the rest
Of his body for swellings
   and lumps.

A. A. MILNE
(1882–1956)

PEDIATRIC EXAMINATION

CHAPTER 19

Science is essentially a matter of observation, inference, verification, generalization. The mind of Sydenham, interested in a sick child and humanely preoccupied with its cure, did not, insofar as it functioned scientifically, operate differently from that of Galileo, interested in cosmic physics. Both alike observed, reflected, verified, generalized.

ABRAHAM FLEXNER
(1866–1959)

The child is not a miniature adult. Characteristics and measurements outlined in this chapter constitute important references with regard to both history and physical examination and serve as guides in evaluating normality or abnormality. Always remember that in contrast to the nearly static adult, children are everchanging organisms.

ANATOMY AND NORMALS

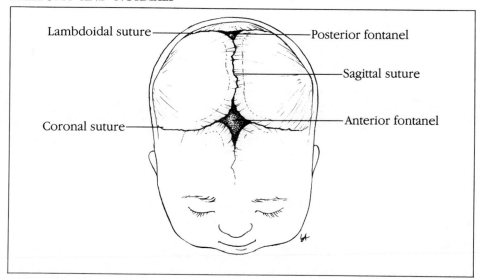

FIGURE 19-1
Skull of the child.

I'll just have to save him. Because, after all, A person's a person, no matter how small.

"DR. SEUSS" (THEODOR S. GEISEL)
(1904–   )

TABLE 19-1. Weight and Height Percentile Table: Boys (Birth to 18 Years)

Weight in Pounds			Weight in Kilograms			Age	Height in Inches			Height in Centimeters		
10%	50%	90%	10%	50%	90%		10%	50%	90%	10%	50%	90%
6.3	7.5	9.1	2.86	3.4	4.13	Birth	18.9	19.9	21.0	48.1	50.6	53.3
8.5	10.0	11.5	3.8	4.6	5.2	1 mo	20.2	21.2	22.2	50.4	53.0	55.5
10.0	11.5	13.2	4.6	5.2	6.0	2 mo	21.5	22.5	23.5	53.7	56.0	60.0
11.1	12.6	14.5	5.03	5.72	6.58	3 mo	22.8	23.8	24.7	57.8	60.4	62.8
12.5	14.0	16.2	5.6	6.3	7.3	4 mo	23.7	24.7	25.7	60.5	62.0	65.2
13.7	15.0	17.7	6.2	7.0	8.0	5 mo	24.5	25.5	26.5	61.8	65.0	67.3
14.8	16.7	19.2	6.71	7.58	8.71	6 mo	25.2	26.1	27.3	63.9	66.4	69.3
17.8	20.0	22.9	8.07	9.07	10.39	9 mo	27.0	28.0	29.2	68.6	71.2	74.2
19.6	22.2	25.4	8.89	10.7	11.52	12 mo	28.5	29.6	30.7	72.4	75.2	78.1
22.3	25.2	29.0	10.12	11.43	13.15	18 mo	31.0	32.2	33.5	78.8	81.3	85.0
24.7	27.7	31.9	11.2	12.56	14.47	2 yr	33.1	34.4	35.9	84.2	87.5	91.1
26.6	30.0	34.5	12.07	13.61	15.65	2½ yr	34.8	36.3	37.9	88.5	92.1	96.2
28.7	32.2	36.8	13.02	14.61	16.69	3 yr	36.3	37.9	39.6	92.3	96.2	100.5
30.4	34.3	39.1	13.79	15.56	17.74	3½ yr	37.8	39.3	41.1	96.0	99.8	104.5
32.1	36.4	41.4	14.56	16.51	18.78	4 yr	39.1	40.7	42.7	99.3	103.4	108.5
33.8	38.4	43.9	15.33	17.42	19.91	4½ yr	40.3	42.0	44.2	102.4	106.7	112.3
35.5	40.5	46.7	16.1	18.37	21.18	5 yr	40.8	42.8	45.2	103.7	108.7	114.7
38.8	45.6	53.1	17.6	20.68	24.09	5½ yr	42.6	45.0	47.3	108.3	114.4	120.1
40.9	48.3	56.4	18.55	21.91	25.58	6 yr	43.8	46.3	48.6	111.2	117.5	123.5
43.4	51.2	60.4	19.69	23.22	27.4	6½ yr	44.9	47.6	50.0	114.1	120.8	127.0
45.8	54.1	64.4	20.77	24.54	29.21	7 yr	46.0	48.9	51.4	116.9	124.1	130.5
48.5	57.1	68.7	22.0	25.9	31.16	7½ yr	47.2	50.0	52.7	120.0	127.1	133.9
51.2	60.1	73.0	23.22	27.26	33.11	8 yr	48.5	51.2	54.0	123.1	130.0	137.3
53.8	63.1	77.0	24.4	28.62	34.93	8½ yr	49.5	52.3	55.1	125.7	132.8	140.0
56.3	66.0	81.0	25.54	29.94	36.74	9 yr	50.5	53.3	56.1	128.3	135.5	142.6
58.7	69.0	85.5	26.63	31.3	38.78	9½ yr	51.4	54.3	57.1	130.6	137.9	145.1
61.1	71.9	89.9	27.71	32.61	40.78	10 yr	52.3	55.2	58.1	132.8	140.3	147.5
63.7	74.8	94.6	28.89	33.93	42.91	10½ yr	53.2	56.0	58.9	135.1	142.3	149.7
66.3	77.6	99.3	30.07	35.2	45.04	11 yr	54.0	56.8	59.8	137.3	144.2	151.8
69.2	81.0	104.5	31.39	36.74	47.4	11½ yr	55.0	57.8	60.9	139.8	146.9	154.8
72.0	84.4	109.6	32.66	38.28	49.71	12 yr	56.1	58.9	62.2	142.4	149.6	157.9
74.6	88.7	116.4	33.84	40.23	52.8	12½ yr	56.9	60.0	63.6	144.5	152.3	161.6
77.1	93.0	123.2	34.97	42.18	55.88	13 yr	57.7	61.0	65.1	146.6	155.0	165.3
82.2	100.3	130.1	37.29	45.5	59.01	13½ yr	58.8	62.6	66.5	149.4	158.9	168.9
87.2	107.6	136.9	39.55	48.81	62.1	14 yr	59.9	64.0	67.9	152.1	162.7	172.4
93.3	113.9	142.4	42.32	51.66	64.59	14½ yr	61.0	65.1	68.7	155.0	165.3	174.6
99.4	120.1	147.8	45.09	54.48	67.04	15 yr	62.1	66.1	69.6	157.8	167.8	176.7
105.2	124.9	152.6	47.72	56.65	69.22	15½ yr	63.1	66.8	70.2	160.3	169.7	178.2
111.0	129.7	157.3	50.35	58.83	71.35	16 yr	64.1	67.8	70.7	162.8	171.6	179.7
114.3	133.0	161.0	51.85	60.33	73.03	16½ yr	64.6	68.0	71.1	164.2	172.7	180.7
117.5	136.2	164.6	53.3	61.78	74.66	17 yr	65.2	68.4	71.5	165.5	173.7	181.6
118.3	137.6	166.8	53.89	62.41	75.66	17½ yr	65.3	68.5	71.6	165.9	174.1	182.0
120.0	139.0	169.0	54.43	63.05	76.66	18 yr	65.5	68.7	71.8	166.3	174.5	182.4

Source: From G. H. Lowrey, *Growth and Development of Children* (7th ed.). Chicago: Year Book Medical Publishers, 1978.

TABLE 19-2. Weight and Height Percentile Table: Girls (Birth to 18 Years)

Weight in Pounds			Weight in Kilograms			Age	Height in Inches			Height in Centimeters		
10%	50%	90%	10%	50%	90%		10%	50%	90%	10%	50%	90%
6.2	7.4	8.6	2.81	3.36	3.9	Birth	18.8	19.8	20.4	47.8	50.2	51.0
8.0	9.7	11.0	3.3	4.2	5.0	1 mo	20.2	21.0	22.0	50.4	52.8	55.0
9.5	11.0	12.5	4.1	5.0	5.8	2 mo	21.5	22.2	23.2	53.7	55.5	59.6
10.7	12.4	14.0	4.85	5.62	6.35	3 mo	22.4	23.4	24.3	56.9	59.5	61.7
12.0	13.7	15.5	5.3	6.2	7.2	4 mo	23.2	24.2	25.2	59.6	61.0	64.8
13.0	14.7	17.0	5.9	6.8	7.7	5 mo	24.0	25.0	26.0	60.7	64.2	67.0
14.1	16.0	18.6	6.4	7.26	8.44	6 mo	24.6	25.7	26.7	62.5	65.2	67.8
16.6	19.2	22.4	7.53	8.71	10.16	9 mo	26.4	27.6	28.7	67.0	70.1	72.9
18.4	21.5	24.8	8.35	9.75	11.25	12 mo	27.8	29.2	30.3	70.6	74.2	77.1
21.2	24.5	28.3	9.62	11.11	12.84	18 mo	30.2	31.8	33.3	76.8	80.9	84.5
23.5	27.1	31.7	10.66	12.29	14.38	2 yr	32.3	34.1	35.8	82.0	86.6	91.0
25.5	29.6	34.6	11.57	13.43	15.69	2½ yr	34.0	36.0	37.9	86.3	91.4	96.4
27.6	31.8	37.4	12.52	14.42	16.96	3 yr	35.6	37.7	39.8	90.5	95.7	101.1
29.5	33.9	40.4	13.38	15.38	18.33	3½ yr	37.1	39.2	41.5	94.2	99.5	105.4
31.2	36.2	43.5	14.15	16.42	19.73	4 yr	38.4	40.6	43.1	97.6	103.2	109.6
32.9	38.5	46.7	14.92	17.46	21.18	4½ yr	39.7	42.0	44.7	100.9	106.8	113.5
34.8	40.5	49.2	15.79	18.37	22.32	5 yr	40.5	42.9	45.4	103.0	109.1	115.4
38.0	44.0	51.2	17.24	19.96	23.22	5½ yr	42.4	44.4	46.8	107.8	112.8	118.9
39.6	46.5	54.2	17.96	21.09	24.58	6 yr	43.5	45.6	48.1	110.6	115.9	122.3
42.2	49.4	57.7	19.14	22.41	26.17	6½ yr	44.8	46.9	49.4	113.7	119.1	125.6
44.5	52.2	61.2	20.19	23.68	27.76	7 yr	46.0	48.1	50.7	116.8	122.3	128.9
46.6	55.2	65.6	21.14	25.04	29.76	7½ yr	47.0	49.3	51.9	119.5	125.2	131.8
48.6	58.1	69.9	22.04	26.35	31.71	8 yr	48.1	50.4	53.0	122.1	128.0	134.6
50.6	61.0	74.5	22.95	27.67	33.79	8½ yr	49.0	51.4	54.1	124.6	130.5	137.5
52.6	63.8	79.1	23.86	28.94	35.88	9 yr	50.0	52.3	55.3	127.0	132.9	140.4
54.9	67.1	84.4	24.9	30.44	38.28	9½ yr	50.9	53.5	56.4	129.4	135.8	143.2
57.1	70.3	89.7	25.9	31.89	40.69	10 yr	51.8	54.6	57.5	131.7	138.6	146.0
59.9	74.6	95.1	27.17	33.79	43.14	10½ yr	52.9	55.8	58.9	134.4	141.7	149.7
62.6	78.8	100.4	28.4	35.74	45.54	11 yr	53.9	57.0	60.4	137.0	144.7	153.4
66.1	83.2	106.0	29.98	37.74	48.08	11½ yr	55.0	58.3	61.8	139.8	148.1	157.0
69.5	87.6	111.5	31.52	39.74	50.58	12 yr	56.1	59.8	63.2	142.6	151.9	160.6
74.7	93.4	118.0	33.88	42.37	53.52	12½ yr	57.4	60.7	64.0	145.9	154.3	162.7
79.9	99.1	124.5	36.24	44.95	56.47	13 yr	58.7	61.8	64.9	149.1	157.1	164.8
85.5	103.7	128.9	38.78	47.04	58.47	13½ yr	59.5	62.4	65.3	151.1	158.4	165.9
91.0	108.4	133.3	41.28	49.17	60.46	14 yr	60.2	62.8	65.7	153.0	159.6	167.0
94.2	111.0	135.7	42.73	50.35	61.55	14½ yr	60.7	63.1	66.0	154.1	160.4	167.6
97.4	113.5	138.1	44.18	51.48	62.64	15 yr	61.1	63.4	66.2	155.2	161.1	168.1
99.2	115.3	139.6	45.0	52.3	63.32	15½ yr	61.3	63.7	66.4	155.7	161.7	168.6
100.9	117.0	141.1	45.77	53.07	64.0	16 yr	61.5	63.9	66.5	156.1	162.2	169.0
101.9	118.1	142.2	46.22	53.57	64.5	16½ yr	61.5	63.9	66.6	156.2	162.4	169.2
102.8	119.1	143.3	46.63	54.02	65.0	17 yr	61.5	64.0	66.7	156.3	162.5	169.4
103.2	119.5	143.9	46.81	54.2	65.27	17½ yr	61.5	64.0	66.7	156.3	162.5	169.4
103.5	119.9	144.5	46.95	54.39	65.54	18 yr	61.5	64.0	66.7	156.3	162.5	169.4

Source: From G. H. Lowrey, *Growth and Development of Children* (7th ed.). Chicago: Year Book Medical Publishers, 1978.

TABLE 19-3. Average Head Circumference of American Children

Age	Mean		Standard Deviation	
	Inches	Centimeters	Inches	Centimeters
Birth	13.8	35.0	0.5	1.2
3 mo	15.9	40.4	0.5	1.2
6 mo	17.0	43.4	0.4	1.1
12 mo	18.3	46.5	0.5	1.2
18 mo	19.0	48.4	0.5	1.2
2 yr	19.2	49.0	0.5	1.2
3 yr	19.6	50.0	0.5	1.2
4 yr	19.8	50.5	0.5	1.2
5 yr	20.0	50.8	0.6	1.4
6 yr	20.2	51.2	0.6	1.4
7 yr	20.5	51.6	0.6	1.4
8 yr	20.6	52.0	0.8	1.8
10 yr	20.9	53.0	0.6	1.4
12 yr	21.0	53.2	0.8	1.8
14 yr	21.5	54.0	0.8	1.8
16 yr	21.9	55.0	0.8	1.8
18 yr	22.1	55.4	0.8	1.8
20 yr	22.2	55.6	0.8	1.8

Source: From G. H. Lowrey, *Growth and Development of Children* (7th ed.). Chicago: Year Book Medical Publishers, 1978.

TABLE 19-4. Some Developmental Milestones*

Age	Activity
1 mo	Head sags when in sitting position Smiles Regards faces
3 mo	Holds head erect when in sitting position Follows large objects with head and eye
6 mo	Rolls over Reaches and grasps objects
8 mo	Sits erect "Talks" jargon and imitates vowel sounds
10 mo	Effects finger-thumb grasp Pulls self to standing position Says and means ma-ma and da-da
12 mo	Walks with one hand held or alone Releases cube in cup after demonstration Helps in dressing
18 mo	Walks up stairs with support Builds tower of three or more cubes Follows simple verbal directions

* These are examples of developmental stages that will be accomplished by more than half the children in an average population. What is important is the individual's making steady progress with advancing age.

TABLE 19-5. Secondary Sexual Characteristics in American Children

Characteristic	Age
Female fat deposition about pelvis	8–10 yr
Initial breast hypertrophy	9–11 yr
Mature breast development	14–18 yr
Female pubic hair	9–12 yr
Female axillary hair	10–13 yr
Enlargement of penis and testes	10–13 yr
Male pubic hair	10–13 yr
Male axillary hair	11–15 yr
Male facial hair	12–15 yr

TABLE 19-6. Pediatric Vital Signs

Variations in Respiratory Rates (quiet breathing)

Age	Rate per minute
Premature	40–90
Newborn	30–80
1 yr	20–40
2 yr	20–35
4 yr	20–35
10 yr	18–20
Adults	15–18

Average Heart Rate at Rest

Age	Rate per minute
Birth	130–150
1–6 mo	120–140
6–12 mo	110–130
1–2 yr	110–120
2–4 yr	90–110
6–10 yr	90–100
10–14 yr	80–90

Normal Blood Pressure for Various Ages (mm Hg)

Age	Systolic	2 S.D.	Diastolic	2 S.D.
1 mo	86	20	54	18
6 mo	90	26	60	20
1 yr	96	30	65	25
2 yr	99	25	65	25
4 yr	99	20	65	20
6 yr	100	15	60	10
8 yr	105	15	60	10
10 yr	110	17	60	10
12 yr	115	19	60	10
14 yr	118	20	60	10
16 yr	120	16	65	10

Source: From G. H. Lowrey, *Growth and Development of Children* (7th ed.). Chicago: Year Book Medical Publishers, 1978.

HISTORY
Infants do not cry without some legitimate cause.

FERRARIUS
(16th Century)

GENERAL

For several reasons this chapter could be conveniently divided into three parts—the infant, the young child, and the older child and adolescent. The physician approaching the infant must rely totally on the parents for the history of illness, and in his physical examination he must depend almost entirely on objective methods. Although observation of behavior is an essential part of this examination, he cannot obtain the verbal responses that are of such value in an older patient. In the preschool and younger school-aged child some history may be obtained directly, but the physician must still rely on the parent. Fear of the doctor and of what he may do will influence the child's responses during the history taking as well as during the examination. In the older child and adolescent, considerable faith can be put in the responses obtained, although anxiety may still modify their responses to a large extent.

In dealing with children the physician has an advantage in that he is usually confronted with facts unchanged by theories or imaginary ills. Symptoms and physical signs are true and dependable when elicited from the child. Nevertheless the examiner must be even more alert to note the wince that indicates tenderness, the facial expression associated with nausea, the position or posture of greatest comfort, and the presence or absence of a smile in response to an appropriate stimulus, to list just a few examples.

In interviewing children the physician should carefully select his words to be understood. His method of questioning should be slow and deliberate, and his attitude should convey real interest in what the patient says. In very young children a few minutes of play of a casual type may be most helpful in "breaking the ice."

The child and the parents who seek help are often worried and anxious and sometimes feel negligent or guilty. These feelings should be respected and their potential influence in giving information must be considered. Questions or attitudes that are either judgmental or condescending should be avoided. Use openended questions as much as possible. It is important for the adolescent to have an opportunity to talk to the examiner in the absence of parents or other caretakers.

The outline of the history given below will vary in order and in detail depending on what is desired in terms of completeness or on the nature of the patient's illness. The history of a 2-year-old who appears to be retarded would require considerable detail in data relating to the course of pregnancy, method of delivery, birth weight, early feeding problems, times of accomplishing the developmental milestones, and similar elements. The family history relative to genetic factors would be important. Conversely, the history of a 12-year-old who has had no previous problems but now has a fever and a sore throat would require relatively little information about his birth and neonatal history.

The history of a sick child should indicate the background of the child and his family and should answer to some degree the question "In what sort of a child did this sickness develop?" As with the adult, the informant may be guided by the examiner, but he or she should be given the freedom to give a complete record in his or her own words.

History Form

Name _____   Informant _____
Birth date _____   Reliability _____

Chief complaint:

Usually a single symptom in the informant's own words, duration.

Present illness:

Initial symptoms, date of onset, subsequent symptoms chronologically, pertinent negative data by direct questions.

Past history:

1. Birth and neonatal: prenatal care, mother's illnesses during pregnancy; gestation time; labor, delivery (position, instruments, etc.); birth weight; immediate cry, cyanosis (duration, therapy); jaundice (duration, therapy); days hospitalized; early feeding (breast, bottle, difficulties); early weight gain.
2. Developmental milestones (examples are given in Table 19-4): toilet training, grade in school, school difficulties and progress. Do parents consider the child either unusually easy or difficult to manage?
3. Feeding history (mainly for young children): breast feeding (duration, etc.); formula (ingredients, changes in formula and why); schedule, duration and quantity per feeding (apparent cause of prolonged feeding time); weight at various ages; solids (when started and how received); vomiting (relation to feeding, character of material, projectile, etc.); stools (frequency, quantity, color, consistency).
4. Immunizations (reactions): pertussis, tetanus, diphtheria, poliomyelitis, measles, rubella, mumps, others (include boosters).
5. Illnesses (frequency, severity, complications, operations, fractures, accidents, allergies, etc.).
6. Habits (sleep, naps, bowel and bladder, nail biting, tics, behavior with other children, etc.)

Family history:

Many complaints about a child may result from problems within the family. Examples are parental conflicts, chronic or recurrent absence of one or both parents, intense sibling rivalry, rigidity of discipline or disagreement of parents in the methods or use, unrealistic expectations of the child's performance. Since many of these factors may not be recognized or may be suppressed by either parent or child, a direct question concerning them is often unrewarding. Clues may be obtained from remarks about changes in behavior, withdrawal from friends, poor schoolwork, etc. In addition to these aspects the usual family history as previously outlined should be recorded.

Social history:

Because of its influence on the child this may be very important—type of home, own room for child or shared, number of people in home, income, interfamily relations, etc.

Systems review:

Similar to that for the adult.

COMMON SYMPTOMS IN PEDIATRIC PATIENTS

FEVER

This is probably the most common symptom experienced in childhood. Throughout the early part of a child's life his febrile response is usually considerably higher than that of the adult to a similar case. Most often the fever is due to an infection in the respiratory tract. Infections of other systems or a generalized infection (as in septicemia) may cause fever. The premature and newborn infant may have little or no fever even with very severe infections, and such reactions as an irregular temperature course, poor appetite, vomiting, and irritability may be the only symptoms. Prolonged or recurrent fever with no apparent cause may result from neoplasms, leukemia, rheumatoid arthritis (initially there may be no joint involvement), hypersensitivity reactions, and diseases of the central nervous system. Chills, delirium, and convulsions often accompany high fever in children.

ABDOMINAL PAIN

This is often difficult to evaluate in children, as some degree of periumbilical discomfort or pain is associated with many illnesses not directly involving abdominal contents. In young children, all abdominal pain tends to localize in the umbilical area. In infants one should suspect such pain in persistent screaming and crying, often associated with flexion of the thighs on the abdomen, grunting respiration, and vomiting. *Colic,* a condition seen in the first few months of life, is characterized by crying and some degree of gaseous abdominal distention and is often relieved by feeding. It tends to recur at the same time of day or night. One has to consider many possible causes of the symptom of abdominal pain in children: appendicitis, intestinal obstruction due to intussusception or volvulus, pancreatitis, peptic ulcer, and urologic diseases, especially infection. Such pain is also observed at the onset of many acute infectious diseases. Discovering and analyzing associated symptoms, such as vomiting and nature of the vomitus, diarrhea or constipation and nature of the stools, is important.

VOMITING

Like abdominal pain, vomiting often accompanies disturbances unrelated to the intestinal tract or central nervous system, the two areas most frequently involved in serious disease. In young children vomiting is frequently associated with acute infections, indiscretion in diet, fear or severe anxiety, and pain. *Regurgitation* is a nonforceful vomiting of small quantities, often seen in early infancy. Occasionally this kind of vomiting may persist, as in the ruminating child. Esophageal atresia is manifested by vomiting shortly after birth and by the presence of large amounts of mucus in the baby's mouth. Choking and cyanosis indicate aspiration. In the newborn period, vomiting of bile-containing material always indicates bowel obstruction until proved otherwise. Vomiting caused by pyloric stenosis in infants is associated with visible peristaltic waves in the upper abdomen and becomes increasingly projectile, but since there is no nausea, refeeding is easily accomplished. In vomiting secondary to lesions of the central nervous system, nausea is often present. In the very young subject, this may be possible to detect only by the facial expression or the preceding "stomach cough." Excessive dosage of any drugs, most commonly salicylates, will produce nausea and vomiting. Many metabolic disturbances may cause vomiting, including diabetes mellitus with acidosis,

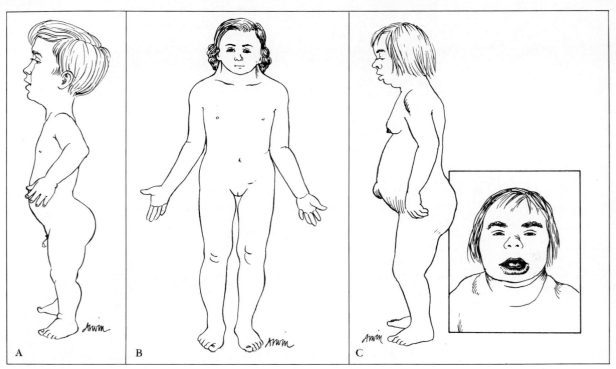

FIGURE 19-2
A. Achondroplasia. B. Turner's syndrome. C. Hypothyroidism.

galactosemia, adrenogenital syndrome with salt loss, excessive hydration resulting in cerebral edema, and dehydration with its opposite effect on the brain.

FAILURE TO GAIN WEIGHT AND LOSS OF WEIGHT

These symptoms are important, since infants and young children normally show a progressive though somewhat variable weight gain (see Tables 19-1 and 19-2). Even the older child and adolescent, except when purposely dieting, will show only brief periods when weight is not gained. Obviously any of the causes discussed under vomiting will result in failure to gain weight if the condition persists. Malnutrition, with or without economic privation, will produce the symptom. Defects in assimilation of food, as in cystic fibrosis of the pancreas and the various malabsorption syndromes, lead to a failure to gain. Most chronic disease will eventually result in failure to gain, because of loss of appetite as well as other less obvious factors, including fever, pain, infection, and impairment of organ function, such as heart failure. Failure to progress in normal statural growth will frequently accompany poor weight gain, as in *hypothyroidism, hypopituitarism, achondroplasia,* and *hereditary dwarfism* (Fig. 19-2 and Table 19-7). The abused ("battered child") or emotionally neglected infant or child may show profound weight loss or failure to grow. Observation of the mother's handling and feeding of her child may be most helpful in determining the proper cause for a failure to thrive. Obviously a careful investigation of the kind and quantities of food ingested is important and, where appropriate, a detailed analysis of formula preparation.

TABLE 19-7. Some Causes of Short Stature*

Constitutional slow growth (delayed adolescence)

Psychosocial (emotional deprivation)

Intrauterine dwarfism
Extreme prematurity
Multiple births
Maternal infection
Maternal drug ingestion (e.g., drug abuse, therapeutic drugs, alcohol, smoking)
Placental dysfunction

Malnutrition (primary or secondary)

Genetic
Racial (pygmies)
Familial short stature
Chromosomal abnormalities (e.g., Down's syndrome, Turner's syndrome)

Chronic disease
Infection (e.g., parasites, malaria, cystic fibrosis)
Renal failure
Heart disease (especially congenital)
Metabolic (e.g., glycogen storage disease, mucopolysaccharidosis, galactosemia, diabetes mellitus)

Endocrine
Hypopituitarism (isolated growth hormones or multiple deficiencies; may involve hypothalamic releasing factors or end-organ response)
Hypothyroidism
Sexual precocity (rapid early growth, but early puberty reduces potential)
Hypothalamic dysfunction

Skeletal diseases
Bone dysplasias (many types including achondroplasia, osteochondrodystrophy, osteopetrosis congenita)
Rickets

Iatrogenic
Corticosteroid therapy
Others

---

* Difficulty arises in any such listing, since there is considerable overlap of categories; for example, cystic fibrosis may cause growth retardation from both malnutrition (malabsorption) and lung infection.

STRIDOR

This is a harsh, high-pitched crowing noise that is most distinct during inspiration. In contrast to wheezing it originates high in the respiratory tract, usually in the trachea or larynx. It indicates obstruction of the airway and may be combined with cough, dyspnea, hoarseness, retractions of the chest wall with respiration, and tachypnea. The small size of the infant airway is conducive to increased frequency and severity of obstruction. Slight stridor with crying is normal in some babies. In the newborn period, congenital structural abnormalities are the most common cause. These include flaccidity of the epiglottis, laryngeal web, cysts, and defects in the tracheal cartilaginous rings. In the older child, acute spasmodic laryngitis (croup) is the most common cause and typically has its onset suddenly and at night with little or no fever. Stridor may also be caused by laryngeal edema due to serum sickness, irritation due to smoke or chemicals, and obstruction by a foreign body. Extrinsic factors, such as a neoplasm or abscess in surrounding tissue, can result in obstruction.

SLOW DEVELOPMENT (MENTAL RETARDATION)

This may be suspected by parents at any age (the most severe forms at an early age), by comparing their children to siblings or other children. The presence of some physical stigmata (mongolism, microcephaly, hydrocephaly, and some of the chromosomal defects) may be important clues. One cannot outline the developmental diagnosis for each age in a brief space, but it can be emphasized that delay in appearance of normal achievements in several areas of behavior is almost always significant (see Table 19-4). The areas of behavior are divided into motor, language, adaptive (reaction to environment and manipulation of it), and personal-social. These areas overlap to a considerable extent. Mental retardation is a symptom with many causes. Any physician who deals with children should become adept at recognizing the child with mental retardation; the degree of impairment may then be determined by a trained psychologist.

DYSPNEA

Labored respiration, or dyspnea, is a symptom that must be discussed in relation to the age of the subject. We have noted the changes in respiratory rate with age (see Table 19-6). In the premature infant a periodic pattern of breathing is normally encountered with short periods of apnea. Gradually this pattern disappears. In the newborn period, dyspnea may be associated with atelectasis, the respiratory distress syndrome (most common in premature babies and those born to diabetic mothers). Aspiration of amniotic fluid, and congenital anomalies such as lung cysts and diaphragmatic hernia, are often associated with dyspnea. Labored breathing may also be seen with congenital heart disease, with or without failure. Later in life, dyspnea is more apt to be caused by pulmonary infection and asthma. *Hyperventilation,* which is seen in diabetic acidosis, fever or any cause, aspirin poisoning, and occasionally with intracranial lesions, must be distinguished from dyspnea.

CONVULSIONS

Convulsions form another symptom complex that varies in causation with age. In the newborn infant, intracranial damage or congenital defects of the brain are nearly always combined with definite neurologic abnormalities. *Hypocalcemic tetany* most commonly is seen in the first 2 months of life and is often accompanied by carpopedal spasms and laryngeal stridor. The convulsive seizures of this metabolic abnormality are not easily distinguished from any of the other seizures, regardless of cause. *Epilepsy* is characterized by seizures of great variety, from grand mal to petit mal, and may or may not be associated with other neurologic symptoms or signs between attacks. Their common characteristic is that they tend to recur over a long period of time. Throughout childhood the most common cause of convulsive seizures is high fever, regardless of whether the cause of fever is an infection of the respiratory tract, meninges, urinary tract, or gastrointestinal tract. The threshold for "febrile convulsions" appears to rise with age. Convulsions are occasionally associated with metabolic abnormalities, such as severe electrolyte imbalance, hypoglycemia, and drug intoxication or poisoning.

THE PHYSICAL EXAMINATION

The childhood shews the man,
As morning shews the day.

JOHN MILTON
(1608–1674)

BEGINNING THE EXAMINATION

Sitting by the bed or examining table is often less threatening than standing and leaning over the older infant and young child. During the initial stages of the examination it is advisable to avoid eye contact with children of up to 4 or 5 years of age. Until good rapport is established, looking directly into the eyes is a very threatening experience for this age group.

Respect the child's sense of modesty and level of understanding. In the young child, undressing may be interpreted as a loss of personal identity and is best done in stages. A sheet should be provided for the older child and adolescent, and the undressing should be accomplished in the physician's absence. The examiner must proceed nonchalantly and in a manner of confidence. Especially in children from about 1 to 6 years of age, some resistance is to be expected. A friendly attitude with conversation and casual play at the child's level is helpful, but the physician should never be condescending nor allow the child to take command of the situation. The physician must never convey feelings of either frustration or anger. An explanation of what is to be done and showing the child the instruments to be used beforehand may contribute to his cooperation. Often part or all of the examination may best be accomplished with the patient in the mother's lap (Fig. 19-3). In the hospitalized patient several attempts with utmost patience may be necessary to perform abdominal palpation or some other portion of the examination. Skill in this respect comes with experience, and the student should not be discouraged by initial failures.

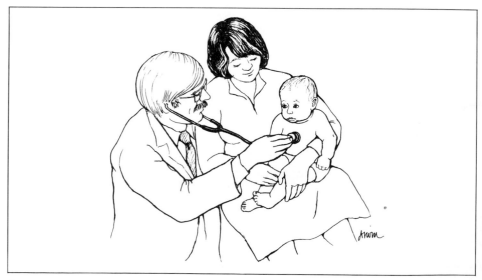

FIGURE 19-3
Examining the child in the mother's lap.

Order of procedure should delay the most objectionable parts until last. It is sometimes desirable to examine first that part of the body from which the chief complaint arises. This is because cooperation is often best early in the examination before fatigue or discomfort is experienced. Listening to the chest or palpating the abdomen before the child frets or cries may be important. Examination of the throat and ears is frequently disagreeable to the infant and young child and may be delayed to the end. The fact that restraint is often necessary in this portion of the examination accounts in part for the patient's objection.

Warm and clean hands and instruments are appreciated by both patient and parent.

These preliminary considerations cannot be emphasized too much. They may mean the difference between a satisfactory and unsatisfactory physical evaluation. Both physician and patient can enjoy the examination, and this attitude should prevail. It might also be emphasized that the short time the examiner spends with the child should not be used as an opportunity to try to correct faults in disciplinary training.

With the very ill child or the smaller premature infant, the physical examination may be carried out in brief stages to permit periods of rest. In the premature infant this may be necessary in order to conserve body temperature and to maintain adequate humidity or oxygen administration in an incubator.

GENERAL APPEARANCE

Observation of the patient during the interview often reveals evidence of mental retardation, parent-child conflicts, parental attitudes concerning discipline, posture related to pain or weakness, and facial expression related to specific questions in the older child. The mother's handling of the infant while dressing or undressing him and while feeding often reveals her level of understanding of and emotional reaction to the infant; it may also indicate errors in feeding techniques. Ambulation, relative to the age of the child, is an important observation that is too often neglected in the usual examination. Giving the child objects with which he can play will also help in the examination of general dexterity and his developmental level.

Height and weight measurements are always a routine part of the examination. Together they have great value in estimating the state of nutrition, general health, and some aspects of endocrine balances and maturation. Often the first recognized sign of disease is either failure to gain normal increments in weight or stature or an actual loss of weight (see Tables 19-1 and 19-2). In the final analysis of the growth of a child, the expected rate of gain is of greater value than any single measurement.

Speech and cry are very important. Hoarseness is often present with laryngitis, hypothyroidism, and tetany. A high-pitched, piercing cry in the infant may indicate increased intracranial pressure. Pharyngeal paralysis due to poliomyelitis or diphtheria will influence speech, producing a nasal quality. A monotone type of verbalization may indicate hearing loss.

Posture, muscle tone, and coordination may be observed during the history taking. Pain in the abdomen can result in flexion of the thighs on the abdomen in infants and younger children. *Opisthotonos* is indicative of meningeal irritation (Fig. 19-4). A "position of protection" is often assumed in the presence of pain or tenderness. Lack or limitation of motion may indicate paralysis, fracture or disloca-

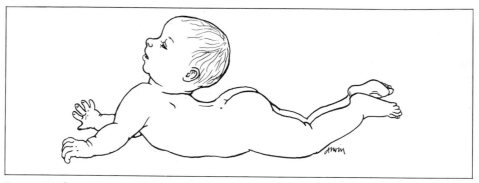

FIGURE 19-4
Opisthotonos. Some causes of opisthotonos are meningitis, tetanus, strychnine, and hysteria.

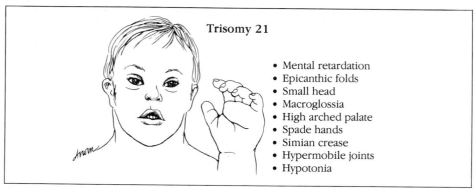

Trisomy 21

- Mental retardation
- Epicanthic folds
- Small head
- Macroglossia
- High arched palate
- Spade hands
- Simian crease
- Hypermobile joints
- Hypotonia

FIGURE 19-5
Down's syndrome.

tion, joint inflammation, or an intracranial lesion. Spasticity, scissors gait, and poor coordination are found as a result of cerebral injury, often present since birth. Many of the muscular dystrophies are first manifested in an abnormal gait and either hypotonicity or hypertonicity. The general lack of tone of all muscle groups characterizes Down's syndrome, or mongolism (Fig. 19-5).

VITAL SIGNS
Temperature is usually obtained rectally until the age of 3 years or over. A normal temperature in infancy and early childhood may be a degree or more above the adult average (98.6°F or 37°C).

Pulse and respiratory rates are more rapid in younger children, and change with age. These rates should be obtained when the child is quiet. Both of these are fairly sensitive measures of fever, increasing about 15 to 20 percent with each degree rise in temperature. The respiratory rate and depth of breathing may increase with either respiratory or metabolic acidosis, and such changes are often the initial physical findings of the underlying abnormality. Cardiac and pulmonary diseases are also reflected by deviations from the normal.

Blood pressure also changes with age. A cuff of proper width is necessary for accurate readings. It should cover approximately one-third to one-half of the upper arm. Most children need to be reassured that the procedure will not be very uncomfortable, and the readings should be considered true values only when the subject is quiet and emotionally undisturbed.

Changes (with age) in normal temperature, respiratory rates, and blood pressure are presented in Table 19-6.

SKIN

The skin and subcutaneous tissues reflect the general state of hydration and nutrition. The status of *tissue turgor* in the infant and child is of particular importance, and it is best demonstrated by picking up a fold of abdominal skin between the thumb and index finger. Normally on release the skin rapidly returns to its former position. In states of dehydration or undernutrition the skin remains creased and raised for a varying period of time.

In the premature and newborn infant the skin appears thin and almost transparent. It is red and wrinkled under normal conditions. Small red patches (nevus vasculosus), which are not raised and which blanch with pressure, may be present over the occiput, forehead, and upper eyelids. These patches are commonly seen in the newborn. The soft, moist, white or clay-colored material covering all newborn infants is the *vernix caseosa*. Some flaky desquamation occurs shortly after birth and varies in degree with individuals. For the first few weeks of life, very small, white to yellow, raised lesions that are discrete are present normally in groups, especially over the face. They are caused by plugging of the as yet poorly functioning sebaceous glands, and collectively they are known as *milia*. *Miliaria* is the red "prickly heat" rash noted during the summer or in overly dressed infants.

A blotchy blue appearance of the hands and feet (*acrocyanosis*) is normal in early infancy but is not a constant finding. Bluish, irregularly shaped areas that are not raised and vary greatly in size are sometimes present over the sacral and buttock areas of the darker complexioned infants and are called Mongolian spots. These spots occur frequently in dark-skinned individuals, such as Africans and Orientals. They gradually decrease in intensity and disappear with increasing age. They have no pathologic significance.

Physiologic *jaundice* is present to a mild degree in many infants, starting after the first day of life and usually disappearing by the eighth or tenth day. Jaundice that appears during the first 24 hours of life usually indicates excessive hemolysis, *hemolytic disease of the newborn,* due to the presence of maternal antibodies against the infant's red cells. If jaundice persists and gradually becomes more intense over the first few weeks of life, congenital anomalies of the biliary tree with obstruction should be suspected.

Cradle cap, or *seborrheic dermatitis,* in the newborn is characterized by a greasy yellowish scale over the scalp that sometimes involves other areas of the head, especially behind the ears. Another common dermatitis of childhood is *tinea capitis,* or ringworm of the scalp. Hair on the involved area is broken off close to the scalp. Edema, reddening, and crusting are usually present.

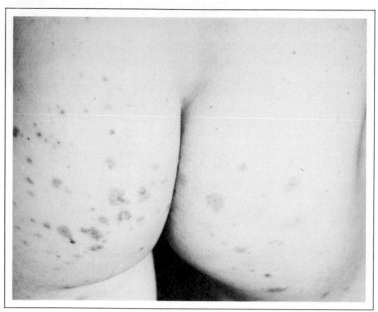

FIGURE 19-6
Henoch-Schönlein purpura.

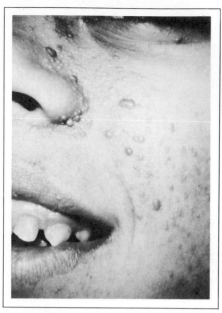

FIGURE 19-7
Adenoma sebaceum.

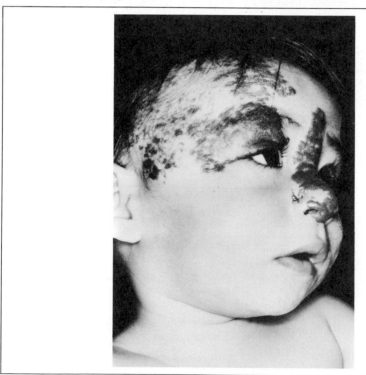

FIGURE 19-8
Hemangioma.

LYMPH NODES

The lymph nodes have a distribution in children similar to that in adults but are more prominent up to the time of puberty. They are easily palpable as shotty, small, bean-sized nodules, and usually undergo considerable hypertrophy in response to infections throughout childhood.

HEAD

SIZE AND SHAPE

Head size is relatively larger in children than in adults; the younger the child, the more this is evident. Head circumference measurements have a relatively narrow range for any age and are directly related to intracranial volume; they therefore permit an estimation of brain growth. Rate of growth is of vital importance in patients with suspected hydrocephalus or microcephalus. The measurement is obtained by passing a tape measure over the occipital protuberance and just above the supraorbital ridges (Fig. 19-9; see Table 19-3). The importance of this measurement can be appreciated when one realizes that more than 85 percent of children with a circumference of more than 2 standard deviations below or above the mean will be mentally retarded or have other neurologic abnormalities.

The head of the newborn often undergoes some distortion in shape as it passes through the birth canal. There may be overlapping of the large flat bones, which are easily palpable. Depending on the degree of *molding,* as this process is called, a few days to a few weeks may pass before normal anatomic relationships are reestablished. Soft tissue molding of the scalp at the time of birth results in *caput succedaneum,* a soft, poorly outlined swelling that pits on pressure from the edema present. It may overlie the suture lines.

Asymmetry of the head may result from premature closure of some of the sutures. It may also be seen in the normal infant who always lies in the same position, since the bones at this time are very soft. Flattening of a portion of the cranium may occur in normal infants but is more often associated with certain pediatric diseases, such as torticollis or mental retardation, due to the tendency for such children to maintain a constant position. *Cephalohematoma* is a swelling resulting from bleeding beneath the periosteum of the cranium and is therefore limited to a single cranial bone. Palpation usually reveals a small firm elevated margin of the lesion, which is becoming organized into a clot and later may be calcified. This and the superficially similar-appearing caput succedaneum are limited to the newborn period.

Careful and frequent measurements of head circumference constitute an important method of appraisal when compared with tables for normal growth rates (see Table 19-1). The posterior fontanel is closed to palpation in a few months. The anterior fontanel varies greatly in size throughout early infancy but is usually palpable only as a slight depression by 12 to 18 months of age. Normally, until they close, some arterial pulsation is transmitted through the fontanels.

Head control and movement of the head are important in evaluation of neuromuscular development. By 2 months the head is held relatively steady when the baby is supported in an erect position, and he can raise it from a prone position. By 4 months head control is good, with no unsteadiness.

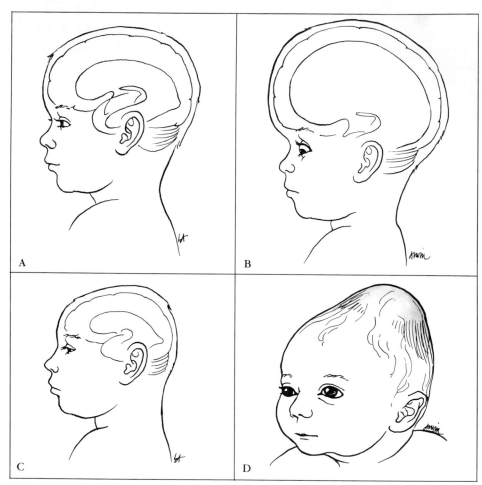

FIGURE 19-9
Some cephalic shapes. A. Normal. B. Hydrocephalus. C. Microcephalus. D. Molding.

Separation of the sutures, which have previously been approximated, and the bulging with tenseness of the anterior fontanel are indicative of increased intracranial pressure, regardless of cause. Prominence of the veins over the head may also be present in such cases. Microcephaly, a head circumference more than two standard deviations below the normal for a given age, may indicate premature synostosis but is more commonly an associated finding in mental retardation with an underlying brain defect. Transillumination of the head is a valuable method of examination in infants. It is done in a dark room with a bright flashlight fitted with a soft rubber collar to ensure a lightproof fit against the scalp. In severe *hydrocephalus* and *anencephaly,* nearly the whole skull will transmit light. In *hygroma,* a localized subdural collection of fluid, a sharply delineated area of transillumination is obtained on the side of the lesion.

FACE

The face is examined for shape and symmetry. Paralysis may be elicited only by making the child smile or cry. Thickening and puffiness of the features may be present with edema or hypothyroidism. *Chorea* is associated with uncontrolled grimacing and must be differentiated from tics and habit spasms. Epileptic seizures may be localized to the face or begin in this area in children. A lack of expression is characteristic of severe mental retardation.

EYES

The eyes of the newborn may be difficult to examine since they are tightly closed most of the time, and often a mild chemical conjunctivitis from silver nitrate instillation is present. Holding the baby upright usually results in at least a brief opening of the eyes; if he is then slowly rotated, the eyes follow in that direction. A bright light shined in the eyes will cause blinking and some dorsiflexion of the head. These two procedures permit examination of the sclerae, pupils, irides, extraocular movements, and light perception. The corneal reflex is present in all normal infants. The red reflex is elicited by setting the ophthalmoscope to "O" and viewing through the pupil at 10 to 12 inches' distance. The normal red-orange color may be distorted if there are lesions of the cornea, anterior chamber, lens, or retina. The pupillary reflex is present at birth.

Conjugate eye movements are present shortly after birth, but true tracking movements may not be present for several days to a few weeks. Conjugate fixation on a large object (e.g. the human face) is often present at birth. Searching nystagmus normally appears for brief periods in the first few days and then normally disappears. Intermittent alternation of convergent strabismus may be observed in normal infants for the first 4 to 6 months of life. Divergent strabismus should always be considered a sign of pathologic significance. By 2 to 3 months, accurate coordinated following of moving objects is present.

In early childhood, before age 6 years, the most important part of the eye examination is to determine the condition of amblyopia ex anopsia. If detected after that age, therapy may be unable to prevent serious loss of visual acuity. The usual causes are weakness of extraocular muscles or a refractive error in one eye resulting in disparity. If muscle weakness causes medial deviation it is termed *esotropia;* if lateral, *exotropia.* Two useful and simple tests to detect muscle weakness of strabismus are outlined. Both require some cooperation but are not difficult to accomplish.

1. The *cover test* has the subject look at a light source held at midforehead of the examiner. Then alternately each eye is "covered" by placing the thumb or fingers in front of one and then removed. Each eye is observed for movement both before and after covering. If either eye moves, strabismus is present. Analysis of the results permits a differential diagnosis of the strabismus, if present (see details in Chap. 8).

2. The *Hirschberg test* also has the child look at the light in the same position as noted for the cover test. The position of the light reflection in the cornea is noted, and then the child's head is slowly turned to the right and then left. The reflection in each cornea normally will be symmetrical in all positions. If strabismus is present the reflections will be asymmetrical, and analysis of the resulting pattern will indicate whether esotropia or exotropia is present.

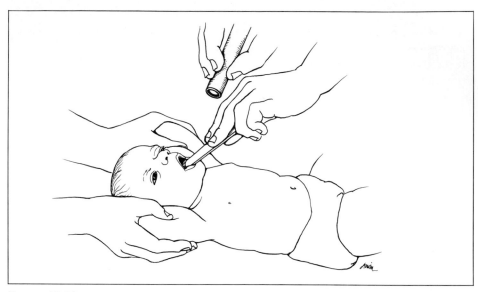

FIGURE 19-10
Examination of the throat. Note how the child's head is immobilized by using its own arms as a "vise."

Visual testing with a *Snellen E* or other appropriate chart can be accomplished by age 2$\frac{1}{2}$ to 3 years. Prior to that time parental observation of the child's awareness of surroundings, exploration, and developmental milestones may indicate normal or abnormal visual response.

Dilation of the pupils may be necessary for adequate funduscopic examination. Many neurologic diseases in infancy and childhood have retinal manifestations (e.g., toxoplasmosis, subdural hematoma, Tay-Sachs and Niemann-Pick diseases, generalized systemic candidiasis).

EAR, NOSE, AND THROAT

The ear, nose, and throat examination is best delayed to the last in the infant and young child, as restraint is often required (Figs. 19-10, 19-11). Small, simple, deformed and low-set external ears (auricles) may indicate other congenital anomalies, such as renal agenesis or chromosomal abnormalities involving multiple systems. For a few days after birth the ear canal is filled with vernix caseosa, obscuring the tympanic membrane. In early infancy the light reflex in the membrane is less sharply delineated than later. Because middle ear infections are so common in early childhood, the physician who will be caring for this age group should use every opportunity during his training to observe normal and pathologic conditions and become familiar with the use of the pneumatic otoscope.

Hearing in infancy can be tested by response to sound ranging in loudness from a small bell to a sharp clap of the hands. Responses may vary and may include cessation of activity, turning head toward the sound, blinking, or even verbal response. Defective or absent hearing may not be apparent for several months and should be suspected if there is a delay in vocalization or diminished smiling and laughing;

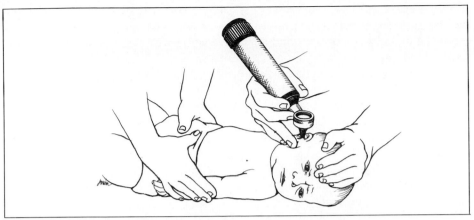

FIGURE 19-11
Examination of the ear. Note that the examiner's hand, holding the otoscope, rests on the child's head so that any sudden movement will be transmitted to both the hand and the instrument, minimizing trauma to the external canal.

what vocalization is present may be monotonal and unmodulated. Extreme visual and tactile attentiveness may be suggestive symptoms.

The tonsils and adenoids, as are all other lymphoid tissue, are relatively large and cryptic in many children. The presence of enlarged tonsils does not necessarily indicate chronic infection. With acute *pharyngitis* in children, the tonsils are nearly always involved. They may have small areas of whitish membrane that is usually not difficult to distinguish from the large, confluent, gray membrane of *diphtheria.*

CHEST

Asymmetry of the chest with bulging over the heart may be present in children with prolonged cardiac enlargement.

The chest in the infant and young child has a relatively greater anteroposterior diameter than in the adult. The chest wall is so thin that diseased underlying structures may be more easily discovered by auscultation and percussion than in the adult. Small nodular breast hypertrophy is found in most newborn infants and may be associated with small amounts of milklike secretion for a few days. Some breast hypertrophy, not always symmetrical, is usually present transiently in adolescent boys. Obese children often have apparent breast hypertrophy; however, this is due to adipose tissue and not to glandular hypertrophy.

Because of the thinness of the chest wall in young children, auscultation reveals breath sounds that normally are loud, harsh, and somewhat bronchial in character as compared with the adult. Pathology is actually more readily apparent than in older subjects, once the physician has gained experience by listening to the normal chest. Percussion note over the lung fields is more resonant in the child and even approaches being tympanic in quality. In the infant, respiration is largely under control of the diaphragm, with little or no intercostal movement. This leads to the so-called abdominal type of respiration that lasts for about the first 6 years of life. Examination of the chest in a crying infant or child has considerable value and should not be considered as meaningless. Deep respiratory sounds are actually enhanced. Even slight changes in position of the infant, such as turning the head, may influence the relative positions of the intrathoracic structures and therefore the intensity of breath sounds or the degree of resonance.

Rhonchi transmitted from the trachea or large bronchi often confuse the student who is listening to the chest of an infant. Their character, position, and differentiation may be facilitated by holding the stethoscope an inch or two from the infant's mouth or nose and comparing these sounds to those heard over the chest.

The heart in early life fills relatively more of the thoracic cavity than in later life, and the apex is one or two intercostal spaces above that which would be considered normal in the adult. *Sinus arrhythmia* is a physiologic phenomenon prominent throughout infancy and childhood. This finding is so constant that its absence suggests cardiac abnormality.

The heart sounds during childhood are of a higher pitch and shorter duration with greater intensity than during later years. Until adolescence the pulmonary second sound is regularly louder than the aortic. *Functional murmurs* are the rule during childhood. They are less common in the newborn than later. Between the ages of 6 and 9, over one-half of the children have murmurs that are obvious to the examiner. The most common areas of maximum intensity in the order of frequency are the third to fourth intercostal area at the left border of the sternum, the pulmonic area, and the apex. *Parasternal murmurs* become less frequent as adolescence approaches, while pulmonic ones become more prevalent. These murmurs usually are of grade III intensity or less well localized, and are either blowing or vibratory in character. Change in intensity or complete disappearance may follow a change in position. A *venous hum* is also common in childhood. It is a continuous purring sound that is best heard either above or below the clavicles. It is accentuated in the upright position. It should not be confused with the murmur of patent ductus arteriosus. With the exception of the venous hum, all the functional or innocent heart murmurs are systolic in time, are rarely transmitted to areas beyond the point of maximum intensity, and do not obscure other normal heart sounds.

Abdomen

The abdominal examination, because a child may cry, may be somewhat more difficult to perform here than in the adult. If the child is frightened, repeated attempts may be necessary. Distraction from the examining hand can often be accomplished by conversation of interest to the child or by attracting his attention with a toy.

The liver edge is often palpable in infancy and childhood, and the spleen is normally palpable on deep inspiration in some children.

Inspection of the abdomen of the crying child may best demonstrate hernia, diastasis recti, or localized bulging due to regional paralysis. Palpation is sometimes done with the child in a prone position, because he relaxes best if he is not looking directly at the examiner. In the infant, relaxation may be obtained during bottle feeding. This procedure may also be used to demonstrate peristaltic waves and for the palpation of a tumor such as that found in hypertrophic pyloric stenosis. *Umbilical hernia* (Fig. 19-12) is particularly common in infants, especially in association with hypothyroidism and mongolism.

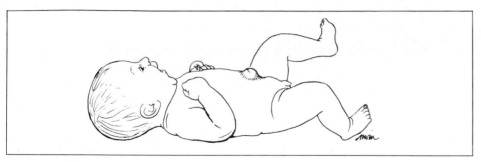

FIGURE 19-12
Umbilical hernia.

GENITALIA

The size of the genitalia must be evaluated in relationship to age and not necessarily to body size. The penis and scrotum often appear disproportionately small in obese boys. It must be remembered that throughout most of childhood or until the increased release of pituitary gonadotropins with the onset of puberty, there is virtually no increase in size of the penis or testes.

The precocious appearance of sexual hair may be caused by adrenal lesions (in early infancy by congenital *adrenal hyperplasia*), brain lesions, gonadal tumors, and a few other rare conditions. Delayed appearance or absence of sexual hair may be found in pituitary, thyroid, or gonadal insufficiency and in certain chronic illnesses. Some degree of retarded growth is usually an accompaniment. Tufts of hair over the spine may indicate an underlying *spina bifida.*

Actual enlargement of the penis or clitoris, often accompanied by the appearance of pubic hair, is seen as a result of virilizing adrenal lesions or other causes of precocious development. Partial fusion of the labia minora is common in prepubertal girls. Because of the patency of the inguinal canal and the sensitive cremaster reflex, several examinations should be carried out before diagnosis of undescended testicle is made.

Secondary sexual development shows great individual variation as to the time of onset. Table 19-5 gives averages of the range for normal American children. Conditions associated with abnormal sexual development are outlined in Table 19-8.

RECTAL EXAMINATION

The rectal examination is an extremely important part of a child's checkup. Digital examination must be done with adequate lubrication, slow and steady pressure with the finger until it passes the sphincter, and the use of the little (fifth) finger in infants and young children. A nasal speculum may be used for examining the anal region in infants.

MUSCULOSKELETAL SYSTEM

The extremities are comparatively short during the first few years of life (the span of the outstretched arms is less than the standing height until approximately age 10 years in boys and 14 years in girls). These proportions, plus the abundant subcutaneous fat, give the infant a rotund appearance. Going into the second and third

TABLE 19-8. Abnormal Sexual Development

Conditions associated with delayed onset of puberty
    Hypopituarism, usually with short stature (i.e., multiple deficiencies)
    Hypothyroidism
    Hypogonadism (agenesis, e.g., Turner's syndrome, atrophy, surgical or traumatic
        castration; may be incomplete as in testicular feminization syndrome)
    Hypothalamic syndromes
    Any severe chronic illness

Conditions associated with precocious sexual development
    Hyperadrenalism
        1. Congenital adrenal cortical hyperplasia
        2. Adrenal cortical tumors
    Hypothalamic lesions
    Pineal gland tumors (predominately in boys)
    Gonadal tumors
    McCune-Albright syndrome (polyostotic fibrous dysplasia)
    Exogenous source of sex hormones

years the child normally becomes more linear and lean. Recognition of these changes is important in counseling worried parents and avoiding feeding problems precipitated by parents who desire to maintain the plumpness, mistaking it for an indication of good health.

The muscular and skeletal systems are examined as in the adult, taking into account the fact that ambulation is not present in the early months of life. Lack of motion, weakness, and distortion of normal relationships must be looked for in the child even more carefully than in older subjects. Congenital dislocation of the hip, brachial plexus injuries, osteochondrosis, rickets, scurvy, amyotonia congenita, and other muscular dystrophies are particularly important in the child. The spine is more flexible in the infant and child than in the adult. Some degree of lordosis and "pot belly" is natural until midchildhood.

NEUROLOGIC EXAMINATION

The neurologic examination will often evaluate the expected behavior and responses to certain stimuli as well as the more formal elicitation of reflexes, muscle tone, and sensation. For example, what the 9-month-old infant does with three cubes or blocks may be as important as his Achilles reflex. Does he grasp firmly, reach accurately, transfer from hand to hand, use fingers as well as palm in grasping?

The changing pattern of *reflex behavior* in early infancy is important in estimating neurologic integrity. At birth, tonicity and activity are equal bilaterally. The premature newborn has decreased tonicity and activity compared to the normal infant. The premature infant lies in a flaccid position with hands open. The full-term infant assumes a flexed position with hands fisted, and efforts to straighten out the extremities meet considerable resistance. When the baby is supported by one hand under the abdomen in a horizontal position, he raises his head and legs toward the plane of his body. This *Landau reflex,* which is normally easily elicited in the newborn, may be absent in the premature infant. The full-term infant firmly grasps an object (e.g., a finger) placed in its palm and can be lifted up so that most or all of its weight is supported. The greater the degree of prematurity, the less strong this grasp reflex becomes. Under 36 weeks of gestation the response may be absent or very weak. Sucking is vigorous on a finger placed in the mouth. When the cheek is lightly stroked the infant turns his head toward the stimulated side and the lips may protrude in preparation for sucking. This reaction is termed the *rooting reflex.* The newborn responds to sudden change in position, jarring, or loud noises by the *Moro reflex.* This is characterized by a tensing of muscles, a wide embracing motion of the upper extremities, and some extension of the legs. Normally this reflex disappears by 2 months of age, and its persistence beyond that time indicates neurologic abnormality.

Blinking, sneezing, gagging, and coughing to appropriate stimuli are easily elicited in the full-term infant and in all but the smallest of those born prematurely. Although a typical *Babinski reflex* is seldom demonstrable in the newborn, dorsiflexion of the great toe to the usual stimulus is present in most infants and may persist throughout much of the first year. Due to the often relaxed Achilles tendon from fetal positioning, the ankle jerk may not exist, but all other deep tendon reflexes are present at birth. All the superficial reflexes—abdominal, anal, and cremasteric—are present at birth, although they may be somewhat difficult to elicit.

In early infancy there may be insufficient development of the nervous system to give reliable neurologic signs. Meningitis in this age group may not be associated with obvious nuchal rigidity, Brudzinski or Kernig signs. Lethargy, anorexia, vomiting, and other symptoms and signs of seemingly less specific significance may be the only findings to indicate meningeal irritation.

EXAMINATION OF THE NEWBORN

If she find it warm, not black, she should blow into its mouth; but if, as sometimes happens, the anus is closed by a little skin, she should cut it with a sharp knife. . . .

PAULUS BAGELLARDUS
(1472–   )

Because no other period of life carries as great a risk of morbidity and mortality as the first weeks of life, it is appropriate to devote special emphasis to the examination of the newborn infant. The 1-minute and 5-minute *Apgar scores* are a general indication of the viability of the infant and the effects of labor (Table 19-9). Scores of 6 or less indicate actual or potential problems.

A limited examination that includes a search for major defects should be done immediately. If no problems are apparent a more complete evaluation can be delayed for several hours. Auscultation of heart and lungs and palpation of the abdomen can best be accomplished while the infant is quiet or asleep. At birth or soon thereafter the umbilicus should be examined for the presence of a single artery. Normally there are two arteries and one vein. A single artery is often associated with anomalies of the heart, central nervous system, and gut.

Not all infants of low birth weight (under 2,500 gm) are premature. A significant number have had full-term gestation but suffered intrauterine malnutrition from maternal disease or poor placental function. An attempt should be made to correlate the baby's gestational age and birth weight. The premature infant is vulnerable

TABLE 19-9. Apgar Score for the Newborn*

	Score		
Signs	0	1	2
Heart rate	Absent	<100	>100
Respiratory effort	Absent	Weak	Good
Muscle tone	Limp	Some flexion	Well-flexed extremities
Response to stimulus to feet	None	Some motion	Motion and crying
Color	Pale or blue	Acrocyanosis	Completely pink

* The score is computed at 1 and 5 minutes following delivery by assigning 0, 1, or 2 to each item. A total score of 10 indicates optimum. A total score of 0 indicates a moribund infant.
Source: From V. Apgar, D. A. Holaday, L. S. James, I. M. Weisbrot, and C. Berrien. Evaluation of the newborn infant: Second report. *J.A.M.A.* 168:1985, 1958. Copyright 1958, American Medical Association.

to *sepsis* and *hyaline membrane disease* (respiratory distress syndrome). He will also show organ immaturity, such as hyperbilirubinemia with jaundice. The malnourished baby is particularly susceptible to hypoglycemia. Unusually large babies (over 3,800 gm) are often born to mothers with diabetes mellitus or to prediabetics.

Since menstrual histories are often inaccurate, more objective means of estimating gestational age are required. These include the following: Before 36 weeks, only one or two transverse creases are present on the sole of the foot, the breast nodule is less than 3 mm in diameter, no cartilage is present in the earlobe, and the testes are seldom in the scrotum, which has few or no rugae. By 40 weeks, many creases are present on the sole, the breast nodule exceeds 4 mm, cartilage is present in the earlobe, and the testes have descended into the scrotum, which is covered with rugae. Increasing muscle tone with assumption of a posture of predominantly flexed extremities is another sign of increased maturity.

The premature infant often has brief periods of apnea lasting up to 20 seconds. Respiratory distress is indicated by an increased rate, grunting, retraction of intercostal and subcostal spaces and suprasternal notch, seesaw sinking of the chest with rising abdomen in contrast to the normal synchronous motions, and flaring of the nostrils.

Airway patency can be assured if a soft catheter will pass through the nose, pharynx, and esophagus into the stomach. The resting newborn is an obligatory nose breather, so obstruction, such as atresia of choanae, syphilis, or reserpine therapy in the mother, may result in serious respiratory difficulty. Passing the tube into the stomach can eliminate the possibility of esophageal obstruction. Excessive collection of mucus in the nose and mouth characterizes atresia of the esophagus.

Visual inspection of the oral cavity as well as palpation with a gloved finger will rule out such defects as a cleft palate or an aberrant thyroid at the base of the tongue. Thrush (candidiasis) is an infection of the mucous membranes with slightly raised dull white patches and can be easily distinguished from Epstein's pearls, which are pearly white nodules limited to the palate.

It is important to remember that respiratory distress, with or without cyanosis, is not limited to intrinsic lesions of the lungs at this period. Intracranial lesions, including anomalies, hemorrhage, or damage due to anoxia, may be responsible.

Congenital heart disease and diaphragmatic hernia are further possibilities to be ruled out and often require a chest x-ray for definitive diagnosis.

Some breast hypertrophy at birth, occasionally with small secretions of "milk," is not uncommon and is transient.

The genitalia should be carefully examined for anomalies such as hypospadias, hydrocele, hernia, and ambiguous development indicating possible abnormal sexual development secondary to endocrine influences. Failure to pass meconium or urine within 24 to 48 hours requires investigation as to cause.

Evaluation of the central nervous system depends on observations of spontaneous alertness and activity, strength and character of the cry, response to stimuli, vigor of sucking and feeding, and postural tone. Head measurements and examination have been described earlier in this chapter, and some of the reflexes also have been mentioned.

CONCLUSION

Lucy: Don't tell me you took that blanket to school today?
Linus: Sure, why not? It calms me down and helps me get better
       grades.
Lucy: But don't the other kids laugh at you?
Linus: Nobody laughs at a straight "A" average!

CHARLES M. SCHULZ
(1922–   )

In this chapter an attempt has been made to emphasize some of the important differences between the child and the adult. The fact that the child is a changing organism is important to remember and is extremely helpful in evaluation of the history and the physical findings. Failure to grow in stature or weight is always significant. Delay in both physical and mental maturation as well as in growth may indicate endocrine or deficiency disorders or chronic infectious disease. Fortunately fever, emotional response, fatigue, general behavior, intestinal upsets, and the like are more labile in the child than in the adult and therefore are important indicators of disease. Special attention to behavior and facial expression before and during the actual examination is of the utmost importance. If these facts are kept in mind, the examination of the infant or child can be an exciting and rewarding experience for the physician.

INJURED PATIENT   CHAPTER 20

Though the experienced practitioner may, by a process of apparently in-
stinctive "short circuiting" achieve a diagnosis so swiftly that he seems to
be guided by something called "clinical instinct," we may be quite sure
that, as a matter of fact, the processes actually involved are observation,
elimination of the irrelevant, inference—in other words induction—
even though the pace has been so rapid that the several steps are indis-
tinguishable.

ABRAHAM FLEXNER
(1866–1959)

GENERAL PRINCIPLES

The aim of this textbook is to present the principles of examination and diagnosis.
The first aim of the examining physician is the preservation of life. When dealing
with acute trauma it is often impossible to separate diagnostic and therapeutic measures; indeed, it would be improper to dissociate completely these features. The
care of the acutely injured patient imposes certain important restrictions on the
examiner. It may be impossible to obtain a detailed or even cursory history from
the patient. The examiner is often forced to rely heavily on physical findings for
diagnosis. The initial examination is as likely to be performed in the field or beside
a highway as in a well-equipped hospital emergency room.

When confronted with an acutely injured patient you should ask yourself the following questions, in rapid order:

1. Is the airway patent?
2. Is there significant hemorrhage?
3. Is there serious or potential brain or spinal cord injury?
4. Is there a fracture?
5. Is there a chest injury?
6. Is there acute intra-abdominal injury?
7. Is there injury to the urinary tract?
8. Is there peripheral nerve injury?

The most urgent requirement is the evaluation of the patient's **airway**. Death may
ensue in minutes if adequate ventilation is not possible. The problem may be compounded by unconsciousness, by aspiration of blood or vomitus, or by serious injuries to the chest wall or lung parenchyma. In evaluating the status of the patient's
airway, the patient should be turned on his side or facedown with the head in the
dependent position to minimize the danger of aspiration. It may be necessary to
exert traction on the tongue to maintain an oral airway. If tracheal obstruction
exists, an emergency tracheostomy may be indicated. If ventilation is inadequate,
mouth-to-mouth resuscitation should be initiated without hesitation. Prompt recognition of this need may be life-saving. It may be necessary to combine these measures with closed-chest cardiac massage. It has been demonstrated that an adequate

peripheral circulation can be maintained by this technique. Unless ideal circumstances exist in an operating-room environment with intratracheal intubation and anesthesia apparatus, open-chest cardiac massage will seldom be indicated.

The second important threat to life is **massive hemorrhage.** In the patient with an injured extremity, the steady oozing of blood is best controlled by constant pressure. This may have to be maintained manually. Elevation of the limb will help to control blood loss. Only in exceptional instances will arterial blood loss be a major problem. In these rare circumstances a tourniquet should be applied proximal to the wound. The limb should be observed carefully; the tourniquet should be loosened occasionally to permit an attempt at reconstructive surgery. By the time the patient reaches operating-room facilities, continuous slow, steady oozing of blood may have seriously depleted the circulating blood volume in an insidious manner. It is easy to underestimate this type of blood loss unless one is alert to this possibility.

When adequate airway and ventilation are ensured and hemorrhage is controlled, it is time to perform a rapid physical examination to assess the extent of coexisting injuries. This should be initiated as soon as possible and, though brief, should be thorough and systematic. Failure to carry out this kind of survey will lead to errors in diagnosis and management that may have serious consequences or may result in loss of life. The information obtained by this preliminary examination provides valuable baseline data by which to follow the patient's progress and also aids subsequent management.

The examination should rule out the possibility of **spinal injury,** since if such a patient is moved roughly or improperly, sudden paralysis may occur. Pain medication should be withheld until a clear indication for it exists and brain injury is ruled out. If narcotics are given before the examination is completed, diagnostic evaluation becomes clouded and neurologic signs are difficult to interpret. When given, the analgesic should be administered intravenously because of the uncertainties of absorption associated with hypotension, which often accompanies massive trauma.

There is a great tendency, based on our natural curiosity, to probe, explore, and investigate **open wounds,** but in most instances this should be avoided. In general, except to control hemorrhage, open wounds should be explored only in the operating room. Anesthesia should be adequate to permit thorough study, cleansing should be performed with copious amounts of sterile saline, and sterile technique should be strictly observed. Anything short of this fosters an incomplete and inadequate examination, is likely to lead to infection, and may result in failure to find foreign bodies. The ideal method of early management calls for application of a dry, sterile (or at least clean) dressing to prevent additional soilage. Definitive care should be given as soon as conditions permit without the controlled environment of the operating room.

RADIOLOGIC EXAMINATION

X-ray examination is a valuable adjunct to the physical examination in evaluating the extent of injuries. Selected studies often provide information that may be obtained in no other way. In addition, a standard-size *chest film* is worth obtaining. In many ways physical examination of the heart and lungs is limited, and every physician realizes that the x-ray is sometimes more accurate and effective in detecting subtle pulmonary, mediastinal, and cardiac changes.

A flat film of the *abdomen* is also important if abdominal trauma has occurred. In addition to the specific studies cited above, free air from a perforated viscus may be detected by an upright or lateral decubitus film.

X-ray examination of the *skull* is an important part of the evaluation of patients with head injury. It is important, however, to select the proper time for x-ray study. To obtain satisfactory films it is usually necessary to enlist the cooperation of the patient. This frequently is not possible in the early state of injury, and the manipulation of such a patient may be attended by considerable hazard. In most instances such films may best be obtained when the patient's condition is stable. Furthermore the types of intracranial hemorrhage requiring prompt surgical treatment will be detected by observation of vital signs and by neurologic examination rather than on the basis of an x-ray study. The principal value of skull films lies in the recognition of skull fracture, which requires specific treatment. As a general rule, radiologic studies should be completed as soon after head injury as the general condition of the patient permits.

Common sense should dictate when radiologic studies will contribute to successful management. Under certain urgent circumstances, early operative intervention is more important than obtaining a complete set of films. In this type of situation, only films that vitally affect decisions are indicated.

HEAD INJURIES

CEREBRAL TRAUMA

Patients with head injury frequently will have airway obstruction or ventilatory problems. This requires primary attention. The neurologic examination may then be performed. The three aims of emergency neurologic evaluation are (1) to determine whether the patient is in need of emergency surgical intervention, (2) to establish the diagnosis of any existing head injury, and (3) to obtain baseline neurologic information for comparison purposes later.

A time-consuming, detailed, elaborate neurologic examination is not appropriate for the early care of patients with head injury. On the contrary, a few carefully selected studies may be obtained using simple equipment. The state of consciousness should be evaluated. The patient's response to painful stimulation should be recorded, for example, response to supraorbital pressure, pinprick, or pressure on the sternum with the knuckles. The condition of the pupils, their relative size, equality, and response to light should be observed and recorded. Small contracted pupils that do not respond may be associated with midbrain damage. This lack of pupillary response may be misleading, however, if the patient has been medicated, or has used alcohol. Dilated fixed pupils have a poor prognosis. Inequality of the pupils may reflect local brain damage. Unilateral dilation of the pupils occurring under observation is strongly suggestive of intracranial hemorrhage.

CHARACTER OF RESPIRATION

Irregular or depressed respirations may accompany severe intracranial injury. If this situation exists in the presence of an adequate airway the prognosis is grave.

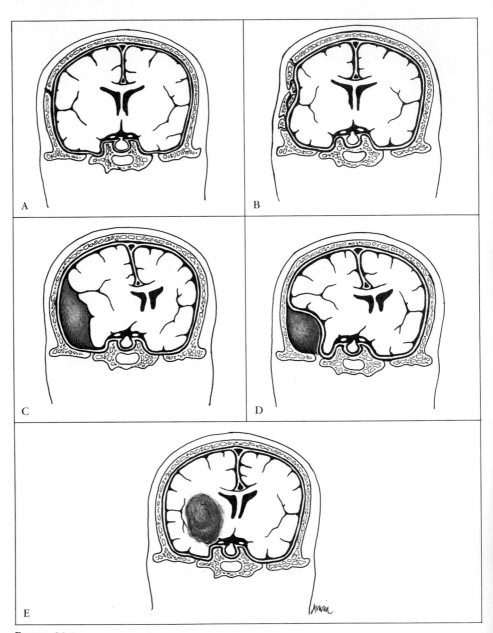

FIGURE 20-1

Some types of head injury. A. Linear skull fracture. B. Depressed skull fracture. C. Subdural hematoma. D. Epidural hematoma. E. Intracerebral hematoma.

DEGREE OF MOTOR ACTIVITY

If the patient is conscious, motor activity may be appraised by having him squeeze the examiner's hands or by testing his ability to resist passive motion of the extremities. In the comatose patient the degree of flaccidity may be evaluated by lifting the extremity and letting it drop. It is important to examine both sides of the patient. This permits comparison and provides baseline information should his condition deteriorate under observation. Extensor rigidity of all extremities implies a bad prognosis. Although alcoholism or drug intoxication may confuse this observation, complete flaccidity and areflexia usually indicate severe central nervous system damage.

BODY TEMPERATURE

In the presence of intracranial injury, the development of hyperthermia to temperatures of 103°F or above may be associated with a bad prognosis.

EVALUATION OF DEEP TENDON REFLEXES

A detailed examination may be inappropriate at first. Study of the triceps, biceps, radioperiosteal, plantar, knee, and ankle reflexes, together with the test for the presence of ankle clonus, should be adequate for initial evaluation.

TYPES OF HEAD INJURIES

A simple linear skull fracture may be of minor importance and should not in itself alter the overall program of management. The importance of this finding will depend on the central nervous system signs and symptoms detectable in the individual patient. Depressed skull fracture occurs from direct trauma with an instrument or missile. Here, too, the resulting brain damage is extremely variable, and no general statements are possible. When dealing with lacerated or contused wounds of the scalp, one should suspect a possible depressed fracture, and careful neurologic examination should be performed. Depressed skull fracture is usually an indication for prompt surgical treatment. Failure to provide it may be associated with the progression of neurologic signs or infection.

Penetrating wounds of the skull may be misleading, since extensive intracranial injury may be associated with a small wound of entrance. Early surgical exploration and debridement are indicated.

Cerebral concussion is associated with a loss of consciousness and memory regarding the accident. The patient may appear to be well when seen initially, but observation is important, since there is the possibility of delayed intracranial hemorrhage.

Extradural or subdural hemorrhage is associated with head trauma. Characteristically a brief period of unconsciousness may be noted, followed by a "lucid interval." Confusion, drowsiness, and progressive coma then supervene. With extradural hemorrhage, the sequence of events tends to be fairly rapid, developing over a matter of hours. With subdural hemorrhage the course of the condition may be extended over several weeks or months. In either event the presence of lateralizing neurologic signs, asymmetric dilation of the pupils, and alteration in the deep tendon reflexes and motor responses should be sufficient reason to prompt emergency neurosurgical intervention.

EXAMINATION FOR FACIAL INJURIES

In accidents in which intracranial injury occurs, fractures of the facial bones are common. Fracture of the nose is often obvious because of deviation from the normal contour. Edema and discoloration of the skin, however, may render the diagnosis difficult. The patient should be examined from above as well as from the front if minor degrees of asymmetry are to be detected. Bimanual palpation and intranasal speculum examination may also be of help.

A blow on the cheek may produce a **fracture of the zygoma**. This fracture is frequently associated with considerable edema and subcutaneous hemorrhage, diplopia, subconjunctival hemorrhage, and anesthesia below the eye due to injury of the second division of the trigeminal nerve.

Fractures of the facial bones do not constitute surgical emergencies although they may be associated with some degree of airway obstruction. Operative treatment may be delayed for several days if necessary to permit adequate treatment of the patient's other injuries.

INJURIES OF THE SPINE

Fractures or fracture dislocations of the spine result from violent trauma. These may occur as a result of automobile accidents, football injuries, and diving accidents. It is essential to complete the diagnosis and transport the patient for initiation of treatment without producing injury to the spinal cord. The cervical spine, because of its mobility, is particularly susceptible to injury. For this reason, in moving a patient gentle traction should be exerted on the head in the long axis of the spine. The patient should not be allowed to flex his neck. A general rule is to permit the patient as little motion as possible and to transport him in the prone or supine position, depending on the circumstances, without permitting rotation, flexion, or extension of the spine.

Injury of the spinal cord is evaluated by asking the patient to move his legs and toes. If he is able to do this he has escaped major cord damage. If, however, the legs are paralyzed but the patient can move his hands, the cord lesion is located below the cervical region. If arm function is interfered with, cervical spine involvement is suggested. It is possible to confirm the location of cord injury by testing for loss of sensation to pinprick.

INJURIES OF THE CHEST WALL

FRACTURES

Rib fractures are common injuries. They may or may not be associated with intrathoracic damage. To permit proper examination the patient should be stripped to the waist and asked to take a deep breath. In the presence of rib fracture there is usually limitation of motion associated with pain on the affected side. The palpation of each rib in order should be carried out to rule out the possibility of subcutaneous emphysema. Compression of the chest cage in an anteroposterior direction and laterally may elicit pain when rib fractures are present.

Percussion and auscultation of the chest should be performed in every instance to detect the presence of intrathoracic injury. It is well to omit compression of the chest cage if physical signs of pleural effusion, pneumothorax, or mediastinal shift are present.

Fractures of the sternum are usually secondary to considerable violence and may occur in steering-wheel injuries. This fracture is usually associated with considerable pain and rapid, shallow respiration. The sternum may show a visible depression and subcutaneous hemorrhage may be prominent. Characteristically, the patient is seen to hold his head forward and rigid. This lesion is often associated with a contusion of the heart, hemopericardium, or injury to the intrathoracic aorta. Cardiac arrhythmias or murmurs may be present.

CRUSH INJURIES

With severe crush injuries of the ribs, resulting in multiple fractures, a portion of chest wall may become freely movable. This condition is known as **flail chest**. With inspiration the mobile portion of the chest wall is sucked inward, resulting in decreased ventilation. In effect, the involved side ceases to function in ventilatory exchange. The result is shunting of blood through the affected lung (physiologic shunt). Diagnosis is not difficult, since respiration is associated with exquisite pain, dyspnea, and cyanosis. The chest wall is seen to move paradoxically. It is imperative to achieve prompt stabilization of the chest wall. Intrapulmonary hemorrhage, or "wet lung," may also be present. Tracheostomy may be indicated to reduce dead space and permit adequate intratracheal toilet.

NONPENETRATING WOUNDS

Nonpenetrating wounds of the chest wall should be distinguished from crush injuries. They show the characteristics of soft tissue wounds in general. Penetrating closed wounds of the chest are usually associated with some degree of intrathoracic visceral damage. The possibilities include hemothorax, tension pneumothorax, subcutaneous or mediastinal emphysema, and cardiac tamponade.

With an open wound of the chest there is free communication between the pleural space and the outside. This is usually associated with great distress and signs of asphyxiation. Cyanosis and hypotension with a rapid and thready pulse are usually present. Inspiration is labored and accompanied by an audible sucking sound. Expiration is forced and often accompanied by frothy serum or blood issuing from the wound (Fig. 20-2). Subcutaneous emphysema is common. A large sucking wound of the chest is a surgical emergency that demands immediate treatment. It can usually be closed by applying a clean dressing. This should be carried out immediately, using materials at hand without regard to sterility. Ventilation may then be improved by having the patient lie on his injured side.

HEMOTHORAX

The physical signs of hemothorax are those of pleural effusion—diminished breath sounds at the base posteriorly on the involved side and dullness to percussion. The mediastinum may be shifted, and this may be detected by percussion and palpation of the trachea for shift. All degrees of hemothorax may occur, depending on the site of hemorrhage. Hemothorax may also be associated with pneumothorax if the parenchyma of the lung is involved. In this situation, increased resonance and

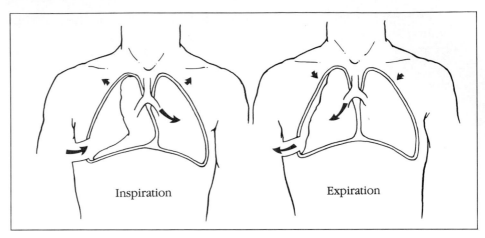

Inspiration   Expiration

FIGURE 20-2
Intrathoracic dynamics in patient with sucking wound of the chest. Note shifts in lung and
mediastinum with inspiration and expiration.

absent breath sounds will be present above the area of dullness. The physical signs
of pneumothorax tend to obscure the signs of pleural effusion.

PNEUMOTHORAX

Physical signs of pneumothorax depend on the amount of air present. Small
amounts of pneumothorax are difficult to identify, but one of any significant size
should be readily recognizable. Respiratory rate is increased and dyspnea is
present. The chest wall on the affected side shows decreased movement, and cyanosis may be present. Percussion may indicate a shift of the heart and mediastinum.
This may be confirmed by palpation of the trachea. The percussion note over the
involved side is characteristically increased in resonance and is tympanitic.

TENSION PNEUMOTHORAX

Tension pneumothorax occurs when injury involves pulmonary parenchynma or
bronchi. It may develop when an open sucking wound of the chest is closed by
packing or strapping, or it may be spontaneous due to rupture of a pulmonary bleb.
This injury is serious and demands prompt surgical treatment. With each inspiration air enters the pleural space on the involved side, increasing the collapse of the
lung and pushing the mediastinum toward the uninvolved side. This further reduces the function of the good lung. Clinically the situation is characterized by pronounced dyspnea and cyanosis. Vascular collapse with hypotension and a rapid
thready pulse are due to decreased venous return to the heart. It is important to
differentiate between circulatory collapse secondary to hemorrhage or shock elsewhere in the body, and that which is secondary to tension pneumothorax. The trachea and heart will be shifted toward the uninvolved side, and the percussion note
is usually hyperresonant and tympanitic. It is possible, however, for tension pneumothorax to exist with minimal signs of hyperresonance and tympany. The mediastinal shift toward the uninvolved side may also be detected by percussion. Breath
sounds on the involved side are generally absent or muffled. Emergency treatment,
consisting of aspiration of the trapped air, should be instituted promptly and may

be of life-saving importance. Sufficient air should be aspirated to produce relief of symptoms. The patient should be followed carefully to prevent recurrence.

SUBCUTANEOUS EMPHYSEMA

Subcutaneous emphysema occurs when air gains access to tissue planes around the wound or injury. Considerable subcutaneous spread is possible and is characterized by local swelling, edema, and crepitation on compression. This is a common accompaniment of compression injuries to the chest involving rib fractures. It may also be seen in rupture of the parenchyma of the lung with dissection beneath the visceropleura into the mediastinum. It may then spread rapidly to produce swelling of the neck, face, and chest wall, and it may even extend to the abdominal wall and scrotum. It may be associated with minimal respiratory distress. If, however, dyspnea and cyanosis are present, one should suspect a coexisting tension pneumothorax. With tension pneumothorax it is possible to develop sufficient mediastinal pressure to embarrass the venous return to the heart. On auscultation over the base of the heart the characteristic crackling "mediastinal crunch" may be detectable.

Blunt Or Penetrating Chest Wounds

These wounds may produce an accumulation of blood within the pericardium that results in progressive compression of the heart with obstruction of the great veins. Cardiac filling is impaired and is reflected in a decreasing cardiac output. This may progress to death unless aspiration of the pericardium is carried out. **Cardiac tamponade** is associated with a high venous pressure. This may be recognized by distention of the neck veins and will be accompanied by dyspnea and cyanosis. If tamponade occurs rapidly the area of cardiac dullness may not be increased, and the diagnosis may be missed on percussion or even on fluoroscopy. On auscultation the heart sounds are distant and rapid. Systemic blood pressure is low, with a narrow pulse pressure created as systolic pressure falls and diastolic pressure rises. A paradoxic pulse is present and may be demonstrated by maintaining the blood-pressure cuff pressure at the level at which systolic sounds are first heard. With each inspiration the systolic sounds disappear. Fluoroscopy will demonstrate decreased cardiac pulsations, and echocardiography will confirm effusion. Treatment consists of aspiration of blood from the pericardium.

With blunt injury of the chest it is sometimes possible to encounter extensive pulmonary damage in the presence of an intact chest wall. An **intrapulmonary hematoma** is one consequence and may be associated with hemoptysis, or frothy sputum, and dyspnea. On percussion, dullness may be noted, whereas on auscultation breath sounds will be diminished and may be associated with coarse, bubbling rales. X-ray examination is an important diagnostic measure, and a high temperature may be present in the postinjury state.

Pulmonary edema may occur secondary to reflex stimulation from the intrathoracic viscera or from fluid overload. This may produce "traumatic wet lung." The physical findings consist of cyanosis, dyspnea, and production of frothy white or blood-stained sputum. Coarse rhonchi may be palpable, and moist rales may be heard on auscultation.

Contusions of the heart may be associated with cardiac irregularities or syncope. The heart may have associated valvular damage or rupture.

Injuries of the aorta may accompany steering-wheel trauma. Delayed rupture of the aorta may occur in the postinjury period. The site of rupture is usually located in the descending aortic arch in the region of the left subclavian artery. Frequent x-ray examination of the chest should be employed to detect early signs of enlargement at this point. These injuries are difficult to manage and many have a fatal outcome.

ABDOMINAL INJURIES

As a general rule, penetrating wounds of the abdomen require surgical exploration. If treatment is to be successful, early operation is an absolute necessity. If more than 8 hours elapse from time of injury to time of exploration, even simple wounds are associated with a high mortality rate. Hypotension occurring early after injury is likely to be associated with blood loss, whereas hypotension developing after several hours' delay may indicate widespread infection or peritonitis.

A complete examination is extremely important. It must take into account the type of agent inflicting the wound and the position of the patient at the time of injury. When the physician is faced with multiple wounds it is easy to be misled and to overlook small wounds of entrance. The buttocks, perineum, and anal canal should be carefully inspected as a general routine. The appearance of the wound may provide information regarding the nature of the injury. For example, the presence of intestinal contents or bile may denote specific visceral injury. Under these circumstances prompt exploration is indicated, and little is to be gained from prolonged detailed physical examination. Where wounds of entrance are small, however, detailed examination is important. This is particularly true when the wounds are located in such a way that intra-abdominal damage is not definitely established. Careful physical examination will then be directed toward eliciting evidence of even minor degrees of peritoneal irritation. This should certainly include rectal examination and may include sigmoidoscopy without the use of air insufflation. Injection of stab wounds with water-soluble contrast medium (Hypaque) is often helpful in determining peritoneal or visceral penetration. X-rays are taken in lateral and oblique projections. A favored policy is to do exploratory operation on patients with peritoneal penetration. The contrast injection technique should not to be used on patients with gunshot wounds or multiple stab wounds of the abdomen, or on patients with stab wounds of the chest. It should be remembered that spinal cord injuries may produce abdominal pain, rigidity, and hypotension. The neurologic examination in such instances is an important part of the evaluation process.

INTRA-ABDOMINAL HEMORRHAGE

Intra-abdominal hemorrhage may be produced by laceration of the liver, spleen, mesenteric vessels, or retroperitoneum. The development of pallor, sweating, restlessness, and thirst within a few hours of the time of injury is significant. Hypotension ensues, and the pulse becomes rapid in rate and thready in quality. Dyspnea or "air hunger," shifting dullness, and rebound tenderness may be present. With massive hemorrhage the abdomen becomes progressively swollen and full. When intra-abdominal hemorrhage is not massive, normal blood pressure may be maintained for several hours. Under these circumstances it becomes necessary to follow the pulse pressure and pulse rate with care. The course of these indices is more important than the actual initial value. With slow continued bleeding, progressive abdominal tenderness and spasm may become evident; with sustained slow blood loss, decompensation and hypotension may occur rather suddenly. A rising pulse rate may indicate impending decompensation.

With perforation of a hollow viscus, abdominal pain and vomiting may occur and will rapidly become associated with a rigid, tender, silent abdomen. These features are most prominent if some time has elapsed following injury. The early signs may be overlooked in the presence of multiple injuries or if analgesics or sedatives have been administered. If shock develops after 8 to 12 hours or more after injury, it may be caused by generalized peritonitis. Shock may be accompanied by tachypnea and characteristic anxious facies.

Several abdominal wounds are commonly associated with hypotension. Pain and syncope may contribute, but blood loss and massive peritonitis may rapidly contribute to "irreversible shock." Although the time period necessary for this to develop may vary, it is worth noting that therapy should not be withheld on the premise that the observed hypotension is irreversible. It is also true, however, that if blood pressure fails to rise after adequate replacement transfusion, a poor prognosis is indicated. It is equally important to be certain that some remediable lesion is not contributing to the patient's poor clinical condition. For example, tension pneumothorax or cardiac tamponade may occur in association with intra-abdominal injury. The physician should be prepared to reevaluate the patient completely at frequent intervals to be certain that his working diagnosis is accurate.

BLUNT ABDOMINAL INJURY

The liver, stomach, intestines, spleen, and pancreas are all subject to severe injury of a blunt or nonpenetrating nature. The injury may occur when the viscus is crushed against the vertebral column. Frequent examination of the abdomen is of considerable importance. If there is reasonable doubt about the possibility of intraperitoneal injury, exploratory celiotomy should be indicated. This is a matter of judgment, since the severity of other associated injuries must be weighed against the possibilities of a negative exploration.

Laceration of the liver results in intraperitoneal hemorrhage, which may vary in extent. With a sizable lesion, exsanguination and death may result. With minor degrees of laceration, bile peritonitis may occur. In either event the physical signs will be those of peritoneal irritation, possibly with shifting dullness, rebound tenderness, and generalized peritonitis.

Splenic rupture is a common injury and should be suspected following blows on the left flank or the lower left chest. The clinical picture is characterized by abdominal pain, pain in the left shoulder, and shock. On physical examination, peritoneal irritation will usually be present and will be more marked in the left upper quadrant. Pain in the left shoulder and dyspnea may result from diaphragmatic irritation. Diagnosis may be exceedingly difficult with minor lacerations of the spleen. Careful clinical evaluation is required.

Mild trauma may produce a *subcapsular hematoma of the spleen* that may rupture several days or weeks later with shock, intraperitoneal hemorrhage, and rebound tenderness. The problem may be difficult to diagnose. Lateral abdominal x-rays may be of help in differentiating this from retroperitoneal tumor masses. An upright film of the abdomen after the patient has drunk a carbonated beverage may reveal irregular hematomas in the gastrosplenic mesentery.

In some diseases, such as malaria, leukemia, or infectious mononucleosis, splenomegaly is a prominent feature of the disease. In these patients the spleen may rupture spontaneously or following minor trauma.

Forcible compression of the small intestine may lead to laceration. The most common location is just distal to the ligament of Treitz or in the terminal ileum, close to points of fixation. The duodenum in its position anterior to the spine is susceptible to rupture. When this occurs, however, bowel contents leak out and peritonitis develops posteriorly. The associated physical signs may appear late. Spasm and abdominal rigidity will be delayed.

Rupture of the large intestine is not common. However, lacerations of the large-bowel mesentery may occur, and necrosis and gangrene may result. The patient will present with considerable abdominal pain but usually without signs of peritonitis. The diagnosis may be extraordinarily difficult to make.

INJURY OF THE URINARY TRACT

Injuries of the kidney are usually seen in association with injury of the abdominal viscera, either the blunt or the penetrating type. Flank pain and hematuria are fairly constant findings. Blood loss may be considerable but is rarely exsanguinating. Extravasation of urine may occur into the renal fossa and flank. The combination of hemorrhage and urinary extravasation may produce muscle spasm, tenderness, and flank fullness. A mass may be palpable and may even be noted on inspection. Other physical signs include ecchymoses in the flank, nonshifting dullness in the flank, and a positive psoas sign secondary to extravasation of blood and urine overlying the psoas muscle.

It may be difficult to distinguish between injury of the spleen or liver and a damaged kidney. If the patient's condition warrants and he is not in shock, an intravenous pyelogram is helpful. This examination provides information regarding the involved kidney as well as the functional state of the uninvolved side.

Bladder and urethral injuries are usually associated with fractures of the pelvis. In evaluating the possibility of this type of injury it is important to establish when the bladder was emptied prior to the accident. If the patient had not voided for some time and the bladder was known to be full at the time of the accident, rupture of the bladder is much more likely than if the bladder had been empty. The passage of bloody urine following injury helps establish the diagnosis of bladder or urethral injury. If the patient successfully voids clear urine after the accident, it is safe to assume that no serious injury to the lower urinary tract has resulted. If there is evidence of injury of the bladder neck or membranous urethra, catheterization should be performed by a skilled urologist who is prepared to assume complete surgical management. Damage may be compounded by unskilled attempts to pass the catheter in the presence of urethral damage.

Intraperitoneal rupture of the bladder occurs only if the bladder was full at the time of injury. Physical findings on examination consist of deep tenderness, muscle spasm, and peritoneal irritation. Rectal examination demonstrates tenderness and a normal prostate and membranous urethra. On completion of these initial diagnostic steps, catheterization may be performed. If bloody urine is obtained, urinary tract damage should be suspected. A cystogram may be diagnostic.

Injury of the bladder neck or membranous urethra results in extravasation of urine into the tissues surrounding the bladder and lower abdominal wall. The extravasation extends laterally, and the area is markedly tender to gentle pressure. Rectal examination is important in localizing the area of injury. Damage to the prostatic urethra results in the presence of a boggy, tender mass that obscures the prostate gland. With laceration of the urogenital diaphragm, urine and blood extravasate into the perineum and perivesical space. These physical findings are indications for early surgical intervention.

Injuries to the lower urinary tract usually occur in conjunction with pelvic fractures. Lateral compression of the pelvis helps to make this diagnosis, although an x-ray will be helpful in determining the extent of the injury.

PERIPHERAL NERVE INJURIES
Wounds in the extremities that include peripheral nerve injuries are encountered in military experience where extensive wounds of soft tissues and long bones occur. Peripheral nerve damage involves lower motor neuron axons, resulting in a flaccid type of paralysis. As a late result muscles distal to the lesion undergo atrophy, sensory loss, and autonomic changes. The skin distally becomes thinned, smooth, and pale or mottled. Sweating is absent. Fingernails and toenails become brittle. These latter signs are, however, late in appearance, and early diagnosis will depend on loss of voluntary muscle power or absence of perception of pinprick.

Some peripheral nerve injuries are commonly encountered in civilian medical practice. For example, the radial nerve may be injured with fractures of the shaft of the humerus; the ulnar nerve may be damaged in association with fractures about the elbow; common peroneal nerve involvement may be found in connection with fractures, soft tissue wounds, or the use of tight casts that produce pressure about the knee. The sciatic nerve may be injured when dislocations or fractures of the hip occur. Lacerations about the wrists may produce damage to the median or ulnar nerves, and traction on the upper extremity may produce brachial plexus damage.

Partial damage to a peripheral nerve may be followed by a characteristic type of pain termed *causalgia,* which may develop rapidly after injury or may require several days to make its appearance. Causalgia is characterized by constant, intense, burning pain. It is made worse by moving, touching, minor trauma, excitement, and often by temperature change. The sciatic and median nerves are those most commonly involved. On neurologic examination the peripheral nerve injury is usually not complete. The skin of the involved member tends to be shiny and glossy, although not invariably so. Anesthetic block of the related sympathetic pathways characteristically produces prompt relief of the pain. This observation is of value in diagnosis.

EXAMINATION OF THE MUSCULOSKELETAL SYSTEM
FOLLOWING ACUTE TRAUMA
GENERAL
The circumstances under which the injuries sustained by an accident victim are first determined usually require a different examination sequence and technique from that used in diagnosing less urgent musculoskeletal problems in the outpatient

clinic or private office. In a modern community, patients who may have severe injuries are usually not seen by a physician until after they have been rushed by ambulance to an emergency department. By the time the doctor sees them they have already been placed in a recumbent position on a stretcher. Following the initial evaluation only a limited degree of repositioning should be performed while x-rays or other special diagnostic studies are completed. Time may be very critical. Adequate functioning of vital organ systems must be established as soon as possible. Only then can attention be given to examination and management of other systems and regions. Frequently no medical history can be obtained from either the patient or any other source; there is no useful information on the magnitude and direction of forces involved in the accident, and the patient may be totally unable to cooperate with the examiner.

Under these circumstances the examiner requires an examination plan that can be executed swiftly, almost instinctively. The plan should first identify malfunction of the most critical organ systems, then determine the existence of any significant injury, and finally clarify the details of any injury. It should involve minimum handling of the patient and allow for the concomitant initiation of urgent therapeutic measures. Such an examination sequence will be described in the last part of this chapter.

Fortunately the symptoms and signs of acute bone or joint injury are few and are easy to detect. Also, although bone and joint injuries involve adjacent soft tissues, the anatomy of each region is conducive to unique patterns of injury that are easily identified by the experienced examiner. For example, the shoulder may sustain either a fracture through the humeral neck, with associated soft-tissue injuries, or a scapulohumeral dislocation; similarly, the elbow may sustain either a supracondylar fracture or an ulnohumeral dislocation.

For quick determination of precisely which injury has occurred, routine x-ray studies are more reliable than the physical examination. Even the most experienced clinician cannot be certain of all details without x-ray studies. Therefore, attempts to distinguish injuries within a given region by lengthy clinical examination should be avoided, especially when the examination requires diagnostic manipulations that might further injure the soft tissues. In the initial survey, on the other hand, a good screening physical examination is more reliable than x-ray films in disclosing regions of injury. X-ray studies should not be performed, therefore, until all suspiscious regions have been identified.

Frequently the treatment of the injuries should be started during the course of the examination. As soon as a presumptive diagnosis of a fracture or dislocation is established, the involved region should be immobilized by splinting in order to minimize further damage to the soft tissues during subsequent examination and x-ray procedures. These splints should not be disturbed either during or following the x-ray examination until definitive treatment has been started.

POSITIONING THE PATIENT

For the initial examination, the accident victim should, if possible, be lying supine on a stretcher. Since moving an injured patient is hazardous, the stretcher frame should be detachable, so that the patient can be lifted to a table and x-rayed or operated on while he is still on the stretcher. Although no single position allows complete inspection of the patient, full supination offers the greatest latitude for both examination and treatment. Turning an accident victim onto his back without regard for a possibly broken spine or other serious fracture, is, of course, fraught with grave risks. On the other hand, if his condition requires immediate airway clearance or closed cardiac massage, there is no choice but to turn him.

In less critical cases the patient should be questioned for location of pain and his limbs quickly inspected for evidence of deformities that might indicate fractures or dislocations. He should be asked to move his fingers and toes; the presence or absence of paraplegia or quadriplegia is thereby established. If the patient has pain in his neck or back, the presence of a vertebral injury should be presumed until confirmed or refuted by x-rays.

If the findings suggest a vertebral injury, it is possible to turn the patient, if necessary, by straightening his back or neck and carefully avoiding any bending or twisting. The patient should be rolled with someone holding his head and turning it in harmony with the rest of his body, with care to see that his arms are extended along the sides of his body. It is remotely possible that straightening an injured vertebral column may aggravate an injury, but this possibility must be accepted since completion of the examination and treatment ultimately require a supine position.

If a limb bone injury is suspected, the patient should be turned with an attendant supporting the injured limb and turning it in gentle harmony with the rest of the body. Although splinting a limb prior to turning has been advocated, splints are most easily applied with the patient supine and are of relatively little value in maintaining fracture alignment during turning. After turning has been accomplished, splinting will afford protection during further maneuvers.

General Types of Fractures
The broken bone, once set together, is stronger than ever.

John Lyly
(1554–1606)

Fracture and break are synonymous terms, classically defined as "a dissolution of continuity of a solid structure," for example, a bone. If there are more than two fragments, the fracture is said to be *comminuted*. Self-explanatory terms, such as *transverse, oblique, spiral, T, Y,* are frequently used to describe the orientation of a fracture line. A fracture line may enter one side of the bone and then divide and extend across the remainder of the bone in two diverging branches, creating an extra piece of bone imaginatively denoted as a *butterfly* fragment.

When a long bone is subjected to bending force, the portion that is under the greatest tension usually breaks apart first. This type of break is similar to that of a broken piece of chalk. The fragments can move apart easily. In the body, the surrounding soft tissues restrain the fragments from displacement. Displacement and deformity are relative to the degree of soft tissue disruption, particularly of the periosteum. In adults the periosteum is thin; therefore, widespread displacement and severe deformity are likely. In children the periosteum is thick and is frequently torn on only one side of the bone, thereby allowing only angular deformity with little or no displacement. In either age group, if the periosteal disruption is sufficiently severe, the ends of the fragments may displace. If the fracture line is oblique or spiral, or if sufficient lateral displacement occurs in a transverse frac-

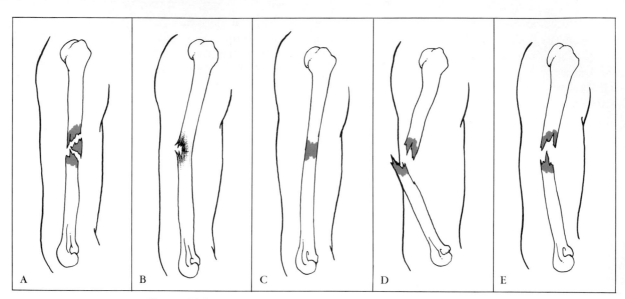

FIGURE 20-3
Some types of fractures. A. Comminuted. B. Greenstick. C. Torus. D. Compound (open). E. Simple (closed).

ture, some overriding of the fragments and consequent shortening of the limb are likely. One fragment may twist with respect to the other (malrotation). Any degree of angulation may occur. The ultimate position of the fragments and the external appearance of the limb are determined by the effects of neighboring muscles as well as by the effects of gravity and the direction and magnitude of the fracture force. Although shortening of a limb is commonly observed immediately after a fracture, lengthening almost never occurs.

Since children's bones are less brittle than adults', only one side of the bone may pull apart; the other side bends. This *incomplete fracture* is referred to as a *greenstick* fracture. It exhibits only an angular deformity. Occasionally, when a child's long bone is subjected to a bending or an axial compression force, it may buckle on the compressed side of the bone. This usually occurs in the flared (metaphyseal) area. The opposite cortex of the bone appears normal on an x-ray and the limb exhibits no deformity, merely localized pain and tenderness to palpation. This type of *incomplete* fracture is referred to as a *torus* fracture.

Fractures near the ends of children's long bones have special significance. If a fracture either crushes or splits an epiphysis and its underlying epiphyseal (growth) plate, a growth disturbance may occur. More frequently, fractures in this area pass transversely along the metaphyseal side of the epiphyseal plate and then deviate into the metaphysis. The terminal fragment then consists of the epiphysis with the epiphyseal plate and a small piece of metaphysis. Although displacement of this composite fragment may be wide, little or no damage has been done to the epiphyseal plate, and an ultimate growth disturbance is unlikely.

If there is a wound extending from the skin surface to the fracture site, there is grave risk of infection of the injured bone regardless of whether this skin is pierced by a bone fragment from within or by a foreign body from without. Such fractures are termed *open* or *compound*. It is essential that any skin wound, however small, that might communicate with the fracture site be recognized and promptly treated. The blood in a fracture hematoma quickly darkens and contains visible globules of fat from the marrow. A skin wound in the neighborhood of a fracture that oozes fluid of this type is therefore one that communicates directly with the fracture. Any fracture, no matter how comminuted, that does not communicate with a skin wound is referred to as a *closed* or *simple* fracture. Because of frequent confusion in the designations *compound* and *simple,* the terms *open* and *closed* are now preferred in standard use.

Small bones, such as those of the spine, ankle, and wrist, may be split or crushed by the forces of trauma. Displacement of the fragments is usually minor compared with that of fragments of long bones. Deformity is seldom evident if the bones are deep beneath the skin, as in the case of vertebral fractures; however, because of their proximity to the spinal cord and nerve roots, even minor displacements of vertebral fractures may produce signs of nerve damage. Fractures of small bones in the ankle and wrist seldom exhibit deformity unless displacement is severe, but they may alter the range of motion of associated joints, as indicated by pain on local palpation or attempted motion. Fractures extending into joints cause bleeding into the joints. Motion is painful and if the joint is a superficial one, such as the knee or elbow, swelling eventually occurs.

In summary, the cardinal symptom of a fracture is pain, which is usually most severe at the fracture site. Tenderness may be evoked by palpation directly over the fracture or by moving the bone fragments. The former technique is safe and reliable; the latter is hazardous. Motion of the fragments is also likely to cause audible or palpable crepitus. The patient may be able to report that he felt or heard his bone snap at the time of injury and has felt the grating of fragments when he has been moved. The examiner should not attempt to elicit crepitus. Instability is usually obvious, but occasionally a fracture may be quite stable, and the fact that a patient can use his injured limb does not rule out fracture. Visible or palpable deformity may or may not be present. Swelling, ecchymosis, and increased local heat occur to a variable extent with all fractures but are late signs.

GENERAL TYPES OF DISLOCATIONS

If the articular surface of one bone is totally displaced from the articular surface of its partner, the joint is *dislocated*. A joint may be dislocated and spontaneously reduce itself, or the bones may be trapped by the surrounding structures and special maneuvers required for reduction. A *subluxation* is a partial dislocation; contact between the articular surfaces is less than normal. This term is best applied to certain malformed joints and is seldom applicable to traumatized joints. In trauma the joint either is or is not dislocated; there are no intermediate possibilities.

As with a fracture, the cardinal symptom is pain, and there is local tenderness to palpation or motion. The range of motion is altered and usually reduced; in fact, the joint seems locked in an abnormal position. The examiner should not attempt to elicit motion but should take the word of the patient on this point. Deformity of adjacent structures is evident in a superficial joint. The posture of the limb distal to the joint is usually abnormal. Dislocation of some joints, such as the shoulder, increases the overall length of the limb. Swelling, ecchymosis, and heat are late signs. Ideally diagnosis should be established and the dislocation reduced before these have been allowed to develop.

X-rays should not be delayed in an effort to establish the details of a joint injury by physical examination, since films are far more reliable. Two points, however, should be quickly determined: the presence of a wound into the joint, since an *open* or *compound* dislocation is as vulnerable to infection as an open fracture, and the presence of vascular or neurologic insufficiency in the limb distal to the injury.

LIGAMENTS, TENDONS, AND MUSCLES

The ligaments of interest in this chapter are those that span joints and thus stabilize and control the motion of the involved bones. In the joints of the arms and legs, motion is possible primarily within a single plane; strap ligaments on either side of the joint allow very limited lateral or medial motion (abduction and adduction). With excessive leverage improperly applied to the joint, a ligament may be ruptured, torn transversely, or separated from one of its points of attachment. In any case, the point of maximum pain and tenderness to digital palpation coincides with the point of injury. If the most tender spot lies over ligament rather than bone, a ligament injury is more probable than a fracture. If x-rays at this time indicate that no fracture is present, it is safe to test the ligament for partial or total disruption by carefully abducting or adducting the joint. If a ligament is totally divided, and if the patient is able to relax his muscles, excessive motion will be found in the joint. Such an examination is sometimes too painful for a patient to endure, and either an anesthetic must be administered or the joint allowed to "cool off" for a couple of weeks in some form of protective immobilization, such as a cast. *Strain* and *sprain* are words frequently used imprecisely. *Strain* is correctly used to refer to a stretch or partial tear; *sprain* is correctly used to refer to a total tear or avulsion. A dislocation cannot occur without serious tearing or avulsion of ligaments.

A tendon forms the connection between muscle and bone, converting the contraction of the muscle into motion of the bone. Tendons, musculotendinous junctions, and occasionally even muscles can be torn apart if the bone is prevented from moving or is forced to move in opposition to a strong muscle contraction. In children, avulsion of a piece of bone at the point of tendon attachment is more common than a tear in the tendon or musculotendinous junction. The opposite is true in adults. Common examples of tendon tears in adults occur in the tendons of the long head of the biceps, the tendon of the supraspinatus, and the tendoachilles of the calf. These injuries are identified by correlating the site of pain with weakness or absence of function in a specific muscle. There may be a palpable soft-tissue defect at the point of pain and enlargement of the muscle indicating its uncontrolled recoil. X-rays that are taken for soft-tissue detail can sometimes confirm a clinical impression of tendon tear.

ARTERIES

Fractures or dislocations may impair distal arterial blood supply by compressing or lacerating the artery at the site of injury. This occurs most frequently at the knee and elbow but can occur with bone or joint injuries in many other regions. Therefore the quality of the peripheral circulation in all four limbs should always be clearly determined and recorded during the initial examination, before any splint is applied or x-rays taken. Early signs of arterial insufficiency are lowered skin temperature, absence of wrist or foot pulses, and pallor. Later signs include hyperesthesia and paralysis. At the site of arterial injury there may be a large and pulsatile swelling, indicating massive extravasation of arterial blood; however, this is a relatively infrequent complication.

NERVES

Wherever nerves lie close to bone, fractures can injure them. The region of greatest concern, of course, is the vertebral column. Elements of the lumbosacral plexus are occasionally damaged by fractures of the pelvis. A significant percentage of posterior dislocations of the hip damage the sciatic nerve and paralyze the dorsiflexors of the foot (footdrop). Severe knee injuries and fractures of the upper end of the fibula may damage the peroneal nerve, producing a footdrop. Fractures and dislocation of the shoulder joint are occasionally associated with injury to the axillary nerve, resulting in a weak abduction. Fractures of the shaft of the humerus, especially at the junction of the middle and distal thirds, may injure the radial, median, or ulnar nerves; radial palsy signified by inability to dorsiflex the wrist (wristdrop) is most common. Elbow injuries may be complicated by the same types of nerve injuries. At the wrist, compression of the median nerve in the carpal tunnel, with resulting numbness over the first two fingers, is common. To determine whether nerves have been injured, the motor and sensory function distal to any fracture must be evaluated and recorded on initial examination.

SPECIFIC FRACTURES AND DISLOCATIONS
VERTEBRAL FRACTURES AND DISLOCATIONS

Paralysis and sensory loss signify spinal cord or nerve root damage with a vertebral injury. Analysis of the level of motor or sensory loss will reveal the level of vertebral injury. Charts of sensory dermatomes and muscle innervations are helpful but are not necessary if the examiner has memorized the nerve supply to a few key regions and muscles. If the patient is comatose or stuporous, the determination is difficult but not impossible. Usually such a patient will move those regions that are not paralyzed in response to painful stimuli. If coma is profound, normal muscle tone as well as response to painful stimuli may be absent. Usually, however, if one foot is raised and dropped directly over the other, the descending heel will not strike the other foot unless the falling limb is paralyzed. The upper limb of an unconscious patient can similarly be tested by dropping the patient's hand toward his face. When innervation is intact, the falling hand will usually either deviate to the side or decelerate just before impact.

Pain in the back or neck of an accident victim should be considered an indication for spinal x-ray. The film should include several vertebrae above and below the painful area, since pain is frequently referred below the level of injury and occasionally above. Palpation of the spinous processes for an area of maximum tender-

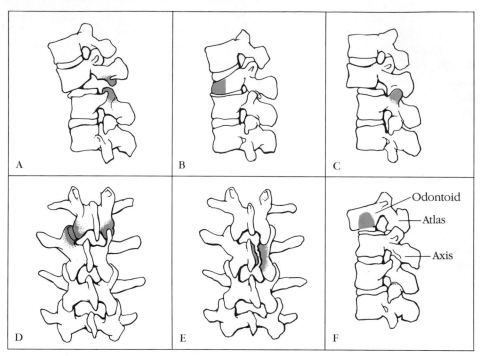

FIGURE 20-4
Common types of vertebral injury. A. Subluxation. B. Compression fracture. C. Bilateral facet joint dislocation. D. Unilateral facet joint dislocation. E. Posterior arch fracture. F. Odontoid fracture.

ness may facilitate precise localization of injury but should not be performed if it requires turning the patient.

Because of the deep position of the vertebral column in the body, external or palpable deformity is rare. Either pain or neurologic deficit is adequate evidence for diagnostic x-rays, and the examiner should not look for deformity or abnormal vertebral motion.

X-rays may show any of the following types of vertebral injuries occurring individually or in combination: subluxation, body fracture, unilateral or bilateral facet joint dislocation, or fracture of the arch, odontoid, spinous process, or transverse process (see Fig. 20-4).

Subluxation of an upper vertebra on a lower one is best seen in a lateral projection of the cervical spine in a neutral or forward flexed position. The interspinous ligament and sometimes the capsular ligaments of the posterior facet joints have been torn by the upper vertebra traveling too far forward on the lower, and sometimes the intervertebral disc space is narrowed. This condition represents a sprain and is an example of the so-called whiplash injury.

A vertebral body fracture is usually caused by compression forces, and the consequent reduction in height of the involved vertebral body is most conspicuous on lateral x-rays. Frequently pieces of the centrum are displaced and may impinge on the spinal cord. Compression of a thoracic vertebra into a wedge, with the nar-

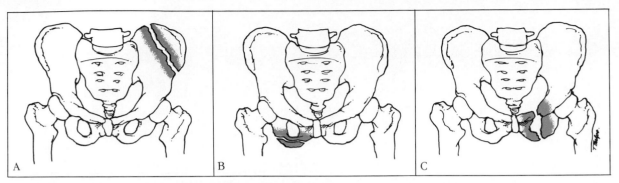

FIGURE 20-5
Benign fractures of the pelvis. A. Shear. B. Avulsion. C. Stable crack.

rower portion anterior and no resulting neurologic deficit, is a common finding in middle-aged and elderly persons with osteoporosis.

Dislocated posterior facet joints are rare except in the cervical spine. When unilateral dislocations occur, the vertebrae are locked in slight malrotation. For this reason the anteroposterior x-rays show a shift in the alignment of the spinous processes, with those above the dislocation shifted about ¼ inch toward the side of the dislocated facet joint. No such rotation occurs with bilateral facet joint dislocations, but the extreme forward shift of the upper on the lower vertebra is likely to cause severe spinal cord injury, in contrast to the minor neurologic deficit following a unilateral dislocation. The articular processes of dislocated facet joints can best be seen in lateral or oblique projections.

A posterior vertebral arch may sustain a fracture through the lamina, which is best visualized on an anteroposterior or oblique x-ray as a faint line near an articular facet. Usually when a ring of bone such as a vertebra is broken in one place, there is a second fracture through another part of the ring, which may be difficult to demonstrate on the x-ray. These fractures should be strongly suspected when there is a slight lateral shift of one spinous process. They may be associated with any degree of neurologic deficit. They may result from a hyperextension injury or a direct blow and are likely to be associated with significant instability of the vertebral column. Hyperextension of the spine should be carefully avoided in handling these cases.

An odontoid fracture represents a perilous injury in view of potential instability of C1 on C2 and the limited space available to the spinal cord if displacement occurs. When cord injury does occur at this level, there may be immediate paralysis of all respiratory muscles and quick death. This fracture is usually best seen on an open-mouth anteroposterior view as a line across the waist or base of the odontoid. The overlying shadow of an upper incisor tooth frequently obscures the true outline of the odontoid in a manner that simulates a fracture. Congenital malformation of the odontoid with incomplete ossification may also confuse the findings. For a reliable diagnosis the x-ray findings must be correlated with the nature of the injury and physical symptoms.

The distal tip of a spinous process, frequently at C7 or T1, may be the site of fracture. These processes are easily palpated and are very tender if fractured. If

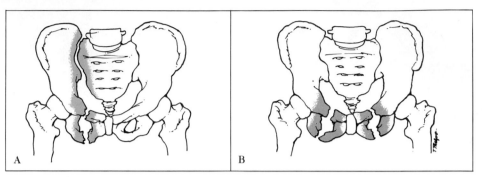

FIGURE 20-6
Unstable fractures of the pelvis. A. Malgaigne. B. Straddle.

there are no other vertebral fractures, the stability of the column is not compromised. These fractures are usually best seen on lateral x-ray projection.

Transverse processes on the lumbar vertebrae serve as points of attachment for the psoas muscles and may be fractured by avulsion. Retroperitoneal hemorrhage may occur, producing abdominal tenderness. The lateral edge of the psoas muscle may be obscured on the x-ray. The fractured transverse processes are best seen on an anteroposterior x-ray of the lumbar spine. Congenital malformation with incomplete ossification is common and may lead to a false diagnosis of fracture. Structural stability of the vertebral column is not impaired.

PELVIC FRACTURE

When evaluating the possibility of fracture, the examiner should think of the normal pelvis as a symmetric ring of bone with various projections serving as points of attachment for muscles. The projections may be sheared off by a direct blow or avulsed by strong muscle action. An example of a shearing injury is a fracture of the iliac crest caused by impingement of the handlebar grip of a motorcycle against the wing of an iliac bone as the rider is hurled forward in a collision; local contusion and loss of normal pelvic contour are apparent. An example of avulsion is the fracture of an ischial tuberosity by a sprinter as he forcibly contracts his hamstrings while pushing away from the starting blocks at the beginning of the race. Pain and tenderness at the point of a specific muscle attachment and on contraction of the involved muscle are diagnostic signs (Fig. 20-5).

Because of the elasticity of the symphysis pubis, the pelvic ring may be broken at only one point, but simultaneous fracture in two separate areas is more likely and also more serious because of the resulting instability. Weak areas are present near the sacroiliac joints, at the ischiopubic junctions, and through the symphysis pubis. A fracture through one sacroiliac joint and the ischiopubic junctions on the same side (Malgaigne fracture) creates a large lateral fragment to which the entire lower limb is attached (Fig. 20-6). This fragment is frequently displaced proximally by the trunk muscles. It may be tilted medially or laterally. Pelvic asymmetry and shortening of the lower limb are present and easily detected. Motion on gentle compression or distraction of the iliac crests is a conclusive finding of this injury. A fracture through the ischiopubic junctions bilaterally creates an anterior fragment that may be associated with bladder rupture. If the symphysis pubis can be moved by gentle pressure, the diagnosis of this fracture is confirmed. This injury is frequently caused by falling astride some large, rigid object. Contusion of the perineum may be present and the scrotum becomes distended with blood. In any of these injuries the abdomen may be tender to palpation and exhibit signs of retroperitoneal hemorrhage. Various branches of the lumbosacral plexus may be injured, producing hyperesthesia or muscle weakness.

HIP JOINT AND UPPER FEMUR

Among the types of fractures sustained by the upper femur are those with stability adequate to permit ambulation initially but that ultimately separate with unpleasant consequences. Significant events in the history are a fall or misstep followed by pain in the hip. Objective physical findings may be entirely negative. Good quality x-rays are necessary to establish the diagnosis, which may be that of a crack from greater to lesser trochanter, or a fracture across the neck of the femur just beneath the impacted femoral head. Although a fracture through the upper femur (broken hip) may occur at any age, it is more common among elderly persons, especially women, and more especially those with osteoporosis. Typically the limb lies in external rotation. The distance between knee and the iliac crest is reduced and any motion of the hip joint is painful.

The fractures are classified according to their anatomic location as determined by x-rays. Proceeding from proximal to distal, commonly used terms are subcapital, high cervical, midcervical, low cervical, intertrochanteric, and subtrochanteric. Since the capsule of the hip joint is attached to the femur near the base of the neck, fractures proximal to this line are intracapsular and those distal to it are extracapsular. This is an important point, since most of the blood to the head of the femur is supplied by vessels that approach the femur in the capsule, travel along the surface of the neck, and finally enter the bone in the subcapital area. Blood supply to the femoral head may therefore be interrupted by displacement of an intracapsular fracture but not by an extracapsular one.

Fractures of the acetabulum are frequently caused by forces that drive the femoral head into it. The femoral head may or may not be displaced medially and/or cephalad with the acetabular fragments. This is termed a *central fracture-dislocation* of the hip (Fig. 20-7). Frequently, however, this injury can be distinguished from an intracapsular femoral fracture only by x-rays.

If a person is in a sitting position with his hip in flexion and adduction at the moment of impact of a force on his knee, the femoral head may be driven over or through the posterior rim of the acetabulum and come to rest against the sciatic nerve just behind the socket. This is known as a posterior dislocation (see Fig. 20-7). Paralysis of foot dorsiflexors (footdrop) from sciatic nerve injury is common. The posture of a patient with this type of dislocation is unique. He lies with his involved limb in adduction, flexion, and internal rotation. He prefers to lie on his uninjured side and resists any attempt at normal positioning of his leg. Two other relatively uncommon dislocations of the femoral head occur—one into the *obturator* foramen, and the other into the region of the *inguinal* ligament. The former is an inferior dislocation and the latter, an anterior one. Both of these are caused by excessive abduction. A patient with an anterior dislocation lies in moder-

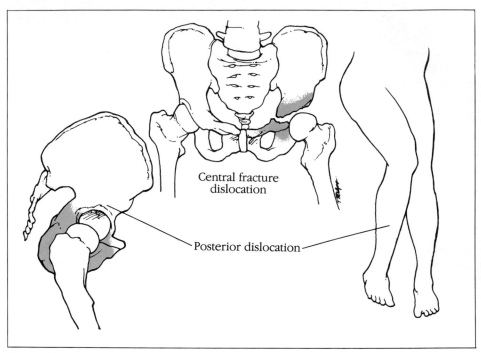

FIGURE 20-7
Central fracture-dislocation of hip and posterior dislocation of hip.

ate abduction and external rotation and the head is palpable beneath the inguinal ligament. A patient with an inferior dislocation lies in extreme abduction and external rotation and the head is not palpable.

SHOULDER JOINT (SCAPULOHUMERAL) AND UPPER HUMERUS

The shoulder is designed to facilitate placement of the hand in an unlimited number of positions in space. This is accomplished by a very shallow socket (glenoid) in the head of the scapula, articulating with the head of the humerus. The clavicle has a sinusoidal curve and is commonly fractured by a compression force applied longitudinally. Such a force may be applied directly by a blow on the tip of the shoulder or indirectly by a fall on the outstretched hand. This injury is one of the most common fractures in children and also in adults. The sternoclavicular joint can be disrupted by a similar force, with the result that the medial end of the clavicle dislocates medially and behind or in front of the sternum. An abrupt force downward on the tip of the shoulder can dislocate the acromioclavicular joint. Any of these injuries is easily detected by inspection and palpation, since the structures lie close beneath the skin. Dislocation of the medial end of the clavicle behind the sternum may create a sensation of airway obstruction due to pressure on the trachea. Clavicular fractures are frequently associated with a sizable subcutaneous hematoma and, rarely, with injury to elements of the brachial plexus and even the apex of the lung.

The common *dislocated shoulder* is an anterior or anteroinferior scapulohumeral dislocation (Fig. 20-8). When the humerus is abducted to the limit of its nor-

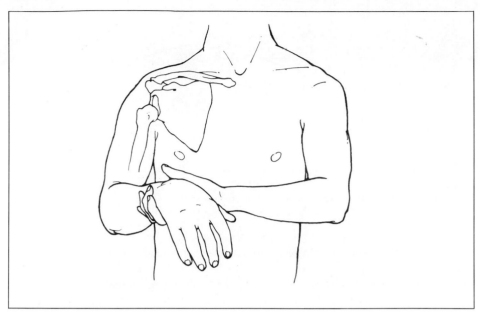

FIGURE 20-8
Anterior dislocation of scapulohumeral joint.

mal range of motion, it impinges against the outer edge of the acromion. If abduction is forced beyond this limit, the head of the humerus is levered over the anteroinferior edge of the rim of the glenoid. The patient is then unable to bring his arm in against his side or to rotate it internally. This type of dislocation frequently recurs. The first episode is extremely painful, but each recurrence is less painful, and the patient may learn to reduce the dislocation himself. The patient's appearance is unique. The deltoid bulge is flattened and the acromion is unusually prominent. The distance between the acromion and olecranon on the afflicted side is greater than on the opposite side. Sometimes it is possible to palpate the humeral head high in the axilla.

Fractures of the head or neck of the humerus can occur from a fall on the outstretched hand. They may be found in any age group but are more common in the elderly. Any active motion of the humerus is painful. In contrast with dislocations, the deltoid bulge is accentuated by displacement, or overriding, of the fragments, and by accumulation of extravasated blood. The distance between acromion and olecranon is unchanged or decreased.

Although these injuries can be identified by physical examination, this should not be done if adequate x-ray facilities are available. The initial examination of a specific area should be limited to determining that a skeletal injury exists; x-rays of that area are then indicated as soon as all other areas have been checked.

SHAFT OF FEMUR AND HUMERUS (SINGLE-BONE SEGMENTS)
Since the thigh segment of the lower limb and the arm segment of the upper limb each contains a single long bone, fracture of the shaft of that bone creates such conspicuous instability of the segment that diagnosis is usually obvious. Palpation

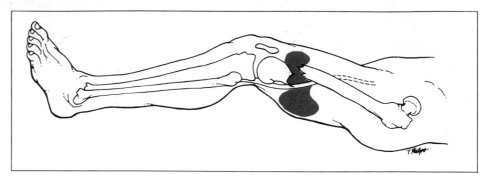

FIGURE 20-9
Injury to femoral artery by supracondylar fracture of femur.

of the bones may be difficult because of the thick muscles in these areas, but motion at the fracture site is revealed by any attempt to move the limb. The tone of the muscle tends to cause overriding of the fragments and therefore a decrease in length of the segment. If overriding is present or a hematoma has accumulated, the girth of the limb is enlarged. The ends of the sharp fragments may injure the neighboring soft tissues. In the femur, one or more of the deep veins may be torn, causing internal hemorrhage. The fractured humerus frequently damages the radial nerve, producing a wristdrop. Open fractures of these bones are especially serious injuries, and a careful circumferential check of the skin for any wound should always be made.

KNEE AND ELBOW

In the knee and elbow, bone fragments may easily be displaced; therefore no diagnostic manipulations should be performed on a deformed or painful joint until x-rays have been examined and found negative.

These joints link single-bone segments with double-bone segments; thus, each articulation involves three long bones. The motion of both joints is primarily within a single plane of flexion and extension. Each joint has a bony prominence that increases the mechanical advantage of the extensor muscle. For the knee this prominence is the patella; for the elbow it is the olecranon. The knee, which is subjected to high compression forces in many positions, has two semilunar wedges of cartilage called the menisci, which function as lubrication wedges, shock absorbers, and shims. Neurovascular structures lie close to the flexor aspects of distal humerus and femur (Figs. 20-9 and 20-10).

Fractures that jeopardize the arteries in these areas occur just above, between, or through the condyles and are termed *supracondylar, intracondylar,* and *condylar,* respectively. Such fractures of the humerus are especially common in children. One of the fragments, usually the distal, may be tilted by the flexor muscles toward the artery. Deformity of the elbow may range from insignificant to severe. Sometimes it may simulate a "gunstock," with medial or lateral deviation, a fullness in the upper part of the antecubital space, and a depression posteriorly just above the olecranon. Supracondylar fractures of the femur are more common in adults. There is an increase in the circumference of the thigh just above the knee. The fracture causes hemorrhage into the knee joint with consequent swelling. The dis-

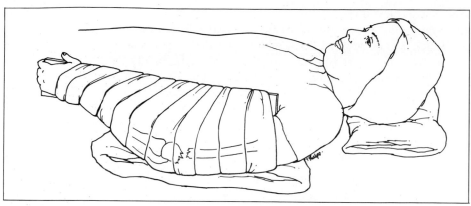

FIGURE 20-10
Supracondylar fracture of humerus.

tal end of the shaft fragment may penetrate the skin near the patella. In view of the strong possibility of arterial injury, circulation to the limb beyond the fracture must always be verified.

Both the olecranon and the patella are vulnerable to fractures from direct blows and from avulsion by muscle action. The former fractures are more often comminuted.

The patella can dislocate to the lateral side of the knee, a condition that is easily diagnosed by inspection and palpation. Dislocations of the tibia on the femur, or vice versa, cause extensive injuries that are usually accompanied by neurovascular injury. Deformity is severe and the diagnosis is self-evident.

An unfractured olecranon can dislocate only in association with the rest of the ulna, which may be displaced posteriorly and sometimes laterally. The deformity seen with posterior dislocation resembles that of a supracondylar fracture of the humerus.

If either the elbow or knee is subjected to excessive abduction or adduction stress, either the ligament fails on the side subjected to tension forces, or the bone crumbles on the side subjected to compression forces. Such fractures in the knee are called tibial plateau or tibial condyle fractures. In the elbow the counterpart of such an injury is a fracture of the radial head or neck. These fractures produce pain at the fracture site, pain on joint motion, and joint swelling. Ligament and meniscus injuries produce similar symptoms. Fractures should always be ruled out by x-rays before subjecting a joint to abduction or adduction stresses in order to ascertain ligament rupture.

If a meniscus is torn, the free part of it may become trapped between the femur and tibia and obstruct joint motion. This obstruction may be unyielding or it may be limited and variable. To detect the obstruction it may be necessary to flex and extend the joint with it twisted internally or externally and abducted or adducted. Such manipulation should never be performed if the possibility of fracture exists. A small area of acute tenderness to palpation is frequently present at the joint line close to a meniscus tear. Joint swelling is likely with this or any other knee injury and of itself may limit joint motion.

MONTEGGIA'S FRACTURE-DISLOCATION

This injury consists of a fracture of the ulna and a dislocation of the proximal end of the radius. It is usually caused by a blow on the ulnar side of the forearm near the elbow. The force breaks the ulna and then acts on the radius. If the radius does not break, the proximal radioulnar articulation is pulled apart. The annular ligament is broken and the proximal end of the radius is displaced from its normal position of articulation against the lateral condyl (capitellum) of the humerus. The existence of this injury may be presumed if a fracture of the ulna is identified and there seems to be pain or limitation of motion of the elbow. Diagnosis is confirmed by x-rays of both the elbow and forearm.

LEG AND FOREARM (DOUBLE-BONE SEGMENTS)

The thin soft tissue covering of the bones in the leg and forearm facilitates detection of an undisplaced fracture by palpation for point tenderness directly over the bone. This technique is especially valuable in establishing the possibility of an incomplete fracture of the torus or greenstick type. Only the radius cannot be palpated throughout its length. In the proximal one-third of the radius, where this bone is covered by the extensor muscles, a fracture should be presumed if tenderness is produced by pronation or supination.

Instability may not be conspicuous if only one of the bones is broken or if both bones are broken at different levels.

Fracture of both bones in a double-bone segment is more common than fracture of only one bone. Since these fractures may occur at a considerable distance from each other, x-rays should always be taken to include the entire length of the segment.

COLLES', BARTON'S, AND SMITH'S FRACTURES

Falling on a dorsiflexed and outstretched hand may fracture the radius just proximal to the wrist joint. The distal fragment is pushed proximally and may override or impact on the proximal one. The ulnar styloid process may be avulsed, but the rest of the ulna remains intact. The hand is forced into radial deviation. The distal radial fragment is usually tilted backward and the volar edge of the end of the shaft fragment crowds the flexor tendons or median nerve where they enter the carpal tunnel. The volar side of the wrist is abnormally prominent. Abraham Colles described the deformity associated with this particular fracture as resembling a dinner fork (Fig. 20-11). Sometimes the main mass of the radius remains intact and only the prominent dorsal margin of the articular surface is broken off, permitting the carpus to dislocate posteriorly. The fracture-dislocation is called a Barton's fracture. The clinical deformity is similar to a Colles' fracture. A fracture that might be defined as a Colles' fracture, except that the distal radial fragment is tilted toward the volar rather than the dorsal side, is called a Smith's fracture.

ANKLE INJURIES (POTT'S FRACTURE)

As with the shafts of the tibia and fibula, the thin, soft tissue covering of the malleoli facilitates detection of an undisplaced fracture by palpation for point tenderness directly over the bone. When maximum tenderness to palpation is over the medial or lateral ligaments or anterior capsule, the injury is more likely due to sprain than a fracture. No other diagnostic manipulation should be performed until fractures are ruled out by x-rays. X-rays may confirm that one malleolus or both is broken. In

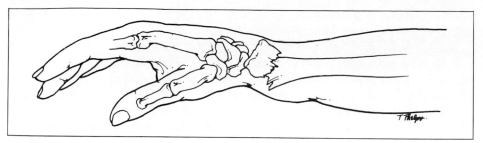

FIGURE 20-11
Colles' fracture of the wrist.

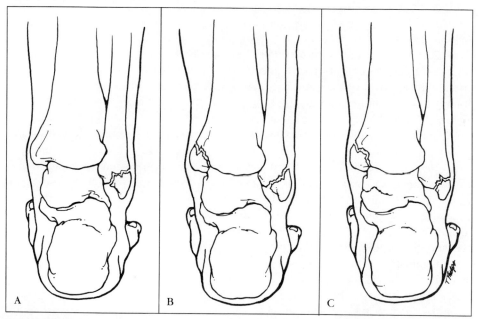

FIGURE 20-12
Some fractures of the ankle. A. Lateral malleolar fracture. B. Medial and lateral malleolar fracture. C. Trimalleolar fracture.

association with these fractures, the talus may be displaced medially or laterally. Sometimes the posterior articular margin of the tibia is also broken and displaced proximally (trimalleolar fracture). If the posterior fragment includes more than one-quarter of the articular surface of the tibia, the talus also dislocates posteriorly. Pott's fracture is a generic term for ankle fractures in general (Fig. 20-12).

FOOT AND HAND
Whereas displaced fractures or dislocations of the bones of the feet and hands are easy to recognize on inspection, x-rays are necessary to identify certain undisplaced fractures, especially those of the carpal and tarsal bones. Fractures of the calcaneus are usually caused by a blow on the bottom of the heel, as when an accident victim strikes the ground in a standing position after falling from a ladder or scaffold. Ver-

tebral compression fractures are commonly associated with this injury and should not be overlooked.

Fist fights result in broken knuckles and Bennett's fractures. The involved knuckle is usually depressed. The fracture is through the metacarpal neck, and the metacarpal head is tilted down into the palm. If a first metacarpal is driven proximally with excessive force, a fracture dislocation of the metacarpomultangular joint is sustained. This is called a Bennett's fracture. The thumb is shortened, and pain is greatest at its base. Thumb abduction and extension are painful and limited.

A blow sustained on the tip of an outstretched finger may forcibly flex the tip before the extensor tendon can be relaxed. The insertion of the extensor tendon is avulsed and the patient is unable to lift the tip of his finger.

CRASH PLAN

The CRASH PLAN mnemonic facilitates examination of an accident victim with injuries of unknown extent in a sequence that is easily remembered, requires minimum manipulation of the patient, is sufficiently complete to detect any significant injury, and is capable of expansion or acceleration as individual circumstances may require (Table 20-1).

Evaluation of **cardiorespiratory function** may be started as one walks toward the patient. If he is talking, he is doubtless circulating oxygen to vital centers, and consideration of immediate cardiac compression or forced pulmonary ventilation may be abandoned. On arrival at the patient's side, vital signs are checked and details of pulmonary exchange, cardiac function, and thoracic injuries are noted. Attention is then given to examination of the **abdomen** for signs of a ruptured viscus or hemorrhage. By this point in the examination there will be some indication of appropriate therapeutic and diagnostic steps, such as tracheal intubation or tracheotomy intravenous infusion, central venous pressure monitoring, electrocardiography, gastric intubation, and catheterization.

After evaluation of the abdomen and while life-supporting measures are being instituted, attention should be directed toward the **central nervous system** as signified in the mnemonic by reference to the *s*pine and *h*ead. The presence or absence of pain along the spine and any gross motor or sensory loss are determined. The state of consciousness should be noted, and the head should be inspected for evidence of fractures.

The possibility and extent of a **pelvic fracture** should be established by the technique described earlier in this chapter. The **limbs** should then be inspected for fractures, dislocations, or other serious injuries; lacerations should be noted for subsequent treatment.

When limb bone fractures might be present, it is particularly important to include in the emergency examination verification of the **arterial pulses,** or at least of the adequacy of circulation in the hands and feet.

At least one of the functions of each of the major **peripheral nerves** should be checked and the result recorded. The following tests are easily applied and interpreted: The patient is asked in sequence to abduct his shoulder (axillary nerve), flex his elbows (musculocutaneous nerve), dorsiflex his wrists (radial nerve), lift his thumbs up away from his palms (median nerve). Since standard muscle tests for

TABLE 20-1. CRASH PLAN

Suggested systematic approach to assessing the injured patient. This system follows a descending order of priorities.

CR = Cardiorespiratory
 A = Abdomen
 S = Spine
 H = Head, including state of consciousness
 P = Pelvis
 L = Limbs
 A = Arteries
 N = Peripheral Nerves (upper and lower extremities)

ulnar nerve function are easily misinterpreted, detection of light touch or pinprick over the ulnar aspect of the little fingers is a desirable alternative.

A similar test sequence for the function of the three major peripheral nerves of the lower limbs is performed by asking the patient to extend his knees (femoral nerve), dorsiflex his toes (peroneal nerve), and plantarflex his toes (tibial nerve).

A quick check for detection of light touch and pinprick over both upper and lower limbs indicates the extent of a suspected major nerve lesion.

SECTION VIII

THE ART AND SCIENCE OF MEDICINE

CHAPTERS

Faith T. Fitzgerald

Richard D. Judge

He's the best physician that knows the worthlessness of the most medicines.
BENJAMIN FRANKLIN
(1706–1790)

DIFFERENTIAL DIAGNOSIS

CHAPTER 21

As soon as a patient utters the chief complaint, experienced clinicians begin a process called differential diagnosis—that is, a consideration of all of the possible different causes of that complaint. It is this process of differential diagnosis, directed by a combination of knowledge and experience, that dictates the course of further historical questioning and physical examination.

The logic on which clinicians structure differential diagnostic thought falls into three basic categories: anatomic, physiologic, and etiologic.

ANATOMIC

One can consider the different causes of a complaint by considering in sequence each of the anatomic structures that, if dysfunctional, might be responsible for that complaint.

If a patient is jaundiced, what are the anatomic structures involved in the biologic handling of bilirubin that might be faulty? The *red cells* may be breaking down excessively (hemolytic jaundice), or the *hepatocyte* may be unable to handle normal amounts of hemoglobin products (hepatitis). The excretion of bile formed in the liver can be impeded at the *canaliculi,* along the *bile ducts,* and at the level of the *gallbladder,* the *common duct,* the *pancreas,* and the *duodenum.* By knowing the clinical characteristics and associations (syndromes) of jaundice originating in each site of anatomic suspicion, the diagnostician, by careful questioning and physical examination, narrows the range of possibilities to one or two major probabilities.

PHYSIOLOGIC

All physiologic systems are in balance in health. Disease may occur if that homeostasis breaks down. Differential diagnosis in the physiologic thought system follows the order of the normal production-metabolism-excretion/destruction of any product, touching upon its sites of possible derangement.

Jaundice may occur if *too much* bilirubin is produced by excessive hemolysis, or if intrahepatic *metabolism* is impaired by inflammation of the hepatocytes (hepatitis), or enzyme deficiencies (Gilbert's disease). If bilirubin is normally produced and metabolized, it may still rise in the blood if its *excretion* is faulty (intra- and extrahepatic obstruction).

ETIOLOGIC

A firm grounding in pathology can give the diagnostician one of the most valuable of the logical constructs on which to hang differential diagnostic thought. A useful mnemonic is *CIT-N-VIT.* It is a categorization of disease:

Congenital
Infectious
Traumatic
Neoplastic
Vascular
Immune-idiopathic
Toxic-metabolic

Jaundice may be caused by congenital-genetic disease (sickle cell anemia, poly-cystic liver), infections (e.g., viral hepatitis, parasitism), trauma (reabsorption of a large hematoma), neoplasm (with liver metastases), immune (chronic active hepatitis), or toxic (e.g., alcohol) liver disease, among others.

Obviously certain disorders lend themselves best to differential diagnostic analysis by the anatomic technique (pain, for example), others to the physiologic (biochemical upsets, or anemia). The etiologic thought process may be applied to any problem but requires a broader base of clinical knowledge to work well. As you progress in your ward work, and as your knowledge of disease expands, you will find that your histories will be more organized and pertinent (you will know what to ask), and your physical examinations will be more directed (you will know what to look for).

In the meantime, in order to facilitate the diagnostic process, the following special examinations are given as examples. You must avoid applying these "workups" to everyone. There is no single "fever workup," for example, that is appropriate to all patients with fever. Both you and your patients will benefit if you rely less on cookbook workups and more on the logical pathophysiology on which they are based. Then when your patient, an individual man or woman, varies from the classic, you will be able to modify your approach accordingly.

None of the three workups presented in the following sections is comprehensive. They should be used only as a pattern, not a rule. They have been chosen to illustrate the three differential diagnostic approaches, using as chief complaints (1) a symptom—shortness of breath, (2) a sign—fever, and (3) a laboratory finding—anemia.

WORKUP OF A SYMPTOM—SHORTNESS OF BREATH
GENERAL
This is one of the most frightening of all complaints, especially if acute (see Chap. 11).

DEFINITION
Dyspnea is a sense of labored or difficult breathing.

PATHOPHYSIOLOGY
The respiratory centers in the brain may be affected by metabolic changes in the blood (hypercarbia, hypoxemia, acidosis, toxins) to stimulate breathing. Chest disease of any sort may also give shortness of breath. Heart disease, by virtue of the heart's intimate connection with the lungs, is a common cause.

DIFFERENTIAL DIAGNOSIS

The symptom of shortness of breath may be logically approached *anatomically*.

I. Central nervous system
   A. Stroke
   B. Tumor
   C. Acidosis
   D. Hypercarbia
   E. Hypoxemia
   F. Profound anemia
   G. Carbon monoxide
   H. Salicylates
   I. Uremia
   J. Hepatic failure
   K. Sepsis
   L. Anxiety
II. Chest wall
   A. Trauma
   B. Weakness
   C. Pain
   D. Restriction of movement (as with bindings)
III. Pleura
   A. Pleurisy
   B. Pleural effusion
IV. Lungs
   A. Airway
      1. Obstruction
      2. Bronchospasm
   B. Parenchyma
      1. Infection
      2. Destruction (emphysema, fibrosis, tumor)
      3. Collapse
   C. Vasculature
      1. Pulmonary embolism
      2. Congestive heart failure
      3. Intrapulmonary bleeding
V. Diaphragm
   A. Elevation (ascites)
   B. Paralysis

HISTORY

Generally the rapidity and completeness of your history will depend on how distressed the patient is and on how obvious is the cause of the shortness of breath. Your patient, if wheezing severely, for example, should have the quickest of histories directed to the things that can lead to bronchospasm (allergies, inhaled toxins, aspiration, bronchitis, pulmonary embolism, pulmonary edema), omitting queries about other, rarer causes until the acute situation is in hand. Likewise, in acute situations a rapid pertinent physical examination of the respiratory and cardiovascular systems generally serves until therapy is begun. When the patient feels better, a more complete history and physical examination may be done. Ask about:

I. Duration and severity of the shortness of breath
   A. If acute or severe, ask about
      1. Known diabetic acidosis, hepatic or renal failure
      2. Known exposure to toxins (smoke, chemicals, aspirin)
      3. Chest wall injury
      4. Pleuritic pain, fever
      5. Asthma or allergies in past, aspiration
      6. Fever, pain, purulent sputum suggestive of infection
      7. Known lung disease (chronic bronchitis, emphysema)
      8. History of past pneumothorax, penetrating injury
      9. Pleuritic pain, hemoptysis, thrombophlebitis suggestive of pulmonary embolism
     10. Known heart disease, heart attack, angina, use of digitalis or diuretics
   B. If chronic or less severe, ask all of the questions listed under (A) above and those below in II through IV.
II. Characteristics of shortness of breath
   A. Associated with exertion? How much exertion?
   B. Postural associates (orthopnea? paroxysmal nocturnal dyspnea?)
   C. Temporal associates (at work only? seasonal? at night only?)
III. Associated symptoms
   A. Chest pain
   B. Hemoptysis
   C. Sputum production
   D. Fever, chills
   E. Wheezing
   F. Calf pain or tenderness
IV. Predisposing features
   A. History of diabetes in patient or family
   B. Symptoms of uremia
   C. Symptoms of liver failure
   D. History of bleeding or anemia
   E. Urinary tract symptoms
   F. Smoking, alcohol, illicit drug use
   G. History of anxiety attacks

PHYSICAL EXAMINATION

On the directed physical examination in patients with shortness of breath, you are looking for physical findings of two sorts: those associated with respiratory distress (AS) and those that give clues to the diagnosis (DX).

Vital signs: Tachycardia (AS and DX), tachypnea (AS and DX), hypotension (DX), fever (DX).
General: Agitated (AS and DX), sweaty (AS).

Skin: Cyanosis (DX), pallor (DX), uremic frost (DX), jaundice (DX).

HEENT: Dry mucous membranes mouth (AS), fruity odor breath (DX), musky or uremic odor breath (DX), fetid odor breath (DX).

Neck: Distended neck veins (DX), neck muscles used as accessory muscles of respiration (AS and DX).

Chest: Barrel shape (DX); decreased excursion, unilaterally or bilaterally (DX); regional dullness to percussion (DX); diffuse tympanitic percussion note (DX); low diaphragms by percussion (DX); rales, rhonchi, wheezes, rubs, regional decrease breath sounds (DX).

Heart: Tachycardia (AS or DX); diffuse PMI (DX); murmurs, gallops, rubs (DX).

Breast: Masses (DX).

Abdomen: Ascites (DX), hepatomegaly (DX), tenderness (DX).

External genitalia: Scrotal edema (DX).

Musculoskeletal: Clubbing (DX), sacral edema (DX), extremity edema (DX).

Neurologic: Anxiety and disorientation (AS and DX); focal neurologic signs (DX).

LABORATORY FINDINGS

1. Chest x-ray
2. Arterial blood gases on room air } Necessary in almost every case
3. CBC, urine analysis, sputum examination by Gram stain, ECG, sputum culture, pulmonary function studies, lung scan, hepatic and renal function, etc., as directed by history and physical examination.

WORKUP OF A SIGN—FEVER

GENERAL

This is one of the most common clinical findings. Its origin may range from trivial to deadly.

DEFINITION

An oral temperature of 100° to 101°F (or higher) in an adult, in the absence of known external cause of temperature elevation, is generally acknowledged to be a fever.

PATHOPHYSIOLOGY

Almost anything may cause fever, but all causes have as a common pathway the action of a pyrogen on the hypothalamic thermoregulatory centers (Chap. 5).

DIFFERENTIAL DIAGNOSIS

Since fever is a constitutional sign and symptom (i.e., it is neither localized to any anatomic region nor the result of a single physiologic mechanism), it is best approached *etiologically* (*CIT-N-VIT*).

1. *Congenital* or genetic fevers have been described (e.g., familial Mediterranean fever).
2. *Infection*—which may be viral, rickettsial, bacterial, spirochetal, fungal or parasitic—is the most common cause of fever.

3. *Trauma* may release pyrogens from necrotic tissue.
4. *Neoplasm* is a classic cause of fever, either by predisposition to concurrent infection or—especially in lymphoreticular malignancy—by itself.
5. *Vascular* disease, with distal ischemia or infarct, may generate pyrogens in damaged tissues.
6. *Idiopathic-immune* disease, such as lupus, rheumatoid arthritis, inflammatory bowel disease, and innumerable other ill-understood disease processes commonly present with fever.
7. *Toxic-metabolic* causes of fever include therapeutic drugs, poisons, hyperthyroidism, adrenal insufficiency, and others.

HISTORY

The patterns and associates of fever may give broad hints to diagnosis. As in other diagnostic problems, a carefully taken history is the most important "test" the physician may obtain. Ask about:

I. The fever itself
   A. Onset
   B. Pattern
   C. Precipitating and relieving factors
   D. Severity
   E. Duration
II. Associated symptoms
   A. Nonspecific (with many kinds of fever); myalgias, arthralgias, mild headache, chilliness, sweats, anorexia
   B. Suggestive of a diagnosis
      1. Chills (rigors)
      2. Night sweats
      3. Weight loss
      4. Clubbing
      5. Polyarthritis
      6. Rash
      7. Pain
      8. Cough
      9. GI dysfunction
      10. GU dysfunction
      11. Swelling
III. Predisposing features
   A. Past history of infection, trauma
   B. Use of medications, intravenous drugs, exposure to toxins
   C. Exposure to other sick individuals or animals
   D. Use of alcohol or tobacco (both carcinogens as well as predisposing to infection)
   E. Family history of fevers, cancer, endocrine or arthritic disease
   F. Immunosupression (diabetes, steroids, poor nutrition)

PHYSICAL EXAMINATION

On the directed physical, you must document the temperature and look for physical findings of two sorts: Those associated with fever itself (AS) and those to give clues to the diagnosis (DX).

Vital signs: Tachycardia (AS and DX), wide pulse pressure (AS), tachypnea (AS and DX).

General: Sweat (AS), anxiety (AS), cachexia (DX).

Skin: Rash (DX), erythema (AS and DX), pigmentation (DX).

Nodes: Regional or systemic enlargement (DX).

Head: Coryza (DX), pharyngitis (DX), otitis (DX), tooth tenderness (DX), funduscopic infarcts (Roth's spots) (DX).

Neck: Meningismus (DX), thyroid enlargement (DX).

Chest: Rales, rhonchi, rubs, dullness, egophony (DX).

Heart: Murmurs (AS and DX), gallops (AS and DX), rubs (DX).

Breast: Masses (DX).

Abdomen: Tenderness (DX), masses (DX), visceromegaly (DX).

Genitourinary: Tenderness (DX), masses (DX), discharge (DX).

Musculoskeletal: CVA tenderness (DX), spinal tenderness (DX), arthritis (DX), myositis (DX), trauma (DX), clubbing (DX), calf tenderness (DX).

Neurologic: Toxic state (AS and DX), focal neurologic signs (DX).

LABORATORY FINDINGS

The studies obtained are, as usual, directed by the history and physical examination but often include the following:

1. CBC with white cell count and differential. Peripheral smear is examined for abnormal cells (leukemia? virocytes?).
2. Urinalysis.
3. Chest x-ray.
4. Sputum, urine, CSF examined for pus and bacteria as indicated; cultures as indicated.

WORKUP OF A LABORATORY FINDING—ANEMIA

GENERAL

Though not a common spontaneous complaint, anemia is a common finding in patients seen in clinic, office, and hospital, with or without a variety of other disorders.

DEFINITION

Anemia is a deficiency of hemoglobin. Normal values for hemoglobin are

Children	13 ± 1 gm/dl
Men	16 ± 2 gm/dl
Women	14 ± 2 gm/dl

PATHOPHYSIOLOGY

The generation of hemoglobin occurs mainly in the marrow of the long bones in adults, under the modulation of erythropoietin and sex hormones. Adequate production depends on a sufficiency of the basic building blocks of hemoglobin (iron and proteins), enzymes (vitamins), membranes (lipids, phosphorus), and adequate marrow space, all under appropriate stimulus. Once released into the circulating volume, red cells may be destroyed or lost in excess of production and, by so doing, produce anemia.

DIFFERENTIAL DIAGNOSIS

The *physiologic approach* to differential diagnosis lends itself well to anemia. Red cells may not be made, or destroyed, or lost.

I. Suppression of production
   A. Inadequate substrate
      1. Iron deficiency
      2. Protein deficiency
      3. Vitamin deficiency (folate, B^{12}, B^6)
      4. Phosphorus deficiency
      5. Copper deficiency
   B. Abnormal production
      1. Erythropoietin deficiency
      2. Thyroid deficiency
      3. Toxic suppression (alcohol, drugs, illness)
   C. Marrow inadequacy
      1. Fibrosis
      2. Radiation, other toxins
      3. Malignancy
      4. Infection
II. Normal production, increased breakdown (hemolysis)
   A. Abnormal red cells (e.g., sickle cell, spherocytosis, G6PD)
   B. Red cell toxins (bacterial hemolysins, immune complexes)
   C. Vascular disease (microangiopathic hemolysis)
III. Increased loss (bleeding)
   A. GI tract (most common cause of anemia in men)
   B. Uterus (most common cause of anemia in women)
   C. Externally (trauma, phlebotomy)
   D. Kidneys (hematuria)
   E. Nose (epistaxis)
   F. Lungs (hemoptysis)

HISTORY

Generally an acute anemia manifests itself as volume loss and symptoms of tissue hypoxemia. The more usual, chronic anemias are less obvious and require more historical perception to define. Ask about:

1. Causes of anemia
   A. Diet, including starch or clay ingestion (binds iron in the gut).
   B. Bleeding (especially GI bleeding and menstrual pattern).
   C. Toxins (alcohol, benzene, drugs). Aspirin induces bleeding.
   D. Chronic infections, renal or hepatic dysfunction.
   E. Family history (pernicious anemia, sickle cell, etc.)
   F. Symptoms of malignancy (swelling, weight loss, pain, etc.)
2. Symptoms of anemia
   A. Weakness, dizziness, shortness of breath, fatigue, palpitations.
   B. Pica (craving for ice or certain foods due to iron deficiency). Another form of pica—the ingestion of laundry starch and clay—is not uncommon in American southern black women and is a *cause* of iron deficiency.
   C. Pruritus (due to iron deficiency as well as other causes associated with anemia).

PHYSICAL EXAMINATION

Again, the physical examination of the anemic patient should be directed to findings suggestive of anemia itself (AS) and of the possible diagnostic causes of that anemia (DX).

Vital signs: Tachycardia (AS), orthostatic BP changes (AS), fever (DX).

General: Pallor (AS), cachexia (DX).

Skin: Jaundice (DX), telangiectasia (DX), petechiae/purpura (DX)

HEENT: Conjunctival pallor (AS), Roth's spots (AS and DX), choroidal tubercules (DX), epistaxis (DX), smooth tongue (DX), pigmentation of mucous membrane (DX), bleeding gums (DX), fetor hepaticus or uremic breath (DX).

Neck: Goiter (DX), scar (DX), masses (DX).

Chest: Change in breath sounds or percussion note suggestive of mass or consolidation (DX), rales (DX).

Heart: Murmurs (DX or AS), gallops (AS).

Breasts: Masses (DX).

Abdomen: Tenderness (DX), organomegaly (DX), masses (DX), splenic rub (DX).

Rectal: Mass (DX), occult blood in stool (DX).

Genitourinary: Mass (DX), tenderness (DX).

Musculoskeletal: Arthritis (DX), myositis (DX), wasting (DX), trauma (DX), clubbing (DX).

Neurologic: Confusion (AS and DX), loss vibratory sense (DX).

LABORATORY FINDINGS

In many cases of anemia, the cause—after careful history and physical examination —is evident. Rarely it is obscure, and the diagnosis is established in the laboratory.

1. CBC with peripheral smear (examination of the smear by physician personally is mandatory in all cases of anemia).
2. Reticulocyte count.

3. If hemolysis is suggested: LDH, bilirubin, haptoglobin, Coombs' test.
4. If iron deficiency is suggested: serum iron, iron-binding capacity.
5. If vitamin deficiency is suggested: serum folate, B_{12} levels.
6. Bone marrow aspiration and examination.

With a firm base in anatomy and physiology, even the beginning student should be able to elaborate logical differential diagnoses. The mark of the finest clinicians is that they can explain almost every historical complaint, understand the origin of each physical finding, and predict each abnormal laboratory result in terms of the pathophysiology of each. This skill is a result not of memorization but of knowledge of fundamental biologic principles and a logical deductive thought process. Only by developing your clinical acumen in this way—rather than by studying lists of signs, symptoms, and therapy—will you be able to master the enormous range of biologic variables that each individual patient represents. Moreover, development of this talent takes clinical medicine out of the category of rote study and into the realm of exciting art.

USE OF THE CLINICAL LABORATORY

The advent of multichannel automated screening of blood samples, newer nuclear diagnostic techniques, the technological revolution of computerized axial tomography, and the availability of sophisticated endoscopy have all broadened the range of vision of today's diagnostician. We can now ask questions about the status of our patients that not long ago could be answered only on the operating or autopsy table.

But the armamentarium of modern laboratory techniques is a very mixed blessing. There are dangers in every procedure. It is essential that you have an understanding of the "therapeutic ratio"—that is, the risk involved in the test compared to the potential gain to the patient—of each laboratory or other study you consider ordering. Ask the following questions of each test:

1. **Why am I getting this test?** The best clinicians are directed in their use of the laboratory by carefully thought-out reasoning that underlies everything they do. One may order a glucose on a patient because he or she has polyuria and a family history of diabetes. Or one may want a thyroid function test on a woman with cold intolerance, constipation, and decreased mentation. To order tests "just to be complete" is more comforting to the doctor than it is to the patient; but it is the patient who pays for them, and that payment may be more than monetary. For example, if a man has a uric acid drawn as part of a "routine screening," though he is without complaints suggestive of gout or kidney stones, it is entirely possible that the uric acid test will come back showing a level somewhat over the normal. Now what? Generally the doctor feels compelled to draw another one, "just to check it out." What if this one is just at the upper level of normal? The doctor can draw a third level and average them (this is a very common sequence of events, by the way). Suppose the third level also comes back from the laboratory marginally high. Is an abnormal uric acid level a disease? If so, we have just discovered a disease in a previously healthy man. Should it be treated? Drugs may have complications associated with their administration. What if the doctor in this case gives a drug for the high uric acid, and the patient has an allergic reaction to it? What good has the doctor done the patient? The patient, previously well, has paid for three uric acid tests and for the drug he was prescribed, and has suffered the complications of that drug.

But suppose the routine screening does show a significant abnormality—for example, a very low hematocrit that can be corrected. It is a well-known event on the ward that a test result comes from the laboratory and, on returning to the bedside, the patient now gives a history and has physical findings fully supportive of the abnormality "discovered" in the lab. The anemic patient mentioned above, on direct requestioning, admits to extra heavy menstrual periods. All this means is that the initially taken history and physical examination were incomplete. It is axiomatic that the best clinicians are rarely surprised by any laboratory test. They take pride in knowing that the laboratory usually confirms their clinical impression rather than creates it. The laboratory test has become, in modern hospital practice, the anonymous critic of our clinical acumen.

2. Is this test necessary? Probably the best way to assay whether or not the study under consideration is important for the best care of your patient is to ask yourself "How would I approach this patient differently if the test were positive? Negative? Equivocal?" If your diagnostic or therapeutic approach would *not* be significantly altered by the test, it is probably as well not to do it. In an elderly woman with disseminated terminal cancer, there is evidence of progressive renal failure. Should you get an intravenous pyelogram to evaluate it? Since she is dying and kept comfortable by appropriate analgesics, there is little reason to do the x-ray: It would be of no added benefit to her. Ask yourself, on each occasion, if any study you may want to do is designed to help the patient feel better or if you are treating *your own insecurity* by doing it.

A side note of the "Is this test necessary" question should also be mentioned here: What will you do if the test indicates that what you are doing shouldn't be working therapeutically, but the patient is getting better nonetheless? In a child with a urinary tract infection, you promptly send a urine sample to the laboratory for culture and, before the result of the culture returns, begin therapy with antibiotic A. Two days later, the child feels much better, and your urine analysis shows disappearance of both the pus and the organisms that you had previously noted. The laboratory, however, now reports that the organism growing in the culture of the urine sample is resistant to antibiotic A. Now what do you do? Most experienced clinicians will simply ignore the laboratory result in this circumstance, but students and younger doctors may feel compelled to change to antibiotic B. They do not trust the evidence of their clinical senses.

3. Is this test reliable? There is a considerable amount of "faddism" in medicine. A new test or procedure appears on the horizon, and the published reports are very positive about its sensitivity (ability to detect an abnormality if it is present) and specificity (ability to fail to detect an abnormality if it is not present). It is well to keep in mind that authors seldom publish negative initial results, so that most early reports on any test will tend to be enthusiastic about it. Each physician must learn the inherent fallibility of each test or procedure in his or her own hospital. Even if a certain scan, for example, is marvelous at detecting hidden abscess at one medical center, the same technique in the hands of less practiced individuals at another medical center may be far less reliable.

Although it is difficult for students and house officers to accept, their own clinical judgment is often superior in accuracy to any laboratory test. This is true if only because the individuals caring for the patient have much more information about that patient in his or her entirety than the laboratory physician or technician, who has only a serum sample or a single organ scan. For example, a 38-year-old man presented to his physician with crescendo angina. Because of a normal ECG, he was allowed to go home. Within the next 12 hours he had a massive myocardial infarction and is now crippled by a ventricular aneurysm. One wonders, in this real case, whether the doctor—whose initial impulse was to hospitalize the patient—may not have been falsely reassured by the lack of ECG abnormality. In this instance the test probably delayed proper therapy. So if a test result runs counter to your best judgment, and you have carefully scrutinized all data available to you, trust your judgment.

4. How much does this test cost? Even if you decide that a given test is necessary, reliable, and likely to be helpful, you are obliged to consider it in terms of hard cash. Health insurance covers many laboratory procedures, but it does not pay for them all. And nothing, even health insurance, is free. It costs somebody— usually your patient—in higher premiums. Ask yourself, as you consider ordering a test, whether you personally would be willing to pay for it out of your own pocket. Indeed, as a taxpayer at times you *will* be paying for it out of your own pocket! Keep abreast of the costs of a variety of common diagnostic tests done in your own hospital. It frequently proves astonishing to students to discover that the scan they ordered "for interest" or "for teaching purposes" has a fee of $200 attached to it.

But there is yet another cost attached to the indiscriminate use of the laboratory. It is not uncommon for students to turn to the laboratory to answer questions for them that they had not been able to answer by their own wits. Such students slavishly take their direction from the printed laboratory result sheet, rather than directing the laboratory to specific questions. The cost to these students, and thus to the physicians they will become, is enormous. When doctors rely on the laboratory to tell them what to think, they have surrendered their intellectual autonomy, have given up the excitement of historical exploration and physical diagnostic detection, and have ceased to practice medicine. If you need a chest x-ray to diagnose lobar pneumonia, an ECG to tell you that your patient has had a myocardial infarction, or a panel of liver function tests to turn your attention to the gallbladder, you have become an extension of the laboratory rather than the other way around. And what will you do, as a physician, if the electricity goes off?

PRACTICAL POINTS FOR THE WARDS

CHAPTER 23

Experience is the mother of science.

PROVERB

History and Physical—Examples of Traditional and Problem-Oriented Medical Records

TRADITIONAL WRITE-UP

HISTORY AND PHYSICAL EXAMINATION

Mrs. Jane Doe
Registration #12345
432 Maple Avenue
Babylon, California
Tel. #(123)-456-7899

August 31, 1982
2:00 P.M.

CHIEF COMPLAINT
This 45-year-old married mother of two has had episodic right upper quadrant "knife-like" pain for the past 2 days.

HISTORY OF PRESENT ILLNESS
Mrs. Doe was in her usual good state of health until 2 days ago (August 29) when, having just finished a pork chop dinner, she had severe "knifelike" pain in the right upper quadrant of her abdomen, radiating to her epigastrium. She concurrently felt "sick to her stomach" (without vomiting), "sweaty," and faint (without loss of consciousness). She immediately lay down on her bed and felt better "after a minute." The severe pain grew rapidly less, as did the nausea, but she had a "dull ache" in her right upper quadrant for several hours. She took no medication. Position did not affect the pain. She felt well enough after an hour to clean up the dinner table, and slept well that night. She has had two subsequent almost identical "attacks," the first at lunch yesterday (August 30) following a hamburger and french fries. The most recent episode was at breakfast today after two slices of bacon.

  She's had no fever, chills, vomiting, or diarrhea. She denies past history of similar episodes. She has no current or past history of jaundice, white stools, dark urine, or change in bowel habits. She is unaware of a history of anemia (other than a mild "low blood" associated with her first pregnancy). She has not had tarry or black stools, hematemesis, burning abdominal pain or other "indigestion," kidney stones, polyuria or hematuria, hepatitis, or foreign travel. She has had no cough, shortness of breath, or pleurisy. She has no calf pain. She regularly examines her breasts and has noted no masses. There is a history of breast cancer in her mother. She has no known heart disease. She denies trauma to her chest, back, or legs. Her menses have been normal.

She takes no regular medications and specifically denies the use of antacids, aspirin, clofibrate (Atromid), or alcohol.

She currently feels quite well.

PAST MEDICAL HISTORY

Childhood illness: Mumps and chickenpox as child. No measles, rheumatic fever, scarlet fever.

Adult illness: None significant. Hospitalized only for childbirth (Soma Hospital, Babylon—1961 and 1963).

Trauma: Fractured left clavicle as child. No sequellae.

Surgery: Tonsillectomy as child of 6 (Soma Hospital). Episiotomy with each childbirth.

Allergies: Penicillin—urticarial rash without wheezing, stridor, (last dose 1976, at which time reaction occurred).

Medications: None at present. Has taken occasional aspirin for headache in past.

Travel: Never outside California.

Habits: Has never smoked tobacco or cannabis. Occasional dinner wine (none in past 2 weeks). No illicit drugs. Regular diet, 3 meals a day.

Immunizations: Does not remember childhood shots other than oral polio vaccine in early 1950s. Last tetanus shot 7 years ago.

FAMILY HISTORY

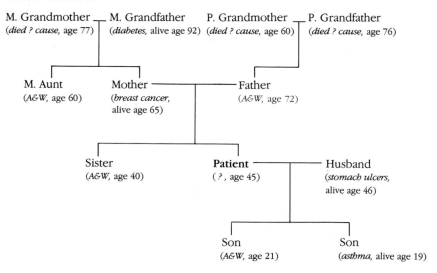

No family history of renal disease, liver disease, hypertension, anemia, tuberculosis.

SOCIAL HISTORY

Mrs. Doe was born and raised in Babylon, where she married her current husband after her graduation from high school in 1955. She worked as a secretary in his construction firm until their first child was born in 1961. She remained at home to raise her two sons, both of whom are college students (majoring in art and mathematics, respectively), and has recently returned to night school to gain college credits herself. She describes her life as full and her marriage as happy. Activities include housekeeping, gardening, and reading "romantic novels." Her husband's medical coverage extends to her, and she is not worried about money. She does admit to some unhappiness at not having gone to college as a young woman, but "is making up for it now." She is worried that her pain may represent an illness that will interfere with her studies, and she has "a test coming up next week." She is also fearful of cancer, as her mother has metastatic cancer of the breast, which is painful and emotionally draining on Mrs. Doe, who visits her in a nursing home every day.

REVIEW OF SYSTEMS

General: See HPI. No weight change.

Head: Occasional "stress" headache. No dizziness. "Faintness" with her recent attacks as described in HPI.

Eyes: Last tested 1 year ago at 20/20. No blurring, double vision, pain, discharge.

Ears: No decreased hearing, tinnitus, pain. Otitis media once as child (R ear).

Nose: No epistaxis, sinusitis.

Throat and mouth: Teeth in good repair. Infrequent sore throats.

Chest: See HPI. No wheezing, hemoptysis, sputum. Chest x-ray normal on screening exam 1 year ago. Negative TB skin test 1 year ago.

Heart: No pain, palpitations, orthopnea, cyanosis, edema. No history hypertension.

GI: See HPI.

GU: See HPI. No dysuria, frequency, urgency, incontinence. No history venereal disease or urinary tract infection.

Menstrual: Menarche age 13. Periods light flow for 3 days every 28 days and regular, with slight cramping on 1st day of flow. Last period normal, ended August 19, G2P2A0.

Neuromuscular: Faintness as in HPI, without syncope. No vertigo, dysesthesias, seizures. No history emotional disease.

PHYSICAL EXAMINATION

August 31, 1982
2:30 P.M.

General: Mrs. Doe is a slightly obese pleasant 45-year-old white woman who is somewhat anxious but in no acute distress.

Vital Signs: BP R arm Sitting: <u>140/90</u>   P85 regular R 12

　　　　　　　L arm sitting: <u>148/92</u>

　　　　　　　　　　　　　　T 99° F orally

　　　　　　　L arm standing: <u>155/95</u>

　　　　　　　　　Weight: 132 lb   Height: 5'6"

Skin: Warm and dry. No petechiae, purpura, excoriations. Anicteric. Hair and nails normal. No cutaneous lesions or rashes.

Nodes: No cervical, supraclavicular, epitrochlear lymphadenopathy. <u>1 × 1 cm, soft, nontender, mobile node R axilla. Scattered shotty inguinal nodes bilaterally.</u>

Head: Normocephalic, without trauma. No scars, tenderness, bruits.

Eyes: Conjunctivae normal. <u>Slight scleral icterus bilaterally.</u> Lids without lesions. Pupils equal, round, and react to light and accommodation. Vision grossly normal (reads newspaper). Visual fields full to confrontation. Extraocular motions full, without strabismus or nystagmus. Fundus shows normal discs and vasculature. No arteriovenous nicking, silver-wiring, hemorrhage, or exudate.

Ears: External ears normal. Tympanic membranes normal bilaterally. Weber midline. Air conduction greater than bone bilaterally.

Nose: Nasal mucosa normal, without inflammation, obstruction, or polyps.

Mouth: Lips, buccal muscosa without lesions. Tongue well papillated, pink, midline. Teeth in good repair. Uvula midline. Oropharynx without inflammation or lesions.

Neck: Supple. Trachea midline. Thyroid not enlarged and without nodules. Jugular veins flat. Venous pulses normal. Carotids 4+ without bruits, normal pulse contour bilaterally.

Chest and lungs: Chest wall contour normal, with symmetrical full expansion. No rib tenderness to palpation. Tactile fremitus normal. Diaphragmatic excursion 5 cm bilaterally. No percussion dullness. Lungs are clear to auscultation save for an isolated musical wheeze on forced expiration at the right base posteriorly. There is no egophony over this area. No rubs heard.

Heart: No visible lifts, PMI palpable 8 cm from the L sternal border in the 6th intercostal space, tapping in quality. No palpable thrills, lifts, heaves. Rhythm regular, rate 80. S_1 normal, S_2 physiologically split. There is no S_3, but a soft S_4 at the apex. There is a $^2/_6$ systolic ejection murmur at the L sternal border, without radiation. No rubs, no diastolic murmurs.

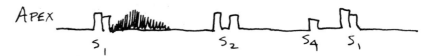

Breasts: R breast slightly larger than L. No retractions, visible dimpling or skin changes. Nipples normal, everted. 2×2 cm cystic, mobile, nontender mass without skin fixation in upper outer quadrant R breast. No nipple discharge.

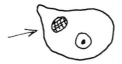

Abdomen: Slightly protuberant. No scars or visible masses. Venous pattern normal. Bowel sounds normal. No hepatic or splenic rubs. No bruits. Liver is 15 cm to percussion, and is 3 cm below the right costal margin. Liver edge is smooth and tender to palpation, with positive Murphy's sign. No epigastric tenderness. Spleen and kidneys not palpable. No shifting dullness or fluid wave. No hernia.

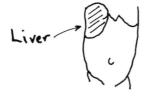

Pelvic and rectal: External genitalia normal, including Bartholin's and Skeine's glands. Vaginal vault without lesions or discharge.
Cervix parous, without lesions or discharge. Pap smear taken.

Bimanual: Fundus normal in size & position. No tenderness. Ovaries and broad ligament felt and are without masses or tenderness.

Rectovaginal: Confirms bimanual

Rectum: No anal lesions. Sphincter tone normal. No ampullary masses. Stool is clay-colored and negative for occult blood.

Extremities: Pulses full and symmetrical, without bruits. Skin and hair normal on extremities.

Pulses:

		Carotid	Supra-clavicular	Radial	Brachial	Aorta	Femoral	DP	PT
4+ = Nl	R	4+	3+	4+	4+	0	4+	4+	4+
	L	4+	3+	4+	4+	0	4+	4+	4+

No clubbing, cyanosis, or edema. No swelling, redness, tenderness, limitation of movement of joints. No visible variocosities. No calf tenderness or cords. Muscle mass normal bilaterally.

Back: Slight cervical kyphosis. No spinal tenderness, CVA tenderness, or sacral edema. Full range of motion spine.

Neurologic:

Mental status: Alert, oriented. Memory, judgment, mood normal.

Cranial nerves: I—Not tested.
                        II—Pupils react to light. Reads newspaper.
              III,IV,VI—No strabismus. EOM normal.
                         V—Corneal reflex intact.
                       VII—Face Symmetrical.
                      VIII—Hearing normal.
                      IX,X—Uvula elevates symmetrically. Gag normal bilaterally.
                        XI—Trapezius, sternomastoid normal.
                       XII—Tongue protrudes midline.

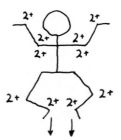

Cerebellar: Gait, finger-nose, and heel-shin normal.

Station and gait: Romberg negative. Heel-toe walk normal.

Motor: Muscle mass normal. Good strength in arms, legs.
       Deep tendon reflexes: 2+ = Nl
       No pathologic reflexes.

Sensory: Normal to touch, pinprick, vibration.

LABORATORY FINDINGS

Hemogram: Hgb 14.2, Hct 45%, WBC 8500, Polys 65, Bands 5, Monos 10, Lymphs 19, Eos 1, Baso 0.

Peripheral smear: Normocytic, normochromic RBCs. No fragments, targets, nucleated RBC. WBC morphology normal. Platelets abundant on smear.

Urine: Clear, dark yellow. SG 1015. *Dipstix* neg. heme, protein, glucose, ketones. 3+ for bilirubin. pH = 6. *Micro:* 0–1 WBC, 0 RBC, no organisms per high-power field. No crystals, casts.

Serologies:

Electrolytes: Na = 140, K = 4.2, Cl = 100, CO_2 = 28, Ca = 10, P = 3,4, Albumin = 4.0, Glob = 3.5, SGOT = 123, SGPT = 85, Alk P'tase = 210. Bili: total = 4.0, direct = 3.5. Amylase serum = 236, GI = 123. Cr = 1.0, BUN = 10.

Chest X-ray: Bones normal, without blastic or lytic lesions. Heart shows slight straightening L heart border. Parenchyma clear except for slight linear atelectasis R base posteriorly (R lower lobe, basal seg.). No evident effusion.

KUB: Bones normal. Psoas shadows seen. Nephrograms show normal-size kidneys. Bowel gas normal. No evident ascites. <u>Speckled calcification medial RUQ in area gallbladder.</u>

ECG: Rate = 80, rhythm = sinus, PR = .15, QRS = .10, QT = .32, axis = +30. P waves normal. QRS normal. No T wave flattening or ST segment abnormalities. No LVH by voltage. Impression—normal ECG.

IMPRESSIONS
1. RUQ pain
   a. <u>R/O cholecystitis with cholelithiasis.</u> This is supported by the historical relationship of RUQ sharp pains associated with fatty foods, scleral icterus, hepatomegaly, and + Murphy's sign, clay-colored stools, and laboratory findings of bilirubinuria, abnormal liver function studies with an obstructive pattern, hyperamylasemia, and calcifications on KUB that might represent gallstones. The RLL atelectasis on chest film is not inconsistent with an intra-abdominal process.
   b. <u>R/O carcinomatosis of the liver.</u> With her family history of breast cancer and the breast mass and axillary node on physical examination, this diagnosis must be considered. The episodicity of her pain, the lack of nodularity of the liver, and the absence of evident disease elsewhere makes this less likely.
   c. <u>R/O pulmonary embolism.</u> Though unlikely, the RLL wheeze on P.E. and atelectasis on chest film could represent the site of lodgment of pulmonary embolism from the legs (for which there is no local evidence of phlebitis) or peripelvic (she has had 2 children) areas. The liver disease in this circumstance would represent congestive hepatopathy from transient right heart failure of pulmonary embolism.
   d. <u>R/O myocardial infarction or ischemia.</u> This is very improbable with her history, but should be considered in light of her recent stress in classes and the association of her pain with eating. Her hypertension, though mild, could predispose her. In this circumstance, her liver disease would be transient congestive hepatopathy.

   Although other diagnoses are possible (infective pneumonia, pancreatitis, peptic ulcer, infective or toxic hepatitis), there is little to support them in the history or physical examination.

PLAN
1. RUQ pain
   Plan: I will hospitalize her today and obtain an ECHO of her gallbladder and biliary tree, as the most immediately available and least invasive of studies. Should this prove nondiagnostic, I would proceed to prepare her for an oral cholecystogram.
       I will ask the surgeon to see her today, should another attack occasion the need for emergency surgical intervention.
       Serial physical examination, urine bilirubin testing, and serum liver function tests will allow monitoring of her progress.
2. Right breast mass and axillary node with FH cancer of the breast
       Although the cystic lesion of the breast probably does not represent a malignancy, her FH and deep concern are troublesome.

   Plan: Mammography and probably biopsy of the mass are in order. These can be done on this hospitalization.
3. Hypertension
       Although this might be due to anxiety, the presence of the S_4 and the straightening of the left heart border on chest film suggest a fixed hypertension rather than a labile one.

Plan: I will monitor her pressures in hospital. Should they remain elevated, salt restriction, weight loss, and probably diuretic therapy will be instituted.

4. Allergy to penicillin

   Her urticarial response could presage anaphylaxis.

   Plan: I will instruct the nurses to flag her chart as allergic to penicillin. On discharge, Mrs. Doe should obtain a Medic-Alert to the effect that she is allergic to this drug.

5. Systolic heart murmur

   This is probably a flow murmur.

   Plan: Observe.

J.H. Galen MD

I. H. Galen, M.D.

The history and physical examination detailed above are a *full and formal,* written H and P. Other situations (emergency visits, trauma, pregnancies, readmissions to hospital, etc.) will demand less broad detail, or other emphases. How "long" a written history and physical "needs to be" (a frequent question asked by students) depends on a judicious balance of the patient's need and the clinician's time available. In all cases, the written history and physical examination *needs to be* as long as is necessary to convey pertinent data clearly and completely. Moreover, as in other fields of science, the clinician need not *say* (or write) everything he knows—but he should *know* everything he says.

PROBLEM-ORIENTED MEDICAL RECORD (POMR)

On the following pages are examples of the various components of a Problem-Oriented Medical Information System. This is not an actual record and all names are fictitious. This example is taken from an exhibit "The Problem-Oriented Medical Information System" prepared for the American Heart Association and the American College of Cardiology by J. Willis Hurst, M.D., Robert C. Schlant, M.D., W. Dallas Hall, M.D., and H. Kenneth Walker, M.D., all of the Department of Medicine, Emory University School of Medicine, Atlanta, Georgia.

Smith, Mr. John 000–001	**Complete problem list** Permanent Part of Medical Record	
Date problem entered	Active	Inactive
11–13–82 *1.	Coronary atherosclerotic heart disease	
	a. Acute anteroseptal myocardial infarction	
	b. Left ventricular dysfunction	
	c. Mitral regurgitation $\xrightarrow{11-14}$ pap. muscle dysf.	
11–13–82 2.	Adult onset of diabetes mellitus (1962)	
	a. Peripheral athero– sclerosis	
11–13–82 3.		Herniorrhaphy, R Ing. (1964)
11–13–82 4.		Depression, situational (1980)
11–13–82 5.		Left BK amputation (1979)
11–15–82 6.	Diabetic retinopathy, as $\longrightarrow$	

* Reason for admission

Patient Identification _____ Smith, Mr. John 000-001 _____ Date __11-13-82__

CHIEF COMPLAINTS:

"Indigestion"

HISTORY OF PRESENT ILLNESS:

57-year-old male who noted epigastric-lower sternal burning type of indigestion while climbing stairs at work 2 weeks ago. Took Tums and pain was lessened after 5-10 minutes. Does not recall any sweating, weakness or palpitations. Pain did not radiate above mid-sternum or to arms, neck or shoulder. It did not recur until—
    Today while mowing the lawn he developed severe lower substernal "indigestion" discomfort that radiated to both elbows and was associated with nausea, weakness and a cold sweat. The pain has persisted over the past 3 hours and was not relieved by 2 Tums and 2 Alka-Seltzer tablets. He has noted some progressive shortness of breath since the onset of pain.

> **Instructions:** Circle positive responses and comment appropriately. Underline negative responses. Leave unaltered if information not available.

PAST MEDICAL HISTORY:

Pediatric and adult illnesses: (mumps), (measles), (chickenpox), rheumatic fever, arthritis, rheumatism, chorea, scarlet fever, pneumonia, tuberculosis, diabetes mellitus, heart disease, renal disease, hypertension, jaundice.

Immunizations: All intact

Hospitalizations: None

Trauma: None

Transfusions: None

Current medications: Only as in present illness

Allergies: None

Habits (drugs, alcohol, tobacco): Drinks one 6-pack beer/weekend
Smokes 2 packs cigarettes daily for 18 years (36 pack-years)

Note: Positive responses are circled and elaborated on. *Negative* responses are underlined or crossed out. No alteration is made when information is not obtained—e.g., when the patient is comatose or when data must come from other sources; then "incomplete data base" becomes a "problem" requiring written plans.

FAMILY HISTORY (Diagram pedigree if indicated):

Diabetes mellitus, tuberculosis, cancer, stroke, hypertension, renal disease, deafness, gout/arthritis, anemia, heart disease.

—Mother (65) controlled by diet

—Brother died of myocardial infarction age 44

SYSTEMS REVIEW:

General: weakness, fatigue, change in weight __+ 2 lb__, appetite, sleeping habits, chills, fever, night sweats.

Integument: color changes, pruritus, nevus, infections, tumor (benign/malignant), dermatosis, hair changes, nail changes.

Hematopoietic: anemia, abnormal bleeding, adenopathy, excessive bruising.

Central nervous system: headache, syncope, seizures, vertigo, amaurosis, diplopia, paralysis/paresis, muscle weakness, tremor, ataxia, dysesthesia.

Eyes: vision, glasses/contact lenses, date of last eye exam __none__, scotomata, pain, excessive tearing.

Ears: tinnitus, deafness, other.

Nose, throat and sinuses: epistaxis, discharge, sinusitis, hoarseness, thyromegaly.

Dentition: caries, pyorrhea, dentures.

Breasts: masses, discharge, pain.

Respiratory: cough (productive/~~nonproductive~~), change in cough, amount and characteristics of sputum, duration of sputum production __1 year__ __36__ pack-years of tobacco usage, wheezing, hemoptysis, recurrent respiratory tract infections, positive tuberculin test.

—Has smoked 2 packs cigarettes daily for the past 18 years; in the past year has noted a frequent cough, productive of small amounts of whitish sputum in the mornings.

SYSTEMS REVIEW (Continued)

Cardiovascular: chest pain, typical angina pectoris, dyspnea on exertion, orthopnea, paroxysmal nocturnal dyspnea, peripheral edema, murmur, palpitation, varicosities, thrombophlebitis, claudication, Raynaud's phenomenon, syncope, near-syncope.

See description in present illness; unable to recall any chest symptoms prior to 2 weeks ago.

Gastrointestinal: nausea, vomiting, diarrhea, constipation, melena, hematemesis, rectal bleeding, change in bowel habits, hemorrhoids, dysphagia, food intolerances, excessive gas or indigestion, abdominal pain, jaundice, use of antacids, use of laxatives.

See present illness

Urinary tract: dysuria, hematuria, frequency, polyuria, urgency, hesitancy, incontinence, renal calculi, nocturia, infections.

Genitoreproductive system:
Male: penile discharge, lesion, history of venereal disease, serology, testicular pain, testicular mass, infertility, impotence, libido.
Female: (Not applicable).

Gynecologic history:
Age of menarche _____, last menstrual period _____, age at menopause _____, post menopausal bleeding, abnormal menses, amount of bleeding, intermenstrual bleeding, postcoital bleeding, leucorrhea, pruritus, history of venereal disease, serology, last PAPs _____, results _____.

Obstetric history:
Full-term deliveries _____
Pregnancies _____
Abortions _____
Living children _____
Complications of pregnancies, infertility, libido.

Methods of contraception:

SYSTEMS REVIEW (Continued)

Musculoskeletal:
   Joints: <u>pain</u>, <u>edema</u>, <u>heat</u>, <u>rubor</u>, <u>stiffness</u>, deformity.

   Muscles: <u>myalgias</u>.

Endocrine: goiter, <u>heat intolerance</u>, <u>cold intolerance</u>, <u>change in voice</u>, <u>polyuria</u>, <u>polydipsia</u>, <u>polyphagia</u>.

Psychiatric: <u>hyperventilation</u>, <u>nervousness</u>, <u>depression</u>, <u>insomnia</u>, <u>nightmares</u>, <u>memory loss</u>.

Additional historical data:

PHYSICAL EXAMINATION:

Vital signs:
   Pulse _____96_____ reg./~~irreg.~~ Respirations ____22____ Temp. ____99°____ oral/~~rectal~~

   Blood pressure

      supine R arm __130/80__ L arm __128/80__ Leg __145/90__
      sitting R arm _____
      standing R arm _____

   Weight __195__ (scales used)

   Height __71"__

General:

Integument: <u>turgor</u>, <u>texture</u>, <u>pigmentation</u>, <u>cyanosis</u>, <u>telangiectasia</u>, <u>petechiae</u>, <u>purpura</u>, <u>ecchymosis</u>, <u>infection</u>, <u>lesions</u>, <u>hair</u>, <u>nails</u>, <u>mucous membranes</u>.

Lymph nodes: <u>cervical</u>, <u>postauricular</u>, <u>supraclavicular</u>, <u>axillary</u>, <u>ulnar</u>, <u>inguinal</u>.

Skull: <u>trauma</u>, <u>bruits</u>, other.

PHYSICAL EXAMINATION (Continued)

Eyes: lacrimal glands, cornea, lids, sclerac, conjunctivae, exophthalmos, lid-lag.

Fundi: discs, arteries, veins, hemorrhages, exudates, microaneurysms.

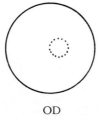   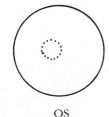

OD   OS

Ears: tophi, tympanic membranes, external canal, hearing, air conduction ___>___
bone conduction, lateralization __no__.

Mouth, nose, and throat: definition, gingiva, tongue, tonsils, pharynx, nasal mucosa,
nasal septum, sinuses.

Neck: mobility, scars, masses, thyroid, salivary glands, tracheal shift, bruits.

Breasts: masses, discharge, nipples, asymmetry, gynecomastia.

Chest:
    Respiratory rate __22__/min   Amplitude: Shallow
                                        Deep
                                      (Normal)

    Respiratory rhythm:(regular)
                        irregular
                        periodical
                        inspiration/expiration ratio

    Chest wall: deformities
                motion
                lateral motion:(good,) fair, absent
                use of accessory muscles: yes, no

PHYSICAL EXAMINATION, Chest (Continued)

Auscultation: rales, wheezes, rhonchi.
breath sounds: increased, decreased, (normal.)
other:

(diagram location of abnormal breath sounds, transmitted voice, or abnormal percussion).

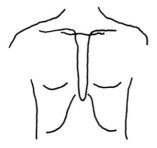 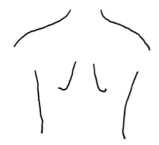

Cardiovascular system:

External jugular veins are distended to ___4___ cm above the angle of Louis at ___45___ degrees of truncal elevation from supine.

Point of maximum impulse is in the ___4th___ ICS ___5 cm lat to LLSB Palpable___ S_4 and S_3; late systolic bulge (see below)

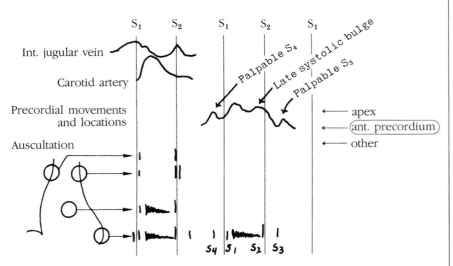

S_1 = Single, slightly diminished in loudness

S_2 = Normal intensity and splitting (not paradoxical)

Gallops = S_4 (atrial) and S_3 (ventricular) at LLSB and apex

Systolic murmur = Blowing mid-late decrescendo systolic grade 3/6 murmur at apex with radiation toward LSB; no change with inspiration

Diastolic murmur = None

Other = No palpable thrill

PHYSICAL EXAMINATION, Cardiovascular System (Continued)

Peripheral pulses:

	Carotid	Brachial	Radial	Aorta	Femoral	Popliteal	DP	PT
R	3^+	3^+	3^+	2^+	2^+	2^+	1^+	1^+
L	3^+	3^+	3^+		2^+	1^+	0	0

0 = absent; 1^+ = thready; 2^+ = decreased; 3^+ = normal; 4^+ = hyperactive.

Extremities: edema, cyanosis, stasis, ulceration, hair distribution, clubbing.

left lower leg amputation   Male pattern baldness; absent
                                   hair on toes of right foot

Abdomen: obesity, contour, scars, tenderness, CVA tenderness, masses, rebound, rigidity, fluid wave, shifting dullness, frank ascites, bruits, hernia, venous collaterals.

Bowel sounds: normal, absent, hyperactive, hypoactive, obstructive.
Organomegaly: liver, spleen, kidneys, bladder, gall bladder.
Liver size ___9___ cm (total dullness)
Liver tenderness: absent, increased
Liver edge: smooth, irregular, nodular.

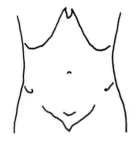

Male:
  genitalia: penis, scrotum, testes, epididymis, masses, other.

  rectal: ⎫ perineum, hemorrhoids, sphincter tone, prostate, bleeding, masses.
  stool: ⎭ ___deferred___.

Female:
  external genitalia: labia, clitoris, introitus, urethra, perineum, other.
  internal genitalia: vagina, cervix, adnexa, cul-de-sac, discharge.
  PAPs: done, omitted.
  rectal: hemorrhoids, sphincter tone, bleeding, masses.
  Stool: _____.

PHYSICAL EXAMINATION (Continued)

Joints: deformity, rubor, calor, tenderness, edema.

    range of motion: fingers, wrists, elbow, shoulder, hips, knees, ankles.

    spine: deformity (kyphosis, lordosis, scoliosis), thoracic excursion.

Neurologic:

    Cerebral function: (alert wakefulness), lethargic, obtunded, stuporous, semi-comatose, comatose.

    Mental status: Intact; oriented to time, person, and place.

    Cranial nerves:

        I. (list test materials) Not tested.

        II. discs, papilledema, venous pulses, optic atrophy, visual fields, acuity.

    III, IV, VI. ptosis, palpebral fissure.
        Pupils: R ____4____ mm L ____4____ mm Shape ____R____

        Reaction to light: R = L
        Consensual reaction: R to L ⌣ L to R ⌣
        Reaction to near vision: R ⌣ L ⌣

        Extraocular movements: (full), abnormal, doll's-eyes, cold calories, gaze preference, nystagmus, opticokinetic nystagmus.

        V. Sensory: 1st division   2nd division   3rd division

                 R corneal   L corneal

        Motor: masseters, pterygoids, temporalis.

        VII. (intact), R-L central, R-L peripheral.

        VIII. (intact)

      IX, X. dysarthria, gag, phonation, uvula, soft palate, swallowing, (intact)

        XI. sternocleidomastoids, trapezii.

        XII. tongue in midline, deviation to R-L, atrophy, fasciculations.

PHYSICAL EXAMINATION (Continued)

Gait and station: (Not tested)

    walking: normal, abnormal, heel walking, toe walking, tandem walking.

    truncal ataxia:

    Romberg: present, absent, R-L.

    involuntary movements:

Cerebellum: rapid alternating movements, finger-nose, finger-finger, heel-shin, past-pointing, rebound, posturing.

Sensory: pain, temperature, light-touch, joint-position, vibratory, two-point discrimination, stereognosis.

Associative functions: speech, writing, reading, apraxia, agnosia, other.

Motor: tone, mass, fasciculations, tremor

    ___0___ hemiparesis   ___0___ hemiplegia.

Reflexes:

	Bi	Tri	Br	F	K	A	Plantar	Abdomen		Snout	Grasp	Jaw Suck
R	2^+	2^+	2^+	1^+	2^+	2^+	↓	+	+	0	0	0
L	2^+	2^+	2^+	1^+	2^+	2^+	↓	+	+	0	0	

    0 = absent c̄ facilitation; tr = trace; 1^+ = decreased; 2^+ = normal; 3^+ = hyperactive; 4^+ = sustained clonus.

LABORATORY DATA (This defined Data Base requires that the following examinations be done on every patient):

Hematology:

    WBC   13,200 mm³   Differential   79 segs, 20 lymphs, 1 band

    Hct   48 vol %   Platelet estimation   Normal

LABORATORY DATA (Continued)

Chemistry:

Na^+ 135 mEq/L   Blood sugar 182 mg %

K^+ 4.5

CO_2 20.0   BUN 18 mg %

Cl 100.0

Urinalysis: 2^+ glucose, negative acetone; otherwise normal

Chest x-ray (diagram if appropriate): ~~routine~~ (portable A-P)

Mild cardiomegaly;
marked pulmonary edema

Electrocardiogram:

rate 96

rhythm Sinus

PR __.18__ QRS __.07__ QT __.28__

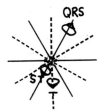

Interpretation: Marked ST elevation and loss of initial forces in V_{1-3}
compatible with acute anteroseptal myocardial infarction; possible
old inferior infarction.

OTHER LABORATORY DATA AVAILABLE (not included in defined Data Base):

pH = 7.46

PCO_2 = 30 mm Hg

PO_2 = 62 mm Hg (room air)

PATHOPHYSIOLOGIC CLASSIFICATION:

I. Heart disease

  A. Classification

    1. Etiologic: Coronary atherosclerosis

    2. Anatomic: Coronary artery narrowing, sclerosis, myocardial infarction

    3. Physiologic: Normal sinus rhythm, acute infarction, left ventricular dysfunction, papillary muscle dysfunction, mitral regurgitation

    4. Functional: Class IV

    5. Therapeutic: Class E

II. Diabetes mellitus

  A. Classification

    1. Etiologic: Congenital predisposition; obesity

    2. Anatomic: Body obesity; pancreas normal to light microscopy

    3. Physiologic: Inadequate beta cell response to stress of obesity

    4. Functional: Not applicable

    5. Therapeutic: Caloric restriction until ideal body weight attained

Note: This page and the next page (Sequence of Events) strictly speaking are not part of the POMR. However, these two items are useful in ensuring that the clinician does not jump too quickly from the raw Data Base to the formulation of a Problem List. In effect, these two features are added as stoplights to encourage the clinician to manipulate and interpret the Data Base with great care.

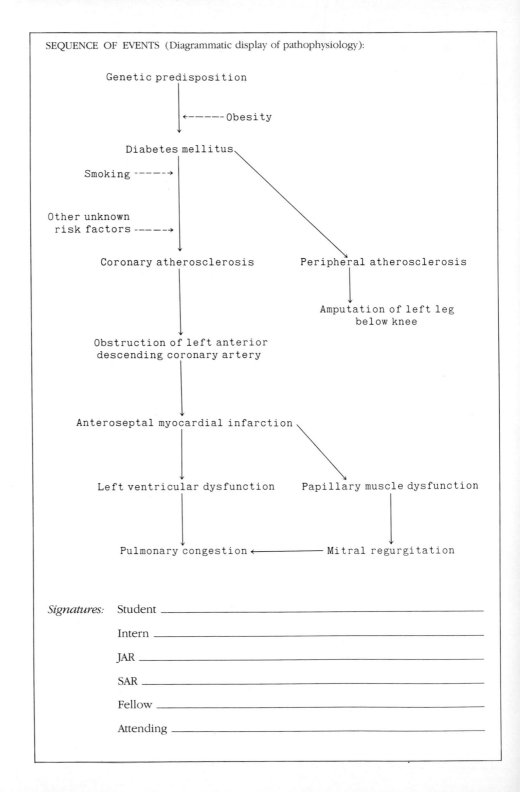

SEQUENCE OF EVENTS (Diagrammatic display of pathophysiology):

Genetic predisposition

←————Obesity

Diabetes mellitus

Smoking ————→

Other unknown
risk factors ————→

Coronary atherosclerosis   Peripheral atherosclerosis

Amputation of left leg
below knee

Obstruction of left anterior
descending coronary artery

Anteroseptal myocardial infarction

Left ventricular dysfunction   Papillary muscle dysfunction

Pulmonary congestion ←————— Mitral regurgitation

Signatures: Student _____

Intern _____

JAR _____

SAR _____

Fellow _____

Attending _____

Smith, Mr. John 000–001 Patient Identification	Initial plans
Problem #1	Coronary atherosclerotic heart disease a. Acute anteroseptal myocardial infarction b. LV dysfunction c. Mitral regurgitation
Diagnostic plans:	Established by history and admission ECG; no other tests required currently; later lipid profile in follow–up period
Therapeutic plans:	Strict bed rest except bedside commode privileges Diet, Na restricted and 1,400 calories split for hs feeding CCU monitoring with prn rhythm strips; rpt ECG and portable chest x–ray in A.M. Slow IV drip of D_5W to keep vein open in case of emergency Colace to help prevent constipation and Valsalva Nasal prong O_2 at 4 L/min flow Measure urine output Diuretic agents for pulmonary congestion Digitalize cautiously (see orders) Slow IV morphine prn pain; watch for bradycardia Elastic stockings to prevent peripheral thrombophlebitis
Educational plans:	Pt and family told of "heart attack" and that the monitor wires, etc., are routine and for early detection of any problems. Explained to him that we will later go into rehabilitation, etc.

(**Initial Plans** are listed for each problem identified on admission, according to Problem Title and Number. Each plan contains three elements: Diagnostic Plans, Therapeutic Plans, Patient Education Plans.)

Smith, Mr. John 000–001 Patient Identification	Initial plans
Problem #2	Diabetes mellitus
Diagnostic plans:	Established by GTT (1962)
Therapeutic plans:	10 U NPH in A.M. with supplementary regular insulin See consultation and 10 P.M. progress note Fractional urines at 7–11–4–9 Fasting plasma glucose in A.M.
Educational plans:	Explained to pt why he may get regular insulin in addition to NPH tomorrow, and why we will need to draw frequent blood sugars for the first few days.

	Ordered			Discontinued

Treatment orders

Hospital Policy:
1. The signature of a physician must accompany all orders.
2. Narcotics, hypnotics, sedatives, anticoagulants, and amphetamines require new orders every 48 hours.
3. Antibiotics require new orders every 7 days.

Smith, Mr. John

000–001

(Reserved Space)

Date & Hour	Doctor	Nurse		Date & Hour
11–13–82			Prob. #1a. Acute Anteroseptal	
7:30 P.M.			Myocardial Infarction	
			— Bed rest with bedside commode	
			— CCU monitoring with rhythm	
			strip q1h and prn	
			— Urine output q4h	
			— Elastic stockings	
			— Keep IV open with slow drip of	
			D_5W	
			— Colace, 50 mg PO bid	
			— Repeat EKG and portable chest	
			X–ray in A.M.	
			— Serum enzymes in A.M.: SGOT,	
			LDH, CPK	
			— Morphine, 5 mg slowly IV q2h	
			prn pain; call me if required	
			more than twice	
			Prob. #1b. LV dysfunction	
			— Digoxin, 0.5 mg PO stat	
			— Diuril, 0.5 gm PO stat	
			— O_2 via nasal prongs, 4 L/min	
11–13–82			Prob. #2 Diabetes	
9 P.M.			— 1,485 cal. ADA diet divided	
			3/10, 3/10, 3/10, 1/10	
			— Urine fractional at 7–11–4–9;	
			have pt empty bladder 30–45	
			min before obtaining sample.	
			— Plasma glucose tomorrow at	
			7 A.M. and 4 P.M.	
			— NPH insulin, 10 U SC in A.M.	
			— 10 U regular insulin IV stat	

Progress Notes	Smith, Mr. John
	000-001
Doctor	(Reserved Space)

Date	Notes
11-13-82	#1 <u>Anterior myocardial infarction</u>
8:06 P.M.	S: Some continued substernal aching pain despite 5 mg
	morphine an hour ago
	O: BP fall to 106/80 in past hour
	Monitor strip (7:50 P.M.) shows coupled PVCs
	S_3 and S_4 remain prominent; murmur unchanged
	A: Hypotension from worsening LV failure; ventricular
	irritability
	P: Watch monitor closely
	Draw up lidocaine
	Page Dr. Wilson stat
11-13-82	#1 <u>Ant. MI</u>
8:17 P.M.	S: As above; also has a "smothering" sensation
	O: New rhythm strip shows occ. runs of 4 PVCs as well as
	couples. BP now 112/80
	A: As above; intermittent ventr. tachy.
	P: Begin lidocaine
	Repeat PO_2 at 4 liter flow
	Monitor hourly urine output
11-13-82	#2 <u>Diabetes</u>
9 P.M.	S: None
	O: Repeat plasma glucose 360 mg% at 8:30 P.M. 1 hr after
	starting D_5W: Urine fractional 3^+/neg.
	A: Worsening hyperglycemia due to acute stress
	situation plus IV drip to keep vein open
	P: 10 U IV regular insulin; repeat plasma glucose at
	midnight
	Key: S = subjective; A = assessment; O = objective; P = plan.

Consultation

To ___Endocrinology___ Date Submitted ___11–14–82___ Hospital No. ___000–001___

Ward ___600 A___ Patient ___Smith, Mr. John___

Problem number and title   *Specific questions*

#2 Diabetes mellitus   Please advise re management of
                                        patient's diabetes. Should we
                                        continue NPH or switch to
                                        regular insulin?

Consultation requested by:

CONSULTANT'S REPORT (date and hour answered: ___11–15–82 10 A.M.___)

For each numbered problem categorize and state:
Conclusions and recommendations
Discussion (display the data used to formulate the conclusions and recommendations)
New problems (with subjective and objective findings)

Conclusions and recommendations:

—Continue NPH insulin in decreased dosage, 10 U q A.M. Supplement with
  regular insulin, 5–10 U as needed based on plasma glucose levels bid
  (7 A.M. and 4 P.M.).
—Continue diet as ordered, 1,485 calories with 90 gm P, 180 gm C, and
  45 gm F divided 3/10; 3/10; 3/10; 1/10 until reaches ideal weight of 172
  lb when diet should be revised to maintain weight.
—Watch insulin requirements closely (a) after acute stress of infarct
  subsides and (b) as weight declines.

Discussion:

The combination of obesity and diabetes undoubtedly has contributed to
his accelerated atherosclerosis. Although we cannot reverse the large
blood vessel damage that has already occurred, hopefully we can slow
the progression by returning his metabolic status to a more normal
state. The most important treatment from this standpoint is to reduce
body weight. He is currently 71" tall with a medium frame and weight
of 195; predicted ideal body weight is 172. After being on the diet for
about 3 months, he should have a repeat lipid profile. Insulin
requirements will probably decrease as weight declines and physical
activity increases.

New Problem: #6 Diabetic retinopathy, OS →

S: No visual complaint
O: 3 small punctate hemorrhages characteristic of background diabetic
   retinopathy in the posterior fundus in the macular region OS. No
   proliferative changes seen but pupils somewhat constricted
   (morphine) and fundus exam not entirely satisfactory.

When the back of the
page is needed, be certain
to rearrange carbon
paper so that the duplicate
copy will be complete.
Send copy of consultation
to chairman of your
department.

Hospital Record Audit

Cardiovascular condition audited: ___Acute Myocardial Infarction (AMI)___

Patient name: ___Smith, John___   Hospital: ___GMH___

Hospital number: ___000-001___   Date of audit: ___11-27-82___

Patient team: ___600 A CCU, Team B___   Audited by: _____

___Physicians and Nurses___

I. Data base
  A. Does the history include data regarding the presence or absence of the following:

		YES	NO
1. Present Illness			
a. Pain compatible with AMI		x	
b. Radiation of pain		x	
c. Duration of pain		x	
d. Time at onset of pain			x
e. Activity at onset of pain		x	
f. Dyspnea		x	
g. Sweating		x	
h. Palpitation		x	
i. Marked weakness		x	
j. Severe apprehension			x
k. Nausea or vomiting		x	
l. Syncope			x
m. Time from onset to reaching hospital			x
n. Time from reaching hospital to CCU		x	
o. Prodromata within preceding 3 weeks		x	

  B.
  C.

II. . . . V.

VI. Plans for correction:

The 73% score on present illness is acceptable; however, this is the 2nd consecutive time the same deficiencies have been noted in this team's Data Base. I have notified Dr. Randall (CCU Cardiac Resident) who has planned to discuss the relevance of syncope and importance of timing in the first 24 hours in caring for patients with acute myocardial infarction.

Standard Orders

GENERAL

1. Follow a systematic sequence (see below) to ensure completeness.
2. Write legibly. A misinterpreted word or drug may harm your patient.
3. Be sure to review your orders frequently and to specifically cancel the old order before a new one is entered.
4. Consider prn orders as generally undesirable but occasionally necessary. Be certain to review prn orders regularly (every other day).
5. Do not order things that your patients do not need (e.g., sleeping pills should not be routine).
6. Record date, time, and legibly sign *all* orders. If an order is immediate or important, discuss it with the responsible nurse.

AN ORDER FOR ORDERS

1. Admitting diagnosis.
2. Patient's condition (critical, poor, fair, good).
3. Known allergies, if any.
4. Activity permitted (e.g., bed rest, or bathroom privileges, up ad lib.).
5. Diet (e.g., 2 gm sodium, low potassium).
6. General orders
   a. Weights (how often).
   b. Fluids (input and output).
   c. Turning (if bedridden).
   d. Precautions (e.g., seizures, confused, myocardial infarction).
7. Vital signs: frequency, and specifics for which you want to be called (e.g., "Notify MD if temp. greater than 102°F").
8. Medications and IV fluids
   a. Specific to diagnosis (1) IV solution and rate. (2) Antibiotics. (3) Cardiac drugs, etc.
   b. General: Drugs for fever, bowels, sedation, etc.
9. Specimens and tests: e.g., "Please obtain sputum for MD and for culture" or "Draw glucose in morning before breakfast."

Sign _____

Print name _____

Common Abbreviations

Although this glossary has potential value to the beginning student when he is first translating and understanding medical records, the authors present it to you with a certain reluctance.

Abbreviations are said to be useful in saving the writer's time. What you will discover is that they may waste the reader's time if he cannot understand them. Moreover, abbreviations—unstandardized and subject to misinterpretation (note below how often the same symbol represents several widely different things)—may obscure rather than clarify the chart. We fervently hope that no student using this appendix will do so for any purpose other than translating *back* into plain, lucid English most of the codelike abbreviations he encounters. To adopt the habit of using all of the abbreviations listed below would be to invite error deliberately. If you do abbreviate, and some abbreviations *are* useful, be certain to define your more specialized abbreviations at least once in the written workup. Since this sort of terminology is extremely variable from place to place, not all terms could be included, and the list below is both imprecise and incomplete.

A—anorexia, aorta, artery, auscultation, albumin

a—ante (before)

A_2—aortic second heart sound

AA—Alcoholics Anonymous, arteries

AAA—abdominal aortic aneurysm

AAL—anterior axillary line

ab—abortion

ABE—acute bacterial endocarditis

ABD—abdomen, abduction

ABG—arterial blood gas

ABO—classic blood type system

AC—air conduction

ac—ante cibum (before meals)

ACTH—adrenocorticotropic hormone

ad—to or toward

ADA—American Diabetes (or Dental or Dietetic) Association

ADH—antidiuretic hormone

ADL—activities of daily living

ad lib.—at liberty, as the patient desires

AF—atrial fibrillation, aortofemoral

AFB—acid-fast bacillus

AHF—antihemophilic factor

AI—aortic insufficiency

AIHA—autoimmune hemolytic anemia

AJ—ankle jerk

AKA—above-the-knee amputation

ALK P'tase—alkaline phosphatase

ALL—acute lymphocytic leukemia

ALS—amyotrophic lateral sclerosis

AMA—against medical advice, American Medical Association

AMI—acute (or anterior) myocardial infarction, acute mitral insufficiency

AML—acute myelogenous leukemia, acute monocytic leukemia

AMML—acute myelomonocytic leukemia

Ao—aorta

AP—anteroposterior, angina pectoris, acid phosphatase

Appy—appendix, appendectomy

ARDS—adult respiratory distress syndrome

ARF—acute rheumatic fever, acute renal failure

AS—aortic stenosis, arteriosclerosis

ASA—aspirin

ASAP—as soon as possible

ASCVD—atherosclerotic coronary (or cerebral) vascular disease

ASD—atrial septal defect

ASH—asymmetric septal hypertrophy

ASPVD—atherosclerotic peripheral vascular disease

AV—arteriovenous, atrioventricular

AVM—arteriovenous malformation

AVN—atrioventricular node

AVR—aortic valve replacement

A&W—alive and well

B—bacillus, black, bruit, basophil

B-I and B-II—Billroth's operations (I = gastroduodenostomy, II = gastrojejunostomy)

BA—brain abscess

Baso—basophil

BB—bundle branch

BBB—bundle-branch block, blood brain barrier

BC—blood culture, bone conduction

BCG—bacille Calmette-Guérin (tuberculosis vaccine)

BCP—birth control pills

BE—barium enema, bacterial endocarditis

bid—bis in dies (twice a day)

bili—bilirubin

BF—black female

B + J—bone and joint

BJP—Bence Jones proteins

BKA—below-the-knee amputation

BM—bowel movement, black man, black male

BO—body odor

BOA—born out of asepsis

BP—blood pressure

BPH—benign prostatic hypertrophy

BRB—bright red blood
BRBPR—bright red blood per rectum
BRRB—bright red rectal blood
BRP—bathroom privileges
BS—bowel sounds, breath sounds, blood smear, blood sugar
BSO—bilateral salpingo-oophorectomy
BSU—Bartholin's glands, Skene's glands, and urethra
BUN—blood urea nitrogen
BW—black woman

C—constipation, Celsius
$\bar{c}$—cum (with)
CA—cancer, cardiac arrest
Ca—calcium
CAB—coronary artery bypass
CAD—coronary artery disease
CAH—chronic active hepatitis
CAT—computed axial tomography (an x-ray)
CBC—complete blood count
CBDE—common bile duct exploration
CBS—chronic brain syndrome
cc—chief complaint, cubic centimeter
CCCR—closed-chest cardiopulmonary resuscitation
C/C/E—clubbing/cyanosis/edema
CCJ—costochondral junction
CDB—cough and deep-breathe
CF—Caucasian female, cystic fibrosis
C&F—chills and fever
CHD—congenital heart disease
CHF—congestive heart failure
CHO—carbohydrate
Cl—chloride
CLL—chronic lymphocytic leukemia
CM—Caucasian man, Caucasian male
CML—chronic myelogenous leukemia
CMV—cytomegalovirus
c/o—complains of
Coags—tests of coagulation function of the blood
COLD—chronic obstructive lung disease
COPD—chronic obstructive pulmonary disease
Cor—heart
CP—chest pain, cerebral palsy
CPAP—continuous positive airway pressure
CPC—clinicopathologic conference
CPR—cardiopulmonary resuscitation

CR—cardiorespiratory
Cr—creatinine
CRA—cardiorespiratory arrest
CRD—chronic respiratory disease
CRF—chronic renal failure
C&S—culture and sensitivity
CSF—cerebrospinal fluid
CT—computerized tomography
CV—cardiovascular
CVA—costovertebral angle, cerebrovascular accident
CVP—central venous pressure
CW—Caucasian woman
CXR—chest x-ray
Cysto—cystoscopy

D—diarrhea, diabetes, dead, developed, day, diastole
d—deciliter
D. bili—direct bilirubin
D/C—discontinued, discharged
D&C—dilation and curettage
Ddx—differential diagnosis
DH—dermatitis herpetiformis
DI—diabetes insipidus
Dig.—digitalis
DIP—distal interphalangeal
DJD—degenerative joint disease
DKA—diabetic ketoacidosis
DL&B—direct laryngoscopy and biopsy
DLCO—diffusional capacity lungs to carbon monoxide
DM—diabetes mellitus
D/NS—dextrose and normal saline
DOA—dead on arrival
DOB—date of birth
DOCA—deoxycorticosterone acetate
DOE—dyspnea on exertion
DP—dorsalis pedis (pulse)
DPH—diphenylhydantoin (phenytoin) (Dilantin)
DPT—diphtheria, pertussis, tetanus immunization
DS—disease
DSS—dioctyl sodium sulfosuccinate
DTRs—deep tendon reflexes
DTs—delirium tremens
DU—duodenal ulcer
DVT—deep venous thrombosis
D&W—dextrose in water
Dx—diagnosis

E—edema, exudate, eosinophils

E&A—evaluation and admission

E → A—designates egophony

EBL—estimated blood loss

ECG—electrocardiogram

ECHO—echocardiogram, or sonography of abdomen.

ECT—electroconvulsive therapy

EDC—estimated date of confinement

EDTA—ethylenediamine tetra-acetic acid (a chelating agent)

EEG—electroencephalogram

EKG—electrocardiogram

EM—erythema multiforme

E&M—endocrine and metabolic

EMG—electromyogram

EMT—emergency medical treatment (or triage, or technician)

EN—erythema nodosum

ENG—electronystagmogram

ENT—ear, nose, and throat

EOM—extraocular motions (EOMI = EOM intact; EOMF = EOM full)

EOS—eosinophils

ER—emergency room

ERBF—effective renal blood flow

ERCP—endoscopic retrograde cannulation pancreas

ERPF—effective renal plasma flow

ERV—expiratory reserve volume

ES—(heart)—extra sound, ejection sound

ESR—erythrocyte sedimentation rate

ETOH—alcohol

ETT—exercise tolerance test

EW—emergency ward

F—fever, female, Fahrenheit

FB—foreign body

FBS—fasting blood sugar

Fe—iron

FEV—forced expiratory volume

FG—fasting glucose

FH—family history

FLK—funny-looking kid (used in children with odd appearance, suggesting genetic disease, but not yet diagnosed as such)

F → N—finger to nose

FROM—full range of motion

FSH—follicle-stimulating hormone

FTA—fluorescent treponemal antibody test

FTSG—full-thickness skin graft

FTT—failure to thrive

FUO—fever of unknown origin

FX—fracture

G—growth, glucose, gravida, globulin, gallop

GA—general anesthesia

GB—gallbladder

GBD—gallbladder disease

GBS—gallbladder series

GC—gonorrhea

Gen—generally, genitalia

Gent—gentamycin

GFR—glomerular filtration rate

GH—growth hormone

GI—gastrointestinal

Gl—gland, glucose

Glob—globulin

gm—gram

GNP—glomerulonephritis

GOT—glutamic-oxaloacetic transaminase (= SGOT)

GP—general practitioner, general paresis (tertiary neurosyphilis)

GPT—glutamic-pyruvic transaminase (= SGPT)

GSW—gunshot wound

G.T.T.—glucose tolerance test

Gtt—guttae (drops)

GU—genitourinary

GYN—gynecology, gynecologic

H—history, hypertrophy, hyperopia, hydrogen, hormone, hemorrhoids

HA—headache

HASCVD—hypertensive arteriosclerotic cardiovascular disease

HBab—hepatitis B antibody

HBag—hepatitis B antigen

HBP—high blood pressure

HBR—His bundle recording

HBs—hepatitis B surface antigen

HCG—human chorionic gonadotropin

Hct—hematocrit

HCTZ—hydrochlorothiazide

HD—heart disease

HEENT—head, ears, eyes, nose, throat

Heme—blood, hematology

Hg—mercury

Hgb—hemoglobin
HH—hiatal hernia
HHD—hypertensive heart disease
5-HIAA—5-hydroxyindoleacetic acid
HJR—hepatojugular reflex
HMR—histiocytic medullary reticuloen-
dotheliosis
HNKDC—hyperosmolar nonketotic dia-
betic coma
HNP—herniated nucleus pulposus
HO—house officer
H&P—history and physical
HPI—history of present illness
HR—heart rate
H → S—heel to shin
HS—hour of sleep (at bedtime)
HTN—hypertension
HVD—hypertensive vascular disease
Hx—history

I—iodine, intake
IADH—inappropriate antidiuretic hor-
mone
IASD—interatrial septal defect
IBD—inflammatory bowel disease
I. bili—indirect bilirubin
ICP—intracranial pressure
ICS—intercostal space
ID—infectious disease
I&D—incision and drainage
Ig—immunoglobulin
IgEP—immunoglobulin electrophoresis
IH—infectious hepatitis
IHSS—idiopathic hypertrophic subaortic
stenosis
IM—intramuscular
IMV—intermittent mandatory ventilation
IND—investigational new drug
INH—isoniazid
I&O—intake and output
IP—intraperitoneal, interphalangeal
IPPB—intermittent positive pressure
breathing
IRDM—insulin-requiring diabetes mel-
litus
ITP—idiopathic thrombocytopenic pur-
pura
IU—international unit
IUD—intrauterine device
IV—intravenous
IVC—intravenous cholangiogram, inferior
vena cava

IVP—intravenous pyelogram
IVPB—intravenous piggyback
IVSD—interventricular septal defect

J—jaundice
JAR—junior assistant resident
JD—joint disease
JOD—juvenile onset diabetes
JRA—juvenile rheumatoid arthritis
JVD—jugular venous distention
JVP—jugular venous pressure

K—potassium, ketones
K-F—Kayser-Fleischer (ring)
kg—kilogram
KJ—knee jerk
KOH—potassium hydroxide
KUB—kidneys, ureter, bladder (a plain
film of the abdomen [x-ray])
KW—Kimmelstiel-Wilson (diabetic) renal
disease

L—left, lymphocyte, lung, lobe
LA—left atrium, left arm, left anterior
L&A—light and accommodation
LAD—left axis deviation, left anterior de-
scending (coronary artery)
LAH—left anterior hemiblock
LAP—leucine aminopeptidase, leukocyte
alkaline phosphatase, laparotomy
LBBB—left bundle-branch block
LBCD—left border cardiac dullness
LBP—low back pain
LDH—lactate dehydrogenase
Le—Lewis (blood group)
LE—lupus erythematosus, left eye, lower
extremities
LES—lower esophageal sphincter
LFT—liver function test
LGV—lymphogranuloma venereum
LH—luteinizing hormone
LHF—left heart failure
LHM—left homonymous hemianopia
Li—lithium
LIM—left inguinal herniorrhaphy
LKS—liver, kidney, spleen
LLL—left lower lobe, late latent lues
LLQ—left lower quadrant
LMCA—left main coronary artery
LMD—local medical doctor
LMP—last menstrual period

LN—lymph nodes
LOA—level of activity, leave of absence
LOC—loss of consciousness
LP—lumbar puncture
LPN—licensed practical nurse
LS—lung scan, lumbar spine
LSB—left sternal border
LUL—left upper lobe
LUQ—left upper quadrant
LV—left ventricle
LVH—left ventricular hypertrophy
LVN—licensed vocational nurse

M—mother, murmur, muscle, melena, mononuclear cell
MAL—midaxillary line
MB—myocardial band of creatinine kinase
MBD—minimal brain dysfunction
MCL—midclavicular line
MD—physician, muscular dystrophy
MEA—multiple endocrine adenomatosis
MEN—multiple endocrine neoplasia
MG—myasthenia gravis
Mg—magnesium
mg—milligram
MI—mitral insufficiency, myocardial infarction
MICU—medical intensive care unit
ML—midline
MM—multiple myeloma, muscles
MMCP—measles, mumps, chickenpox
MOD—maturity onset diabetes
MOM—milk of magnesia
Mono—mononucleosis
MP—metacarpophalangeal
MR—mitral regurgitation, mental retardation
MS—mitral stenosis, multiple sclerosis, morphine sulphate
MSL—midsternal line
MVA—motor vehicle accident
MVR—mitral valve replacement

N—nausea, nitrogen, nerve
NA—no answer, not applicable
Na—sodium
NAD—no acute distress, no active disease
NAS—no added salt
NC—no change
NF—Negro female
NG—nasogastric

NK—not known, nonketotic
NKA—no known allergies
Nl—normal
NM—Negro man, Negro male
NMT—nebulized mist treatments
NN—nerves
NPO—nothing by mouth
NPH—neutral protein Hagedorn insulin
NR—nonreactive, not relevant
NS—not sufficient
NSR—normal sinus rhythm
NT—nasotracheal
NTG—nitroglycerin
Nullip—nulliparous
N&V—nausea and vomiting
NVD—nausea, vomiting, diarrhea
NW—Negro woman

O—oxygen
OB—obstetrics
OBS—organic brain syndrome
OCG—oral cholecystogram
OD—overdose, right eye (oculus dexter)
OM—otitis media
ONC—oncology
OOB—out of bed
OPD—outpatient department
Ophthy—ophthalmology
OR—operating room
ORIF—open reduction internal fixation
Ortho—orthopedics, orthostatic
OS—opening snap, mouth, left eye (oculus sinister)
OT—occupational therapy, oxaloacetic transaminase (SGOT)
Oto—otology

P—phosphorus, parent, pupil, pulse, para, penicillin, platelet, percussion, polymorphonuclear leukocyte
P_2—pulmonic component second heart sound
$\bar{p}$—post (after)
PA—posteroanterior, physicians' assistant, pulmonary artery, pernicious anemia
P&A—percussion and auscultation
PAB—premature atrial beat
PABA—para-aminobenzoic acid
PAC—premature atrial contraction
PAF—paroxysmal atrial fibrillation (or flutter)

PAN—polyarteritis nodosa

PAP—pulmonary artery pressure, Papanicolaou (cervical) smear

PAR—postanesthesia recovery room

PAS—para-aminosalicylic acid, periodic acid-Schiff

PAT—paroxysmal atrial tachycardia

PAW—pulmonary artery wedge

PBC—primary biliary cirrhosis

pc—post cibum (after meals)

PCN—penicillin

PCV—packed cell volume

PDA—patent ductus arteriosus

PDR—*Physicians' Desk Reference*

P.E.—pulmonary embolism, physical examination

PEEP—positive end-expiratory pressure

PEG—pneumoencephalography

PEN—penicillin

PERRLA—pupils equal, round, react to light and accommodation

PF—pulmonary function

PFTs—pulmonary function tests

PH—past history, pulmonary hypertension

PHx—past history

PI—principal investigator, pulmonic insufficiency

PID—pelvic inflammatory disease

PIP—proximal interphalangeal (joints)

PKU—phenylketonuria

PM—post mortem

PMI—point of maximum impulse

PMN—polymorphonuclear leukocyte

PMR—polymyalgia rheumatica, physical medicine and rehabilitation

PND—paroxysmal nocturnal dyspnea

PNH—paroxysmal nocturnal hemoglobinuria

PO—per os (by mouth)

Post—autopsy (used as noun)

PPD—purified protein derivative (tuberculosis skin test), percussion and postural drainage, pack per day (smoking)

prn—as necessary (pro re nata)

PRV—polycythemia rubra vera

PS—pulmonic stenosis

PSS—progressive systemic sclerosis (scleroderma)

PSVT—paroxysmal supraventricular tachycardia

PT—physical therapy, pyruvate transaminase (SGPT), prothrombin time

Pt—patient

PTA—prior to admission

PTH—parathyroid hormone

PTT—partial thromboplastin time

PUD—peptic ulcer disease

P&V—pyloroplasty and vagotomy

PVB—premature ventricular beat

PVC—premature ventricular contraction

PWP—pulmonary wedge pressure

PZI—protamine zinc insulin

q—quaque (every)

Q̇—perfusion

qd—every day

qh—every hour

qid—four times a day

QNS—quantity not sufficient

qod—every other day

Quad—quadriplegic

R—resistance, respirations

RA—rheumatoid arthritis, right atrium, right arm, right anterior

RAD—right axis deviation

RAI—radioactive iodine

RBBB—right bundle-branch block

RBC—red blood cell

RC—Roman Catholic, respirations ceased (died)

RDS—respiratory distress syndrome

RE—regional enteritis, right eye

RF—rheumatic fever, renal failure, respiratory failure, releasing factor

RFT—renal function test

RHD—rheumatic heart disease

RICU—respiratory intensive care unit

RLL—right lower lobe

RLQ—right lower quadrant

RML—right middle lobe

RND—radical neck dissection

ROM—range of motion

ROS—review of systems

RPGNP—rapidly progressive glomerulonephritis

RPT—registered physical therapist, repeat

RR—respiratory rate

RSB—right sternal border

RT—respiratory therapy

RUL—right upper lobe

RUQ—right upper quadrant

RV—right ventricle, residual volume

RVD—rheumatic valvular disease
RVH—right ventricular hypertrophy
Rx—therapy, treatment

S—systole, sound
S_1—first heart sound
S_2—second heart sound
S_3—third heart sound
S_4—fourth heart sound
$\bar{s}$—sans (without)
SA—sinoatrial, septic arthritis
SAN—sinoatrial node
SAR—senior assistant resident
SBE—subacute bacterial endocarditis
SBO—small bowel obstruction
SBFT—small bowel follow-through
SC—subcutaneously
SCCA—squamous cell carcinoma
SCM—sternocleidomastoid
SG—specific gravity
SGOT—serum glutamic oxaloacetic transaminase
SGPT—serum glutamic pyruvic transaminase
SI—sacroiliac
SIADH—syndrome of inappropriate ADH
SICU—surgical intensive care unit
SOB—shortness of breath
S/P—status post (after)
SPEP—serum protein electrophoresis
SQ—subcutaneously
SSA—sickle cell anemia
SS Hgb—sickle cell hemoglobin
SSKI—saturated solution of potassium iodide
SubQ—subcutaneously
SVC—superior vena cava
SVT—supraventricular tachycardia

T—temperature, time
T_3—triiodothyronine
T_4—tetraiodothyronine
T&A—tonsillectomy and adenoidectomy
TA—therapeutic abortion
TAb—therapeutic abortion
TAH—transabdominal hysterectomy
TB—tuberculosis
T&C—type and cross (blood)
TFA—fluorescent treponemal antibody
TFT—thyroid function test
TH—thyroid hormone

TI—tricuspid insufficiency
TIA—transient ischemic attack
TIBC—total iron-binding capacity
TICU—thoracic intensive care unit
TLC—total lung capacity, tender loving care
TM—tympanic membrane
TMJ—temporomandibular joint
TP—total protein
TPR—temperature, pulse, respirations
TR—tendon reflex
TS—tricuspid stenosis
TSH—thyroid-stimulating hormone
TTP—thrombotic thrombocytopenic purpura
TURP—transurethral prostatic resection

U—upper, ulcer, unit
UA—urinalysis, uric acid
UC—ulcerative colitis
UE—upper extremities
UGI—upper gastrointestinal
UGIB—upper gastrointestinal bleeding
UH—university hospital
UQ—upper quadrant
URI—upper respiratory tract infection
UTI—urinary tract infection
UV—ultraviolet

V—ventricle, vomiting, very, vision, vagus, valve, vein, vancomycin
VA—Veterans Administration, visual acuity
VAH—Veterans Administration hospital
VB—ventricular beat
VC—vena cava, vital capacity, color vision
VD—venereal disease
VDRL—Venereal Disease Research Laboratories (test for syphilis)
VF—ventricular fibrillation
VG—very good
V-gram—venogram
VH—ventricular hypertrophy
VHD—valvular heart disease
VMA—vanillylmandelic acid
VNA—Visiting Nurse Association
VO—verbal orders
$V/\dot{Q}$—ventilation/perfusion ratio
VS—vital signs
VSD—ventricular septal defect
VSS—vital signs stable
VT—ventricular tachycardia

VV—veins

W—with, well, white
WA—white adult
WAP—wandering atrial pacemaker
WB—white boy
WD—well developed
W/D—withdrawal
WF—white female
WG—white girl

WM—white man, male
WN—well nourished
WNL—within normal limits
W/O—without
WPW—Wolff-Parkinson-White

X—times, for

Y—year
y/o—year-old

Commonly Used Laboratory Values

The values given for the variety of tests below are the average normals in current units for a variety of hospitals. Since both the average values and the units may differ from laboratory to laboratory, it is essential that the student obtain local information on these tests as soon as possible.

HEMATOLOGY

Hematocrit: men 42–52%
                 women 37–47%
Hemoglobin: men 14–18 gm/dl
                 women 12–16 gm/dl

RBC count: men $5.4 \pm 0.8 \times 10^6$/dl
           women $4.8 \pm 0.6 \times 10^6$/dl

  Leukocytes 5,000–10,000 (may be lower than 5,000 in normal blacks)
    juvenile neutrophils (bands) 3–5%
    segmented neutrophils 54–62%
    lymphocytes 25–33%
    monocytes 3–7%
    eosinophils 1–3%
    basophils 0–1%
  Platelets 150,000–450,000/dl
Red blood cell indices:
  Mean corpuscular hemoglobin 27–31
  Mean corpuscular hemoglobin concentration 32–36
  Mean corpuscular volume 81–99
Bleeding studies:
  Prothrombin time 70–100% of control
  Partial thromboplastin time 24–36 seconds

BLOOD/PLASMA/SERUM

Electrolytes:

Sodium	136–145 mEq/L	Chloride	100–106 mEq/L
Potassium	3.5–4.5 mEq/L	Bicarbonate	24–32 mEq/L
Calcium	9.0–11.0 mg/dl		
Phosphorus	3.0–4.5 mg/dl		
Creatinine	0.6–1.3 mg/dl		

Blood urea nitrogen (BUN) 10–23 mg/dl
Glucose (plasma, fasting) 60–110 mg/dl
Total protein 6.5–8.5 gm/dl
Albumin 3.5–5.5 gm/dl
Bilirubin: total   0.3–1.3 mg/dl
             direct 0.1–0.4 mg/dl
Lactic dehydrogenase (LDH) 110–250 mU/ml
Transaminase: SGOT 10–40 mU/ml
             SGPT   5–35 mU/ml
Alkaline phosphatase 30–95 mU/ml
Uric acid 4–8 mg/dl
Cholesterol 165–310 mg/dl

Common Drugs, With Brand Names and Uses

It is much easier to write upon a disease than upon a remedy. The former is in the hands of nature and a faithful observer with an eye of tolerable judgment cannot fail to delineate a likeness. The latter will ever be subject to the whim, the inaccuracies and the blunders of mankind.

WILLIAM WITHERING
(1741–1799)

In taking the history and reviewing the medical records, the student will discover that most patients are on more than one medication and not infrequently are unaware of the purpose of any.

The student should make frequent reference to pharmacology texts, the *Physicians' Desk Reference,* and other sources (including the hospital pharmacologist or pharmacist) to learn as much as possible about these drugs, their good and their harm.

Common Brand Name	Generic Name	Family of Drug
Aldactone	spironolactone	diuretic
Alkeran	melphalan and L-phenyl-alanine mustard	cancer therapeutic
Amethopterin	methotrexate	cancer therapeutic
Amphojel	aluminum hydroxide	antacid
Amytal	amobarbital	barbiturate
Anturane	sulfinpyrazone	uricosuric, antiplatelet
Ara-C	cytosine arabinoside	cancer therapeutic
Aramine	metaraminol	vasopressor
Arfonad	trimethaphan camsylate	hypotensive
Aristocort (Aristogel, Kenalog)	triamcinolone acetonide	corticosteroid
Aventyl	nortriptyline hydrochloride	antidepressant
Azulfidine	sulfasalazine	sulfa and salicylate (used in inflammatory bowel disease)

Common Brand Name	Generic Name	Family of Drug
Bactrim (Septra)	trimethoprim-sulfamethoxa-zole	antibacterial, antiproto-zoal
Benadryl	diphenhydramine	antihistamine
Benemid	probenecid	uricosuric
Benisone	betamethasone benzoate	corticosteroid
Benoxyl (Benzagel)	benzoyl peroxide	topical antibacterial and drying agent (acne therapy)
Bentyl	dicyclomine hydrochloride	anticholinergic
Bicillin	benzathine penicillin G	penicillin antibiotic
Blenoxane	bleomycin sulfate	cancer therapeutic
Burow's solution	aluminum acetate	topical antiseptic
Butazolidin	phenylbutazone	anti-inflammatory
Calcimar	calcitonin	hypocalcemic
Celestone	betamethasone	corticosteroid
Colace	dioctyl sodium sulfosuccinate	stool softener
Compazine	prochlorperazine	phenothiazine
Cordran	flurandrenolide	corticosteroid
Cort-Dome	hydrocortisone	corticosteroid
Co-Salt	KCl, NH$_4$, Cl, choline, lactose	salt substitute
Cosmegen	dactinomycin	cancer therapeutic
Coumadin	sodium warfarin	oral anticoagulant
Cuemid	cholestyramine	binding resin
Cytomel	sodium liothyronine	thyroid hormone
Cytoxan	cyclophosphamide	immunosuppressive cancer therapeutic
Dalmane	flurazepam	sedative
Darvon	propoxyphene hydrochloride	analgesic
DBI	phenformin	oral hypoglycemic
Decaderm	dexamethasone	corticosteroid
Decadron	dexamethasone sodium phosphate	corticosteroid
Delta-Cortef	prednisolone	corticosteroid
Demerol	meperidine	narcotic analgesic
Diabinese	chlorpropamide	oral hypoglycemic
Dilantin	phenytoin sodium	antiepileptic
Dilaudid	dihydromorphinone hydro-chloride	narcotic analgesic
Diuril	chlorothiazide	diuretic
Doriden	glutethimide	sedative
DTIC	dimethyl-triazenoimidazole carboxamide (dacarbazine)	cancer therapeutic
Dulcolax	bisacodyl	laxative
Dymelor	acetohexamide	oral hypoglycemic
Dyrenium	triamterene	diuretic
Edecrin	ethacrynic acid	diuretic

Common Brand Name	Generic Name	Family of Drug
Efudex	5-fluorouracil	cancer therapeutic (skin)
Elavil	amitriptyline hydrochloride	antidepressant
Epsom salts	magnesium sulfate	cathartic
Equanil	meprobamate	sedative
Euthroid	liotrix	thyroid hormone
Flurobate	betamethasone benzoate	corticosteroid
Furacin	nitrofurazone	topical antibacterial
Furadantin	nitrofurantoin	urinary antibacterial
Gantrisin	sulfisoxazole	antibacterial
Gelusil	aluminum hydroxide, magnesium hydroxide, and simethicone	antacid
Hydrea	hydroxyurea	cancer therapeutic
HydroDiuril	hydrochlorothiazide	diuretic
Hydromox	quinethazone	diuretic
Hygroton	chlorthalidone	diuretic
Hytone	hydrocortisone	corticosteroid
Imferon	iron dextran	iron
Imuran	azathioprine	immunosuppressive
Inderal	propranolol hydrochloride	beta blocker
Intropin	dopamine hydrochloride	vasopressor, cardiotropic
Iosel	selenium sulfide	antifungal (topical)
Ismelin	guanethidine sulfate	hypotensive
Isuprel	isoproterenol	vasopressor, cardiotropic
Kaon	potassium gluconate	potassium
Kaopectate	—	antidiarrheal
Kayexalate	sodium polystyrene sulfonate	K^+-binding resin
Kenacort	triamcinolone	corticosteroid
Kenalog	triamcinolone acetonide	corticosteroid
K-Lyte	potassium bicarbonate	potassium
Kwell	gamma benzene hexa-chloride	antiectoparasite therapy
Lasix	furosemide	diuretic
Letter	sodium levothyroxine	thyroid hormone
Leukeran	chlorambucil	immunosuppressive cancer therapeutic
Levophed	levarterenol	vasopressor
Librium	chlordiazepoxide hydro-chloride	sedative
Lidex	fluocinonide	corticosteroid
Lomotil	diphenoxylate hydrochloride	antidiarrheal
Lotrimin	clotrimazole	antifungal (topical)
Luminal	phenobarbital	barbiturate

Common Brand Name	Generic Name	Family of Drug
Maalox	magnesium hydroxide	antacid
Mandelamine	methenamide mandelate	antibacterial (urine)
Marplan	isocarboxazid	MAO inhibitor
Matulane	procarbazine hydrochloride	cancer therapeutic
Medrol	methylprednisolone	corticosteroid
Mellaril	thioridazine	phenothiazine
Meltrol	phenformin	oral hypoglycemic
Mercuhydrin	meralluride	diuretic
Mestinon	pyridostigmine bromide	cholinesterase inhibitor
Metahydrin	trichlormethiazide	diuretic
Meticortelone	prednisolone	corticosteroid
Meticorten	prednisone	corticosteroid
Miltown	meprobamate	sedative
Mobidin	magnesium salicylate	anti-inflammatory
Motrin	ibuprofen	anti-inflammatory
Mustargen	mechlorethamine hydro- chloride	cancer therapeutic
Mutamycin	mitomycin-C	cancer therapeutic
Mylanta	magnesium hydroxide	antacid
Myleran	busulfan	cancer therapeutic
Myochrysine	gold sodium thiomalate	antiarthritic
Nalfon	fenoprofen calcium	anti-inflammatory
Naqua	trichlormethiazide	diuretic
Narcan	naloxone hydrochloride	narcotic analgesic
Nardil	phenelzine sulfate	MAO inhibitor
Nembutal	pentobarbital	barbiturate
Neo-Synephrine	phenylephrine	decongestant
Nipride	sodium nitroprusside	hypotensive
Nitro-Bid	nitroglycerin	antiangina
Noludar	methyprylon	sedative
Norpramin	desipramine hydrochloride	antidepressant
Oncovin	vincristine sulfate	cancer therapeutic
Orinase	tolbutamide	oral hypoglycemic
PanOxyl	benzoyl peroxide	topical antibacterial and drying agent
Parnate	nonhydrazine tranylcypro- mine sulfate	MAO inhibitor
Pentothal	thiopental sodium	barbiturate
Permitil	fluphenazine hydrochloride	phenothiazine
Persantine	dipyridamole	antiplatelet
Pertofrane	desipramine hydrochloride	antidepressant
Phenergan	promethazine hydrochloride	antihistamine
Placidyl	ethchlorvynol	sedative
Plaquenil	hydroxychloroquine sulfate	antimalarial, antiarthritic
Pro-Banthine	propantheline bromide	anticholinergic
Prolixin	fluphenazine hydrochloride	phenothiazine

Common Brand Name	Generic Name	Family of Drug
Proloid	thyroglobulin	thyroid hormone
Pronestyl	procainamide	antiarrhythmic
Prostigmine	neostigmine	cholinesterase inhibitor
Purinethol	6-mercaptopurine	cancer therapeutic
Questran	cholestyramine	binding resin
Regitine	phentolamine	alpha-blocker
Riopan	magnesium hydroxide	antacid
Robinul	glycopyrrolate	anticholinergic
Senekot	extract of senna	laxative
Solganal	gold thioglucose	antiarthritic
Sparine	promazine hydrochloride	phenothiazine
Stelazine	trifluoperazine hydrochloride	phenothiazine
Stimex	paramethazone	corticosteroid
Surfak	dioctyl calcium sulfosuccinate	stool softener
Synalar	fluocinolone acetonide	corticosteroid
Synthroid	sodium levothyroxine	thyroid hormone
Tacaryl	methdilazine hydrochloride	phenothiazine
Tagamet	cimetadine	antacid
Talwin	pentazocine	analgesic
Tandearil	phenylbutazone and oxy-phenbutazone	anti-inflammatory
Tapazole	methimazole	antithyroid
Temaril	trimeprazine	phenothiazine
Tensilon	edrophonium chloride	cholinergic
Thiomerin	mercaptomerin	diuretic
Thorazine	chlorpromazine	phenothiazine
Thyrolar	liotrix	thyroid hormone
Tindal	acetophenazine maleate	phenothiazine
Tinver	sodium thiosulfate	topical antifungal
Tofranil	imipramine	antidepressant
Tolectin	tolmetin sodium	anti-inflammatory
Tolinase	tolazamide	oral hypoglycemic
Trilafon	perphenazine	phenothiazine
Urecholine	bethanechol chloride	cholinergic
Valisone	betamethasone valerate	corticosteroid
Valium	diazepam	sedative
Vasoxyl	methoxamine hydrochloride	alpha-adrenergic
Velban	vinblastine sulfate	cancer therapeutic
Vivactil	protriptyline hydrochloride	antidepressant
Xylocaine	lidocaine hydrochloride	antiarrhythmic, topical anesthetic
Zaroxolyn	metolazone	diuretic
Zyloprim	allopurinol	hypouricemic

GLOSSARY

BREAST

GYNECOMASTIA: Hypertrophy of breast tissue in the male patient, which causes resemblance to a female breast.

MASTITIS: Inflammation of the breast, usually due to pyogenic infection.

MASTOPATHIA CYSTICA (CHRONIC CYSTIC MASTITIS): Inflammatory condition of the breast characterized by diffuse nodularity and cystic changes.

PAGET'S DISEASE: Excoriating or scaling lesion of the nipple associated with an underlying carcinoma.

CARDIOVASCULAR SYSTEM

ANEURYSM: Saccular dilatation of an artery or cardiac chamber.

ANGINA PECTORIS: Literally, strangulation of the chest; a paraoxysmal, constricting substernal pain of brief duration, which frequently accompanies myocardial ischemia.

APEX (CARDIAC): Pointed, most lateral portion of the heart, usually located near the left fifth intercostal space.

ARRHYTHMIA: Any variation from the normal, regular rhythm of the heart.

ATRIAL FIBRILLATION: Grossly irregular ventricular rhythm associated with rapid, uncoordinated movements of the atria.

ATRIAL FLUTTER: Cardiac arrhythmia associated with rapid (about 300 per minute), regular, uniform atrial contractions and a ventricular rate and rhythm that vary with the grade of AV block.

ATRIAL TACHYCARDIA: An arrhythmia arising in the atria, usually characterized by rapid, extremely regular beating of the entire heart.

AV BLOCK: Slowing or interruption of impulse conduction from atria to ventricles.

BASE (CARDIAC): Region of the aortic and pulmonic outflow tracts; the second and third intercostal spaces parasternally.

BRADYCARDIA: Slow heart beat (less than 60 per minute).

BRUIT: Extracardiac blowing sound heard at times over peripheral vessels, usually arterial.

CORONARY HEART DISEASE: Heart disease resulting from narrowing or occlusion of one or more coronary arteries.

COR PULMONALE: Heart disease secondary to pulmonary disease.

CYANOSIS: Bluish discoloration of the skin produced by inadequate oxygenation of the blood.

DIASTOLE: Dilatation; period of "relaxation" during which ventricles fill with blood; technically ends with the onset of the first heart sound.

DYSPNEA: Difficult or labored breathing.

EDEMA: Presence of abnormal amounts of interstitial fluid in soft tissue or lungs.

EMBOLISM: Sudden occlusion of a vessel by clot or other obstruction carried to its place by the current of blood.

FRICTION RUB: Characteristic grating adventitious sound, usually pericardial or pleural, simulating noise made by friction between two rough surfaces.

GALLOP RHYTHM: Characteristic cadence produced by three heart sounds (first and second heart sound with one or more extra sounds) in conjunction with tachycardia.

HYPERTENSION: Persistent elevation of arterial blood pressure.

INFARCTION: Ischemic necrosis of tissue resulting from interference with its circulation.

MURMUR: Adventitious sound resulting from turbulent blood flow within the heart or great vessels.

ORTHOPNEA: Inability to breathe comfortably when supine.

PALPITATION: Awareness of the heart beat.

PAROXYSMAL: Sudden, unexpected.

PRESYSTOLIC: Immediately preceding the first sound; occurring in the latter one-third of diastole.

PROTODIASTOLIC: Immediately following the second sound; occurring in the initial one-third of diastole.

PULSE: Expansile wave felt over an artery. It is propagated at a speed approximately ten times that of the actual flow of blood in the system.

RAYNAUD'S PHENOMENON: Paroxysmal pallor or cyanosis of a distal extremity, induced by chilling or emotion.

SHOCK: Acute circulatory collapse, with pallor, hypotension, and coldness of the skin (also, a palpable heart sound).

SYNCOPE: Temporary unconsciousness due to cerebral ischemia.

SYSTOLE: Contraction; period of contraction during which the atria or ventricles eject blood; *ventricular systole* includes the first and second sounds and the period between them; when the term *systole* or *diastole* is used alone, it is assumed to refer to the ventricles.

TACHYCARDIA: Rapid regular heart beat (over 100 per minute in adults).

THRILL: Palpable vibrations (palpable murmur).

VARICOSE: Dilated.

VENTRICULAR TACHYCARDIA: Arrhythmia originating in the ventricles, characterized by rapid, relatively regular heart beat.

ENDOCRINE SYSTEM

ACROMEGALY: A disorder in the adult resulting from an excess production and secretion of growth hormone by the pituitary gland, characterized by overgrowth of bony, cartilaginous, and soft tissues, especially noticeable in acral parts.

ADDISON'S DISEASE: A disorder resulting from chronic underproduction of cortisol and aldosterone by the adrenal cortex, characterized by hyperpigmentation, asthenia, and low blood pressure.

CUSHING'S SYNDROME: A disorder resulting from chronic overproduction of cortisol by the adrenal cortex, characterized by thinned skin and wasted muscles, accumulation of fat on the trunk, easy bruising, plethora, and high blood pressure.

EXOPHTHALMOS: Prominence or protuberance of the eyes, frequently associated with hyperthyroidism.

GOITER: Enlargement of the thyroid gland.

GRAVES' DISEASE: A disorder characterized by exophthalmos, goiter, and overproduction of thyroid hormone, the latter producing thyrotoxicosis.

HIRSUTISM: A state of increased amounts of body and facial hair, especially in the female.

HYPERPARATHYROIDISM, HYPOPARATHYROIDISM: Overproduction of parathyroid hormone and hypercalcemia in the former state; underproduction and hypocalcemia in the latter. Both are characterized by abnormalities in neuromuscular excitability as well as by abnormalities of the eye and of bone.

HYPOGONADISM: Absent or reduced function of the testis or ovary characterized by diminished germ cell production and/or maturation and by decreased production of sex hormones. Underdevelopment of secondary sexual characteristics or regression of developed secondary sexual characteristics results.

MYXEDEMA: A disorder resulting from underproduction of thyroid hormone, characterized by puffiness of soft tissues, slowing of body movements, and deepening of the voice.

OBESITY: The accumulation of an excessive amount of fat.

VIRILISM: A state of masculinization in the female.

EYE

AMBLYOPIA: Decreased vision of an eye from any cause.

ANISOCORIA: Inequality in size of the pupils.

ANTERIOR SEGMENT: Anterior portion of the eye.

ARCUS SENILIS: A white ring around the limbus of the cornea occurring in elderly persons.

ASTHENOPIA: Discomfort related to use of the eyes.

AV NOTCHING: Indentation of a retinal vein by an overlying retinal artery in arteriosclerosis.

CATARACT: Opacity in the crystalline lens of the eye.

CONJUNCTIVITIS: Inflammation of the conjunctiva.

DIPLOPIA: Double vision.

ECTROPION: Eversion of the lid border.

ENTROPION: Inversion of the lid border.

EPIPHORA: Overflow of tears down the cheek.

EXOPHTHALMOS: Protrusion of the eyeball.

FUNDUSCOPY: Examination of the interior of the eyeball using an ophthalmoscope.

GLAUCOMA: Increased intraocular pressure as well as the disease resulting from such pressure.

HYPHEMA: Presence of blood in the anterior chamber of the eye.

HYPOPYON: Presence of pus in the anterior chamber, often with a horizontal fluid level.

IRITIS: Inflammation of the iris.

MIOSIS: Constriction of the pupil; a drug that constricts the pupil is called a *miotic.*

MYDRIASIS: Dilation of the pupil; a drug that dilates the pupil is called a *mydriatic.*

NYSTAGMUS: Irregular jerking movement of the eyes.

O.D.: Abbreviation for the right eye (oculus dexter).

O.S.: Abbreviation for the left eye (oculus sinister).

OPTIC ATROPHY: Loss of tissue of the optic nerve due to prior disease, usually making the optic disc appear whiter in color under the ophthalmoscope.

PAPILLEDEMA: Swelling of the optic nerve head.

PHORIA: Latent tendency to deviation of the visual axes, which is held in check by the fusion reflex.

PHOTOPHOBIA: Sensitivity to light that is usually associated with corneal disease.

POSTERIOR SYNECHIAE: Adhesions between the iris and the lens.

PRESBYOPIA: Diminution of the power of accommodation of the eye due to the aging process.

PROPTOSIS: Forward displacement of the eyeball.

PTOSIS: Drooping of the upper lid (*blepharoptosis*).

TROPIA: Deviation of the visual axes from parallelism that is not overcome by the fusion reflex.

VISUAL FIELD: Area of vision of each eye measured while the eye is directed straight ahead.

YOKED MUSCLES: Muscle pairs, one on each eye, that lead in a specific diagnostic position; for example, the right lateral rectus and the left medial rectus in gaze to the right side.

FEMALE GENITOURINARY SYSTEM

ABORTION: Interruption of pregnancy before the fetus becomes viable (26 weeks).
ADNEXA: Ovaries and adjacent fallopian tubes.
AMENORRHEA: Absence of menses.

CYSTOCELE: Hernial protrusion of the urinary bladder through the vaginal wall.

DYSMENORRHEA: Painful menstruation.

HYPERMENORRHEA (MENORRHAGIA): Abnormally increased volume of menstrual flow.

MENARCHE: Beginning of the menstrual function.
MENOPAUSE: Termination of menses at the end of a normal reproductive span of years.
MISCARRIAGE: Nonmedical term for premature expulsion of a fetus.
MULTIPARA: Woman who has borne more than one viable child.

POLYMENORRHEA (METRORRHAGIA): Abnormally increased frequency of menstrual flow.
PRIMIGRAVIDA: Woman pregnant for the first time.
PRIMIPARA: Woman who has borne one viable infant.

RECTOCELE: Hernial protrusion of part of the rectum into the vagina.

GASTROINTESTINAL SYSTEM

ANOREXIA: Loss of appetite.
ASCITES: Free fluid within the peritoneal cavity.

BORBORYGMI: Audible bowel sounds due to active peristalsis. Not necessarily a pathologic sign.

CACHEXIA: Profound malnutrition and weight loss.
COLIC: Acute, cramping abdominal pain occurring in waves or surges.
CONSTIPATION: Difficult evacuation of stool because of firm consistency. Should be distinguished from simple infrequency of bowel movements.

DEGLUTITION: Swallowing.
DIARRHEA: Passage of frequent stools of watery consistency.
DYSCHEZIA: Painful defecation.
DYSPEPSIA: Indigestion, usually with uncomfortable abdominal fullness, belching, and nausea.
DYSPHAGIA: Difficulty in swallowing.

FLATULENCE: Passage of gas from the lower bowel.

GUARDING: Involuntary spasm of the abdominal muscles, frequently localized to an area of underlying pain and tenderness.

HEMATEMESIS: Vomiting of blood.

ILEUS: Intestinal obstruction with dilation of the bowel and obstipation. May be on a mechanical or paralytic basis.

JAUNDICE: Yellow coloration of the skin, mucous membranes, and sclera, due to accumulation of bilirubin pigments in serum and tissues. Also referred to as *icterus*.

MALABSORPTION: Inadequate and disordered absorption of intestinal nutrients.
MELENA: Passage of black stool, which is darkened by altered blood. The blood may be deep maroon or black and tarry in appearance.

NAUSEA: An unpleasant sensation of impending vomiting, frequently localized to the epigastrium.

OBSTIPATION: Persistent failure to pass any stool.

PREPRANDIAL AND POSTPRANDIAL: Before and after a meal.

REBOUND: Abbreviated term for rebound tenderness; abdominal discomfort on sudden withdrawal of the palpating hand.

SCAPHOID: A thin, concave-shaped abdomen. Literally "shiplike," derived from the Greek.

STEATORRHEA: Excessive fat in the stool.

STOMATITIS: Inflammation of the mouth.

TENESMUS: The sensation of the need to evacuate the bowels, but without result.

TYMPANITES: Distention of the abdomen due to presence of gas or air in the intestine or peritoneal cavity.

XEROSTOMIA: Dryness of the mouth.

HEAD

APHONIA: Loss of the voice.

DEGLUTITION: Act of swallowing.

DYSPHAGIA: Difficulty in swallowing.

DYSPHONIA: Difficulty or pain in speaking.

EPIPHORA: Tearing.

EPISTAXIS: Nasal hemorrhage.

LARYNGOPHARYNX: Lower pharynx extending from the lingual surface of the epiglottis to the trachea and esophagus.

MUCOCELE: Intrasinus cyst arising from mucosal lining.

NARES: The openings into the nasal cavity.

NASOPHARYNX (EPIPHARYNX): Upper pharynx extending from the choanae to the inferior border of the soft palate.

ODYNOPHAGIA: Painful swallowing.

OROPHARYNX: Portion of pharynx directly behind the oral cavity extending from the inferior border of the soft palate to the lingual surface of the epiglottis.

OTALGIA: Pain in the ear.

OTITIS: Infection of the ear.

OTORRHEA: Discharge from the ear.

PYOCELE: Infected mucocele.

RHINORRHEA: Nasal discharge.

STRIDOR: Noisy respiration.

VALLECULA: Space between the base of the tongue and the lingual surface of the epiglottis.

VESTIBULE: Of the ear, the oval cavity in the middle of the bony labyrinth; of the nose, the area just inside the nares.

HEMATOPOIETIC SYSTEM

AGRANULOCYTOSIS: Acute reduction in the number of circulating polymorphonuclear leukocytes.

ANEMIA: Reduction in the number of circulating red blood cells and/or hemoglobin with respect to age and sex.

EPISTAXIS: Nosebleeds.

ERYTHROCYTOSIS: Increase in the number of circulating red blood cells with respect to age and sex.

HEMATOPOIETIC: Blood forming.

HEMOLYSIS: Accelerated dissolution or destruction of red blood cells in vivo.

INFECTIOUS MONONUCLEOSIS: Systemic infection associated with enlargement of lymph nodes and spleen, and eliciting a specific peripheral blood response.

LEUKEMIAS: A group of disorders of the blood-forming organs characterized by excessive proliferation and/or failure of differentiation of one of the types of white blood cells.

LEUKOCYTOSIS: Increase in the white blood cell count above normal.

LEUKOPENIA: Decrease in the white blood cell count below normal.

LYMPHADENOPATHY: Any lymph node enlargement.

LYMPHOMA: General term for neoplasms originating from the lymphoid reticulum.

MYELOID: Pertaining to the bone marrow.

PETECHIAE: Pinpoint-size hemorrhages.

POLYCYTHEMIA: Erythrocytosis.

POLYCYTHEMIA, SECONDARY: Erythrocytosis secondary to chronic hypoxia and other rarer causes, such as renal tumors.

POLYCYTHEMIA VERA: Primary or idiopathic erythrocytosis, in which there is leukocytosis, thrombocytosis, and splenomegaly.

PRURITUS: Itching.

PURPURA: Purplish discolorations caused by bleeding into the skin and visible mucous membranes, that is, "black and blue spots."

SPLENOMEGALY: Enlargement of the spleen.

THROMBOCYTOPENIA: Reduction below normal in the number of circulating platelets.

THROMBOCYTOSIS: Increase above normal in the number of circulating platelets.

MALE GENITOURINARY SYSTEM AND HERNIA

ANURIA: Complete suppression of urinary output.

BACTERIURIA: Presence of bacteria in the urine.

BALANOPOSTHITIS: Inflammation of the glans penis and prepuce.

BULBOCAVERNOSUS REFLEX: Reflex elicited by squeezing the glans penis, which results in constriction of the bulbocavernosus muscle and the anal sphincter.

CHORDEE: Bowing of the penis during erection secondary to fibrotic plaques in the corpora cavernosa, or to congenital absence of the distal portion of the urethra.

CRYPTORCHISM: Failure of one testis or both testes to descend into the scrotum.

CYSTITIS: Inflammation of the urinary bladder.

DYSURIA: Painful micturition.

ENURESIS: Involuntary voiding during sleep.

FEMORAL HERNIA: Type of hernia in which the abdominal wall defect lies along the femoral canal, with the hernial sac presenting deep to the inguinal ligament.

HEMATURIA: Blood in the urine; when blood is detected visually it is called *gross hematuria* and when only microscopically, *microscopic hematuria.*

HYDROCELE: Fluid-containing cystic mass, usually arising as a result of incomplete obliteration of the processus vaginalis; common in infancy and often bilateral; may occur in the scrotum as a hydrocele of the testis or appear anywhere along the inguinal canal as a hydrocele of the cord.

INCARCERATED HERNIA: One in which the contents cannot be returned to the abdominal cavity; no inflammation or interference with blood supply, however, has resulted.

INGUINAL HERNIA, DIRECT: Hernia through weakness in the abdominal musculature, with protrusion through the region of Hesselbach's triangle.

INGUINAL HERNIA, INDIRECT: Hernia through the internal inguinal ring, with the hernial sac descending beside the spermatic cord toward or into the scrotum.

NEPHROCALCINOSIS: Deposition of calcium in the renal parenchyma.

NEUROGENIC BLADDER: Dysfunction of bladder secondary to abnormality of its innervation.

OLIGURIA: Urinary output less than 400 ml per 24 hours.

PARADOXIC INCONTINENCE: Involuntary dribbling of urine secondary to chronic urinary retention.

PHIMOSIS: Tightness of the prepuce so that it cannot be retracted to uncover the glans penis.

PNEUMATURIA: Voiding of urine containing free gas.

POLYCYSTIC KIDNEY: Congenitally abnormal kidney that contains numerous cysts of various sizes.

PRECIPITOUS MICTURITION: Involuntary loss of urine caused by sudden urge to void.

PRIAPISM: Prolonged erection of the penis.

PROTEINURIA: Presence of protein in the urine; *orthostatic proteinuria,* presence of protein in a urine specimen taken while the patient is upright, which is absent from specimen taken while patient is supine.

PYURIA: Presence of leukocytes in the urine.

REDUCIBLE HERNIA: One in which the contents of the hernial sac can be returned to the abdominal cavity.

RESIDUAL URINE: Urine that remains in the bladder after micturition.

RICHTER'S HERNIA: Type of strangulated hernia in which only a small portion of the wall of intestine is caught in the ring of the defect; as a result, local gangrene may appear without the production of the signs or symptoms of intestinal obstruction; usually seen with a femoral hernia.

SCROTAL HERNIA: Inguinal hernia, almost always of the indirect type, of sufficient size to permit the hernial sac and its contents to enter the scrotum together with the contents of the spermatic cord.

SPERMATOCELE: A cystic scrotal mass containing whitish, milky fluid with spermatozoa.

STRANGULATED HERNIA: One in which the blood supply to the viscera within the hernial sac has become obstructed, resulting in necrosis of tissue.

STRESS INCONTINENCE: Involuntary loss of urine during period of increased intravesical pressure, such as can be produced by coughing, straining, or lifting.

VARICOCELE: Dilated veins of the pampiniform plexus in the scrotum.

MUSCULOSKELETAL SYSTEM

ABDUCTION: Motion of a part away from the midline.

ACTIVE RANGE OF MOTION: Limits of motion through which a joint may be moved by those muscles that cross the joint.

ADDUCTION: Motion of a part toward the midline.

ANKYLOSIS: Complete loss of motion of a joint.

ARTHRITIS: Inflammation of a joint.

BURSA: Potential space often filled with fluid between two soft tissue layers that move upon each other.

CALCIFIC TENDINITIS OF THE SHOULDER: Inflammatory condition of a tendon about the shoulder, one stage of which is the deposition of crystals containing calcium within the structure of the tendon.

CAPSULE: The fibrous tissue sheath about a joint.

CARPAL TUNNEL: The potential space on the volar (anterior) aspect of the wrist, the floor of which is formed by the carpal bones, the roof by the transverse carpal ligaments. Within the carpal tunnel travel the deep and superficial flexors of the fingers, the long flexor to the thumb, and the median nerve.

CAVUS FOOT: Foot deformity in which a very high arch is present.

CLUB FOOT (TALIPES EQUINOVARUS): Foot deformity consisting of varus of the heel, equinus of the ankle, and adduction and supination of the forefoot.

CONTRACTURE: Shortening of soft tissues about a joint, which limits normal motion of the joint.

CONTRALATERAL: On the opposite side.

CREPITATION: Grating or cracking sensation produced by motion.

EVERSION: Position achieved by turning a part away from the midline of the body.

INVERSION: Position achieved by turning a part toward the midline of the body.

JOINT EFFUSION: Excessive fluid within a joint.

KYPHOSIS: Angular curvature of the spine, the convexity of which is posterior.

MENISCUS: Fibrocartilaginous structure found between the articular surfaces of certain joints.

PARESTHESIA: Sensation of burning, crawling, or tingling.

PASSIVE RANGE OF MOTION: Limits of motion through which a joint may be moved without use of the muscles that cross the joint.

PRONATION: Position of the forearm achieved by turning the palm down; position of the foot achieved by turning the sole down.

PSEUDOARTHROSIS: Lack of bony continuity after the process of bone repair has ceased.

ROTATOR CUFF OF THE SHOULDER: Common insertion of the subscapularis, supraspinatus, infraspinatus, and teres minor muscles into the proximal humerus.

SPONDYLOLISTHESIS: Forward displacement of a vertebra upon the one below as a result of bilateral defects in the vertebral arch.

SUBLUXATION: Lack of a completely normal relationship between the articular surfaces of two bones that comprise a joint, such that, however, the articular surfaces are still in contact (that is, not dislocated).

SUPINATION: Position of the forearm achieved by turning the palm up; position of the foot achieved by turning the sole up.

SUPINE: Position of lying on the back, face upward.

SYNOVITIS: Inflammation of the lining of a joint.

TENDINITIS: Inflammation of a tendon.

THORACIC OUTLET: Anatomic region between the base of the neck and the axilla through which pass the brachial plexus and subclavian vessels.

VALGUS: Angulation of a part of an extremity away from the midline.

VARUS: Angulation of a part of an extremity toward the midline.

NERVOUS SYSTEM

ANARTHRIA: Inability to articulate words (complete voicelessness) due to disease of the nerves or muscles of speech.

APHASIA: Loss of the power of expression by speech, writing, or signs, or of comprehending spoken or written language, due to injury or disease of the higher cerebral centers concerned with expression and comprehension.

ATAXIA: Failure of muscular coordination; irregularity of muscular action.

ATROPHY: A wasting away of or diminution in the size of a muscle.

BULBAR PALSY: Paralysis and atrophy of the muscles of lips, tongue, mouth, pharynx, and larynx due to degeneration of the nerve nuclei of the floor of the fourth ventricle or of the motor nerves originating from them.

DYSARTHRIA: Imperfect articulation in speech.

DYSMETRIA: Disturbance of the power to control the range of movement in muscular action; a sign of cerebellar dysfunction.

DYSPHAGIA: Difficulty in swallowing.

DYSPHASIA: Incomplete degree of aphasia.

DYSSYNERGIA: Disturbance of muscular coordination; a sign of cerebellar dysfunction.

EXTINCTION (SUPPRESSION): Failure to perceive one of two identical bilateral simultaneous stimuli; if sensory perception is otherwise intact, extinction or suppression may indicate parietal cortex dysfunction.

FASCICULATION: Visible spontaneous contraction of a number of muscle fibers supplied by a single motor nerve filament.

GRAPHESTHESIA: Sense by which figures or numbers written on the skin are recognized.

HOMONYMOUS HEMIANOPIA: Loss of vision in the nasal half of the visual field in one eye and the temporal half in the other.

HORNER'S SYNDROME: Sympathetic paralysis causing ptosis of the upper lid, constriction of the pupil, and decreased sweating, all on one side of the head and face.

LOWER MOTOR NEURONS: Peripheral neurons whose cell bodies lie in the ventral gray columns of the spinal cord and whose terminations are in the skeletal muscles.

NYSTAGMUS: Involuntary repetitive rapid movement of the eyeball.

OPTIC ATROPHY: Pale appearance of the optic nerve head when the nerve has become demyelinated.

OPTIC NEURITIS: Inflammation of the optic nerve that, when acute, produces a swollen appearance of the optic disc similar to that of papilledema.

PAPILLEDEMA: Edema of the optic disc ("choked disc") usually due to increased intracranial pressure.

PARESIS (HEMI-, PARA-, QUADRI-): Weakness or partial paralysis.

PLEGIA: Complete paralysis. *Hemiplegia,* paralysis of one side of the body and the limbs on that side; *paraplegia,* paralysis of the legs and lower part of the body, usually caused by disease or injury of the spinal cord; *quadriplegia,* paralysis of all four limbs.

PROPRIOCEPTION: Perception of movements and position of the body and joints.

PSEUDOBULBAR PALSY: Weakness of the pharyngeal, laryngeal, and facial muscles, simulating bulbar paralysis but due to supranuclear (upper motor neuron) lesions.

PTOSIS: Drooping of the upper eyelid.

QUADRANTANOPIA: Blindness in one of the quadrants of the visual field.

SCOTOMA: Blind or partially blind area in the visual field.

SENSORY "LEVEL": Level below which there is a decrease or loss of sensation corresponding to the level of dysfunction of the spinal cord.

STEREOGNOSIS: Faculty of perceiving and understanding the form and nature of objects by the sense of touch.

UPPER MOTOR NEURON: Neuron that conducts impulses from the motor cortex to the motor nuclei of the cranial nerves or to the motor cells in the ventral gray columns of the spinal cord.

RESPIRATORY SYSTEM

ASTHMA: A disease characterized by hyporeactive airways and usually atopy with acute intermittent airways obstruction and bronchospasm, manifest clinically as wheezing and cough, with a return to or toward normal between episodes.

ATELECTASIS: Partial or complete airlessness with reduction in the volume of the affected segment, lobe, or entire lung; with or without locally obstructed bronchi; chronic or acute. Also refers to diffuse small areas with loss of volume, microatelectasis.

BREATHLESSNESS: Appropriate shortness of breath, e.g., following heavy exercise.

BREATH SOUNDS: Sounds due to the movement of air through the air passages appreciated by auscultation; *asthmatic,* noisy musical respirations due to rhonchi of all types; *bronchial,* abnormal breath sounds, quite similar to tracheal sounds, heard over consolidated lung, also called *tubular; bronchovesicular,* sounds intermediate between vesicular and tracheal, heard over the major bronchi; *tracheal,* normal to-and-fro sounds heard over the trachea; *vesicular,* the normal breath sounds, predominantly inspiratory, heard over most of the lung.

BRONCHIECTASIS: A disease characterized by chronic dilatation of bronchial walls associated with chronic suppuration.

BRONCHITIS: Acute or chronic bronchial inflammation.

CHRONIC BRONCHITIS: A clinical entity characterized by cough and sputum production on most days for at least three months in at least two successive years without a specific cause, usually associated with airways obstruction and a history of cigarette smoking.

CHRONIC OBSTRUCTIVE PULMONARY DISEASE (COPD): A general term describing diseases characterized by diffuse airways obstruction; asthma, chronic bronchitis, and emphysema.

CLUBBING: Deforming enlargement of the terminal phalanges, usually acquired, associated with certain cardiac and pulmonary diseases; it is characterized by loss of the normal angle between the skin and nail base and sponginess of the nail base.

COLLAPSE: Reduction in lung volume, acute or chronic, due to bronchial or parenchymal disease.

COMPRESSION: Mechanical reduction of lung volume by pressure.

CONSOLIDATION: Diffuse replacement of a large zone of pulmonary parenchyma with liquid and solid products of inflammation but only when the associated bronchus is patent. Preferably the term is used as a description of physical rather than pathologic or roentgenographic findings.

CRACKLE: See Rale.

CREPITATION: See Rale.

CYANOSIS: A blue color of the skin and mucous membranes usually due to severe arterial oxygen desaturation, e.g., a hemoglobin saturation of less than 75 percent, a PO_2 of less than 40 mm Hg.

DYSPNEA: The subjective sensation of abnormal or inappropriate shortness of breath or difficulty in breathing.

EMPHYSEMA: A disease characterized pathologically as destruction and dilatation of lung tissue distal to the terminal bronchioles and clinically by dyspnea, a minimally productive or nonproductive cough, airways obstruction, persistent hyperinflation of the lung, and decreased breath sounds; most commonly it is associated with chronic bronchitis; *compensatory emphysema,* a term referring to secondary dilatation of air spaces adjacent to areas of fibrosis; *subcutaneous emphysema,* air or other gas in the subcutaneous tissues.

EMPYEMA: Pus in the pleural cavity; pyothorax.

FORCED EXPIRATORY TIME (FET): The time required to empty the lungs completely with maximal effort from full inspiration to full expiration.

FORCED VITAL CAPACITY (FVC): The amount of air exhaled from the lungs from a maximum inspiration to a maximum expiration, with expiration as rapid and forceful as possible; the volume expired is measured against time.

FREMITUS: A palpable vibration or thrill; *rhonchal fremitus,* vibration due to rhonchi; *tactile* or *vocal fremitus,* voice sound vibration.

FRICTION RUB: Grating sensation, heard or palpated, that arises from inflamed serous surfaces.

HEMOPTYSIS: Expectoration of gross blood, by coughing, from the larynx or lower respiratory tract.

KYPHOSIS: Increased convexity of the spine in the anteroposterior plane.

MÜLLER'S MANEUVER: Production of increased negative intrapleural pressure by an attempt to inhale forcibly against a closed glottis.

PLEURAL EFFUSION: Fluid of any type in the pleural cavity; it includes empyema, hemothorax, and chylothorax. Thoracentesis is required for specific identification.

PLEURISY: Any pleural inflammation; loosely, the pain associated with disease of the pleura.

PNEUMOCONIOSIS: Condition of chronic pulmonary scarring resulting from inhalation of inorganic (mineral) or organic dusts; more broadly, parenchymal pulmonary disease of occupational cause, including reactions to fumes, gases, etc.

PNEUMONIA: Clinical term that most commonly refers to pulmonary inflammation due to infection.

PNEUMONITIS: Any pulmonary inflammation.

PNEUMOTHORAX: Air or other gas within the pleural cavity.

RALE: Abnormal sound that originates from the trachea, bronchi, or lungs; *crepitation, crepitant rale,* a rale of crackling quality, usually applied to moist rales; *consonating rale,* a loud, clear, ringing rale that sounds close to the ear, often associated with pulmonary consolidation; *fine, medium, coarse rale,* classificatory terms referring to loudness, duration, and quality of moist rales; *moist rale,* an interrupted sound arising from alveoli and smaller bronchi—the term *rale* is limited to this variety by some; *rhonchus,* a continuous, coarse sound arising from the trachea or bronchi—also termed *dry* or *musical rale; sibilant rale,* a high-pitched, very musical rhonchus; *sonorous rale,* a low-pitched, snoring rhonchus; *wheeze,* a nonspecific whistling sound associated with obstruction to air flow—applied to both rhonchi and coarse moist rales.

RESPIRATION: Variations in respiration include *apnea,* the absence of breathing; *bradypnea,* breathing at a slow rate; *Cheyne-Stokes,* cyclic breathing in which there is increased depth and rate of respiration between periods of apnea; *hyperpnea,* increased depth and, usually, rate of respiration; *orthopnea,* inability to breathe comfortably while supine, relieved by sitting up; *tachypnea,* increased rate of respiration.

SCOLIOSIS: Lateral deviation of the spine.

STRIDOR: Difficult respiration due to upper airways obstruction, characterized by high-pitched crowing sounds in inspiration.

VALSALVA MANEUVER: Production of decreased negative intrapleural pressure by an attempt, after deep inspiration, to expire forcibly against a closed glottis.

VOICE SOUNDS: The vibrations of the spoken voice transmitted through the lungs and appreciated by auscultation; also called *vocal resonance* and, rarely, *vocal fremitus; bronchophony,* increased intensity of voice sounds; *egophony,* a peculiar bleating nasal quality of voice sounds in which articulated long *e* (ee) simulates long *a* (ay); *pectoriloquy,* transmission of articulate speech; *whispering pectoriloquy,* distinct transmission of whispered sounds.

WHEEZE: See Rhonchus.

SKIN

ALBINISM: A disease of generalized hypopigmentation in which little or no melanin is formed.

BULLA (pl. BULLAE): Loculated fluid in the skin; a large blister.

CAFÉ AU LAIT SPOTS: Sharply marginated brown patches. The presence of one or two such spots is normal.

CAROTENE: A yellow-orange pigment found in many foods.

CRUSTS: Dried or hardened serum proteins on the surface of the skin.

EROSION: Superficial loss of skin.

ERYTHEMA: Redness.

FRECKLES: Sharply circumscribed small brown macules.

KERATIN: The protein product of skin metabolism. Scale is formed by the macroscopic accumulation of keratin.

LENTIGO (pl. LENTIGINES): Sharply circumscribed small brown macules that appear late in life following years of sun exposure.

MACULE: A circumscribed area of color change.

MELANIN: The brown pigment of the skin that is made by melanocytes.

NODULE: A large palpable mass, usually elevated above the skin surface.

PAPULE: A small palpable mass, usually elevated above the skin surface.

PLAQUE: A flat elevated mass, the confluence of papules.

PRURITUS: Itching.

PUSTULE: A cloudy or white vesicle, the color of which is due to the presence of polymorphonuclear leukocytes.

SCALE: The macroscopic accumulation of keratin.

SCLERODERMA: A disease in which the dermal component of the skin is thickened.

SEBORRHEA: Oiliness of the skin due to lipids that originate in the sebaceous gland.

ULCER: As applied to the skin, a deep loss of tissue or large erosion.

URTICARIA: The presence of edema in the skin secondary to histamine release.

VESICLE: A small loculation of fluid in the skin; a small blister.

VITILIGO: Circumscribed areas of pigment loss.

WHEAL: An edematous papule, the primary lesion of urticaria, a "hive."

XEROSIS: Dryness of the skin.

INDEX

INDEX